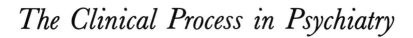

The Clinical Process in Psychiatry

The clinical process in psychiatry

Diagnosis and
management planning

Barry Nurcombe, M.D., F.R.A.C.P.
Rollin M. Gallagher, III, M.D.

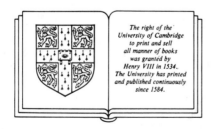

The right of the
University of Cambridge
to print and sell
all manner of books
was granted by
Henry VIII in 1534.
The University has printed
and published continuously
since 1584.

CAMBRIDGE UNIVERSITY PRESS

Cambridge
London   New York   New Rochelle
Melbourne   Sydney

Published by the Press Syndicate of the University of Cambridge
The Pitt Building, Trumpington Street, Cambridge CB2 1RP
32 East 57th Street, New York, NY 10022, USA
296 Beaconsfield Parade, Middle Park, Melbourne 3206, Australia

© Cambridge University Press 1986

Printed in the United States of America

Library of Congress Cataloging in Publication Data

Nurcombe, Barry, 1933–
    The clinical process in psychiatry.

    Bibliography: p.
    1. Psychiatry. I. Gallagher, Rollin M. II. Title.
[DNLM: 1. Mental Disorders—diagnosis. 2. Mental
Disorders—therapy. 3. Psychiatry—methods.
WM 100 N974c]
RC454.4.N87 1985   616.89   85-4171
ISBN 0-521-24741-1
ISBN 0-521-28928-9 (pbk.)

British Library Cataloging-in-Publication Data applied for.

Acknowledgments

The authors are grateful for permission to publish the following copyrighted material.

p. 161, Table 9.6

Reprinted with permission from the American Geriatrics Society and the author, Pfeiffer, E. A short portable mental status questionnaire for the assessment of organic brain deficit in elderly patients. *Journal of the American Geriatrics Society,* 1975, *13,* 441–443.

p. 162, The Set Test

Reprinted with permission from Isaacs, B., & Kennie, A. T. The set test as an aid to the detection of dementia in old people. *British Journal of Psychiatry,* 1983, *123,* 467–470.

p. 163, Table 9.7

Reprinted with permission from Folstein, M. D., Folstein, S. V., & McHugh, P. R. Mini mental state: A practical method for grading the cognitive state of patients for the clinician. *Journal of Psychiatric Research,* 1975, *12,* 189–198. Copyright 1975, Pergamon Press, LTD.

p. 191, quote (McIntyre & Romano, 1977, p. 1150)

Reprinted with permission of the publisher and author from McIntyre, J. S., & Romano, J. Is there a stethoscope in the house (and is it used).'' *Archives in General Psychiatry,* 1977, *34,* p. 1150. Copyright 1977, American Medical Association.

pp. 407, 408, Table 19.1, Table 19.2, Table 19.3

Reprinted by permission of the publisher and author from McKegney, F. P., King, J., & McMahon, T., The use of DSM-III in general hospital consultation service, *General Hospital Psychiatry,* 5(2), 115–121. Copyright 1983 by Elsevier Science Publishing Co., Inc.

For
Alison and Diane

Memory is a net; one finds it full of fish when he takes it from the brook; but a dozen miles of water have run through it without sticking.

Oliver Wendell Holmes

ALICE: Would you tell me please which way I ought to go from here?
THE CAT: That depends a good deal on where you want to get to.

Lewis Carroll

διαγνωσις

Dia: through, right through, asunder, to the end, utterly, thoroughly, out and out.

Gignosko: to learn, know, perceive, mark, discern, distinguish, observe, form a judgment on a matter, judge, think, understand, determine.

Diagnosis: a distinguishing, discernment, power of discernment, a resolving or deciding.

(Liddell, H. G. *An Intermediate Greek-English Lexicon.* Oxford: Oxford University Press, 1889.)

Contents

PART IV Diagnosis and planning

PART V Special situations

Preface

When we were medical students, we learned facts, concepts, and techniques. Our instructors were less successful, however, in teaching us how to solve problems. Although we were enthralled by their expert medical detective work, few of our seniors told us how they actually reached a diagnosis and few of them were explicit about how they designed complex management plans.

In the wards and clinics, our mentors praised us for compiling interminable histories, reciting lengthy differential diagnoses, and leaving no investigative stone unturned. They, themselves, solved medical problems by rapidly matching patterns, juggling alternative diagnostic hypotheses and generating probing lines of inquiry. They had learned to do this without formal instruction. Consequently, they could neither reflect upon nor convey the elements of their skill, and they were prone to ascribe it to "art" or "intuition."

This book attempts to make explicit the art of clinical work. In it we review the basic information and procedures required to generate and test diagnostic hypotheses. We describe the progression of clinical reasoning from the beginning of the diagnostic encounter to the termination of treatment, and we then apply the generic model of problem solving to particular clinical situations.

The book evolved from our collaborative efforts to teach psychiatry and primary care medicine at the Medical Center Hospital of Vermont. Barry Nurcombe collaborated with Dr. Ina Fitzhenry-Coor in an investigation of clinical reasoning and the evaluation of a teaching program to promote hypothetic-deductive problem solving. Rollin Gallagher developed a method of organizing biopsychosocial information in such a way as to facilitate diagnosis and planning. Both of us collaborated in the development of a goal-oriented approach to management and record-keeping.

During the past ten years, few funds have been available to support research in medical education. We are grateful to William Luginbuhl, Dean of the Faculty of Medicine, and Sheldon Weiner, Chairman of the Department of Psychiatry, at the University of Vermont, for their consistent support of this project, and to the Psychiatry Education Branch of the National Institute of Mental Health for grant support. We are also indebted to the Education Committee of the Department of Psychiatry, Drs. John Ives, Robert Lenox, Richard Bernstein and Lee Weaver, our colleagues in Family Practice, and to the students who helped us refine our ideas.

A number of colleagues reviewed sections of the book, particularly Drs. Thomas Achenbach, Patrick McKegney, Alan Tisdale, John Cawte, Thomas Gazda, and Jack Modell. Several people helped prepare the manuscript. Marianne Raymond typed and guarded earlier versions of this book. Audrey Racine typed many of the final chapter drafts and compiled the book. Maureen O'Reilly typed several chapters and Elizabeth Beckwith helped with the typing and prepared rough sketches for many of the illustrations.

Like most academic physicians, we were not relieved of our clinical and teaching duties to write this book but used nights, weekends and vacations. Our children, Victor, Stephen, and Lisa Nurcombe and Krysia, Anne, and Loch Gallagher waited patiently for "the book" to be completed. When we flagged, our wives, Alison and Diane, sustained and encouraged us. It is to them that we dedicate our work.

Barry Nurcombe
Rollin M. Gallagher

PART I

Introduction and knowledge base

1

Content and process

This book is about how to think.

Textbooks of clinical medicine are usually of two kinds. One kind classifies diseases; describes their characteristic symptoms, signs, and course; considers etiology, pathology, and laboratory findings; and discusses treatment in a somewhat prescriptive way. Another type of book deals with the application of diagnostic or therapeutic procedures to symptoms and diseases.

Books are banks of information that expand or supplement memory. How can a clinician gain access to these dormant stores? How can static information be activated and transformed into the dynamic knowledge required for clinical practice?

Confronted by somebody who presents a clinical problem, the physician must search memory for disease patterns and treatments; hunt for the abstract, rather idealized information stored in libraries; and apply an understanding of human behavior to the individual. However, nobody ever completely fits the textbook pattern, and no syndrome could possibly describe all a physician should know about a patient. It may be important, for example, to appreciate that the man in bed seven, with subacute bacterial endocarditis secondary to rheumatic scarring of the aortic valve, is a recently divorced, alcoholic engineer who rides a motorcycle. Clinical diagnosis and treatment demand more than a bald categorization of symptoms and signs and the prescription of specific treatment.

Given the complexity of medical practice the educational problem is twofold. How can the student learn to:

1. Match the raw, jumbled, clinical phenomena presented by the patient, with the idealized patterns stored in memory; yet
2. Develop an understanding of the patient sufficiently comprehensive to allow individualized management.

Traditionally, physicians have learned these aspects of their profession in an informal manner, picking them up by trial and error.

Some would say that one cannot teach another person to think and that clinical reasoning is so intuitive, artful, and personal as to defy detailed or general understanding. Others, taking a contrary line, assert that clinicians are so inconsistent that their decisions should be made by machines applying mathematical formulae to codified information with cast-iron reliability.

The essence of medical education is the promotion of decision-making and planning. This book proposes that it is desirable for a physician to think about thinking, since analysis of medical reasoning will foster systematic clinical problem-solving. Clinical reasoning is undeniably hampered if the student has insufficient fundamental knowledge; but the most controversial question in contemporary medical education is how to begin. One approach – the most traditional and familiar in medical schools – is to acquire fundamental information first and then tackle clinical problems. Another, more radical, strategy is to start with clinical problems and be guided to the information needed to resolve them. A third procedure combines the first two, in varying degrees.

This book takes the third approach. It proposes that acquiring clinical skills can be accelerated if the student interweaves the solving of problems with the acquisition of knowledge. Consequently, the book starts with an abbreviated survey of biopsychosocial functioning, next considers the tactics and strategy of clinical reasoning in psychiatry, proceeds to summarize the knowledge and procedures required for the clinical process, outlines a method of systematic planning, describes how the general principles can be applied to different clinical settings, and concludes with a review of empirical research into clinical reasoning. The central theme of the book has been derived from research of this kind.

Some advice to young players

Learning to be a clinician is a little like learning to play golf. Admittedly, golf is a game of motor coordination, whereas psychiatry is a conglomerate of knowledge, procedures, and social skill. Nevertheless, golf and psychiatry each has its own characteristic core of tactics and strategy that is its source of expertise.

No golfer is born a champion. Whatever genetic advantages have been dealt out at conception, the most talented competitor must learn the game. How is the beginner to begin? How can one emulate the power, precision, touch, judgement, coolness, and consistency of an expert?

Go to a coach who disarticulates the fundamental strokes into sequential steps and teaches them in an integrated way. Read books on equipment, stroke-making, and strategy. Watch good players. Practice driving, approaching, and putting until the harmonious flow of their components becomes second nature. Play as often as you can with different opponents. Think about your game and seek criticism from those you respect. Given reasonable potential, you should be playing at least adequately in a few years. As you get older, you may compensate for diminished power by tactical judgement, a keener awareness of an opponent's flaws, and a better sense of strategy.

This book is like a manual on golf. It deals with equipment, strokes, tactics, and strategy. The patients you will meet in the wards and clinics are the game itself. The psychiatrists and residents who teach you are your models and coaches.

Like any complex skill, competence in diagnosis and planning requires detailed knowledge available in books containing abstract, generalized information and acquired from clinical experience. Knowledge is applied through such clinical procedures as history-taking, mental status examination, physical examination, and special investigations. During these procedures, the clinician uses systematic tactics and a strategy of reasoning, both of which aim at establishing a diagnosis. The diagnosis, in turn, is not an end in itself but a guide to rational, comprehensive, and individualized management.

The Clinical Process in Psychiatry does not aim to replace conventional text-books but rather to complement them. It proposes to do so by linking your knowledge, your procedural skills, and the tactics and strategy of your clinical reasoning with the patients you will encounter. The book takes as its central theme a theoretical doctrine that Engel (1978) refers to as **biopsychosocial,** a doctrine proposing that a patient can be adequately understood only if the clinician considers all levels of functioning:

1. Physical
2. Psychological
3. Social

The physical level refers to phenomena associated with peripheral organ systems and autonomic, neuroendocrine, and subcortical controls.

The psychological level denotes a self-conscious inner world that directs the processing of information from, and communication with, the external world. The psychological level also includes internal representations of self, other people, and things in a kind of map of the personal world, together with the urges, motives, taboos, principles, ideals, and aspirations that regulate conduct. At the center of the psychological level is the person or conscious self, the vehicle of self-hood, self-regulation, and individuality.

The social level refers to the personal and impersonal world of people, things, groups, and institutions with, to, or by which the patient lives, relates, and is influenced.

Engel (1978) contends that recent advances in biomedical science have distracted physicians from the whole patient, leading to a nearly exclusive emphasis on the somatic, with cursory attention to psychosocial issues. Patients suffer in a number of ways from the fragmentation inevitable when medical care is restricted by such a narrow perspective. This book aims to counter the contemporary imbalance in medicine by describing the principles, strategy, and tactics the comprehensive physician can use when addressing the problems of the whole patient.

The book also suggests how the psychiatrist of the future might function. We have already considered the trends in medicine that entail fragmentation of diagnosis and care. The same forces are splintering psychiatry. There is a danger that psychiatrists will withdraw into the synapse and leave the rest of the mental health to nonmedical clinicians trained in different aspects of the psychosocial field.

Another future is possible. The psychiatrist could become the physician best able to integrate all levels of the biopsychosocial axis. As an individual, it is likely that the psychiatrist will acquire additional training in therapy or research applicable to a particular level in the systemic dimension. Psychopharmacology, psychoanalysis, behavior therapy, and group therapy are a few of the diverse opportunities available. Prepared to use a reductionist or restricted paradigm in research or clinical work when expedient, the comprehensive psychiatrist will appreciate that such an approach is a utilitarian fiction. In diagnosis, therapy, and research, the psychiatrist will be able to step back from the trees and view the phenomenal terrain before plunging back into the forest.

The psychiatrist's medical training provides the basis for reasoning in the somatic domain. Residency training expands and refines psychosocial knowledge and skills and enhances competence in somatic fields important to clinical psychiatry. Training should emphasize comprehensiveness and integration, particularly since the psychiatrist should be the clinician best suited to coordinate mental health workers who deal with acute, complex, or severe mental disorder.

This book proposes that systematic biopsychosocial problem-solving should be the basis of clinical reasoning in psychiatry (although the tenets propounded are important to all physicians). These concepts are specially useful to psychiatrists in what will become the leitmotiv of their work: comprehensive, multilevel, integrated diagnosis and the kind of individualized management planning calling for a mosaic of different therapies.

The Clinical Process in Psychiatry emphasizes the logical tactics and strategy most frequently used by experts in comprehensive diagnosis and management planning. The book is divided into six parts:

- Part I consists of the introduction, the objectives of the book, and chapters on illness behavior, psychological functioning and neurobiological systems.
- Part II, the heart of the book, outlines the clinical process and the tactics and strategy of clinical reasoning.
- Part III deals with the procedures (history-taking; mental status examination;

physical examination; and special investigations) and knowledge (clinical phenomenology; categorical syndromes; and modes of treatment) required for efficient reasoning.

- Part IV deals with planning (the problem-oriented record; comprehensive diagnosis; and goal-directed management planning).
- Part V applies the general scheme to special situations (outpatient psychiatry; emergency psychiatry; inpatient psychiatry; liaison psychiatry; family practice; and child psychiatry).
- Part VI summarizes research into clinical reasoning and describes an educational program that aims to accelerate it.

The medical student should concentrate upon parts I, II, and III and have a general understanding of part IV. The advanced student may find that selected chapters from part V are helpful, particularly if they relate to his or her clinical experience in inpatient or ambulatory settings. Psychiatric residents and other mental health professionals in training should concentrate on parts I, II, III, IV, and V. Chapter 6 is written for the clinical teacher who seeks an empirical justification for the central principles of the book, and for suggestions on how the principles can be conveyed to students.

After you appreciate the objectives of the book and understand how it fits into the goals of your clinical training in psychiatry, you may start with either part II or part III (or go back and forth between them).

The true test of this book is whether it helps you think systematically about patients. As you read it, refer to your own experiences. As you work with patients and think about them afterwards, keep the tactics and strategy in mind and consider whether they help you to reason more clearly, systematically, and efficiently.

Do not apply the tactics and strategy in a mechanical way. They are not cast-iron formulae or infallible algorithms, but rather are intended to lend structure to your work. If the tactics and strategy described in chapter 7 seem to confine you, reconsider how you are using them. They are meant to be a framework, not a suit of armor.

The same considerations apply to the method of diagnostic formulation and management planning described in chapters 14 and 15. If the precise technique does not suit you, modify it to suit your experience; but keep in mind the need to account for different levels of systemic organization and the full temporal dimension of physical and mental disorder.

2

Objectives

At the end of this book, if you have the opportunity to apply its principles to clinical work, you should have achieved the five objectives discussed in this chapter.

1. Distinguish among illness, disease, illness behavior, abnormal illness behavior, and the sick role. Describe the stages of illness behavior. Discuss the effect on illness behavior of physical, psychological and sociocultural factors. Discuss the interaction of vulnerability, stress, coping, and illness behavior.

2. Define psychological functioning as the executive domain of biopsychosocial functioning. Analyze it in terms of information processing; perceptual-motor and language functions; images, emotions and attitudes; defenses and controls; social competence; the sense of self; and coping techniques. Give examples of how psychopathology can be manifested in developmental delay, disintegration, or disorganization of each of these functions.

3. Discuss the neurophysiology and neurochemistry of psychoimmunology; arousal and sleep; the regulation of drives and emotion; reward, punishment

and pain; learning and memory; and neurotransmission, mental illness, and psychopharmacology.

4. Describe, in order, the stages of the clinical process. Discuss the difference between diagnostic and therapeutic phases and the interpenetration of the two.

5. Describe and define the most prominent psychiatric symptoms and signs in the areas of appearance and motor behavior; affect and mood; sensorium; speech and language; thinking and intellect; and content of thought.

6. List the components of a comprehensive diagnostic formulation. Describe the content and purpose of biopsychosocial assessment; the temporal dimension; the developmental axis; the diagnostic net; and the integrated formulation.

7. Describe the main special investigations likely to aid psychiatric diagnosis: biochemical, hematological, microbiologic, radiological, physiological, and psychological.

8. Describe the nature and purpose of the main modes of therapy in psychiatry: biological, psychological, and social.

Procedures

1. Facilitate an interview by using the following supportive techniques: listening, open-ended probes, nonverbal encouraging, and clarifying questions. Use these techniques to move an interview from inception, through reconnaisance and detailed inquiry, to termination.

2. Take a psychiatric history to elicit: presenting problem; history of present illness; history of past illnesses and habits; developmental, educational, occupational, sexual, and marital history; usual coping mechanisms; family history.

3. Conduct a mental status examination appropriate to the particular case.

4. Perform an appropriate physical examination.

5. Order appropriate special investigations and justify them in terms of expense, discomfort, and relevance to diagnosis.

Tactics

1. Discern and evaluate salient clues from the encounter with patient.

2. Interpret clues when appropriate.

3. Assemble clusters of clues and their interpretations to define a pattern.

4. Generate an array of alternative categorical and dynamic hypotheses to explain the pattern.

5. Develop an inquiry plan with routine and discretionary lines of inquiry based on the array of hypotheses.
6. Search for evidence to disconfirm or support the hypotheses.
7. Revise interpretations or hypotheses if fresh evidence warrants it by adding, refining, deleting, and weighing.
8. Reach a conclusion about which hypothesis is best supported by the evidence.
9. Formulate a comprehensive diagnosis.
10. Design a management plan based on goals derived from the comprehensive diagnostic formulation.

Strategy

1. Keep separate clue and interpretation, observation and inference. Be prepared to cite the clues on which an interpretation is based.
2. Tolerate uncertainty, avoid premature closure, and consider alternative explanations.
3. Give adequate weight to negative evidence and to new evidence appearing later in the interview.
4. Be prepared to revise the interpretations and hypotheses if fresh evidence demands it.
5. Do not go on interminably. Be prepared to commit yourself when enough evidence has been gathered.
6. Be aware of your personal reactions to the patient. Use them as clues. Guard against stereotyping. Try to distinguish between genuine understanding and projecting personal conflict onto the patient.

Application

1. Apply the aforementioned principles to the following clinical situations: outpatient and private office psychiatry, emergency psychiatry, inpatient psychiatry, liaison psychiatry, family practice, and child and adolescent psychiatry.

3

Illness behavior

Disease, illness, and illness behavior

Disease: objective

The terms *disease* and *illness* are often used synonymously. They are better kept separate. **Disease** is an hypothetical construct; it is a classifiable set of symptoms and signs stemming from disturbed bodily function and associated with characteristic paraclinical findings, course, and etiology. **Disorder** refers to a syndrome of somatic or psychological dysfunction less clearly defined than disease generally because the biomedical etiology is not understood.

Illness: subjective

Illness, on the other hand, refers to a subjective perception of being unwell. It is possible to harbor a disease (breast cancer, for example) without feeling ill. It is possible to feel ill (after bereavement, for example), without having a disease. Commonly, the two overlap; somebody who feels ill is found to have a disease. If illness is subjective, disease is relatively objective. You look sick; I feel ill. You have a disease, but I am ill.

The physician's social role

Society has authorized the physician to diagnose and treat people who have sicknesses. The physician does so by evaluating the patient's history, signs, and symptoms, diagnosing a disorder or disease, and prescribing treatment.

The difference between illness and sickness and disease, and the physician's function, can become contentious in the sicknesses that psychiatrists treat. There are several reasons for this:

11

The uncertain reliability of psychiatric diagnosis

1. Although much recent work has been done to improve their reliability, the validity of most psychiatric diagnoses will remain uncertain until the physical dysfunctions underlying certain psychiatric disorders have been clarified (see chapters 5 and 11).

Flaws in the disease model of psychiatric disorder

2. However, it is arguable that the criterion of disturbed bodily function (referred to in the definition of disease) is appropriate to only a minority of psychiatric disorders. Many psychiatric disorders appear to be related to temperament, to distortions of early learning, and to stress. Some commentators contend that certain disorders (for example, mental retardation, specific developmental learning disorders, ego-syntonic homosexuality, and antisocial personality disorder) should not be included in a psychiatric classification. In such debates, philosophical, moral, political, legal, and administrative issues are entangled. They will be considered further in chapter 11.

The psychiatrist as agent of society

3. People other than the patient may define him or her as sick. The patient may resist their definition. A psychiatrist may be called on to give an opinion if the patient is regarded as dangerous to self or others. The psychiatrist thus becomes an agent of society (which may assume responsibility for the patient) rather than the patient's chosen advisor. The contract that traditionally applies between patient and physician is thereby compromised.

The concept of disease in general, and mental disease in particular, will be examined further in chapter 11.

The sick role

Sometimes, therefore, patient, society, and physician disagree about whether the individual is sick. These ambiguities are less troublesome when the patient adopts a sick role. Parsons (1951) has postulated that all social groups make allowances for sick members who are unable to function normally by assigning them to a sick role. The sick role is defined by:

Factors defining the sick role

1. Exemption from normal duties.
2. Exemption from responsibility for the sickness.
3. The desire to get better.
4. An attempt to seek treatment and to cooperate with those providing it.

Flaws in the disease model in regard to antisocial or self-inflicted disorder

Szasz (1963) pointed out how debatable the concept of mental disease becomes when an individual has been involved in antisocial behavior, and the question arises whether the person should be considered criminal or sick, culpable or blameless. Further problems arise when a patient does not accept the sick role (as when a heavy drinker refuses help), when the patient does not cooperate in treatment or appears to prefer the sick role to recovery, when there is a possibility the patient has deliberately assumed the sick role for ulterior purposes, and when a disease could be regarded as self-inflicted.

Illness behavior and compliance

Illness vs. illness behavior

Just as the terms *disease* and *illness* are sometimes used interchangeably, *illness* and *illness behavior* are also often confused. Most research supporting the notion that stressful life events can lead to disease gauges the incidence of illness by the number of times a patient visits a physician, a kind of illness behavior (Rahe, Ryman, & Ward, 1980). But ill people who visit doctors do not necessarily have disease, and those who do are not necessarily more ill than those who do not (Barsky, 1981). If we are to comprehend the clinical process, we must understand not only the concepts disease and illness, but also the concept *illness behavior,* a term referring to an individual's unique responses to the perception of being ill.

Compliance

Disease affects organisms: People fall ill. People determine when and why they will visit a physician and whether they will adhere to prescribed treatment. One aspect of illness behavior, therefore, is compliance with medical care: the degree to which a patient cooperates with a physician in his or her own treatment. Obviously, a patient's compliance influences the outcome of treatment.

The high cost of noncompliance

Noncompliance is a major health problem. One extensive review indicates a 50% rate of noncompliance with health-related appointments and long-term medication regimens (Haynes, Sackett, & Taylor, 1979). The health of 44% of noncompliant patients is seriously threatened by this behavior (Steward & Cluff, 1972). The costs are staggering. Death and disability associated with noncompliance to treatment for hypertension, for example, have been estimated to cost the nation between three and five billion dollars annually (Kanelle, 1974; Kristian, Arnold, & Wynden, 1977).

"Good" patients

Compliant patients tend to get better. Even if they do not improve, they try so hard that those who care for them regard them as good patients.

Case 3.1

■ Lennie, a 23-year-old professional skier, hits a tree during a race. He fractures his spinal column, damaging the spinal cord at the twelfth thoracic vertebra, and partly paralyzing his legs. The surgeons stabilize his spine operatively, hoping that protecting the spinal cord might lead to functional recovery. However, he does not recover the use of his legs.

Despite a growing realization that he might not recover his ability to walk, let alone ski, Lennie remains cheerful and cooperative. He participates in as many activities as his condition permits, shaving, bathing, and feeding himself. He learns to catheterize himself in order to prevent urinary tract infection. He develops sufficient arm strength to become mobile, first on a stretcher, then in a wheelchair. Knowing that he will never race again, he makes plans to finish his college degree and pursue a career in journalism. Little wonder he becomes a very popular patient.

Lennie never does recover the use of his legs. In that sense, surgery has failed; but all the staff, including his surgeons, truly believe that his care is a success.

Before his transfer home to a distant state, the ward staff gives him a party. Six months later, he will drive back to Vermont in his own specially modified car and marry one of the nurses who looked after him. ■

"Bad" patients

Noncompliance drains those who try to help. Noncompliant patients may not improve and are blamed for not trying. If they do improve, they may not credit their physician for it. Thus, they are often regarded as problem or bad patients.

Case 3.2

■   Bill, a 21-year-old unemployed carpenter, fractures his seventh cervical vertebra in an automobile accident. A contusion to the spinal cord partially paralyzes him from the neck down. Initially, he was compliant, though noticeably anxious and irritable. After one week, his fracture is surgically stabilized. Neuromuscular function returns completely. Nevertheless, immobilized on a Stryker frame, Bill repeatedly demands attention and pain medication and joins his family in a chorus of criticism about his care.

After several weeks, Bill is discharged, his neck supported by a brace extending from the shoulders and attached to the skull with pins. He is carefully advised to care for the pins meticulously and to avoid strenuous or risky exercise.

Two weeks later he returns, complaining of headache, fever, pain around the fracture site, and weakness in the left arm. Physical examination reveals infection around the pin sites in his scalp. X-rays show slippage of the surgical repair of the spinal column. Bill's brother reveals that he has been drinking, exercising, and riding motorcycles since discharge. The staff is angry and frustrated. Despite surgical cure, the patient's care is regarded as a failure.   ■

Behavior predicts disease

The high cost of smoking

It is clear that behavior can affect the progress of sickness and disease. It is less apparent, perhaps, that behavior can predict disease. Cigarette smoking is a case in point. The mortality rate of cigarette smokers is 44% to 80% higher than that of nonsmokers (Houpt et al., 1980). The direct cost of medical care, accidents, absenteeism, and loss of productivity due to smoking has been estimated at more than 27 billion dollars annually (Luce & Schitzer, 1978). In fact, five of the six leading causes of death in the United States (disease of heart and blood vessels, cancer, accidents, diabetes mellitus, and hepatic cirrhosis) are related to life-style (Gori & Ritker, 1978).

The stages of illness behavior

Suchman describes the following five stages of illness behavior:

The five stages of illness behavior

1. *Symptom experience:* In the initial stage, patients decide something is wrong because they feel ill. They may choose to medicate themselves or seek help from lay people or folk practitioners. The outcome of this stage is recovery, uncertainty, denial or the acceptance of being sick.
2. *Assumption of the sick role:* At this point patients cease to function normally and seek from associates a validation of their assumption of the sick role.

3. *Medical care contact:* The patient seeks professional advice and negotiates treatment.

4. *Dependent patient role:* The patient accepts and undergoes treatment. Sometimes, however, patients will reject treatment, particularly if they disagree with the diagnosis or plan, or if they do not feel at ease with the physician.

5. *Recovery:* The patient relinquishes the sick role and resumes normal functioning. A less favorable outcome involves persistence in the sick role despite recovery from bodily disease. (Suchman, 1965b, pp. 114–128)

These five stages have been described from the patient's point of view. In chapter 6, they will be considered from the clinician's perspective.

The medical management of illness behavior

It is apparent that understanding behavior in health and illness should be an important goal of medical research and that physicians should be taught to help patients change maladaptive behavior.

Unfortunately, very little medical research and education addresses psychosocial questions, and few doctors have been prepared to cope with their patients' maladaptive illness behavior or life-styles.

How physicians cope with noncompliance

How can a young physician cope with this deficiency in training? At present, the management of illness behavior (as distinct from the management of disease) is determined less by systematic training than by the physician's personality and the emulation of role models. Physicians tend to adopt one or a combination of three clinical roles described here.

The physician as technician

The physician as technician

The physician abdicates responsibility for behavior and retreats behind technology. Noncompliance is very likely.

Case 3.3

■ A 45-year-old executive visits his doctor for the first time in four years with headaches and dizziness of one year's duration. He is found to have moderately severe hypertension. The doctor prescribes appropriate medication and a low-salt diet, telling the patient to take it easy: "You're working too hard."

Despite several return visits, the patient's blood pressure responds only marginally since he has not changed his life-style.

One year later, he suffers a myocardial infarction. In the hospital, he reveals that he thought the medication had slowed him down at work and caused impotence. He had expressed his concern about these side effects to his physician, who did not pursue their impact on compliance. ■

The physician as informant

The physician as
information provider

The physician informs the patient fully of the risks and responsibilities associated with the disorder and its treatment and leaves it to the patient to decide what to do about it. Compliance is more likely in this case, but it can be unstable.

Case 3.4   ■ A 42-year-old obese woman is diagnosed as diabetic. Her doctor recommends diet and a hospital-based nutrition education program describing the relationship between diet and diabetes. The patient successfully loses 20 pounds in 3 months and does not require insulin therapy.

Unable to sustain her weight loss, however, the patient eventually requires insulin to control blood sugar. A review of her recent history reveals that despite a full understanding of the importance of the diet, she abandoned it the first time her daughter and family visited, and has been unable to diet when she has visitors thereafter. ■

The physician as educator

The physician as
educator

The physician helps the patient change risky or noncompliant behavior by intellectual mastery and education. The physician who empathizes with a patient and attempts to help the patient understand and minimize risky behavior will promote compliance and achieve better results.

Case 3.5   ■ A 50-year-old executive with hypertension complains of medication effects slowing him at work and impairing his sexual performance. The doctor inquires further and finds that the patient's job is extremely stressful and that he has been irritable and depressed at home. She informs the patient of the relationship between stress and hypertension, but the patient finds himself unable to change at work or at home.

The doctor recommends a course of stress management and arranges marital therapy to help patient and wife jointly to modify stress. Within a month, the patient is using less medication, experiencing fewer side effects, and beginning to enjoy work and home life. His sexual life has improved considerably. His family doctor maintains him on minimal medication and daily relaxation exercises, seeing him twice yearly to reinforce stress management techniques. Patient and family doctor all feel pride in their successful collaboration. ■

This kind of intervention seems elementary. Why, then, is it exceptional?

Recently, many primary care training programs have included behavioral science in their curriculum. Too often, however, little more is conveyed than elementary interviewing and counseling skills; concepts derived from contemporary psychosomatic and behavioral medicine are omitted.

In an attempt to address these issues, Balint (1957) propounded an approach involving groups of doctors who regularly present problem cases to each

The use of
Balint groups

other with a psychiatrist who acts as discussion leader. Balint groups are popular in Europe and are beginning to be used in the United States (Gallagher & Chapman, 1981; Gazda et al., 1984).

Young physicians often try to get patients to change their behavior but become discouraged when they find their untutored efforts are ineffective. Common sense and good will are not enough. The physician must understand that illness behavior influences the physical, psychological, and social responses of every patient and that these phenomena in turn affect illness behavior. This book addresses the principles of comprehensive medicine and introduces a convenient method of organizing biopsychosocial information for diagnosis and management planning (see chapters 14 and 15).

Biopsychosocial influences on illness behavior

Systems theory

The application of general systems theory to biology by von Bertalanffy (1968) and Weiss (1962) has given medicine a new conceptualization of the influence of different factors on disease and illness.

The person as a
system

Engel (1977, 1980) conceptualizes human experience as an interaction of multiple systems within systems. At the heart of the matrix of systems is the person, an integrating and executive psychological function. Illness behavior is a personal phenomenon influenced by physical, psychological, and sociocultural factors. Let us consider how.

Physical factors in illness behavior

Behavior can be influenced by such endogenous factors as systemic disease and neuropsychiatric disorder or by such exogenous factors as drugs or toxins.

Physical disease and brain dysfunction

Brain dysfunction
affects behavior

Since the central nervous system is the substrate of behavior, a disease process affecting brain function will probably influence behavior.

Case 3.6

■ A physician asks a psychiatrist to evaluate the strange behavior of his 55-year-old aunt. For several years, his aunt's depression has been treated with phenelzine, a monoaminoxidase inhibitor prescribed by another psychiatrist who is out of town. In the last few days, her behavior has changed; she has become emotionally labile, muttering odd phrases and bumping into furniture and bruising herself. Her family think she is worse than ever.

Alerted by the recent onset of this behavior, the psychiatrist completes a brief routine screening neurological examination. The patient has a slight right facial weakness and a tendency to bump into objects on her left. Further history from her daughter reveals the patient had been well until 2 days before, when, after a breakfast of toast and bacon, she complained of sudden, severe headache. Within an hour, the daughter noticed her mother's strange behavior.

The psychiatrist suspects a stroke caused by the acute hypertension of a monoaminoxidase inhibition crisis precipitated by diet. More extensive neurological examination, spinal tap, and CT scan confirm the diagnosis of cerebral hemorrhage. An investigation of the contents of the aunt's refrigerator reveals the bacon is moldy. ■

The brain is exquisitely sensitive to the failure of diseased somatic systems.

Case 3.7
Diseased organs affect the brain

■ A 60-year-old male ex-smoker becomes irritable, depressed, and, at times, slightly confused whenever an upper respiratory infection progresses to bronchitis. His pO_2 falls from 90 mm Hg. to 65 mm Hg. during these episodes. Ironically, at these times he is apt to resume smoking cigarettes. ■

Case 3.8

■ A 45-year-old man has severe liver disease caused by alcoholism and by a bout of hepatitis sustained while taking hard drugs. He has been anxious and depressed. Wishing to help the patient sleep, the physician prescribes 30 mg of flurazepam to be repeated once as needed. Four days later, the patient's wife calls to say that her husband was difficult to rouse that morning and is confused and belligerent now that he is awake. The physician recalls, with chagrin, that flurazepam is metabolized in the liver. ■

Neuropsychiatric disorder

Psychiatric disorder and behavior

Any psychiatric disorder with a biological substrate will affect behavior. It can be a challenge to distinguish the primary manifestations of the disorder in question from illness behavior.

Case 3.9

■ A 45-year-old accountant is a reserved, careful man. He complies meticulously with medical instructions for the care of hypertension. However, during a major depressive episode, he cannot be bothered with salt restriction and medication. His blood pressure escalates out of control and hospitalization is required. Antidepressant therapy successfully resolves the depressive episode, and the patient again complies with his outpatient antihypertension regimen. ■

Medication, toxins, and brain dysfunction

Medications, toxins, and behavior

Exogenous factors can alter central nervous function. Some drugs cross the blood–brain barrier; whereas others affect organ systems with direct and indirect consequences to brain function. Digitalis, for example, can cause confusion either by direct effect on the brain or through cardiac arrythmia, which diminishes cerebral blood flow. By its depressant action on the nervous system, alcohol initially disinhibits brain function, then sedates it. Hepatitis and cirrhosis impede the metabolism of centrally active drugs and natural metabolites, both of which can embarrass brain function. When the physician assesses behavior in the context of physical disease, these factors must be kept in mind.

Case 3.10

■ A 30-year-old woman is brought by her husband to the emergency room because she has been acting strangely in recent weeks. In the past 2 years, she has had migratory polyarthralgia and fever and two spontaneous abortions, the most recent 2 months ago. During the last pregnancy, she was diagnosed as having systemic lupus erythematosus. High doses of corticosteroids have been administered for three months to control the disease. Her husband reports that she has been increasingly irritable and overactive and alternately angry or despondent. Diazepam has been prescribed to calm her.

The consulting psychiatrist generates several hypotheses about this vulnerable woman's psychological symptoms: (1) the effect of steroids on mood; (2) active central lupus; (3) the disinhibiting effects of diazepam on mood and behavior in a patient who has sustained several psychological losses; and (4) combinations of the first three conditions. ■

Psychological factors in illness behavior

Mechanic (1968) described how the following **symptomatic factors** influence a person's response to illness:

The influence of symptoms on behavior

1. Perceptual salience: The more obvious or discomforting a symptom, the more likely it will be acted on (for example, by seeking medical care).
2. Perceived seriousness: The more dangerous a symptom is considered to be, the more likely it will be acted on.
3. Disruptiveness and frequency: The more symptoms interrupt daily life, the more the effect of illness on behavior.
4. Understanding: The patient's response is affected by his or her comprehension of the nature of the sickness.

Psychological factors affect illness behavior, an association too often ignored in practice. Ill people who attend physicians are not necessarily sicker than ill people who do not; the two groups are indistinguishable when number and type of symptoms are compared (Zola, 1972). Psychological rather than physical factors account for this observation.

The patient's personality affects his or her manner of presenting to, and behaving in, a medical setting. The following personality types can be recognized (Kahana & Bebring, 1964):

Personality types and
illness behavior

1. The dependent, demanding patient
2. The orderly, controlled patient
3. The dramatizing, emotionally captivating patient
4. The long-suffering, self-sacrificing patient
5. The guarded patient
6. The patient who conveys a sense of superiority
7. The patient who seems uninvolved and aloof.

These personality types should not be regarded as personality disorders but rather as normal reaction-types manifested in stressful conditions. Physicians who recognize these reactions can use relatively simple tactics to enhance cooperation. For example, it is helpful to schedule frequent visits for the dependent patient.

Dependent patients

Case 3.11   ■ A 30-year-old woman plagues her doctor with multiple minor physical complaints. Never reassured by negative physical and laboratory examinations, she demands an immediate investigation of every new symptom.

Recognizing her need for reassurance and care, the physician decides to schedule her for a regular visit every 2 weeks. Subsequently, the number and scope of her complaints diminish markedly; so does her doctor's frustration. ■

Controlling patients

Prescribe a precise regimen for orderly, controlling patients and provide opportunities for them to exercise control over their own treatment.

Case 3.12   ■ John, a 35-year-old married engineer with disabling panic attacks, has been referred to a psychiatrist. John is critical of an internist who prescribed diazepam, which made him groggy. He was baffled by the inscrutable responses of a nondirective psychotherapist. The psychiatrist, recognizing the patient's obsessional tendencies and need for cognitive mastery, carefully outlines the rationale for a limited course of medication and for 10 sessions of stress management training and biofeedback. John contracts for the treatment program, which successfully modifies his symptoms. Buoyed by his new mastery, he agrees to a longer course of psychotherapy in order to explore the psychodynamic meaning of his symptoms. ■

Dramatizing patients   To a dramatizing patient give close, calm, concerned attention.

Case 3.13   ■ Mary, a 22-year-old mother of a 3-week-old daughter, calls the pediatrician almost nightly, tearfully or frantically presenting her concerns about routine child care problems. During the fifth such call in one week, the annoyed pediatrician reminds her that she (the pediatrician) needs some sleep. Mary hangs up in a huff

After some reflection, the pediatrician calls back and apologizes. She contracts to see Mary and the infant in her office every week and enrolls both parents in a child-care education class. Mary learns to note her questions on a list to show the physician each visit. The inappropriate telephone calls virtually disappear. ■

Long-suffering patients

Appreciate the pluck and grit of the patient who has suffered a burden of complaints but carried on despite it.

Case 3.14

■ A 50-year-old man has spent a lifetime helping others with their problems, despite a chronically painful low-back condition. His family practitioner, unlike other physicians who were frustrated by his complaints, regularly but quietly acknowledges the patient's ability to function despite his suffering. ■

Suspicious patients

Present a calm, matter-of-fact, open demeanor to the suspicious patient.

Case 3.15

■ A 35-year-old woman with major depression fears losing control over her mind and refuses to take antidepressants. The psychiatrist does not argue with her but calmly explains the potential benefits and liabilities of the medication and asks the patient to consider her choices before returning. At the next appointment, she asks a few questions, then agrees to cooperate. ■

Superior patients

Acknowledge the stature of the patient who conveys an air of superiority, exaggerated self-confidence, and self-importance.

Case 3.16

■ A 35-year-old bank vice-president presents to a behavioral medicine service with chronic headaches. During his first meeting with the psychiatrist, he makes disparaging remarks about the inexperience of his last physician, a neurology resident, and criticizes the nurse clinician who has taken his history. The psychiatrist takes pains to let the patient choose an appointment time that is convenient to his busy work schedule. He also briefly mentions the outstanding credentials of the psychologist who will be treating him with a stress management program. ■

Aloof patients

Be considerate but nonintrusive towards an aloof, uninvolved patient.

Case 3.17

■ A 50-year-old woman begins treatment for adult-onset diabetes mellitus at a family practice clinic. While completing a family pedigree, her resident physician enthusiastically encourages her to talk about family relationships. She responds with brief, uninformative answers. He tries harder. She gets quieter.

    During the next visit, he tries again to complete his psychosocial data base; no luck. She cancels her next appointment, with a message that she is returning to her previous physician, who, the resident recalls, rarely inquires about his patients' personal lives. ■

Sociocultural factors in illness behavior

Social factors affect disease incidence and mortality

Biophysical mechanisms mediate the influence of psychologic factors on disease, illness, and illness behavior. Psychologic mechanisms mediate the influence of sociocultural factors. Yet, as mentioned in the section on medical management of illness behavior, medical education gives cursory attention to such matters. It is known, for example, that social factors correlate directly with the incidence and mortality rates of many diseases. A 9-year study of 4,700 adults demonstrated that poor social integration predicted mortality, especially from four conditions: cancer, ischemic heart disease, cerebrovascular disease, and circulatory disease (Berkman & Syme, 1979). These predictions pertained even when allowance was made for the effects of baseline health, social class, obesity, smoking, alcohol consumption, and health practices. Life stress provokes, and social support mitigates, depressive illness, neurotic symptoms, angina pectoris, chronic physical conditions, pregnancy complications, and hypertension (Eisenberg, 1980). Hormonal and immunologic control systems presumably mediate the influence of social factors on vulnerability to disease. (Borysenko & Borysenko, 1982; Locke, 1982). Bereavement, for example, has been associated with indices of impaired immune function (Schleifer et al., 1980; Bartrop et al., 1977). This subject will be further discussed in chapter 5.

Ethnocultural factors

Ethnicity

As mentioned in the discussion of compliance, behavior reflects the influence of social factors on illness and disease. Several studies have investigated the effect of culture on illness behavior. Zborowski (1952), for example, studied the reactions to pain of different ethnic groups. Jewish and Italian patients responded emotionally, emphasizing their distress to the physician. ''Old Americans'' were more stoic and denying. Jews were more concerned about the meaning of pain; whereas Italians were more worried about relief from it.

Zborowski suggested that ethnic differences in pain reaction are the result of different childrearing experiences: Jewish and Italian parents respond with anxiety and protectiveness to their children's pain; Anglo-Saxons and Celts are more likely to expect self-control. Mechanic (1963) found that Jews and Italians are relatively more likely than other ethnic groups to report symptoms. Sternbach and Tursky (1965) compared the reactions of Irish, Jewish, Italian, and Anglo-Saxon housewives to painful electric skin stimulation. Italian women showed the lowest tolerance; Jewish women were intermediate; while Irish and Anglo-Saxon women were more likely to suffer in silence. Although such studies report *relative* statistical differences between large subsamples, the overlap between ethnic groups is marked. There is no support for stereotyping; stoical Jews, emotional Irish, and stolid Italians abound.

Cultural disadvantages to medical care

Ethnic differences and the pattern of symptoms

Nevertheless, Suchman (1964, 1965) found that minority ethnic groups in New York City were likely to be uninformed and skeptical about medical care and to adopt a dependent pattern of behavior when sick. Ethnic differences also affect the pattern of psychiatric symptoms. Opler and Singer (1956) compared schizophrenic New York men of Irish and Italian parentage matched for age, class, education, and intelligence. The Irish men tended to manifest latent homosexual conflicts, repressed hostility to female family figures, and sexual guilt. The Italian men were less prone to sexual guilt and more liable to be emotional, assaultive, destructive, and rebellious and to express open hostility to their fathers. They had less elaborate delusions and were more hypochondriacal.

Other studies document the influence of social groups on illness or symptoms, particularly on pain. Wounded troops request pain medication after trauma much less often than do civilians (Beecher, 1959). To a soldier, a wound is an honorable passport to safety. To a civilian, injury means expense and unemployment.

Family influences

The family has a powerful influence on illness behavior. The tendency to complain of pain has been associated with having been raised in big families (Gonda, 1962). Wooley, Blackwell, and Winget (1978) showed that of all factors, an intact family had the most beneficial influence on maintaining adaptive behavior in patients discharged from a psychosomatic unit.

Case 3.18

■ Because he has an irrational fear of heart attack, Bill, a 32-year-old lawyer, checks his pulse repeatedly. If it is over 100 per minute, for whatever reason, he panics and hyperventilates and usually ends up in a doctor's office or emergency room.

Bill is referred to a behavioral medicine unit, where a psychiatrist prescribes imipramine to block the panic episodes; but despite behavioral psychotherapy, Bill's fear and pulse-checking persist. Further history reveals that Bill's mother died suddenly when he was 12. Bill's wife, a nurse whose father died at 42 years from a heart attack, reveals that Bill has irrational fears that she will leave him. His panic and cardiac anxiety invoke her close attention, to the point at which she will monitor his pulse and verbally reassure him. Made aware of this in therapy, Bill and his wife decide to change their habitual patterns of response and reinforcement. Bill's irrational fears and abnormal illness behavior gradually subside. ■

Social factors related to attitudes to psychiatric care

The tendency to deny, rationalize, minimize, or normalize is greater in psychiatric than in physical disorder, although these defenses are common in both situations. Scheff (1966) found that college students who sought psychiatric help were more likely to have college-trained parents with no definite religious allegiance and to be from an urban background. He suggested that psychiatrically unsophisticated people, in contrast, ignore psychiatric problems until they are overwhelming and seek help only in a crisis.

The adaptation of the social group

The social group is called on to adapt to the individual's illness. Yarrow et al. (1955) described how a wife typically responds to the mental illness of her spouse. First, as she gradually becomes aware of the cumulative change in his behavior, she tries to account for it. She entertains different explanations but cannot decide. Next, she tries to accommodate to his behavior, waiting for more information before she makes up her mind. Her adaptation is likely to involve denial ("He'll snap out of it") or the rationalization of his behavior in physical terms ("He's just exhausted"; "Tired blood"; "Needs a vacation"). She tends toward minimization ("It's nothing") and normalization ("Anyone would be a bit down after all he's been through"), until eventually she must concede that he is mentally ill.

Plaintive set

Shepard, Oppenheim, and Mitchell (1966) found that maternal neuroticism and the tendency to seek advice determined which symptomatic children were taken to a London child guidance clinic. Scott-Henderson et al. (1981) hypothesize a plaintive set, which causes many patients prone to psychological illness to describe their social supports as inadequate.

Sex

Sex has been found to affect the recognition of symptoms. Boys are more stoic than girls (Mechanic, 1964). Women are more likely than men to use medical facilities (Anderson, 1963).

The effect of community coherence

Anthropology hints at the diversity of sociocultural influences on illness behavior. A study of the Hutterites (Eaton & Weil, 1953) demonstrated how a community with close social ties and shared religious values recognize mental disturbance and actively cooperate to help the patient. Depression, for example, is considered the work of the devil: The victim must have questioned God's word. Neighbors congregate to help. The patient is induced to confess transgression publicly, and group solidarity is affirmed.

The Lardil tribe of Northern Australia adopt a comparable approach to depressed or hypochondriacal kinfolk. A tribal practitioner is called on to diagnose the problem. He may attribute the disorder to the transgression of a social taboo (mixing food from land and sea, for example) or to the patient's illegitimate intrusion into a part of the fishing coast belonging to a different clan (with the consequent invasion of the victim's body by the totemic spirit dwelling in that place). The practitioner extracts a confession and exorcises the intrusive spirit with a magical combination of song, spell, body manipulation, and group therapy (Cawte, 1974).

Community tolerance

Aborigines with major mental disorders are identified by their neighbors as "deaf" (unresponsive), "confused," or unpredictable. They are regarded as different from those who are possessed. Nevertheless, psychotic people are tolerated unless they disrupt the camp by shouting at night, lighting fires, or assaulting others.

The adverse effect of a lack of community

Anthropology suggests that people are more likely to tolerate mental illness in those they know, especially those to whom they are kin, and that tolerance is associated with a desire to help. The reverse of this situation is exemplified in Western society by the deinstitutionalized patient shuffling with his or her bags around the metropolis, bereft of family, friends, or social support.

The effect of cultural disadvantage on attitudes to psychiatric disorder

Knowledge, education, and class also affect illness behavior. Psychologically unsophisticated rural people are slow to ascribe mental illness to their family or friends or to recognize it in themselves. They tend to deny, minimize, normalize, or rationalize the problem. Some consult folk practitioners, in accordance with cultural beliefs. Many lower-class patients who are admitted to hospital are referred by the courts, police, or other agencies (Hollingshead & Redlich, 1958). Less sophisticated patients are likely to place more emphasis on symptom relief than on the treatment of a disorder. They are prone to stop treatment prematurely or to abandon medication. Such behavior is of serious consequence to managing psychotic patients who have been discharged from hospital.

It is particularly evident in the poorest, most disadvantaged people who feel alienated and powerless and who make inadequate use of preventive services (Hollingshead & Redlich, 1958).

Competing needs

Factors that delay assuming the sick role

Competing needs in a social group can influence illness behavior. The need to keep working in order to care for a family may incline the patient to deny symptoms for a time or to minimize, normalize, or rationalize them. The perceived stigma of referral to a mental health center may prevent patients and families from seeking assistance or cause them to resist referral.

Accessibility of medical care

Geographical remoteness, lack of finances, difficulty in securing an appointment, and language or cultural barriers can also prevent, delay, or complicate matters. During the past 20 years, some progress has been made toward providing mental health services to the poor, to various cultural groups, to people in remote places, to children, and to the elderly. Much more remains to be done.

Figure 3.1 schematizes the effect of biological, psychological, and social factors on behavior.

Learning and illness behavior

Conditioning

Illness behavior can be considered as learned insofar as it is conditioned by external or internal events that increase or decrease the frequency of the behavior (Wooley, Blackwell, & Winget, 1978). Two forms of conditioning have been described: classical and operant. **Classical conditioning** occurs when one stimulus that leads to a rewarded or punished response is repeatedly paired with another stimulus; the second stimulus eventually produces the same response in absence of the first. There are many examples of this phenomenon in clinical settings. If an injection causes pain and fear and the physician is present during injections, ultimately the presence of the physician alone may be enough to cause fear. To avoid this, many primary care physicians have nurses give injections and are quick to support, encourage, and reward children who come to their offices.

Operant conditioning occurs when the consequences of an action affect its frequency. For example, if a visit to a physician is rewarding, the patient will be more likely to return. If the visit is unhelpful or unpleasant, the patient is less likely to come back. Operant conditioning has been applied to the treatment of

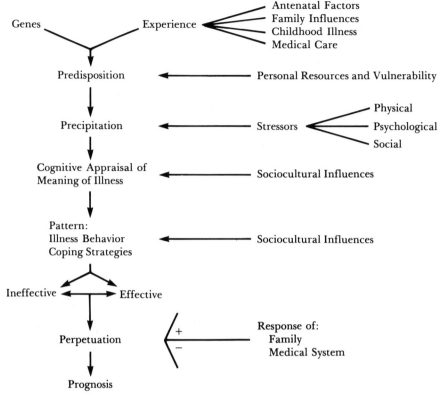

FIGURE 3.1
Biopsychosocial development of illness behavior

chronic pain syndromes (Fordyce et al., 1968) and to other medical disorders (Wooley, Blackwell, & Winget, 1978).

Case 3.19   ■ After suffering severe leg fractures in an automobile accident, Peter, a 24-year-old maintenance man, has a very painful, ischemic left leg. To obtain morphine, he must call for a nurse, but he is not allowed to have medication more often than every four hours. Sometimes he must wait up to thirty minutes before the nurse arrives to give him relief. After a while, he learns that loud complaints of pain and facial grimacing elicit a more rapid response from the nursing staff. He is thus induced to dwell on the pain so much that even though his leg is objectively improving, he acts as though he felt worse. His dose of morphine rises to 70 mg daily, and he refuses to participate in physical therapy.

Called to consult, a psychiatrist recommends the narcotic be given every four hours, whether or not it is requested. The nurses are asked to provide five minutes of attention about every two hours. After physical therapy, the patient is wheeled outside to be with friends on the sundeck.

Peter's complaints subside. Within a week, he is participating actively in his rehabilitation and taking only one or two doses of narcotic daily, usually before a particularly painful experience such as physical therapy. ■

In this case, the staff stopped rewarding Peter's complaints of pain. They gave him medication regularly, not on demand; in addition, they rewarded his adaptive involvement in physical therapy.

Stress and illness behavior

Stressor, stress, distress, and stress response are often confused. A **stressor** is an internal or external physical or psychosocial stimulus that provokes a state of unpleasant arousal called distress. **Stress response** refers to the physiologic concomitants of distress (Cannon, 1934), together with the psychological responses known as coping techniques. Different patterns of psychological response to stressors have been identified (Horowitz, 1975; Horowitz & Wilner, 1976), as shown in Figure 3.2.

As the biopsychosocial model suggests, adaptation to stressors involves all organizational levels – molecular, cellular, systemic, neural, and psychosocial (Engel, 1977). Biomedical research concentrates on the lower levels; behavioral research focuses on the whole organism in its social context. Biomedical and biobehavioral sciences converge when the mechanisms of the stress response are considered.

The mediation of the stress response

It has been known for some time that such peripheral physiologic patterns as an elevation of plasma corticosteroids are characteristic of the stress response. Recent research has implicated central mediating mechanisms in the stress response (Usdin, Kvetnansky, & Kapin, 1980). Neural circuits between midbrain limbic lobe and hypothalamus convey the effects of perceived stress to the endocrine and autonomic nervous systems, which, in turn, affect cardiovascular, gastrointestinal, reproductive, and immune systems. Midbrain circuits, acting in concert with the cerebral cortex, also mediate the adaptive functions of perception, cognitive appraisal, emotional response, and memory. A number of central neurotransmitters function as chemical messengers to specific cellular receptor sites in these circuits. A detailed exposition of how different neurochemical systems relate to specific neuropsychologic functioning and to disorders of the brain and mind is presented in chapter 5.

Stress correlates with disease

Epidemiologic research has demonstrated a strong association between stress and disease. Compared to people with few stressors, individuals with many life problems are at higher risk for serious disorder (Elliot & Eisdorfer, 1982), have more serious sicknesses (Rahe & Arthur, 1978), and seek medical help more often (Mechanic, 1978; Anderson et al., 1977). For example, in a population of 5,000 British widowers, the death of a spouse was associated with a 40% increase in mortality (Young, Bernard, & Wallis, 1963). Among bereaved adults, subjective distress is a better predictor of medical care use than is actual morbidity

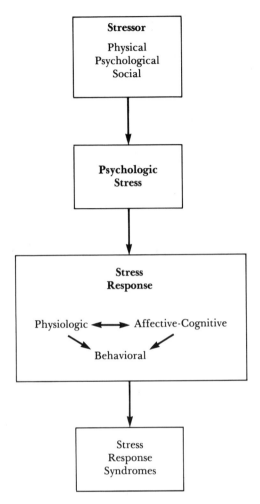

FIGURE 3.2
Stress and illness behavior

Perceived stress, sickness, and illness behavior

(Tessler, Mechanic, & Diamond, 1976). In fact, the extent to which an individual experiences frustration in daily life is a better predictor of sickness and illness behavior than is actual life stress (Karmer et al., 1981).

Emotional distress, disguised or undisguised, may be the primary reason for seeking medical help (Balint, 1957). Distress conduces to medical contact in two ways. It causes people to notice, amplify, and report symptoms they might otherwise ignore and thus to perceive themselves as ill. In addition, people receptive to the sick role are likely to adopt it as a method of coping with distress (Mechanic, 1972).

Coping

Coping techniques and ego defense mechanisms

Coping is a unifying construct linking psychosocial factors and illness behavior. Although the difference is somewhat arbitrary, it is helpful to distinguish between coping techniques and ego defense mechanisms. **Ego defenses,** such as denial, repression, displacement, and projection, serve to ward off, avoid, or divert the awareness of painful or stressful internal or external stimuli. They are never manifest in pure culture but always in combination (see chapter 4).

Case 3.20

■ Henry, a 35-year-old man admitted to a cardiac care unit for myocardial infarction, pulls out his intravenous catheter and walks out of the hospital, accusing the staff of incompetence and blaming his pain on muscle strain. ■

Henry is combining the defenses of denial, projection, and rationalization in order to minimize the psychological threat of a serious illness. He is actually increasing the risk of morbid or mortal complications.

Coping techniques in illness

Coping techniques, on the other hand, are combinations of defenses in action and are best viewed as ways in which individuals adapt to life stress, in the sense of relative competence. Illness is indeed a threat to life, but it can also become a spur to psychological maturation, through the acquisition of more competent coping techniques.

Case 3.21

■ Severely injured in a car accident, a jobless, alcoholic 22-year-old man has sustained permanent loss of function in the right leg. During prolonged hospitalization, he is counselled regularly by a supervised medical student from a psychiatric consultation service. The patient takes up the study of electronics, decides to finish his high school diploma, and subsequently goes to college to complete an engineering degree. ■

Illness can directly threaten the adequacy of an individual's customary coping techniques.

Case 3.22

■ When a 22-year-old college student is stressed by personal relationships or academic demands, he copes by plunging into competitive athletics. Following an ice hockey injury, a bad knee immobilizes him. He finds he is unable to concentrate, and his grades fall. ■

Treatment can impair coping

The treatment of illness can impair coping.

Case 3.23

■ Charles, a 45-year-old executive with major depression, is prescribed antidepressant medication. Accustomed to coping with job demands by working at high speed with great efficiency and unable to tolerate the moderate sedation that is a side effect of the antidepressant, he stops medication. His depression deepens. ■

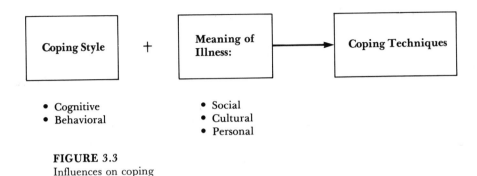

FIGURE 3.3
Influences on coping

Tailor treatment to coping style

In both these cases, a physician aware of the patient's coping style could tailor treatment appropriately. The student might be encouraged to convert to competitive swimming or cycling. The executive could have been prescribed a nonsedative antidepressant. In both instances, the stress of the illness and its treatment interfered with fundamental coping mechanisms.

Coping style

Lipowski (1970) uses the terms *coping style, meaning of illness,* and *coping strategy* to describe the ways people cope with illness.

The meaning of illness affects coping strategies

Coping style refers to a person's enduring disposition to meet challenges and stresses with a particular constellation of attitudes and behavior, as in Figure 3.3.

Cognitive coping style

The concept of coping style refers to two fundamentally different attitudes:

1. Minimization
2. Vigilance

Minimization denotes the tendency to ignore or explain away the significance of an illness. Rigid defenses such as denial are employed. Henry (Case 3.20), the 35-year-old man with myocardial infarction, is a case in point. Despite vigorous education and persuasion, Henry was determined to exercise his heart and walked out of the hospital. More subtle phenomena, such as the selective misrepresentation of an illness, can be used to veil its implications.

Case 3.24

■ A 50-year-old alcoholic salesman, recently discharged from the hospital following an episode of alcohol-induced hepatitis, temporarily moderates his use of alcohol. He tells his friends and family he has suffered an infection of the liver and his doctor has advised him to "take it easy on the booze for a while." ■

Coping styles are on a continuum

Minimization can be viewed as on a continuum, from maladaptive extremes (such as the anosognosia of parietal lobe syndrome or the denial of emaciation in anorexia nervosa) to the adaptive optimism that enables a paraplegic to face an extended rehabilitation.

Vigilance involves persistent attempts to reduce the uncertainty of illness. To feel secure when ill, people using this style try to understand the precise nature, treatment, and progress of their illness. Again, as with all coping styles, *Vigilant focussing* vigilant focusing varies in the extent to which it is used. The hypervigilant patient, for example, exaggerates every twinge and registers every change in the physician's expression, to the extent that effective care is impeded.

Case 3.25   ■ Janice, a depressed 32-year-old teacher, has persistent neurovegetative symptoms and suicidal ideation. After several interviews, the psychiatrist finally persuades her to accept antidepressant medication. She immediately goes to the library, reads the *Physician's Desk Reference* (which lists all possible side effects, however rare) and proceeds to investigate each side effect in other texts in the library. Increasingly concerned about the complications of the medication, she stops it after the first day. Her depression worsens, and she eventually requires hospitalization.   ■

In comparison, another vigilant patient may clearly appraise the nature of an illness and contribute rationally to a therapeutic plan.

Case 3.26   ■ A 35-year-old man presents with low back pain caused by instability of the lower lumbar spine. He studies the relationship of back mechanics and stress to pain and keeps a log of pain-inducing activities. Within several weeks, he and his physician have outlined a program of exercise, weight loss, change of lifestyle, and back hygiene. Surgery and disability are both averted.   ■

Behavioral coping styles   Lipowski describes several behavioral coping styles: tackling, capitulating, and avoidance. **Tackling** denotes an active approach and is usually associated with vigilance. In an exaggerated form, it can worsen the patient's condition; for example, some cardiac patients tackle physical rehabilitation so vigorously that they unduly stress the myocardium, producing a fatal arrhythmia or further infarction. In less extreme form, tackling can foster recovery. For example, a cardiac patient may actively participate in designing and implementing a gradual rehabilitation schedule that leads to full functional recovery and greatly reduces the risk of complication or further infarction.

Capitulating refers to passive, withdrawing, or dependent behavior when confronted by illness. Such patients participate little in their own care and have little initiative to achieve maximum recovery. Some passivity is adaptive during the acute stage of many illnesses; for example, a patient with recent myocardial infarction must accept the need for rest. However, some patients cling to invalidism and become cardiac cripples. The physician can identify pathological passivity by its intensity, duration, and disproportionateness.

Avoiding denotes an active effort to escape the threat of illness and is often combined with minimization. For example, the 35-year-old man who denied the seriousness of his myocardial infarction (Case 3.20) avoided all reminders of the threat by leaving the hospital. Avoiding can be healthy; for

TABLE 3.1
The relationship between behavioral and cognitive coping system

		Behavior		
		Tackling	*Capitulation*	*Avoidance*
Attitude	*Minimization*	I'll be over this in no time.	What, me sick?	I'm getting out of here!
	Vigilance	I'll follow the treatment plan to the letter.	I'm done for!	————

example, patients may actively avoid activities that put them at risk of injury and disease, such as driving while intoxicated, smoking, or overeating.

Table 3.1 provides specific examples of the relationship between these attitudinal and behavioral styles.

The meaning of illness and coping techniques

The meaning of illness

Coping techniques involve the attitudes and behavior that a patient manifests in coping with a particular illness and are influenced by the patient's construction of the meaning of the illness. Meaning is multidetermined and is affected by the following factors:

1. Sociocultural attitudes to illness and the medical system.
2. Family attitudes to illness and the medical system.
3. Personal remembrances of illness and the medical system.
4. The patient's interpretation of the nature and course of the illness in question.

Illness may be interpreted in a number of ways, for example, as threat, punishment, weakness, relief, manipulation, loss, or challenge.

Illness as threat

1. Illness as threat provokes anxiety, fear, and anger. Anxiety and fear can lead to denial, minimization, or overassertiveness. An overassertive attitude can cause disputes with the physician or hospital staff. In extreme cases, it can be associated with paranoid thinking, the patient accusing the staff of incompetence, malpractice, or conspiracy. On the other hand, assertiveness can have adaptive value. For example, in women with breast cancer, a fighting spirit has been associated with a better outcome than has a demeanor of helplessness (Greer, Morris, & Pettingale, 1979). Sometimes the medical system is inert, particularly in hospitals with fragmented care, where the patient is forced to demand information or to insist that inappropriate treatment be changed.

Illness as punishment

2. Illness as punishment may be associated with anger, hostility, or depression. A patient with a capitulating coping style may offer little resistance.

In contrast, a patient who is a tackler may see the illness as an opportunity for atonement or self-sacrifice.

Illness as weakness

3. Illness as weakness is commonly associated with shame, denying illness, and avoiding reminders of it.

Illness as relief

4. Illness as relief is associated with anxiety reduction. The patient may be relieved by illness from personal or occupational responsibilities, or assured thereby of financial security. Conscious or unconscious strategies arising from this interpretation include malingering, conversion, hypochondriasis, and the overuse of medical facilities – all forms of abnormal illness behavior.

Illness as manipulation

5. Illness as manipulation is closely related to illness as relief. It is associated with the need to use illness to manipulate interpersonal relationships. Dependent patients, particularly children or the elderly, may use the sick role to get the care they fear they would not otherwise receive.

Illness as loss

6. Illness as irreparable loss or damage leads to hostility, depression, resistance to care, and even suicide. It is often associated with the sense of losing physical attractiveness.

Case 3.27

■ A 52-year-old married mother of four had a mastectomy following discovery of a malignant breast tumor. Three years later, despite good evidence that there has been no spread of the tumor, the woman remains depressed, reclusive, and emotionally distant from husband, children, and friends. ■

Illness as challenge

7. Illness as challenge or opportunity represents a viewpoint propounded in the popular literature of previous generations. Famous people who had transcended illness and gone on to be more productive than before were often held up as exemplars. Franklin Roosevelt's rising political career was halted by infantile paralysis. At Hot Springs, Georgia, his personal struggle to rehabilitate himself, an experience he shared with similarly afflicted Americans of all backgrounds, attuned him to the plight of the common man. He developed a new political philosophy and his career was rejuvenated.

According to the concept of coping, the stages of an illness can be defined by illness behavior, rather than by the disease process. A patient's reaction to a symptom can be understood as a sequence of linked cognitive and behavioral responses (see Figure 3.4). The different meaning the patient gives to each stage will determine the individual's coping technique. This coping technique will, in turn, affect the timing of the subsequent stage.

Let us apply these concepts to a man with psychiatric illness – the 45-year-old executive with major depressive disorder who stopped medication because he disliked its sedative effect (Case 3.23).

■ Charles interpreted his initial symptoms (fatigue, diminished energy, poor concentration) as signs of weakness and potential danger. He thought, ''I'm getting old. My mind is deteriorating. I'd better not tell anyone or they might sack me. I must work even harder.'' In the past, his characteristic style had been to minimize

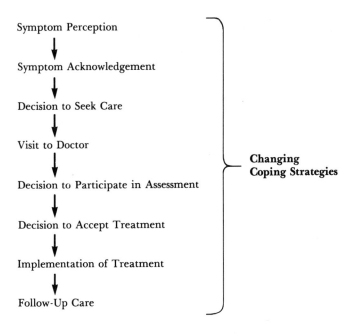

Symptom Perception

Symptom Acknowledgement

Decision to Seek Care

Visit to Doctor

Decision to Participate in Assessment

Decision to Accept Treatment

Implementation of Treatment

Follow-Up Care

**Changing
Coping Strategies**

FIGURE 3.4
Stages of illness

symptoms and tackle what he perceived as their cause. Thus, it was not surprising in the current situation that he worked hard and long, mentioning his symptoms to no one. It was only after his work deteriorated and his wife protested about his restless sleep, emotional withdrawal, and diminished libido that he acknowledged his symptoms were significant and revealed them to her. Consequently, she pressed him to seek medical care.

Unfortunately, he interpreted the sedation caused by medication as further deterioration and responded with familiar coping behavior. Only when the consulting psychiatrist clarified what he was doing and successfully treated the biologic aspects of Charles's depression with nonsedating antidepressants, did he begin to tackle the actual stressors that had precipitated his depressive episode: excessive work and deteriorating personal relationships. ■

Abnormal illness behavior

Under the conceptual umbrella of abnormal illness behavior, Pilowsky (1971, 1978) and Pilowsky, Spence and Waddy (1978) group phenomena as diverse as the denial of illness, the exaggeration of physical complaints, hypochondriasis, psychogenic pain, somatization disorder, conversion disorder, factitious disorder, and malingering.

*Falsification,
exaggeration
or denial*

The physician can detect **abnormal illness behavior** when the patient complains of symptoms in the absence of physical pathology sufficient to explain it or, conversely, when the patient denies, ignores, or fails to report symptoms that would be anticipated in view of existing physical pathology.

*Symptoms can be
conscious or
unconscious*

Abnormal illness behavior involves physical or psychological symptoms. It involves the falsification, exaggeration, or denial of symptoms, and it can be deliberate or unconscious in motivation. **Malingering,** for example, denotes the deliberate falsification of physical symptoms in the absence of physical pathology adequate to explain them. **Psychogenic amnesia,** in contrast, involves the unconsciously determined presentation of psychological symptoms in the absence of pathology of the central nervous system. **Hypochondriasis** involves an unconsciously determined preoccupation with physical symptoms in the absence of physical pathology. In contrast, the stoical middle-aged athlete, determined to finish the marathon despite a pain in his chest, may be manifesting **illness-denying behavior,** which is both consciously and unconsciously determined.

Contrary to expectation, patients with abnormal illness behavior are not relieved when their physicians reassure them they are physically well. In fact, they usually present their symptoms with even more urgency or consult physician after physician, seeking one who is more congenial.

*The family back-
ground of somatizers*

Merskey and Spear (1967a, 1967b) found that patients with somatically focused abnormal illness behavior are likely to have come from large families of lower socioeconomic status. Engel (1959) suggested that such patients have often been exposed to violence, punishment, and suffering in childhood, that they rarely express anger, and that they are prone to be guilty about their sexuality. Bianchi (1973) found that patients with chronic psychogenic pain tended to come from families in which there was much illness and that they had experienced many life defeats.

Iatrogenic factors

It is important to note that physicians can inadvertently train patients to adopt a maladaptive coping style. The patient can learn, for example, to get care and concern in the form of medical attention and medication by presenting such physical or psychological symptoms as pain and anxiety or by being an ''interesting case.''

Case 3.28

■ Following an attack of undiagnosed joint pain and fever, Sue, a single, 25-year-old nurse, has developed writhing movements involving arching of the back, torsion of the trunk, and rotation of the upper limbs.

The initial diagnosis is sydenham's chorea; but the neurological staff, who have assumed responsibility for her care, are puzzled by inconsistencies. Although she is emotionally quite labile, Sue does not exhibit other signs characteristic of chorea. Her grasp, tongue protrusion, and antistreptolysin O titer are normal. Her movements resemble those of torsion dystonia or tardive dyskinesia rather than of chorea; but she has no abnormal family history, no history of taking neuroleptics, and no abnormal eye signs.

Sue's disorder continues for six weeks, without abatement. It is noted that the movements diminish during sleep and intensify during physical examination. One resident comments on their sinuous, erotic quality.

An interview with the patient's family reveals that Sue has always been a shy girl and that she has been depressed for some time about her inability to attract men. Recently, her sister, a strikingly beautiful woman (and like Sue, a nurse), had become engaged to a physician.

The neurologist recommends to Sue that she be interviewed by a psychiatrist, but Sue takes umbrage at the suggestion. Abruptly, the movements cease. Sue packs her bags and walks out, never to return. ■

Most examples of abnormal illness behavior are less dramatic than Sue's case. Often the division between what is a normal variant and what is abnormal is arbitrary and subjective. In clinical practice, it is most convenient to consider illness behavior as on a continuum from healthy to abnormal.

Summary

Disease is a construct, a set of signs and symptoms stemming from disturbed bodily function and associated with a characteristic set of paraclinical findings, course, and etiology. A disorder is a syndrome of clinical features, less clearly defined than a disease. Illness is the subjective perception that one is unwell. Sick role is the social status accorded to a person who feels ill, whose sickness has been validated by others, and who is thereby relieved of responsibilities until better. The physician is authorized to validate the sick role and to diagnose and treat those who assume it. Illness behavior refers to the individual's unique responses to the awareness of being ill.

Compliance refers to the degree to which someone who has assumed the sick role is prepared to cooperate with the medical system. Compliance is affected by the degree to which a physician can understand and educate the patient.

Physical factors such as systemic or central nervous disease and intoxication can affect illness behavior. Neuropsychiatric disorders such as major depression can present with disturbed illness behavior.

Psychological factors affect illness behavior. Personality, for example, influences the way people present illness and respond to being treated. One aspect of personality is coping style, the manner in which an individual characteristically masters (or fails to master) stress, especially illness. Illness behavior and coping are also affected by the meaning of the illness to the patient.

A stressor is a physical or psychological stimulus that provokes a state of unpleasant arousal or stress. The entire biopsychosocial organism responds to stress, leading to a stress response, that is, to the physiological concomitants of stress, combined with psychological coping strategies. The more stressors to which individuals are exposed, the higher the morbidity and mortality. Illness behavior can also be affected by classical or operant conditioning. Pain, in particular, conduces to maladaptive learned response patterns.

Social factors such as the adequacy of social support, family dynamics, ethnic background, social class, and degree of sophistication about health care affect illness behavior. These factors particularly affect the way people present or deny illness and seek or respond to treatment.

Abnormal illness behavior refers to illness behavior that is both outside the normative range and maladaptive. It may be associated with the presentation of symptoms in the absence of adequate somatic pathology or with a denial of, or failure to report, symptoms associated with disease. Abnormal illness behavior may be deliberate and fabricated, as in malingering and self-induced injury, or unconsciously determined, as in hypochondriasis and somatoform disorder. Patients who are prone to dwell upon, exaggerate, or deny physical symptoms are likely to have had life experiences fostering maladaptive coping styles.

The next two chapters, 4 and 5, descend the biopsychosocial staircase, through the psychological level to neurophysiological and neurochemical systems.

Selected Readings

Hamburg, Elliott, & Parron's (1982) report, *Health and Behavior*, assembles the reviews of leaders in the biobehavioral sciences on the relationships between health, disease, illness, and behavior. Houpt et al. (1980) succinctly review how psychiatric problems and psychosocial factors directly influence the practice of medicine. Mechanic (1968) reviews sociocultural factors that influence illness behavior.

Weiner's (1977) *Psychobiology and Human Disease* thoroughly reviews accumulated knowledge about the role of psychosocial factors in seven major diseases and postulates mechanisms underlying the influence of these factors on all illness and disease.

Cox's (1978) *Stress* reviews current concepts and knowledge about stress and health.

4

Psychological functioning

Introduction

Mental structures

This chapter classifies and briefly reviews the psychological functions most relevant to the clinician. The chapter is arranged on a continuum from reception, through processing, to motor expression and communication. The fundamental concept is that behavior is not merely reflexive but organized by hierarchically arranged and **coordinated mental structures.** Mental organization is reflected in behavior as deceptively simple as making eye contact with a friend and as complicated as writing a sonnet.

Inherent structures and learning

Mental organization develops from inherent brain structures that regulate behavior from the earliest days of infancy (see chapter 24). The function of inherent structures is soon affected by experience, according to the principles of learning, for brain maturation and learning are intertwined as psychological functions mature. Eventually, the individual has the capacity to be aware of his or her own functioning and of some of the structures underlying it, even to the extent of deliberately modifying or altering structures to change behavior.

The psychiatrist observes the patient's behavior (see chapter 9) while eliciting from the patient, through verbal and nonverbal communication, the images, emotions, attitudes, sense of self, rules, and aspirations reflected in the patient's behavior (see chapter 8). Diagnostic formulations are articulations of the clinician's comprehension of the patient's biopsychosocial organization over time

The essence of therapy   (see chapter 14). Therapy is an attempt to modify or eliminate the stresses, change the maladaptive responses, or modify the mental structures associated with disordered behaviour (see chapter 12).

We are all interdependent. The survival of the individual depends on the preservation of the social group. We must balance the urgency of our desires against the needs and demands of family, clan, and society and the exigencies of the physical environment. Putting the matter more directly, we must seek and find what we need from ourselves, from others, and from the environment, knowing the group imposes penalties for violating its social prescripts.

The individual and society

Psychological functions   We do so by virtue of a set of **psychological functions** representing the executive level of organismic functioning. Psychological functions are comprised of the coordinated mental operations through which the individual finds and gets what he or she needs without disrupting social cohesion.

Selfhood   At the heart of psychological functioning is the **sense of self,** the individual's awareness of personal existence as an individual who is, nevertheless, part of the group.

Crisis, adaptation and coping

Crises and coping   All individuals face **crises:** life problems that demand exceptional coping. Some people have the constitutional potential and early experiences that favour successful coping; others do not. Psychiatric disorder, psychological dysfunction, and abnormal illness behaviour are ultimately manifestations of:

1. Chronically maladaptive coping techniques.
2. The failure of previously adequate coping techniques in the face of crisis.
3. The development of new but maladaptive coping techniques when habitual techniques have failed.

Adaptation   The terms *adaptation* and *adaptive* denote the capacity to find reasonable satisfaction for personal needs through organized behaviour, without disrupting society. The organism must adapt or perish. The terms *normal* and *normality* are also often used in regard to behaviour and coping strategies. Unfortunately, normal wavers between the following meanings:

Normality

1. Ideal or optimal.
2. Statistically average, modal, usual or conventional.
3. Without structural lesion or pathophysiology.

Maladaptive behaviour   **Abnormal** or **pathological coping** usually refers to behaviour that is suboptimal and maladaptive and also likely to be recognized as eccentric or unconventional by the individuals or others. **Maladaptive coping** is manifested if one or more of the following conditions prevail:

1. The individual persistently expresses personal needs in a heedless, uncontrolled, or unpredictable manner.
2. The needs expressed by the individual are disorganized, immature, or deviant.
3. The needs expressed are self-destructive or dangerous to others.
4. Needs are consistently expressed in a self-defeating manner.
5. The individual is alienated from personal needs.
6. The individual's usual coping techniques are failing in the face of an acute crisis, and the individual is in a state of distress.
7. In the face of crisis, the individual adopts new coping techniques that are poorly controlled, disorganized, deviant, dangerous, frustrating, self-defeating, alienating, or chronically unstable.
8. The individual manifests maladaptive coping techniques as a result of derangement in neurobiologic functioning.

Psychiatric disorder as maladaptive coping

Psychiatric disorder, psychological dysfunction, and abnormal illness behavior are essentially forms of maladaptive coping in the terms of these eight criteria. To understand psychiatric disorder and related phenomena, one must understand coping. To understand coping, one must understand the following concepts:

1. Biopsychosocial integrity
2. Motivation and emotion
3. The levels of biopsychosocial functioning
4. Psychological functions
5. The concept of ego defense
6. The concept of crisis.

Each concept is discussed in this chapter.

Biopsychosocial integrity

Regression and disintegration

Although it can be dissected into component parts or analyzed according to different functions, the organism actually operates in an integrated manner. Serious decline or **regression** from normality is characterized by diminution in structure or reduction of function and also by disintegration. Disintegration allows the reappearance of primitive functions inhibited and superceded earlier in development (see chapter 24).

Case 4.1   ■ The first sign of Bert's presenile dementia was forgetfulness. He was able to deny it for a while, both to himself and his fellow workers, but eventually the decline in his memory was inescapable, since he became subject to sudden rages if he misplaced a tool or could not get his equipment to work properly.

After early retirement, Bert became even more volatile emotionally. His wife had to ask him to stop driving because, although his coordination was reasonable, his road sense had become poor and he was liable to make abrupt, dangerous decisions under stress.

Towards the end of his illness, he became almost mute, had to be fed, and was incontinent. ■

Motivation and emotions

What drives and empowers the organism to behave? What makes people feel hungry, laugh, cry, fall in love, raise children, run marathons, or study medicine?

Instinct theory
Drive theory

Different psychological theories have attempted to answer this perennial question in different ways. Earlier in this century, McDougall postulated a veritable parliament of **instincts.** Later, Hull distinguished **primary drives** of physiological nature from **secondary drives** which he considered arose from social learning. Freud focused on the vicissitudes of **sexuality** and **aggression,** which he viewed as of critical importance in psychological disorder. Both Hullian theory and psychoanalysis conceived of drives as arising from body needs and

Homeostasis

described the organism as seeking **homeostasis** by **drive-reduction.**

Incentives

By the 1950s, it was apparent that some behavior (curiosity, for example) was incompatible with the theory of organic drive-reduction. Scientific attention shifted to **positive** and **negative incentives** in the environment. The concept of homeostasis was replaced by the concept of **optimal arousal:** If the organism's internal state deviates too greatly in either direction from an optimal level, then the organism is motivated to restore itself to the optimal level.

Physical needs

Aside from basic **physical needs** for food, water, and oxygen and for the avoidance of pain, highly evolved social species exhibit complex sets of predict-

Biosocial responses

able biosocial responses associated with mating, parental behavior, attachment, predation, defense of territory and social dominance.

Psychological motives

However, because of a capacity for symbolic thought and social learning, human beings develop an **hierarchy of needs** superimposed on these biosocial responses. The hierarchy is composed of these **psychological motives:**

1. Affiliation: The need to love, to be loved, to be accepted, and to belong.
2. Mastery: The need to feel competent.
3. Exploration: The need to understand.
4. Aesthetics: The need for beauty and harmony.
5. Actualization: The need for fulfillment.

Many of these psychological needs appear to arise from elementary biosystems; affiliation needs are derived from the attachment system, for example. Different social experiences, interacting with different temperaments, probably produce variations of individual psychological needs for power and submission, freedom and control, order and disorder, dependence and independence, and activity and passivity.

The activation of biosocial drive systems

Recent ethological theories have suggested that the different **biosocial need systems** (for example, attachment) depend on internal states and external releasing stimuli for their activation. Once activated, drive systems are goal-directed; that is, they are organized to reach preset goals. The organism continuously monitors its progress towards the set goals of its activated drive systems.

Emotions as part of internal monitoring

Emotions represent a kind of internal monitoring, an awareness of whether one is on track toward a set goal, approaching it, blocked from getting there, or whether one has attained the goal or relinquished hope of doing so. Interest, excitement, anger, triumph, and regret can be explained on this basis. Other more complex emotions could be explained according to the nature of the drive system involved, as well as the individual's progress toward the set goal. For example, romantic interest, erotic arousal, sexual jealousy, ecstasy, and bitterness are all associated with the need to love and to be loved and with differences in the degree to which an erotic set-goal has been attained.

Altruism

Motivation operates at the service of self and species preservation. **Altruistic behavior** (for example, a mother's defense of her infant against predators), even though it involves self-sacrifice, has the ultimate evolutionary result of preserving genetic material, family, and species.

Human motivation (and its accompanying emotions) can be destructive to the self or others in the group, particularly when the individual has lost hope of being loved, of belonging, or of achieving self-respect. Violence and suicide are the fruits of despair.

Biopsychosocial functions

Biopsychosocial functions operate at three levels:

1. Physical
2. Psychological
3. Social

Biopsychosocial functions

Physical functioning refers to all peripheral organ system functions and all autonomic, neuroendocrine, and central nervous functions organized at a subcortical level and therefore automatic and primarily outside conscious awareness.

Psychological functioning refers to the cortical mental processes through which an individual finds satisfaction for personal drives and needs and avoids danger. Many, but not all, of these processes are conscious or potentially conscious. The keystone of psychological functioning is the sense of self.

Social functioning refers to the individual's behavior in relation to family, friends, enemies, authorities, subordinates, and community institutions (school, church, and medical system, for example).

This chapter discusses the following psychological functions:

Psychological functions

1. Information processing and motor skills.
2. Communication.
3. Images, emotions, and attitudes.
4. The sense of self.
5. Social competence.
6. Internal controls, rules, and aspirations.
7. Ego defenses and coping.

Internal processes are inferred from behavior

The distinction between the functions is arbitrary; these internal processes are hypothetical constructs inferred from behavior. Memory, for example, can be detected in another person only if that person exhibits behavior involving the recall of past events. In actuality, one never observes a pure mental operation such as memory; behavior is always the (more or less) integrated expression of a biopsychosocial unit.

Following a discussion of the levels of psychological awareness, each psychological system is considered.

Levels of psychological awareness

Five levels or kinds of awareness can be described:

Conscious level

1. One can become aware of, or direct one's awareness to, many psychological processes such as perceptual scanning, learning, and the retrieval of a memory or current emotion. This is the level of **conscious awareness.**

Preconscious level

2. Other processes are on, or beyond, the periphery of the conscious mind but could be brought to awareness if desired (the buzzing of a fly as you read this book, for example, or what you had for breakfast yesterday). This level is known as **preconscious.**

Automatized level

3. Other processes, such as driving a car, were once conscious (if not self-conscious) but have become **automatized** with practice. Thus, one can listen to the radio and whistle a tune while steering a car along a winding road.

Automatic level

Unconscious level

Automatized processes can usually be brought to awareness, though sometimes only with difficulty.

4. Fundamental psychological processes involving, for example, decoding language, coordinating motor programs, and the perceptual recognition of patterns have always been outside awareness and cannot be the object of scrutiny. These processes are described as **automatic.**

5. Some memories are so disturbing to self-esteem or so anxiety-provoking that they are kept out of awareness. In other words, their retrieval is actively inhibited. These memories are said to be **unconscious.**

Information processing

Information processing involves the reception and interpretation of sense data and the control of the voluntary activity by which an individual orients to, seeks, and finds what is required to satisfy drives and needs.

Information processing involves the following six coordinated functions:

1. Consciousness and orientation
2. Perception
3. Attention
4. Learning and memory
5. Information and comprehension
6. Reasoning and judgment

Consciousness and orientation

Although mental processing can occur during sleep (particularly in the REM state) and outside of awareness, focused thought demands alertness. The mental products of unconscious or disorientated states are likely to be fragmentary, as in the hallucinosis found in delirium (see Case 9.1), whereas the thinking associated with reverie is characterized by its fanciful (though sometimes genuinely creative) quality.

Perception

Perception refers to the interpretation of sensory phenomena. It usually involves the combination of impressions from different sense modalities. Perception is disorganized in a number of conditions such as delirium, psychosis, or heightened emotional arousal, with the appearance of such perceptual distortions as illusions or hallucinations (see chapter 9).

Attention

Attentional processes

Attention requires the capacity to scan the environment for objects relevant to one's needs, to resist distraction by irrelevant stimuli, to maintain concentration on an object, idea, or problem, and to inhibit random or impulsive action until an appropriate response has been chosen. These functions are impeded in such states of emotional arousal as anxiety or fear and in depression, organic brain disorders (see chapter 10), and attention deficit disorder (see chapter 22).

Learning and memory

The infant learns predominantly by conditioning, but during development, increasingly applies general principles to particular problems (see chapter 22).

Schemes, schemas, and structures

These principles are represented by sets of schemes, schemas, structures, scripts, or cognitive maps to which familiar problems are assimilated and that must be altered if new experiences are to be accommodated.

Short-term memory

If attended to, perceptual data are registered and temporarily held in **short-term memory,** which has a capacity of about from five to nine items. If the thinker can group together (chunk) the items to be memorized, short-term memory capacity is expanded.

Long-term memory

Storage and retrieval

Items are transferred from short-term to **long-term memory** by encoding them either as visual or acoustic imagery or as semantic units. Failure of memory is due to a failure of **registration, transfer, storage,** or **retrieval.** Retrieval is facilitated if memories are well organized and if the thinker's internal state resembles that existing at the time of the original encoding (state-dependent learning). Retrieval is impeded by poor memory organization, distraction, and repression (see ego defense mechanisms discussed later in this chapter). The physiology of memory is described in chapter 5 and the clinical phenomenology of disordered memory is described in chapter 9.

Information and comprehension

Imagery

Information is stored as kinesthetic, visual or auditory imagery, or as concepts. Concepts are usually coded as words or mathematical symbols and can be stacked

Symbolic hierarchies

in hierarchies of increasing abstraction, as in the following example:

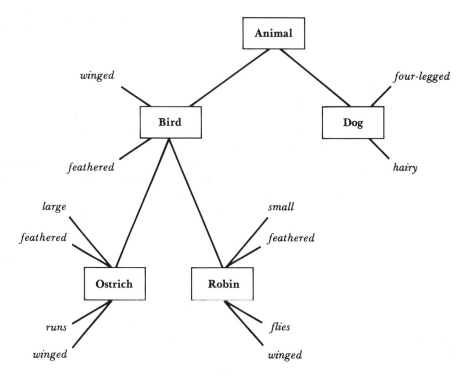

Knowledge and comprehension depend on:

Factors influencing the storage and application of knowledge

1. The amount of information in long-term memory (storage)
2. The amount of information that can be retrieved from long-term memory (retrieval)
3. The arrangement of information in long-term memory (organization)
4. The capacity to apply to problems the schemas, structures, scripts, or maps in long-term memory

For example, the capacity to diagnose patients depends on how much one has learned. Long-term memory is greatly enhanced by organization (e.g., by a hierarchical classification of disease). Diagnostic acumen, for example, is associated with the facility with which one can retrieve learned information and can apply general principles to particular patients who present diagnostic problems. This book aims to enhance the organization and application of clinical knowledge.

Reasoning and judgment

Faced with an unfamiliar problem, the thinker must either adapt old principles to it (sometimes modifying the old principles in the process) or discover novel solutions based on new principles.

Spatial reasoning

Conceptual reasoning

Mechanical reasoning (for example, the skill required to repair an automobile engine or perform plastic surgery) relies, at least in part, on visual and kinesthetic imagery. **Conceptual reasoning** (for example, the ability to generate diagnostic hypotheses), on the other hand, uses words or other codes (such as mathematical symbols). Chapter 7, *The tactics and strategy of clinical reasoning*, describes a form of hypothetico-deductive reasoning that can be applied to problems involving diagnostic concepts. The sequential tactics of clinical reasoning are essentially a set of subgoals coordinated by the superordinate purpose of reaching a diagnostic conclusion. A diagnostic conclusion is itself a subgoal coordinated by the overarching clinical process (see Figure 6.1).

Judicial decision-making, another example of conceptual reasoning, involves sifting the evidence for facts, which are then interpreted in accordance with (a) the law bearing on the issues of a case, (b) the judge's knowledge of human behavior, and (c) the judge's conception of fairness and justice. Settling litigation, determining guilt, and disposing of a case require the judge to apply legal knowledge and an understanding of human nature to conceptual reasoning about the facts that have been determined.

Conceptual reasoning and judgment are the first cognitive processes to deteriorate in acute or chronic brain disorder. They are also distorted in schizophrenia and mania (see Cases 9.2 and 9.3).

Motor skills

Perceptual-motor skill translates intention into action. It is attained by practice and can be enhanced by training. A skill is adaptable and can be attuned to a specific goal. An habitual movement acquired in the course of development (such as walking) can be trained for a specific purpose (such as performing on a tightrope).

The mental processes underlying skilled performance have been described according to four steps, each involving:

The four steps underlying a perceptual skill

1. Sensory input
2. A subgoal
3. Rules of operation
4. A specified output.

Gathering information about the object

Stage I. The first stage involves gathering sensory information about the object involved (e.g., a baseball bat) and a target (e.g., an approaching baseball). The subgoal is to match object to target (i.e., by approximating bat to ball). The rules involve a series of suboperations that determine the output. The output is what needs to be done (with the arms and bat) to meet the demands of the task (hitting the ball).

Gathering information about the motor system

Stage II. Information about the spatial location of the motor system (neck, shoulders, elbows, wrists, hands, hips, legs) is used, given the subgoal to modulate the object (swing the bat). The rules operate to relate changes in the motor system to changes in the object (e.g., to relate changes in the neck, shoulder, arm, back, and hip musculature to the swinging of a bat).

Activating the motor program

Stage III. At this stage, a motor program is activated to coordinate the skilled movement of the object (bat). Proprioceptive feedback is required. By the time the batter has committed to the motor program, a fast baseball has already traveled halfway from mound to plate.

Executing the motor program

Stage IV. Efferent neural signals are transmitted to the muscles, which contract and relax in a coordinated way, governed by muscle spindle servo-control.

Importance of feedback

Automatization

People learn skills by watching others, by practicing, and by assimilating constructive criticism. Criticism can be verbal (e.g., "Good stroke, but keep your eye on the ball"), visual (e.g., from mirror or videotape), or intrinsic (e.g., the way you feel when you have executed a strong backhand). The rules in Stage I and II are often self-conscious and verbal when first acquired (e.g., "Keep your wrist firm"), but they are automatized with practice. Like conceptual reasoning, complex perceptual-motor skills deteriorate early in organic brain dysfunction and in extreme emotional arousal. This is one reason it is dangerous to drive an automobile after an argument.

Communication

Thinking precedes language

Initially separate from, but increasingly interwoven with, information processing is the function of language. The development of language depends in part on cognitive growth: Thinking precedes language. However, by adolescence, advanced conceptual reasoning requires language.

The development of language is described in chapter 24. It is apparent that a native tongue is not acquired primarily by conditioning or parroting. Comprehension requires deciphering the structure, meaning, and context of language into its basic elements. Consider these sentences:

- Mothers love babies.
- Babies are loved by mothers.
- It is mothers who love babies.
- Do mothers love babies?
- Why do mothers love babies?

The deciphering of language to its elementary propositions

Beneath each sentence is an elementary proposition that has to do with an active feeling of one group of persons towards another. Fundamental propositions attribute to an object, objects, or person(s) an activity (e.g., loves), state (e.g., is asleep) or attribute (e.g., is big). Fundamental propositions such as:

- Mothers love babies
- Fathers love babies

can be combined into complex sentences; for example:

- Mothers love babies and so do fathers.
- Mothers and fathers love babies.
- It is babies that mothers and fathers love.
- Babies are loved by mothers and fathers.

Complex sentences are analyzed into their elementary propositions by disimbedding one from the other; for example:

The fox is quick.

+

The fox is brown.

The quick brown fox jumps over the lazy dog   =   +

The fox jumps over the dog.

+

The dog is lazy.

The listener is an intuitive grammarian, breaking down sentences into noun phrases (e.g, *mothers* or *the quick brown fox*) and verb phrases (e.g., *love babies* or *jumps over the lazy dog*). Some statements are ambiguous; for example:

(*These apples are cooking.*)

or

These are cooking apples   =   (*These are apples.*)

+

(*The apples are for cooking.*)

The ambiguity in the first statement arises from uncertainty about which propositional structure is appropriate. When ambiguity occurs, the listener must rely on semantic context to extract the appropriate propositions.

Sentences can be parsed beyond the phrases that compose them; for example:

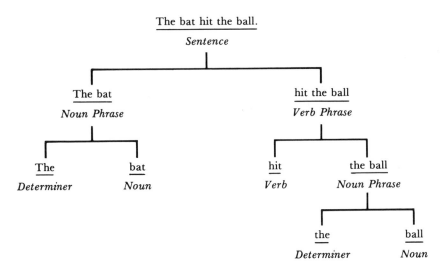

*Hierarchical structures
and sentence*

Even a simple sentence, therefore, breaks up into an **hierarchical structure** of words.

Syntactic rules

Words are comprised of phonemes (for example, *bat* = /b/ + /a/ +/t/) that are blended phonologically in articulation. Just as each language has **syntactic rules** for combining words to form phrases and phrases to form sentences, it

Phonological rules

also has **phonological rules** for combining phonemes; for example, an English speaker would recognize *brek* as phonologically regular (though incomprehensible) but reject *kber*.

Morphemes

Morphemes are the smallest sound-units that convey meaning. To analyze a compound word like *disintegration,* one separates it into smaller units of meaning, or morphemes, in this way:

$$disintegration \ = \ dis \ + \ in \ + \ tegr \ + \ ate \ + \ ion$$

Prepositions, conjunctions, verb endings (-ed, -ing, -en, etc.) and other function words are morphemes that are added to a sentence to convey tense, voice, interrogation, and relation between elements.

Codes

Language has obvious parallels to motor control and conceptual thinking. To convey meaning, one generates propositions and codes them as phonemes, morphemes, words, phrases, and sentences. Language has rules for combining

Rules

sounds, syntactic elements, and meaning and is organized into hierarchical, sequential schemes for translation into speech acts. Comprehension involves the reverse: Speech is decoded phonologically and analyzed into its syntactic elements and fundamental propositions.

In chapter 9, abnormalities of speech and language are described, together with the clinical phenomena related to nonverbal or mimetic com-

Mimesis

munication (facial expression, posture, gesture, etc.). Psychosis and brain disorder are particularly likely to be associated with the disintegration of language, the disarticulation of speech, and the disorganization of communication due to the intrusion of bizarre propositions and eccentric or incongruous facial expressions and gestures.

Images, emotions, and attitudes

From early interaction with parents, siblings, and peers, individuals construct a matrix of **basic assumptions** and **expectations** about themselves, people, and life. The adult's interpersonal world is thus **structured** or mapped according to emotional valences, attitudes, and scripts that are the consequence of key childhood experiences.

The fortunate individual has good genetic potential and matures in a favorable intrauterine and extrauterine physical environment. This person has parents who are available for attachment, provide affection and security, support curiosity and initiative, are good models, provide reasonable limits and guidelines, and convey to the child a sense of being a worthwhile, unique in-

Generic attitudinal structures

dividual. From many experiences, an organized, adaptive set of **attitudes** is assembled. This set is comprised of generic assumptions about the self and others and of basic expectations for the future. The flexibility of these structures allows the healthy individual to assess the world realistically and to assimilate new experiences, even traumatic ones, without resorting to maladaptive, self-protective coping strategies.

Attitudinal structures in the vulnerable individual

In contrast, the vulnerable individual has a set of basic assumptions that impose a rigid, unrealistic or extreme viewpoint on the external world. Such important people as spouse, child, peer, or boss are responded to in stereotypic, self-protective ways. The vulnerable individual is constantly in danger of and on guard against interpersonal threat. This person characteristically views the outcome of important events in fearful, passive, pessimistic, destructive, or inflated terms.

Premorbid personality

Vulnerability and decompensation

Vulnerable attitudes (towards self, others, and the future) are manifest in **premorbid personality traits.** Different sets of images, emotions, and attitudes are characteristic of people vulnerable to some psychiatric syndromes. Tables 4.1 to 4.4 (adapted from Guidano & Liotti, 1983) outline the cognitive features associated with four disorders: depression, agoraphobia, obsessive-compulsive disorder, and anorexia nervosa. The tables are organized according to the following headings:

1. Development: The childhood experiences associated with predisposition to this disorder.
2. Predisposition: The set of assumptions and expectations characteristic of the person vulnerable to this disorder.

TABLE 4.1
Depression: Images, emotions, and attitudes

Depression

Development: Some patients have experienced actual loss during childhood or adolescence, but most have been exposed to parental absence due to sickness, depression, mental illness, divorce, or work. The family stresses success and prestige.

Predisposition: If I am good (dutiful, hard-working, successful), I might avoid failure; but nobody really likes me. You can't rely on others. Nothing lasts. Life is a struggle. Don't hope for too much or you'll be disappointed.

Precipitation: 1. Personal loss or the threat of it. 2. Material loss or disappointment. 3. Disillusionment in a significant person. 4. Change of residence.

Pattern: I am alone and I deserve it because I am bad. They are right to despise me. The future is bleak. It is pointless to do aything; I'm too weak. I give up.

3. Precipitation: The stressors likely to cause decompensation.
4. Pattern: The set of assumptions and expectations associated with the active disorder.

Tables 4.1 to 4.4 present the images, emotions, and attitudes associated with vulnerability and decompensation in the first person. The experienced clinician is alert for patients' comments reflecting these themes. Understanding such key personal themes is essential to planning therapy (see chapter 12).

The sense of self

The psychologically healthy adult has a strong sense of self. This person feels whole, coherent, and distinct from, yet not alienated from, others. He or she can

TABLE 4.2
Agoraphobia: Images, emotions, and attitudes

Agoraphobia

Development: Parents impede the child's attempt to explore the environment because they perceive the child as fragile. ("If you got lost, what would you do?" "Don't play with them; they are bad boys.")

Predisposition: I want freedom, but I need protection. If I control myself, I'll be safe. I don't want to submit to (get close to) anyone. If I lose control (of my life, feelings, erotic excitement), I'll make a fool of myself.

Precipitation: 1. Impending developmental transitions that signify independence (e.g., going to college, marriage). 2. Personal loss. 3. Marital crisis or change in the marital relationship.

Pattern: If I left home (went out), I'd lose control of my life (body, feelings) or get sick; there would be nobody to help me. Strangers are hostile and dangerous. I want you to stay home with me.

TABLE 4.3
Obsessive-compulsive disorder: Images, emotions, and attitudes

Obsessive-compulsive disorder
Development: The dominant parent is inflexible, strict, morally rigid, and orderly. This parent claims to love the child but offers little affection. The expression of sexuality or aggression is proscribed.
Predisposition: He (or she) loves me; he (or she) hates me. I am loveable/unloveable. I am the opposite of what I should be. I must be perfect in all that I do. There is a precise solution to all human problems.
Precipitation: Nonspecific stress.
Pattern: I doubt everthing that I do. I must dwell on minutiae. I must ward off (expiate, atone for, undo) bad actions or thoughts. I try to stop these recurrent thoughts (actions) but cannot.

discriminate between personal feelings and feelings of others and between fantasy and reality.

The sense of self is comprised of the following elements:

The constituents of the sense of self

1. A distinct and realistic image of one's body.
2. An awareness of one's mental functioning.
3. Clear boundaries between the self and the outside world.
4. A healthy defensive barrier against disruptive drives, images, and affects.
5. A normal self-esteem.
6. A sense of personal identity, individuality, and coherence.

The developmental origins of the sense of self

A sense of self evolves from the intimate, empathic, symbiotic relationship between mother and child in the first year of life; from the capacity of the sensitive parent to foster separation and autonomy in the second year; and from the capacity of the environment to promote initiative, industry, and individuation in middle childhood and beyond. The development of a healthy sense of self also

TABLE 4.4
Anorexia nervosa: Images, emotions, and attitudes

Anorexia nervosa
Development: The mother is dependent on her own mother. Mother and daughter are enmeshed. Marital and family problems are denied or camouflaged. Goodness is rewarded; initiative and independence are discouraged.
Predisposition: I do not know who I am. I feel empty. Growing up is frightening because it means being independent. I hate my breasts, thighs, and menstrual periods. Erotic feelings scare me.
Precipitation: 1. Disillusionment with the father. 2. Disappointment in love. 3. Separation from parents. 4. Criticism from peers about secondary sexual characteristics.
Pattern: To be fat is to be rejected. If I don't stop eating my insatiable needs will get out of control. If I lose weight, my figure will be perfect. Starving snuffs out my sexual and aggressive feelings. Refusing to eat is one way of resisting (controlling) my parents. If I don't eat, I can stop time. I have to keep moving to stop thinking.

presupposes that the child has the intrinsic potential to assimilate favorable experiences and that the fit between the parents' personality and the child's temperament is a good one.

Psychopathology of the sense of self

Psychopathology of the sense of self is manifest in one or several of the following ways:

1. Body image: A sense of vagueness, unattractiveness, or defectiveness, or a narcissistic overvaluation, of body image.
2. Mental function: An inability to evaluate or think about one's mental functioning; a sense that one's mental functioning is incompetent; an unrealistic exaggeration of one's mental ability.
3. Ego boundaries: An inability to distinguish between one's own feelings and the feelings of others; the tendency to project one's own feelings onto other people or to be absorbed and confused by the feelings of others.
4. Ego defenses: The tendency for psychic life to be disrupted by the intrusion of alien images, ideas, and feelings from the unconscious, such as illusions, or hallucinations, obsessions, or disturbing fantasies.
5. Self-esteem: A pervasive sense of worthlessness, badness, or hatefulness; or grossly unrealistic feelings of grandiosity and omnipotence.
6. Synthesis and identity: A sense of emptiness, vagueness, incoherence, fragmentation, dissolution, or of being split into a number of selves. The sense of needing to maintain a facade or a false self in order to camouflage the emptiness, incoherence, and fragmentation within.

Many psychiatric disorders are associated with psychopathology in the sense of self. They are alluded to in chapters 9 and 10.

Social competence

The fundamental assumptions and expectations each of us has about others reflect the cognitive structures (scripts) that direct our interaction with them. These structures allow us to infer, predict, or hypothesize about the motives, feelings, and intentions of others. The more flexible and accommodating the structures, the more likely it is the individual will be able to respond in a discriminating way to a wide range of people. On the other hand, the more rigid and stereotypic the structures, the more repetitious and maladaptive the individual's social behavior. Consider the following social stereotypes. Try to imagine the childhood experiences that could lead to them and the behavior that could be their result if any were the central script of a patient's social life:

Stereotypic social attitudes

- Women are humiliating bitches. They should be taught a lesson.
- Men are unpredictable tyrants who must be obeyed.

- Don't trust strangers. Get them before they get you.
- Be very good or your parent (spouse) will leave you.

The development of social cognition is described in chapter 24.

Applying internal social structures to social life depends on more elementary social skills; for example:

Elementary social skills

1. The capacity to recognize and distinguish one's own needs and feelings.
2. The capacity to communicate one's needs and feelings in a socially adroit manner.
3. The capacity to recognize and distinguish the feelings of other people.
4. The capacity to infer the motives and intentions of others.
5. The capacity to reason causally and consequentially about interpersonal events.
6. The capacity to solve interpersonal problems by considering alternative actions.
7. The capacity to make and keep friends.
8. The capacity to gain acceptance by and to influence a peer group.
9. The capacity for leadership, loyalty, and fidelity.

Each capacity is diminished and made rigid by stereotypic internal social scripts such as those already described.

Internal controls, rules, and aspirations

The stimulus barrier

The central nervous system has a threshold beyond which sensory input results in arousal. Repetitive stimulation results in **habituation,** an increase in sensory threshold. This is an example of the self-regulatory aspect of central nervous functioning, the intrinsic controls that come wired-in to the nervous apparatus.

As a result of experience, an individual learns to check the immediacy of personal needs in accordance with the constraints of social life. Consequently, the individual builds up:

Ego defense

1. Layers of internal control involving **unconscious defenses** that block, ward off, or divert basic drives.

Superego

2. Conscious and unconscious taboos, rules, and prohibitions constituting the conscience or **superego.**

Ego ideal

3. The values, ideals, and aspirations comprising the **ego ideal.**

Shame and guilt

4. The **emotions** of pride, anxiety, shame and guilt that signal to the individual the transgression (or possible transgression) of internal prohibitions or the failure to be true to personal standards.

Self-image disparity

The **superego** is deficient in antisocial personality and conduct disorders. It is hypertrophied in obsessive-compulsive disorder and associated with the guilty perception of an irredeemable disparity between self-image and ego ideal (that is, between what one is and what one ought to be).

Different **ego defenses** operating in combination comprise the coping strategies described next in this chapter.

Ego defenses and coping

Ego defenses block, ward off, or divert drives

Disruptive drives, affects, memories, and images are kept out of awareness by **ego defense mechanisms,** alluded to in chapter 3 (with reference to illness behavior). An ego defense mechanism is an unconscious process operating to block, ward off, or divert into indirect channels unacceptable urges, drives, or needs and their associated affects and images.

If the unacceptable motives, affects, and images were to breach, leak through, or circumvent the **defensive barrier,** the individual would experience **anxiety,** a signal that psychological functioning is in danger of being disrupted or overwhelmed.

The unacceptability of certain drives and images

Drives, affects, and images are usually unacceptable because the individual has learned they are socially proscribed or because their expression (or even their entertainment in fantasy) would endanger vital human relationships. Social proscription is especially likely to fall on the unfettered expression of rage or sexuality.

A classification of ego defenses

Ego defenses can be classified according to their maturity, the developmental stage during which they were established, and the degree to which they provide for impulse expression, in contrast to impulse blocking.

1. Primordial defenses: Habituation, withdrawal.
2. Infantile defenses: Blocking, denial, regression, introjection, projection, splitting, distortion, acting out, turning against the self, autistic fantasy, somatization.
3. Neurotic defenses: Repression, controlling, displacement, dissociation, conversion, identification, externalization, isolation, rationalization, reaction formation, counterphobia.
4. Mature defenses: Suppression, renunciation, anticipation, intellectualization, humor, sublimation.

Defenses act in combination

As each defense is described, remember that the distinction between these abstract constructs is arbitrary and that the notion of a pure defense is a convenient fiction. Also remember that aside from some mature ego defenses, these mechanisms are unconscious, the individual being unaware of their motivation or operation.

Primordial defenses

Habituation
Withdrawal

The neonate has the capacity to **habituate** to repetitive stimulation, that is, to dampen responses to stimuli no longer novel. The neonate can also **withdraw** into torpor or sleep in the face of excessive stimulation. These primordial processes may be the biological roots of all defenses that develop later in infancy and childhood.

Infantile defenses

During infancy, the individual develops a number of defenses that, if manifested in adult life, are associated with psychopathology.

Blocking

     Blocking refers to the inhibition of drives and affects as close to their source as possible. It is an inflexible defense, and likely to be maintained only temporarily.

Denial

     Denial is blocking applied to external reality. The individual ignores or refuses to become aware of aspects of the world that are unacceptable or anxiety-provoking. Denial is an important element in some forms of abnormal illness behavior (see chapter 3), as when a woman delays seeking help for a lump in the breast.

Regression

     Regression, a fundamental mechanism, pervades psychopathology. It refers to a dropping back in behavior, with the re-appearance of responses that would be characteristic of an earlier stage of development. Normal regression occurs during illness when a patient takes to bed and wants to be nurtured. Relative to the stress that provoked it, abnormal regression is disproportionate and protracted.

Introjection

     Introjection refers to the tendency to incorporate, or take into the self, parts of the external world, particularly of the mother. The infant thus achieves a partial protection against separation anxiety by establishing within the self aspects of the loved object (introjects).

Projection

     In **projection,** the infant perceives unacceptable aspects of introjects in the external world, especially in significant people. This defense is often associated with the affect of rage. Bad (hostile) parts of the original introjects are split from the good parts and projected onto the external world, a defense which is exaggerated in paranoid disorders.

Splitting

     In **splitting,** the infant keeps apart incompatible (usually good and bad) parts of early introjects (for example, the good and bad aspects of the mother) and the self (the good me and the bad me). Splitting is associated with unresolved **ambivalence** and is characteristic of borderline personality disorder (see chapter 11).

Distortion

     Distortion refers to the misperception or misinterpretation of external reality in accordance with egocentric personal needs. In delusional states, for example, the entire world may be restructured according to psychotic beliefs (see chapter 9).

Acting out

Acting out refers to the unreflective, direct, impulsive expression of unacceptable impulses. Acting out indicates an inability to tolerate the tension and anxiety associated with impulses. This defense is a central feature of antisocial and impulsive behavior (running away, stealing, violence, and suicide, for example).

Turning against the self

Turning against the self refers to passive-aggressive or masochistic behavior whereby an individual turns against the self unacceptable impulses originally directed at loved objects. An extreme example of this defense is seen in adolescents who lacerate their wrists after a disappointment or rejection.

Autistic fantasy

In **autistic fantasy,** the successor to primordial withdrawal, an individual substitutes compensatory fantasy for problem-solving activity. It is seen normally in the imagination of the creative writer, for example; but it is exaggerated, and a serious social impediment, in schizoid personality (see chapter 10).

Somatization

Somatization is associated with the tendency to ignore anxiety by focusing on its physiological concomitants. Patients using this defense are frequently encountered by primary-care physicians (see chapter 19). They may be conceived of as exhibiting abnormal illness behavior (see chapter 3).

Neurotic defenses

Repression

Repression is associated with the purposeful forgetting of or refusal to become aware of warded-off impulses, affects, and images that would otherwise cause anxiety or guilt. It is the keystone of psychoneurotic disorder. When repression fails due to increased strength of impulses, free-floating anxiety arises in an acute distress that sometimes foreshadows a more clearly defined psychiatric disorder.

Control

The **controlling** individual invests much energy in manipulating others in order to ward off potential conflict.

Displacement

In **displacement,** the individual finds substitute expression for a repressed desire through a person or thing actually or symbolically similar to the object of the original impulse. In this manner, although the object is different, the impulse is expressed unaltered. Displacement is an important component of phobic disorders.

Dissociation

Dissociation refers to the tendency for part of psychic life to become separate from the rest and to function autonomously. Dissociation occurs in depersonalization, fugue, and multiple personality (see chapter 11).

Conversion

In **conversion,** unconscious conflict is expressed through physical symptoms referable to voluntary muscles or special senses. The symptom (such as paralysis or anesthesia) usually represents both a warding off and a substitute expression of unacceptable impulses (see Case 3.27).

Identification

Indentification is a sophisticated form of introjection. The individual using this defense patterns the self on someone much admired or loved (identification with the loved object), someone who has been lost (identification with the lost object), or someone who is hostile and feared (identification with the aggressor). Identification with the lost object is integral to normal grief. It is accentuated when the bereaved individual has previously been markedly ambivalent to the person lost.

Externalization

Externalization is a sophisticated form of projection. It refers to the tendency to perceive in other people one's own feelings or characteristics. Externalization is a component of empathy.

Isolation

Isolation refers to the tendency to strip emotionally charged thoughts or impulses of their associated feelings and to think about them in a neutralized manner. Latinate technical terms can be used in this way to sterilize conflictual ideas.

Rationalization

Rationalization provides, for oneself and others, a spurious explanation for behavior that has a baser origin.

Reaction formation

Reaction formation is the tendency to adopt behavior or attitudes toward other people that are the reverse of unconscious attitudes the individual finds unacceptable. The muckraking prurience of some censorious people is an example. Reaction formation is an important component of obsessive-compulsive personality.

Counterphobia

Counterphobic defense is manifest when the individual takes risks to flout a fear. Some stuntmen begin their careers with counterphobia, and it is commonly seen in adolescent dare-taking.

Mature defenses

Mature defenses have the following characteristics:

The characteristics of mature defenses

1. They are less inflexible, automatic, and all-or-none.
2. They tend to discharge impulse rather than block it.
3. They tend to divert impulses into socially acceptable, even desirable, directions.
4. They tend to promote awareness or resolution of conflict, rather than its avoidance or camouflage.

Suppression

In **suppression,** the individual decides not to dwell on something distressing. Instead, the person deliberately keeps it out of mind for the time being. This is an adaptive defense when a problem cannot be resolved at once and other responsibilities must be discharged; but it is a temporary expedient. The problem will have to be addressed at a later time.

Renunciation

Renunciation is necessary when a goal cannot be attained or a loss is irreversible. The individual, aware that further striving would be fruitless, forswears a hope or ambition. Renunciation is a part of normal grief and can be seen in normal aging or in the loss of physical attractiveness after surgery.

Anticipation

The individual who identifies a problem ahead of time, considers alternative ways of handling it, and develops a plan using **anticipation.** Children waiting for elective surgery can be helped to cope with it by preparatory hospital visits, books, and doll play. A psychotherapist can help a patient anticipate problems (for example, when he or she goes on leave from the hospital) and consider how to deal with them ahead of time.

Intellectualization

Intellectualization, in its more adaptive sense, involves using verbal concepts to think about human problems. This book is full of intellectualization. In its more defensive sense, intellectualization refers to a concentration on words and abstraction in order to avoid feeling. It is sometimes encountered during psychotherapy when a patient (who usually has a professional background) tries to involve the therapist in a debate about psychological theory instead of exploring personal conflict.

Humor

Humor involves expressing tension about conflict. Since it is usually a social phenomenon, it permits people to acknowledge and share problems. The physician who appreciates and reciprocates a patient's humor without making illness seem trivial actively contributes to the patient's recuperation. Be alert, however, for the ward comedian who uses humor to camouflage depression or fear and do not use humor at the expense of empathy.

Sublimation

In **sublimation,** impulses that originally had a more egocentric aim are transformed into socially valuable activity. A childless person, for example, may devote a lifetime to the welfare of children. The raw desire to win in competition with others can be transmuted into a fascination with the physiology and training of athletes.

Coping strategies are sets of ego defenses and attitudes used habitually or called on in times of stress. The styles of coping with personal illness described in chapter 3 are combinations of ego defense mechanisms characteristically used by people confronted by sickness.

Crisis

Emotional crisis

During the course of a life, an individual will inevitably encounter a number of **crises.** A crisis is a life problem demanding more than habitual coping. To resolve crisis, the individual must develop new methods of coping or apply existing coping strategies in an original way. Having done so, the individual is strengthened and better able to face future crises. One measure of **ego strength** is the adaptability and capacity of the individual's coping strategies in the face of crisis.

Crises are of two types:

1. Developmental crises
2. Accidental crises.

Developmental crisis

A **developmental crisis** results from a problem that is predictable in that most members of a society are expected to encounter it at a particular developmental point. The following occurrences are examples of developmental crises:

1. Habit training
2. First attendance at school
3. Puberty
4. Leaving home
5. Marriage
6. Having a child
7. Middle age.

Accidental crisis

Accidental crises, on the other hand, are the less predictable life changes or misfortunes that can befall people at any time. Some examples are:

1. Death of a loved one
2. Illness of a loved one
3. Personal illness
4. Losing a job
5. Shifting house
6. Divorce
7. Promotion
8. Taking out a mortgage.

Some events, such as the death of a child, would obviously be stressful for virtually everyone. Other events are stressful only to some people, presumably because the event directly or metaphorically represents a previous trauma or threat to those who are vulnerable. Sometimes, an event that at first appears benign or favorable demands resources the individual does not have.

Case 4.2

■ Arthur, a 42-year-old assembly-line worker, was an exceptionally hard-working, dependable, and cheerful employee who had been with one firm for 15 years. Consequently, it was no surprise when he was elevated to the position of foreman.

Several weeks after promotion, Arthur developed chronic lower back pain, dyspepsia, and palpitations, which he attributed to an impending heart attack, like the one that had killed his father at the same age. Arthur's wife complained that he was a different man; he had changed from an equable, reliable husband into a querulous, insomniac invalid.

Although Arthur could not discuss the matter directly, his family physician hypothesized that the responsibility of the new job was beyond Arthur's personal and intellectual resources. Arthur was advised to return to his old job, on the grounds of ill health. With judicious medication, relaxation exercises, and supportive psychotherapy, he gradually recovered, although he never entirely lost his palpitations. ■

Case 4.3

■ Virginia, an energetic, able, and creative 25-year-old advertising executive was given more and more opportunity by her appreciative superiors. Eventually, a much-coveted new account was added to her portfolio.

Soon afterwards, while driving across a bridge on her way to work, Virginia had a sudden sensation of vertigo, associated with a panicky presentiment that her car would stall, the bridge would break up in the high wind, and her car would tumble into the water.

Nevertheless, though shaken, she got to the office and finished a full day's work. Every morning for the next four days, the same thing happened. Within a week, Virginia had developed an acute phobia of driving and crossing the bridge and was forced to take a taxi to work by a circuitous route.

In exploratory psychotherapy, it became apparent that the hidden threat at work was not the new responsibility (which she was well able to meet) but the need to relinquish one or more of her other accounts. Virginia dreaded disappointing clients and could not cope with the rejection implicit in dropping them. Her extraordinary sense of obligation and duty stemmed from a complex relationship with her successful, demanding, but admiring and appreciative father, whom she had yearned to see more often. He and her mother had divorced when Virginia was a teenager. ■

Anxiety as a motive for confronting crisis

The normal initial response to a critical life change is anxiety, experienced as feelings of worry, strain, and uncertainty. In this circumstance, anxiety is healthy. It is both an alert that something needs to be done and a motive for doing it. Usually, the most adaptive response is to confront the problem, analyze it, consider alternative solutions, decide on one of them, implement it, and see if it works. If the problem cannot be solved but must be borne, the individual must work out how to live with it.

Maladaptive coping responses to crisis involve one or more of the following patterns of behavior:

Maladaptive coping responses to crisis

1. The individual is aware of the problem but flounders in indecision.
2. The individual persists in using old coping strategies that are no longer adaptive.
3. The individual grasps impulsively for the first solution that comes to mind.
4. The individual fails to confront the problem, repressing or denying it.
5. State (4) leads to the development of secondary, maladaptive coping strategies that enable the individual to avoid confronting the problem. Maladaptive coping is manifest in different forms of psychiatric disorder or psychological dysfunction.

The following examples illustrate each of these maladaptive responses:

Case 4.4   ■ A graduate student has been offered two highly desirable postdoctoral positions that in her mind are of equivalent merit. Like the donkey starving between two bales of hay, she is in an agony of indecision. A friend suggests she toss a coin. ■

Case 4.5   ■ Whenever he felt frustrated by his father's authoritarian behavior in their family business, a young man would get drunk with the boys at a local hostelry. After he married, his wife objected to his doing so and told him he was "running away from his problems.'' Incensed by what he saw as her trying to run his life, he stamped out of the house and got drunk. ■

Case 4.6 ■ It is the weekly faculty meeting of an academic department. In conflict with his chairman over a matter of policy, a junior professor angrily threatens to resign unless he has his way. Embarrassed in front of his staff, the chairman cannot back down; neither can the young professor. ■

Case 4.7 ■ In case 4.3, if Virginia, the advertising executive, had not been successfully treated, a different outcome might have resulted. The bridge phobia could have distracted her from facing the underlying problem: her fear of disappointing paternal figures. A continuation and extension of her anxiety could then have produced a housebound agoraphobia, completely incapacitating her. Hypochondria and diazepam dependence might then readily be fostered by inappropriate medical attention. ■

Maladaptive coping patterns are the essence of psychiatric disorder, psychological dysfunction, and abnormal illness behavior.

Summary

Although the organism operates as a biopsychosocial unity, it is possible to delineate a psychological level of functioning. The psychological level is comprised of executive functions allowing an individual to be self-aware while finding satisfaction for physical, biosocial, and psychological motives in a manner that does not disrupt social life. Adaptation is defined by the extent to which an individual can find satisfaction for personal needs without resorting to impulsive, immature, deviant, self-destructive, self-defeating, or dangerous behavior or without manifesting psychological symptoms.

The following psychological functions can be delineated: information processing; perceptual-motor skills; communication; images, emotions, and attitudes; internal controls, rules, and aspirations; ego defenses and coping.

Information-processing involves coordinating consciousness, orientation, attention, perception, learning, memory, comprehension, reasoning, and judgment. Information is stored in long-term memory in a hierarchically organized manner. Perceptual-motor skills involve staged suboperations with continuous feedback.

Language expression involves the transformation of fundamental semantic propositions into the syntactic, phonological, and graphic forms of spoken and written language. Comprehension requires deciphering language into basic propositions. Like memory and motor performance, it is hierarchically organized.

The images, emotions, and attitudes unique to the individual's mental life are organized into sets of cognitive structures comprised of generic assumptions about the self, about others, and about the future. The vulnerable individual is likely to have unrealistic, inflexible attitudinal structures derived from adverse early experience. The sense of self, a subset of attitudinal structures, is affected by the individual's images of his or her body, mind, ego boundaries, ego defenses, self-esteem, and identity. Social competence is also affected by the cognitive structures projected into the social world.

The internal controls, rules, and aspirations of personality make up the superego and ego ideal and the different ego defense mechanisms. Ego defenses, acting in combination, comprise the coping techniques with which the individual faces crises such as personal illness.

If habitual coping strategies are inadequate to a problem, a crisis ensues: The individual must find new strategies or apply old strategies in new ways. If the new coping strategies are maladaptive – that is, if they involve repression, denial, or camouflage of the problem – psychiatric disorder, psychological dysfunction, or abnormal illness behavior arise.

Selected Readings

For a review of the fundamental psychological functions of motivation, orientation, perception, attention, learning, memory, reasoning, language, and motor skills, the reader is referred to an introductory psychology text such as Hilgard, Atkinson, and Atkinson (1979), *Introduction to Psychology*.

The development of psychological functioning is described in chapter 24 of *The Clinical Process in Psychiatry*.

The concepts of stress and coping have already been discussed in chapter 3. The concept of life crisis is developed by Caplan (1964) in *The Principles of Preventive Psychiatry*.

Attitudinal structures are discussed in detail by Guidano and Liotti (1983) in *Cognitive Processes and Emotional Disorders*. Most psychiatric textbooks have excellent descriptions of the ego defense mechanisms and the psychoanalytic concepts of id, ego, superego, and ego ideal. The reader could refer, for example, to the chapter by Meissner, Mack, and Semrad (1975) in Freedman, Kaplan, and Sadock (Eds.), *The Comprehensive Textbook of Psychiatry*.

5

Neurobiological systems

■ It was not the first time Hector had felt like this. Five years before, when he was 30 years old, he had had an attack of depression, as a result of which he entered the hospital, where he was successfully treated with antidepressant medication. The problem was in his family, too: his late mother and her brother had both suffered from recurrent bouts of nervousness and hypochondria, and his maternal grandfather had killed himself with a shotgun at the age of 56.

Nevertheless, this was the worst Hector had ever felt. Two months before, run down as a result of several months of demanding work at the office, he had contracted influenza. Despite several days' rest in bed, he still felt debilitated when he returned to his job. He also had a persistent, hacking cough that worried his wife and irritated his fellow workers.

The trucking company at which Hector was employed as an accountant was in the process of converting its records to a fully automated system. Hector was apprehensive about the change, particularly since it was coordinated by the company's computer expert, a demanding and abrasive man. As a result of the attack of influenza, Hector had fallen behind in his work. A highly conscientious man, he detested this situation but characteristically would not ask for help.

Over the next month, Hector's coughing and fatigue dragged on. He began to have episodes of panic, particularly when he woke up and contemplated the mountain of paper waiting for him at work and the unfinished chores at home. He began to be troubled by nightmares and insomnia. Lying awake in the early morning hours, thoughts of failure and disaster filled his mind.

Never had he felt so low. This feeling was different from the grief and sadness he had experienced when his mother died. He likened his current mood to mental torture, a horrible desolation of the spirit. Coincident with his anguish and fatigue, Hector lost interest in eating and drinking, with the consequence that he now weighed four pounds less than before he became ill. He lost his zest for love-making and his former pleasure in music and gardening. In company, he could keep up a smiling front for a time and even be amused by a joke, but eventually he would become so edgy and preoccupied that he would have to make an excuse and leave. At work he was forgetful, missing appointments and losing his place when he tried to read, as his mind drifted back to gloomy ruminations. It seemed to him as though the whole world was without color or purpose.

Hector's wife had held her tongue up to this point; she knew how touchy he was about people butting into his affairs. But when she found him weeping in the kitchen before breakfast, she insisted he get help. This time, he was not ungrateful she intervened for he had begun to think about doing away with himself.

The family physician referred him to a psychiatrist. Hector was admitted to the local hospital and discharged after a week, apparently improved by rest and an-tidepressant medication. With the psychiatrist's grudging approval, he decided to return to work.

The first day went fairly well; but the second was not as good. On the morn-ing of the third day, he woke at 4 A.M., could not go back to sleep, and lay in bed with mounting agitation. How was he going to cope?

Hiding his panic from his wife, Hector set off in his car. Before getting to work, however, he stopped at a shop for coffee. He can remember only fragments of the next 24 hours, until he was transferred to the psychiatric unit of a teaching hospital. Apparently, he was discovered by a policeman wandering along the street, weeping and asking for his mother. He knew his name and address, but was vague about the date and where he was.

By the time he got to the hospital, his confusion had cleared. Neurological examination, electroencephalogram, and CT scan were all normal. During his stay in the hospital, Hector developed a close relationship with a female psychiatric resi-dent and responded quickly to medication and cautious psychotherapy. His wife was also involved in therapy. After 2 weeks in the hospital and a convalescence of two weeks, he was able gradually to return to work, without recurrence of his former distress.

During the next 6 months, he explored with his therapist how close he had been to his gentle, emotionally fragile mother; how angry he was with the father he could never please; and how resentful he was toward his brother, the father's favorite. He remembered bitter quarrels with his father during adolescence, after his mother died of cancer when he was fourteen years old. Eventually, he coped with his predicament by controlling his anger and plunging into work. Thus, he learned to take pride in the way he could shoulder a load under which most would falter. It was well known that he never refused a new assignment. Only later, in psychotherapy, did he remember how lost he felt as a child when his mother would withdraw from the family in what she referred to as one of her blue spells. ∎

Hector's case history provokes a number of questions common in psychiatry and useful as an introduction to a selective review of neurobiology:

1. What is the relationship between emotional stress and physical illness?
2. What are the neural mechanisms of sleep and arousal?

3. What are the neural mechanisms of hunger, thirst, sex, pleasure, and reward?
4. What are the neural mechanisms of emotion?
5. What are the neural mechanisms of attention and memory?
6. What are the neural mechanisms of learning?
7. Which neurotransmitter systems are involved in different mental illnesses, in what ways are they dysfunctional, and how do antipsychotic drugs exert their therapeutic action?

These questions will be dealt with in the following sections on these topics:

1. Psychoimmunology
2. Arousal and sleep
3. The regulation of drives
4. The regulation of emotion
5. Learning and memory
6. Neurotransmission, mental illness, and psychopharmacology

Psychoimmunology

Stress and physical disorder

Physicians have long suspected a connection between life stress and such physical disorders as infection, cancer, and autoimmune disease. In recent years, a number of correlational and experimental studies have supported this association. What mediates the connection between stress and disease? Recently, this question has stimulated some promising research.

The cell and antibody mediation of immuno-suppression and auto-immune disease

The immune system has two components: one **antibody-mediated** and the other **cell-mediated**. Antibodies are derived from plasma cells, which are converted B-lymphocytes. The cell-mediated component of the immune system consists of macrophages and killer cells. Both systems are activated by antigens and modulated by T-lymphocytes of various types that enhance or suppress other T-lymphocytes, B-lymphocytes, or macrophages. An increased susceptibility to disease is conveyed by immunodeficiency, whereas a hyperactive immune system results in autoimmune phenomena. The scientific problem has been to (1) demonstrate immunologic changes in association with stress, (2) demonstrate similar changes in stress-related disease, and (3) determine the mechanism whereby stress affects the immune system.

Over the past 10 years, a number of studies have in fact demonstrated the connection between a variety of stresses (e.g., spaceflight, bereavement, sleep deprivation, and academic pressure) and different indices of immune function (e.g., depression of lymphoblast transformation, increased interferon production, change in phagocyte or killer cell function, and change in antibody titre following vaccination). Most studies have shown immunosuppression during stress and a rebound immunohyperreactivity after stress is relieved. Several studies have demonstrated an interaction between stress, coping strength or personality, and immune response.

Neurohumoral conse-
quences of stress

The **neurohumoral** consequences of stress are conveyed via the hypothalamus, through the pituitary or adrenal medulla, and thus to other glands. Different stressors, of different duration, interpreted differently by people of different coping capacities produce different endocrine responses. It has been demonstrated that lymphocytes have **receptor sites** for a number of **stress hormones** (such as catecholamines), all of which stimulate adenylate cyclase and generate cyclic adenosine monophosphate (AMP). AMP stimulates immature and suppresses mature lymphocytes. Other cell membrane enzyme systems in lymphocytes have an opposite effect.

Autonomic mediation
of stress

The innervation of lymphoid organs by **autonomic** fibers suggests another mediating mechanism which might operate via **mast cells.** Mast cells are responsive to immunogenic and autonomic agonists and are aggregated in organs susceptible to psychophysiologic disorder. Mast cells are also responsive to endogenous opiates known as **endorphins.**

Arousal and sleep

Biological rhythms

The most prominent of the **circadian rhythms** is the cycle of sleeping and wakefulness. Evidence suggests that circadian and other biological periodicities are not dependent solely on environmental cues (such as sunrise and sunset) but

The neural regulation
of circadian rhythms

on **neural pacemakers.** The **pineal** has been suggested as an important pacemaker. This gland contains high concentrations of serotonin and melatonin, which have a regular diurnal variation synchronized with the light-dark cycle. Serotonin has been implicated in sleep regulation and melatonin in the periodicity of the oestral cycle in mammals. An association has been suggested between psychiatric disorder, particularly depression, and disturbance in the neural regulation of biological rhythms.

Neural arousal systems

Arousal and sleep are not determined solely by the waxing and waning of sensory stimulation. They are regulated by intrinsic brain activity originating in several centers: brain stem, hypothalamus, basal cortex, and limbic cortex.

Neural centers of
arousal

The **reticular activating system** is a diffuse brain stem center that has **ascending** and **descending** divisions. Excited by afferents from the ascending sensory tracts, it projects upward to the diencephalon, thalamus, and cerebral cortex and downward to the spinal cord.

The posterior hypothalamus is associated with arousal and the anterior hypothalamus with inactivity and sleep. The midline thalamus and ventral frontal lobes are involved in the induction of sleep and appear to counterbalance the reticular activating system. The amygdala and surrounding temporal lobe, hippocampus, and septal nuclei also appear to suppress arousal.

The architecture of sleep

Along the continuum from alert wakefulness to deep sleep, different stages with distinctive physiologic characteristics can be recognized, as follows:

Stage	Electroencephalogram
Alert wakefulness: eyes open	Desynchronized electroencephalogram, low amplitude 13–30 c.p.s. beta waves.
Relaxed wakefulness: eyes closed	Electroencephalogram dominated by medium 8–12 c.p.s. alpha waves, which are desynchronized when the eyes are opened.
Stage 1 sleep:	Low amplitude, fast frequency activity.
Stage 2 sleep:	Bursts of 12–16 c.p.s. sleep spindles on a low amplitude, fast frequency background.
Stage 3 sleep:	High amplitude slow waves of 1–4 c.p.s. comprise 20% to 50% of the record.
Stage 4 sleep:	High amplitude slow waves of 1–4 c.p.s. comprise 50% of the record. Heart rate, blood pressure, and respiration are depressed.
Stage 1 rapid eye movement sleep:	Low amplitude, fast frequency pattern with 50–60 c.p.s. bursts of eye movement, decreased muscle tone, myoclonic movements, penile erection, and accelerated respiration and heart rate.

REM sleep

The REM sleep cycle   The first episode of rapid eye movements (REM) occurs about 100 minutes after the onset of sleep. One non-REM–REM sleep cycle lasts about 90 minutes, and four to five cycles occur each night. During each cycle, the sleeper descends from stage 1 sleep through stages 2 and 3 to stage 4 and then ascends back from stage 1 REM sleep through stages 4, 3, and 2. The duration of REM sleep per cycle increases as the night proceeds.

If wakened during REM sleep, the subject will report dreaming. Dreams can also occur during non-REM sleep, but non-REM dreams are more fragmentary. Sleepwalking, sleeptalking, night terrors, and enuresis all occur during stage 4 sleep.

PGO activity and REM sleep

In the cat, characteristic high voltage activity can be detected during REM sleep in the pontine reticular formation, lateral geniculate bodies, and occipital cortex. These **pontogeniculooccipital** (PGO) **waves** appear to trigger and coincide with REM sleep and are associated with hippocampal and cortical activity.

The neurochemistry of sleep and arousal

Serotonin and deep sleep

Drugs that decrease brain serotonin also reduce stage 4 sleep. Serotonin precursors given to a serotonin-deficient animal restore stage 4 sleep. Damage to serotonergic brain nuclei or fibers leads to increased physical activity and decreased sleep.

Acetylcholine and REM sleep

Drugs with anticholinergic effects, such as tricyclic antidepressants, reduce REM sleep. Facilitating noradrenergic transmission reduces REM sleep whereas noradrenergic blockade increases it.

Norepinephrine, dopamine, and arousal

Arousal is associated with the activity of noradrenergic and dopaminergic brain nuclei and tracts. Stimulant drugs such as amphetamine appear to act by facilitating noradrenergic and dopaminergic neurotransmission, particularly in the reticular activating system.

The function of sleep and dreaming

Restoration

Sleep has long been thought to have a restorative function, enabling the body to recuperate after the day's activity. Physical exertion is associated with an increase of stage 4 sleep, whereas selective deprivation of stage 4 sleep causes lethargy.

The purpose of REM sleep and dreaming is unclear. The predominance of REM sleep in the preterm and normal neonate suggests it has a special significance in the immature nervous system. It has been suggested that rapid eye movements are associated with the establishment of depth perception.

REM sleep and memory

Animals selectively deprived of REM sleep have impaired memory for tasks in which they were previously trained. However, human subjects similarly deprived exhibit no impairment of memory. Instead, they experience irritability, poor concentration, and (rarely) hallucinosis. Following REM sleep deprivation for several nights, REM rebound occurs, the total duration of REM sleep being increased for about half the number of nights on which REM sleep deprivation occurred.

REM rebound

Dreaming and unresolved conflict

Freud considered that dreaming protected sleep by acting as a release: Through dreams, the sleeper expresses in symbolic form unresolved old conflicts, which have been reactivated by recent events. Were it not for dreaming, the sleeper would be awakened by such conflicts. The psychoanalytic theory of dreaming has recently been attacked from a number of sources. It has been contended, for example, that dreams are meaningless fragments representing the brain's attempt to make sense of random electrical activation originating in the pons (PGO waves).

Dreaming and the erasure of parasitic modes of thought

Another theory suggests that REM sleep is a mental housekeeping system regulated by electrical activity from the brain stem. Bursts of brain stem activity trigger parasitic modes of cortical activity that would otherwise interfere with rational thought. When these aberrant thought patterns are activated, they are sometimes recalled as dreams. Dreaming, however, is a side effect. The main purpose of activating parasitic modes is to weaken synaptic connections and erase unwanted ideas. How do the aberrant ideas arise? It is suggested that they are an inexpedient by-product of the exuberant associations of waking cognition. This theory suggests that an infant's pervasive REM sleep purges its brain of unwanted mental connections.

Sleep disorders

Insomnia has a number of causes, one of the most important being sedative-hypnotic medication. Pain, discomfort, and worry can cause sleep-onset insomnia or restless sleep. Early morning or mid-cycle waking is associated with major depression (see chapter 10).

The pathophysiology of sleep

Sleep apnea is associated with blockage to the upper airways, as in obesity. **Sudden infant death syndrome** may be associated with sleep apnea.

Narcolepsy is associated with episodes of brief, irresistible but refreshing sleep, cataplexy (falling due to sudden muscular paralysis, often precipitated by emotion), sleep paralysis and hypnagogic hallucinations. Narcoleptic patients plunge into REM sleep without the normal progressive descent through intermediate stages.

Hypersomnia is associated with anxiety and depressive disorders. The **Kleine-Levin syndrome** is associated with hypersomnolence and hyperphagia. The electroencephalogram in this syndrome reveals persistent high amplitude slow activity at 2–3 c.p.s.

The neural regulation of drives

Hunger and thirst

It has long been known that tumors in the region of the pituitary stalk produce genital atrophy and obesity. Experimental lesions of the **ventromedial hypothalamic nucleus** (VMH) produce hyperphagia and obesity; and it was

*The control of
appetite*

originally suggested that the VMH region is a satiety center. Recently, however, it has been discovered that lesions in the vicinity of the VMH have their effect because they coincidentally damage a noradrenergic pathway known as the **central tegmental tract.** This tract arises in the medulla, pons, and subcoeruleus cell group, joins with another noradrenergic tract (the dorsal tegmental bundle) in the **median forebrain bundle,** and terminates in the **paraventricular nucleus of the hypothalamus** (PVH). It is not clear what basic physiological mechanism is disrupted by experimental lesions in the vicinity of the VMH.

*The drives of hunger
and thirst*

In contrast to the obesity caused by ventromedial hypothalamic lesions, destruction of the **lateral hypothalamus** (LH) causes adipsia and aphagia. This effect may be due to coincidental damage to a dopaminergic pathway, the **nigrostriatal tract,** which arises in the substantia nigra and terminates in the caudate nucleus. The earlier concept of a lateral hypothalamic feeding center is probably incorrect.

Other centers in the **mid-lateral hypothalamus, ventral tegmentum,** and **septum pellucidum** activate or inhibit the thirst related to angiotensin secretion or the increase of sodium in cellular fluids following dehydration.

Sexuality

*The priming of sexual
differentiation by fetal
androgenization*

The potential of primordial reproductive tissue to differentiate into male or female organs is known as **sexual dimorphism.** The sex of the fetus is determined by the differentiation of the gonads. In the absence of androgens, nature activates a female. If the fetus does not produce functioning male hormones, it will resemble the female in anatomy, in the cyclicity of gonodotrophic hormone release from the anterior pituitary, and in sexual behavior.

The influence of ovarian hormones on female sexual drive is unclear. It is suggested (though by no means established) that estrogens and adrenal androgens increase female sex drive, whereas progesterone decreases it. However, a deficiency of testosterone results in a reduction of male libido.

*The neural control of
sexual behavior*

Within the central nervous system, seminal emission is associated activity of the **median forebrain bundle,** which conducts catecholaminergic fibers in a caudal-rostral direction from medulla, pons, and tegmentum to the hypothalamus, thalamus, hippocampus, and neocortex. Many locations in the frontal lobe, limbic lobe, preoptic area, and medulla affect sexual behavior in the animal; and clinical associations have been found between temporal lobe dysfunction and disturbed sexuality. The anterior and ventromedial hypothalamus appear to regulate basic sexual reflexes in females. Dopaminergic pathways facilitate male and inhibit female sexual behavior, whereas serotonergic neurones are inhibitory in both sexes. The brain areas for which sex hormones have the greatest chemical affinity are the same in both sexes: the basomedial and preoptic hypothalamus, amygdala, periaqueductal gray matter, neocortex, and hippocampus.

Maternal behavior

The neural control of maternal behavior

The nest building and pup care of rodents are primed by humoral factors (which have not yet been clearly identified). Lesions of the medial preoptic region of the hypothalamus preclude maternal behavior. Lesions of different parts of the limbic system disrupt maternal behavior by scrambling its normal sequence.

Emotion and aggression

Physical feedback and emotion

The **James-Lange theory of emotion,** propounded in the late 19th century, contended that emotions were the subjective perception of reflex bodily changes provoked by environmental stimuli. Evidence from patients with spinal cord injury supports the James-Lange theory: Emotions do depend partly on feedback from the autonomic system. However, most information about regulating emotion is derived from experimental studies of aggression in animals. The only subjective data available is from neurosurgical patients.

Aggression is an overinclusive term applied to the following agonistic behaviors, some of which may be biologically distinct:

Forms of aggression

1. Predation. This set of behaviors may be biologically different from others usually regarded as aggressive. Predation refers to a coordinated series of goal-directed behaviors involved in seeking, detecting, stalking, pursuing, and killing prey.
2. Territorial defense. The animal, usually a male, defends its habitat against the intrusion of another male.
3. Sexual aggression. In some species, the male animal displays attacking or threatening behavior before, during, or after copulation. Sexual aggression is not observed in the absence of testosterone and appears to be primed by an androgen pulse to the fetal or infantile diencephalon.
4. Maternal aggression. The lactating female defends her young against intruders.
5. Self-defense. The threatened animal reacts with fight or flight, attacking another animal when cornered.
6. Irritable aggression. A frustrated animal, particularly one in pain, will sometimes attack another animal or an inanimate object.

The neural control of aggression

Predatory attack, self-defense, and irritable aggression have been provoked by electrical stimulation of the brain. The **periaqueductal gray matter** (PAG) coordinates the contralateral movements involved in self-defense and irritable aggression. Stimulating the **lateral hypothalamus** facilitates predatory attack, whereas the **medial hypothalamus** provokes irritable aggression and the **dorsal hypothalamus,** flight. The hypothalamus appears to inhibit or facilitate midbrain mechanisms that activate aggression.

Stimulation of different parts of the **amygdaloid nuclei** has produced attack and escape behavior and the facilitation or inhibition of predation. Two pathways, the stria terminalis and ventral amygdalofugal tract, connect the amygdala to the hypothalamus through which the amygdala exert their influence on midbrain structures.

Reward and punishment

Intracranial self-stimulation

Animals with intracranial electrodes in a variety of sites will learn to stimulate themselves. Humans undergoing neurosurgery may report pleasure or euphoria following electrical stimulation of the forebrain. Other parts of the brain appear to be associated with aversive stimulation. It is unclear whether rewarding self-stimulation reinforces specific drives or activates a pleasurable nonspecific arousal system that can trigger a number of subsidiary drives. Both mechanisms probably occur.

The following sites are associated with rewarding effects: hypothalamus, median forebrain bundle, limbic system, prefrontal cortex, and different parts of the brain stem. Aversion is associated with the tegmentum, medial lemniscus, and periventricular gray matter.

Evidence suggests that the **mesolimbic dopaminergic system** is important in reinforcement. Cocaine and amphetamine are dopamine agonists and potent reinforcers. The facilitatory effect of these drugs can be blocked by injecting a dopamine antagonist into the nucleus accumbens.

Pain

Central ascending pain tracts

A complex network of neural systems subserves the perception of pain. Nociceptive sensory endings respond to mechanical, thermal, and chemical stimuli in the skin, deep tissues, or viscera. The cell bodies of these neurones are located in the **dorsal root ganglia.** Their central axons synapse with internuncials in the outermost laminae of the **dorsal horns** of the spinal cord. Pain sensation is conveyed via fibers that cross and ascend in the **lateral spinoreticulothalamic tract** to the **posteroventral nucleus of the thalamus** and **postcentral gyrus** of the parietal cortex. The central axones of pain fibers from the face and head, which have their cell bodies in the **trigeminal ganglion,** enter the spinal cord and synapse with internuncials in the **spinal nucleus of the fifth cranial nerve.** Ascending pathways then cross and terminate in the **posteroventral nucleus of the thalamus** via the **trigeminal lemniscus.**

Sharp superficial pain is relayed to the cerebral cortex via the **ventroposteromedial** and **ventroposterolateral nuclei** of the thalamus. Deep pain is conveyed via the **parafascicular** and **intralaminar nuclei.** The emotional component of pain is mediated through the **limbic system** and **prefrontal cortex.**

Two types of ascending pain fiber and at least one system of descending fibers underly the perception of pain.

Fast ascending tracts   1. Small, fast fibers from peripheral nociceptors conduct sensory information via relay neurones to the cerebral cortex, where sensory discrimination occurs.

Slow ascending tracts   2. Large, slow fibers from peripheral nociceptors transmit pain stimuli to the dorsal horn, where *T* cells relay pain stimuli to conscious awareness. The *T* cells form a physiologic **gating mechanism.**

Descending tracts from the PAG   3. Fibers descend from the central sensory-discriminative cortex to the **peri-aqueductal gray matter** (PAG). Stimulated by endorphins, PAG neurones descend and synapse in the medulla in the **nucleus raphe magnus** (NRM). The neurotransmitter involved at the NRM synapse may be glutamate, aspartate, or the peptide neurotensin. Opiates excite PAG and, subsequently, NRM neurones. NRM neurones descend to the outermost laminae of the dorsal horns, where they terminate in serotonergic synapses on internuncial neurones.

Descending tracts from the LC   4. Descending neurones from the **locus coeruleus** (LC) project downward to noradrenergic synapses in the dorsal horn.

Via interneurone synapses on the central processes of dorsal root neurones, or by the nonspecific release of neurotransmitter into the dorsal horn, descending neuronal systems inhibit *T* cells and suppress the primary relays of painful stimuli (see Figure 5.1).

The descending pathways appear to convey the supraspinal analgesia associated with opiates, acupuncture, and transcutaneous nerve stimulation. They may also be involved in placebogenic analgesia. The analgesia of acupuncture and placebo are both blocked by naloxone, an opiate agonist-antagonist. Naloxone also blocks the action of endorphin.

Learning and memory

The difference between short-term memory (STM) and long-term memory (LTM) is discussed in chapter 4. The clinical phenomenology of memory is described in chapter 9. This chapter considers the neuropsychology and physiology of memory, in the following order:

1. Attention and registration
2. Short-term memory
3. Long-term memory
4. The cellular basis of memory
5. The pathology of memory

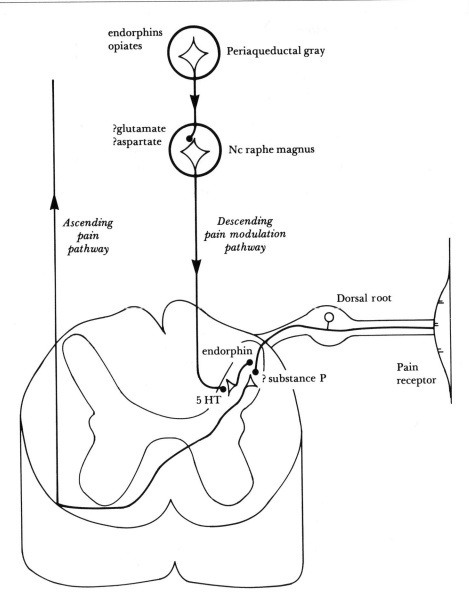

FIGURE 5.1
Schematic representation of descending cord pain modulation pathway.

Attention and registration

People are more likely to remember what they attend to, and the persistence of a memory is related to the duration and intensity of its stimulus. The **reticular activating system** is required to sustain the alertness required for attention, but the direction of attentional focus is regulated by the **hippocampus** and **frontal lobes.**

Short-term memory

The limits to STM

STM includes **immediate memory** (as measured by the digit-span test) and **recent memory** (as measured by the ability to recall items after several minutes). STM can hold a maximum of from five to nine items and is practically synonymous with consciousness or working memory. Without rehearsal, its duration is about 30 seconds. Memories are transferred to, or retrieved from, LTM through STM. STM tags information to be stored in LTM and later matches stimulus cues to the tags in order to retrieve items from LTM.

Different types of STM have different cortical locations; for example:

The loci of STM

STM Function	*Location*
Auditory memory for figures or words	Left supramarginal and angular gyri
Auditory memory for music	Right parieto-temporal cortex
Memory for the serial visual recognition of objects in space	Right parieto-occipital cortex

Thus, different short-term memories are associated with different modalities (visual, auditory, etc.).

Long-term memory

LTM is a more or less permanent record of past events. It has four stages:

1. Transfer
2. Consolidation
3. Storage
4. Retrieval

Transfer and consolidation

Transfer involves the movement of material from STM to LTM. Transfer involves the (en)coding of the material to be stored in categories organized by time,

Rehearsal aids transfer

space, or abstract properties. By focusing attention on an item, rehearsal prolongs STM and aids coding, transfer, and consolidation. **Consolidation,** which takes much longer than transfer, begins .5 seconds after the stimulus is presented.

The locus of consolidation

Bilateral damage to the **hippocampus** eliminates the capacity for consolidation. The left hippocampus is the anatomical substrate for the consolidation of verbal material; the right hippocampus is associated with nonverbal material. STM and retrieval remain intact after bilateral hippocampal damage.

Storage

A permanent memory trace involves a relatively permanent change in brain structure, although initial gradual decay may occur.

The loci of storage

Episodic memory involves information with temporal or spatial coding. **Categorical** or **semantic memory** usually involves the use of words or abstractions. Episodic memory may be associated with the temporal lobe. Verbal memory may be associated with the left anterior temporal lobe and nonverbal memory with the right hemisphere.

Retrieval

Retrieval refers to the location of material stored in LTM. It is the reverse of coding and transfer and can be either automatic or conscious (as in the deliberate search for an elusive memory). In a retrieval search, a number of stimulus cues (a set of symptoms and signs, for example) are associated with a specific item (acute pyelonephritis, for example) or a general area (renal infection, for example). The

Using a pattern of cues to access LTM

cue or set of cues that afford access to LTM are the same as those used originally to code memory.

The STM, LTM storage, and cognitive processing associated with a particular function apparently all operate in the one area of the brain. For example, digit span memory functions are located in the left angular gyrus. Other kinds of registration, storage, and processing are associated with other areas of the brain. Of all memory processes, only consolidation is located in a single brain area – the **hippocampus.**

The cellular basis of memory

STM requires temporary neural activity. LTM storage requires a stable neural change. STM can be disrupted by head trauma, electroconvulsive therapy, anoxia, or other conditions that temporarily suppress neural activity. Material stored in LTM is more resistant to disruption.

STM and reverberating circuits

It has been suggested that STM is associated with reverberating neural circuits or cell assemblies, as between cerebral cortex and thalamus. It is not clear how such circuits could represent external stimuli.

LTM and structural change

Structural changes in synapses could result in the development of cell assemblies that are more likely to be activated by specific cues. Presynaptic terminals could multiply, terminal boutons could enlarge, the synaptic cleft could narrow, the production of neurotransmitter chemicals could be facilitated, or the enzymes involved in degradation could be inhibited. One or more of these processes might be operative. It has been found that the sensitization of effector neurones is due to the presynaptic facilitation of sensory terminals. Facilitatory interneurones terminate on presynaptic cells, where they release serotonin, which increases the level of cyclic adenosine monophosphate in the cell membrane of the sensory neurones. Cyclic adenosine monophosphate acts to increase the influx of calcium ions, possibly by phosphorylation of a membrane channel. Calcium ions then potentiate the release of neurotransmitter from sensory nerve terminals.

Structural change and protein synthesis

Whatever the process, it is probably controlled by protein synthesis. For example, the continuing reverberating electrical activity of a cell assembly could activate nucleotide cyclase enzymes in postsynaptic neuronal membranes. This would result in the phosphorylation of nonhistone proteins in the cell nucleus, the synthesis of messenger RNA, and ribosomal protein synthesis. The synthesized protein could then produce any or several of the structural changes suggested as possibilities.

Disorders of memory

Korsakoff's syndrome

This disorder is associated with impairment of recent memory; disorientation; some loss of remote memory; lack of insight; and confabulation, which patches up the memory gaps. It is most often caused by the thiamine deficiency associated with chronic alcoholism. It can also occur as a result of encephalitis, toxic encephalopathy, head trauma, and cerebrovascular disease. Korsakoff's syndrome is associated with damage to the hippocampus, fornix, mammillary bodies, and dorsal thalamus.

Traumatic amnesia

Closed head injuries can produce a **concussional syndrome** associated with loss of consciousness, anterograde amnesia, retrograde amnesia, and neurological signs. The amnesia shrinks during recovery but does not entirely disappear.

Dementia

Impairment of memory is characteristic in the dementia of degenerative brain disease. Recent memory deteriorates; remote memory is well retained, especially recollections of personal significance.

Pseudodementia

As with Hector (Case 5.1), depression can interfere with recent memory and simulate organic brain disease.

Transient global amnesia

This syndrome is characterized by a (usually) transient episode of anterograde amnesia with some retrograde amnesia, mild confusion and disorientation but with retention of other cognitive processes. It is possibly caused by cerebrovascular insufficiency.

Psychogenic amnesia

Psychogenic amnesia varies from the psychologically determined forgetting of a name to a complete loss of memory for the past. Sometimes an amnestic patient wanders or travels a considerable distance (fugue) or assumes another personality (multiple personality).

It is evident that in psychogenic amnesia, unwanted memories are kept out of consciousness by an active process (repression). Little is known of the physiology of repression, although it is a cornerstone of psychoanalytic theory.

Neurotransmitters

The number of possible central nervous transmitters is more than 40. Why so many? It is likely that chemical coding and patterns of chemical interaction are as important to mental activity as bouton-to-neurone facilitation and inhibition. Axo-axonic connections, for example, can regulate the release of synaptic transmitters presynaptically or can modulate neuronal states postsynaptically, and some chemical transmitters may be released into nervous tissue to diffuse over wide target fields.

Rapid signaling systems

GABA and inhibitory interneurones

Most fast-signaling transmitters are amino acids. γ-aminobutyric acid (GABA), for example, is an inhibitory transmitter found widely in the nervous system, particularly in the short inhibitory interneurones of the brain and spinal cord. It is also found in the axones of cerebellar Purkinje cells and the striatonigral tract. GABA acts by increasing membrane permeability to chloride. **Glycine,** another inhibitor, is concentrated in the dorsal horn of the spinal cord.

Glutamate, aspartate, and excitatory inter-neurones

L-**glutamate** and L-**aspartate** appear to be the most important transmitters for excitatory interneurones (see Figure 5.1). They operate by activating membrane sodium channels.

Diffuse regulatory systems

Neuromodulation rather than rapid transmission

Diffuse regulatory systems are associated with neurones that have elongated, highly branched varicose axones and that release neurotransmitters diffusely from many points along their processes. They are thereby adapted more to diffuse modulation than to rapid transmission.

Acetylcholine

Arousal and REM sleep

Acetylcholine is found in spinal and cranial motoneurones and in the basal ganglia. Cholinergic pathways ascend from the basal ganglia to the hippocampus and cerebral cortex and provide the neural substrate for the **reticular arousal system** and **REM sleep** (see Figure 5.2).

Catecholamines

Two noradrenergic pathways

The three main central catecholamines are **epinephrine, norepinephrine,** and **dopamine.** Epinephrine systems are of minor significance.

The two principal **noradrenergic pathways** (pathways associated with norepinephrine as a synaptic transmitter) are the **central tegmental tract** and the **dorsal tegmental bundle** already described in association with hunger and depicted in Figure 5.3. The central tegmental tract arises from the medulla, pons, and subcoeruleus cell group and terminates in the hypothalamus. The axones of the dorsal tegmental bundle arise in the locus coeruleus and project to medulla, cerebellar cortex, thalamus, hippocampus, and neocortex. In their rostral course, adjacent to the lateral hypothalamus, the noradrenergic pathways unite in the median forebrain bundle.

Two dopaminergic pathways

The two principal **dopaminergic pathways** are the **nigrostriatal** and **mesolimbic systems** (see Figure 5.4). The nigrostriatal system arises in the substantia nigra and projects to the putamen and caudate nucleus of the basal

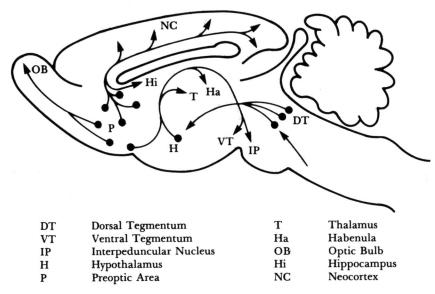

DT	Dorsal Tegmentum	T	Thalamus
VT	Ventral Tegmentum	Ha	Habenula
IP	Interpeduncular Nucleus	OB	Optic Bulb
H	Hypothalamus	Hi	Hippocampus
P	Preoptic Area	NC	Neocortex

FIGURE 5.2
Schematic representation of the principal central cholinergic pathways in the rat brain.

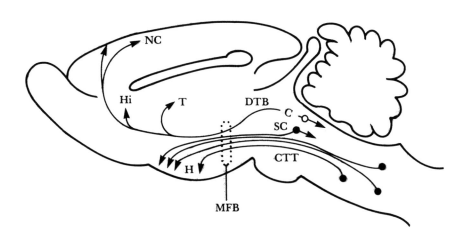

C	Locus Coeruleus	H	Hypothalamus
SC	Subcoeruleus	T	Thalamus
DTB	Dorsal Tegmental Bundle	NC	Neocortex
MFB	Median Forebrain Bundle	Hi	Hippocampus
CTT	Central Tegmental Tract		

FIGURE 5.3
Schematic representation of the principal central noradrenergic pathways in the rat brain.

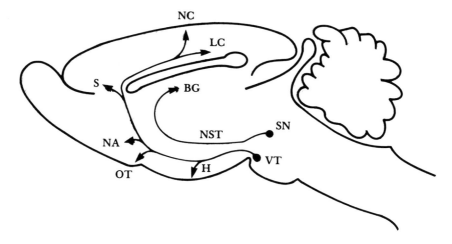

SN	Substantia Nigra	OT	Olfactory Tubercle
VT	Ventral Tegmentum	NA	Nucleus Accumbens
NST	Nigrostriatal Tract	S	Septum
BG	Basal Ganglia	NC	Neocortex
H	Hypothalamus	LC	Limbic Cortex

FIGURE 5.4
Schematic representation of the principal central dopaminergic pathways in the rat brain.

ganglia. The mesolimbic system originates in the ventral tegmental area and projects to the hypothalamus, nucleus accumbens, olfactory tubercle, septum, limbic cortex, and neocortex.

Voluntary movement

Reward

Arousal and attention

The functions of the catecholaminergic pathways are unclear. The dopaminergic nigrostriatal pathway appears to modulate voluntary movement and is antagonistic to acetylcholine-mediated pathways. Dopaminergic and noradrenergic pathways in the limbic system may be associated with reward and reinforcement. The dopaminergic mesolimbic system may be involved in arousal and attention.

Serotonin

Analgesia

Sleep and waking

Temperature and aggression

The indoleamine **5 hydroxytryptamine** (serotonin) system arises in the **brain stem raphe nuclei,** ascends through the median forebrain bundle to the hypothalamus and basal ganglia and descends to the ventral and dorsal horns of the spinal cord (see Figure 5.5). The spinal serotonergic system mediates the central analgesic effects of opiates. The forebrain serotonergic system may control the sleep-wake cycle. Serotonin may also be involved in the control of body temperature and aggression.

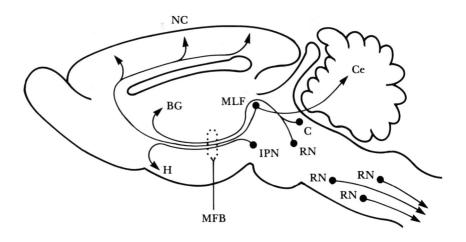

RN	Raphe Nuclei	H	Hypothalamus
C	Locus Coeruleus	BG	Basal Ganglia
IPN	Interpeduncular Nucleus	NC	Neocortex
MLF	Median Longitudinal Fasciculus	Ce	Cerebellum
MFB	Median Forebrain Bundle		

FIGURE 5.5
Schematic representation of the principal central serotonergic pathways in the rat brain.

Neuropeptides

Of the more than 30 neuropeptides described, the opioid peptides (**endorphins**) have been studied in most detail. Endorphins occur naturally in three families: (a) the **enkephalins,** (b) extended versions of **met-encephalin,** and (c) extended versions of **leu-encephalin.** Endorphins are distributed widely in the central nervous system, pituitary, and enteric nervous system and are associated particularly with the primary sensory and *Pain relay system* pain relay systems (see Figure 5.1), basal ganglia, and retina.

Substance **P** is a peptide found in gut and brain. It may be the main excitatory transmitter in the primary relays of pain sensation.

It has been suggested that the analgesia, drinking, and locomotor *Neuromodulators* behavior associated with different peptides are due to their function as neuromodulators rather than as neurotransmitters.

It is now known that some neurones secrete more than one neurotransmitter or neuromodulator. For example, catecholamines and endorphins coexist in the adrenal medulla, and serotonin and substance P are found together in the cells of the raphe nucleus of the brain stem.

Biochemical theories of mental illness

A number of theories relate mental illness to the malfunction of different neurotransmitter systems. None of the theories is satisfactory, and probably all are oversimplified. Nevertheless, they have directed research to potentially fruitful areas; for example, in several instances, they have suggested the structure of new synthetic psychotropic drugs.

The three general approaches to research in the biochemistry of mental illness are:

Pathochemical models

1. To search in the brain or body fluids of mentally ill subjects for a biochemical abnormality that could be related to the metabolism of neurotransmitters.

Pharmacological models

2. To use psychoactive drugs as research tools by determining the sites at which they operate, the neurotransmitters they affect, and the functions they influence. It is of particular interest if one drug can be found to provoke a mental illness (e.g., amphetamine psychosis) and another to combat it (e.g., neuroleptics).

Animal models

3. To develop animal models of mental illness and with them to investigate the biochemistry and pharmacology of mental dysfunction.

Schizophrenia

Dopaminergic systems

Dopamine activation accentuates schizophrenia

The dopamine-blocking effect of neuroleptic drugs has suggested that dopaminergic systems might be dysfunctional in schizophrenia. It has been found that dopamine activation (e.g., by the administration of amphetamine, cocaine, L-DOPA or methylphenidate) accentuates schizophrenic symptoms, whereas dopamine blocking (e.g., with neuroleptics) ameliorates them. However, no abnormality of dopamine metabolism has yet been detected in schizophrenia. The increase in dopamine receptor binding sites found in the schizophrenic brain post mortem is probably secondary to neuroleptic medication. Nevertheless, the possible associations between the ventral tegmental dopamine pathway and attention and between attentional defect and schizophrenia continue to stimulate research.

Noradrenergic systems

Inhibition of noradrenalin release ameliorates schizophrenia

Abnormalities in noradrenergic systems have been suggested by the effects of the noradrenalin release inhibitor, clonidine. After the administration of clonidine, schizophrenics excrete less of the noradrenalin metabolite MHPG than do normal controls. Clonidine also ameliorates psychotic symptoms.

Platelet MAO reduction

Monoamines are degraded by monoamine oxidase (MAO), the activity of which can be studied conveniently in platelets. Platelet MAO levels are reduced in schizophrenia, but MAO is also diminished in depression, perhaps as a result of nonspecific neurohumoral stress factors.

Endorphins

Naloxone, an opiate antagonist, produces a moderate amelioration of schizophrenic symptoms; but the administration of an endorphin precursor has also caused a reduction of schizophrenic symptoms. These findings are contradictory if schizophrenia is thought to be caused by an abnormality of endorphin metabolism.

Depression

The finding that tricyclic drugs and MAO inhibitors enhance the availability of 5-HT and noradrenalin at central synapses stimulated the initial interest in neurotransmitters in depressive disorder. Compared to the insubstantial status of biochemical theory in schizophrenia, research has made more progress in affective disorders.

Serotonergic systems

5-HT breakdown metabolite is reduced in the CSF of retarded depressives

Figure 5.6 represents the metabolism of **serotonin** (5-HT). It can be seen that 5-HIAA is the natural metabolite of 5-HT. Since probenecid blocks the transport of 5-HIAA from the nervous system to the bloodstream, it is apparent that the concentration of 5-HIAA in the cerebrospinal fluid before and after probenecid loading is a rough index of 5-HT turnover in the central nervous system. It has been found that 5-HIAA in the cerebrospinal fluid is reduced in about 50% of the people with major depression, particularly if the depression is associated with motor retardation. Blood platelets from depressive patients demonstrate abnormal cellular uptake of 5-HT and a reduced density of imipramine receptors (the probable uptake sites for 5-HT). It has also been found that when 5-HTP, a precursor of 5-HT (see Figure 5.6), is administered to patients with depression, it has a therapeutic effect.

If these disturbances in 5-HT metabolism are causal, are they necessary but insufficient (predisposing), or necesary and sufficient, in nature? The observations that the 5-HIAA deficiency persists after recovery from depression and that low 5-HIAA is found in the relatives of depressives support the first

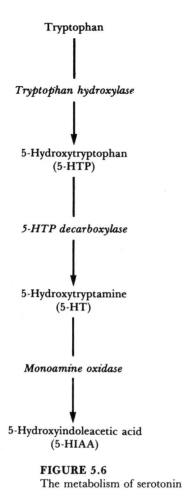

Tryptophan

Tryptophan hydroxylase

5-Hydroxytryptophan
(5-HTP)

5-HTP decarboxylase

5-Hydroxytryptamine
(5-HT)

Monoamine oxidase

5-Hydroxyindoleacetic acid
(5-HIAA)

FIGURE 5.6
The metabolism of serotonin

5-HT deficiency and depression   hypothesis: A persistent 5-HT deficiency predisposes to depression, but is insufficient to account for it entirely.

Noradrenergic systems

The main urinary metabolite of the catecholamines is 3-methoxy, 4-hydroxyphenylglycol (MHPG). Since about 60% of urinary MHPG is of central origin, the 24-hour urinary excretion of MHPG is a crude index of catecholamine turnover in the central nervous system. MHPG excretion is, in fact, reduced in major depression and schizoaffective disorder.

Endocrine studies suppport the hypothesis of a connection between noradrenergic dysfunction and depression. About 50% of people with major

Hypersecretion of cortisol in depression is not suppressed by dexamethasone

depression have an excess of cortisol secretion from the adrenal cortex. This excess results from the failure of ACTH production in the anterior pituitary to wax and wane diurnally. Moreover, cortisol hypersecretion is not totally suppressed by dexamethasone. This phenomenon is the basis of the dexamethasone suppression test for depression (see chapter 10). A diminished growth-hormone response to noradrenergic agonists and insulin and a diminished thyroid-stimulating hormone response to thyrotrophin releasing hormone have also been detected in depression. These findings are consistent with the effect on the anterior pituitary of a hypoactivity in noradrenergic pathways.

Dopaminergic systems

In depression, after probenecid loading, the main metabolite of dopamine is diminished in the cerebrospinal fluid. This finding is particularly likely if the depression is associated with motor retardation (as is also the case with cerebrospinal fluid 5-HIAA, the metabolite of 5-HT).

In summary, a diversity of observations suggests that depression is associated with diminished monoaminergic function, but much more work remains to be done.

Anxiety

Animal models

Anxiolytic drugs suppress experimental conflict

If an animal is electrically shocked whenever it attempts to ingest food or fluids, eating and drinking will be suppressed and the animal will be placed in a state of conflict. Anxiolytic drugs restore eating and drinking in conflicted animals. Suppressed behavior in conflicted animals can also be restored by agents that block the effect of serotonin. Agents that affect dopamine, norepinephrine, and GABA neurotransmission have little effect on conflict behavior. However, no pathochemistry has been found in conflicted animals or in psychiatric patients with anxiety disorders.

Sedatives, convulsants, and GABA neurotransmission

BZ receptors are coupled with GABA receptors and enhance chloride influx

Benzodiazepines enhance the presynaptic and postsynaptic inhibition of GABA. Radioactive diazepam selectively binds to protein in the lipid outer neuronal membrane. These protein sites are known as **BZ receptors,** one moiety of which appears to be related to anxiety and to be concentrated in the amygdala, hippocampus, and prefrontal cortex.

BZ receptors are coupled with **GABA receptors.** When GABA is added to a neurone, the BZ receptor of which is already occupied by a benzodiazepine, the flux of chloride ions is enhanced (usually from outside to inside the neurone) and the neurone is inhibited (by virtue of an increase in its electronegative potential).

Barbiturates enhance chloride influx

In contrast to benzodiazepines, barbiturates may act directly on the chloride channels to facilitate the influx of chloride ions. Other drugs (e.g., convulsants, anticonvulsants, sedatives) apparently act on different parts of the GABA receptor-chloride channel system. Benzodiazepine-like drugs act by enhancing GABA neurotransmission, whereas convulsants impede GABA transmission and neuronal inhibition. Other receptor-activation systems are currently the focus of intense research.

Dementia

Alzheimer's disease

Alzheimer's disease is characterized by progressive dementia and dysphasia. It is associated with deterioration of neurones in the cerebral cortex and less often in the basal ganglia. Alzheimer's disease is associated with a depletion of choline acetyltransferase (ChAT) (the enzyme responsible for the biosynthesis of acetylcholine) and diminished cholinergic activity, especially in the temporal neocortex, septum, amygdala, and hippocampus. A depletion in dopamine-B-hydroxylase has also been identified (see Figure 5.7), along with a loss of cells from the locus coeruleus (the origin of the noradrenergic dorsal tegmental bundle, which projects rostrally to the thalamus, hippocampus, and neocortex).

Depletion of the cholinergic system

The cholinergic system depleted in Alzheimer's disease appears to be part of the ascending arousal system. In experimental animals, it is associated with memory.

Parkinson's disease

Parkinson's disease is characterized by progressive muscular rigidity, tremor, akinesia, and dementia. It is associated with a degeneration of neurones in the substantia nigra and locus coeruleus and with a depletion of dopamine in the substantia nigra and striatum. Dopamine deficiency in the striatum is probably responsible for the motor signs of Parkinson's disease. The cause of the neuronal degeneration is unknown.

Depletion in the nigrostriatal dopaminergic system

Huntington's disease

This hereditary disease is characterized by progressive dementia, chorea, and mental disorder. It begins in adult life. Atrophy and gliosis occur in the cerebral cortex and striatum. There is a marked depletion of GABA and GABA receptors in the striatum and other biochemical abnormalities that are of uncertain significance.

Depletion of striatal GABA

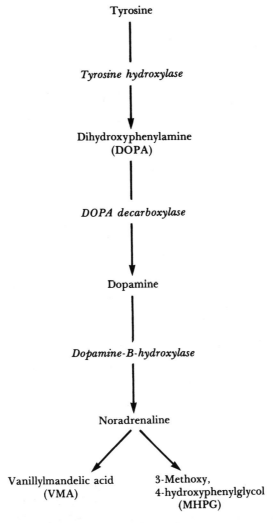

FIGURE 5.7
The metabolism of catecholamines

Psychopharmacology

The mode of action of different psychopharmacologic agents is described in the schematic diagrams of the biochemical pathways of each of the following neurotransmitters:

1. γ-aminobutyric acid
2. Acetylcholine

3. Norepinephrine
4. Dopamine
5. Serotonin

See Figures 5.8, 5.9, 5.10, 5.11, and 5.12.

Summary: an integrative model

In the last three chapters, we have descended the biopsychosocial staircase from sociology, through individual psychology and neurophysiology, to the molecular biology of the neural synapse. At several points, we have explored suggestive links between social, psychological, physiological, and biochemical domains of functioning. A number of glittering theories have been introduced to account for these connections.

Few of these theories are firmly established; empirical behavioral and central nervous data are difficult to measure and control. Nevertheless, research is progressing rapidly. In the words of Cooper, Bloom, and Roth (1981): "Don't blink or you'll miss the next blazing development."

Let us now return to Case 5.1, Hector, the accountant who developed major depression in the aftermath of an attack of influenza. Can we fit together the themes of his life and the levels of his functioning to make sense of what happened to him? To be more specific, what was the soil from which his illness grew? What caused its germination? What kept it growing? Why did it eventually subside?

There is a family history of depression in Hector's kin; one first-degree and two second-degree relatives probably suffered from the disorder. It is reasonable to speculate that Hector, too, inherited a depressive diathesis. But other information about Hector's early life is likely to be significant. In psychotherapy, he recalled his closeness to his mother, his sense of being "lost" as a child during her periodic episodes of depression, and his grief at her death in his early adolescence. Angry and depressed in the wake of bereavement, he came into conflict with his father, a man he could never please. Subsequently, he appears to have coped with the unresolved loss of his mother and his resentment toward his father and brother by developing a meticulous, compulsive, hyperindependent personality.

Such a personality has some adaptive features: honesty, a capacity for hard work, and a strong sense of obligation. However, compulsive people are never satisfied with their achievements. They are likely to feel that although love and appreciation are probably unattainable, they must work harder and harder to satisfy an internal image of a stern, unyielding, dissatisfied parent.

With such a personality, Hector would be highly vulnerable in work situations where his superiors had unreasonable expectations and expressed little appreciation. His natural coping style – to assume more and more responsibility – would eventually exhaust his physical and mental resources. Before the onset of

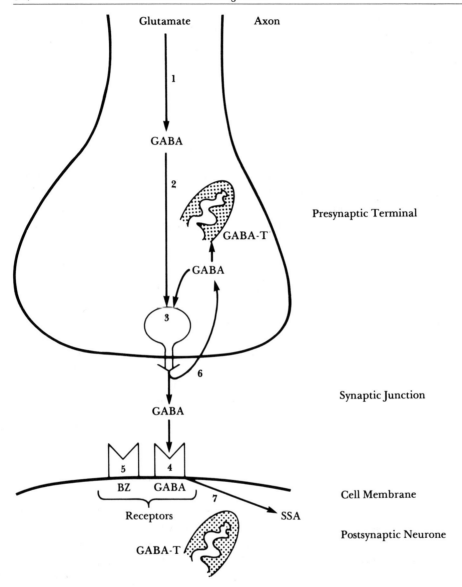

FIGURE 5.8

Possible Sites of Drug Action at Central GABA-ergic Synapses

1. Synthesis of GABA from glutamate is catalysed by the enzyme glutamic acid decarboxylase and can be inhibited by a number of hydrazines.
2. Uptake and storage of GABA in synaptic vesicles have no know facilitator or inhibitor.
3. Release of GABA into the synaptic space depends on Ca^{++}.
4. Postsynaptic receptors for GABA bind GABA and facilitate the influx of Cl^-. GABA receptors are potentiated by barbiturates and blocked by anticonvulsants.
5. The BZ receptor, which is coupled with the GABA receptor, binds benzodiazepines and enhances the receptor function of GABA.
6. Reuptake of GABA into the presynaptic membrane is an active process that depends on Na^+.
7. Degradation of GABA into succinic semialdehyde (SSA) is catalysed by GABA-transaminase (GABA-T) in mitochondria. It can be inhibited by a number of agents.

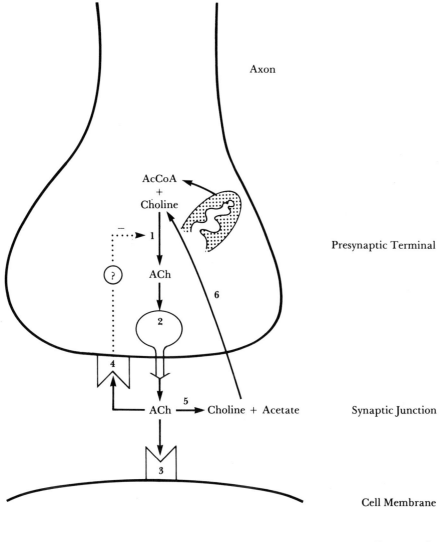

Axon

Presynaptic Terminal

Synaptic Junction

Cell Membrane

Postsynaptic
Neurone

FIGURE 5.9

Possible Sites of Drug Action at Central Cholinergic Synapses

1. Synthesis of ACh from choline is catalysed by choline acetyltransferase.
2. Release of ACh from synaptic vesicles is promoted by black widow spider venom and blocked by botulinum toxin.
3. Postsynaptic receptors are activated by cholinometric drugs and anticholinesterases. Nicotinic receptors are blocked by rabies virus, curare, and decamethonium. Muscarinic receptors are blocked by atropine and scopolamine.
4. Presynaptic receptors are blocked by atropine and scopolamine, which enhance the release of ACh by blocking a negative feedback loop.
5. Degradation of ACh is catalysed by acetylcholinesterase, which is inhibited by physostigmine or DFP.
6. Reuptake of choline can be inhibited by a number of competitive blockers.

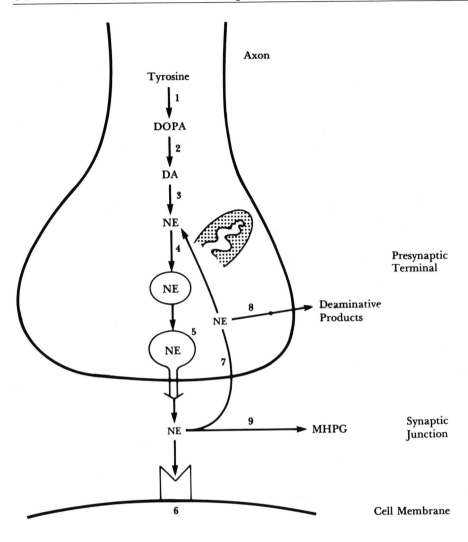

FIGURE 5.10

Possible Sites of Drug Action at Central Noradrenergic Synapses

1. Synthesis of DOPA is catalysed by tyrosine hydroxylase and can be blocked by tyrosine competitors.
2. Synthesis of DA is catalysed by DOPA decarboxylase.
3. Synthesis of NE is catalysed by dopamine-B-hydroxylase and can be blocked by a wide variety of compounds (e.g., copper chelating agents).
4. Uptake and storage of NE in synaptic vesicles can be blocked by reserpine.
5. Release of NE is augmented by amphetamine and may be inhibited by lithium.
6. Postsynaptic receptors for NE can be stimulated by clonidine and blocked by phentolamine, yohimbine, and piperoxane.
7. Reuptake of NE is inhibited by amphetamine and desipramine and may be facilitated by lithium.
8. Degradation of free presynaptic NE is catalysed by MAO in mitochondria.
9. Inactivation of NE in the synaptic space is catalysed via several enzymatic reactions to MHPG. Tropolone inhibits the first of these reactions.

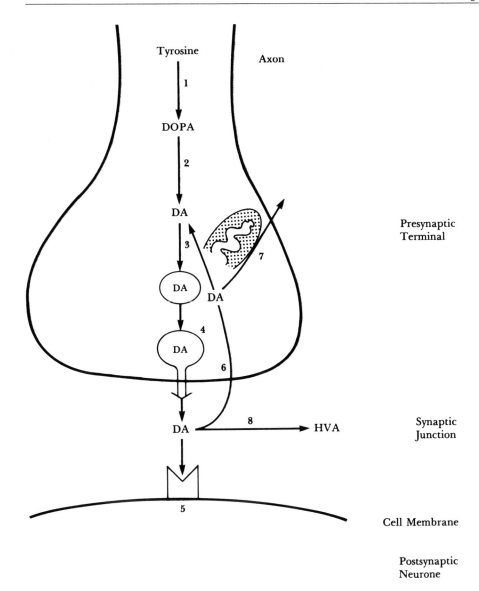

FIGURE 5.11

Possible Sites of Drug Action at Central Dopaminergic Synapses

1. Synthesis of DOPA is catalysed by tyrosine hydroxylase and blocked by tyrosine competitors.
2. Synthesis of DA from DOPA is catalysed by DOPA decarboxylase.
3. Uptake and storage of DA in synaptic vesicles can be blocked by reserpine.
4. Release of DA is augmented by amphetamine (but possibly more because amphetamine blocks reuptake). Release is blocked by γ-hydroxybutyrate because it blocks impulse flow in DA-ergic neurones.
5. Postsynaptic receptors for DA are stimulated by apomorphine and blocked by perphenazine and haloperidol.
6. Reuptake of DA is inhibited by amphetamine and benztropine.
7. Degradation of free presynaptic DA is catalysed by MAO in mitochondria.
8. Inactivation of DA in the synaptic space is catalysed via several enzymatic reactions to homovanillic acid. The first of these is inhibited by tropolone.

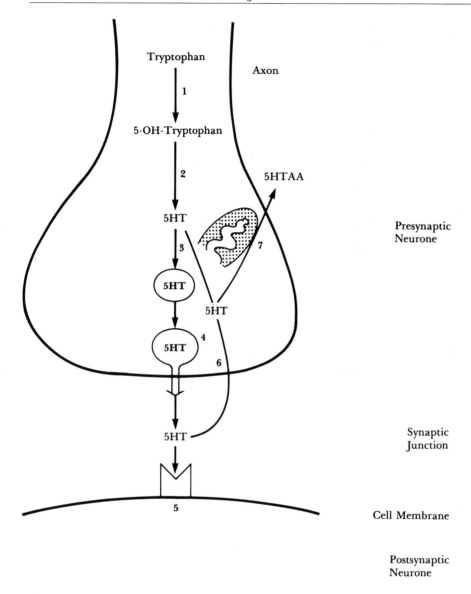

FIGURE 5.12

Possible Sites of Drug Action at Central Serotonergic Synapses

1. Synthesis of 5-OH tryptophan from tyrosine is catalysed by trytophan hydroxylase and inhibited by p-chloraphenylalamine.
2. Synthesis of 5-HT from 5-OH-tryptophan is catalysed by amino acid decarboxylase.
3. Uptake and storage of 5-HT in synaptic vesicles is blocked by reserpine.
4. Release of 5-HT is inhibited by LSD (which blocks impulses in serotonergic neurones).
5. Postsynaptic receptors for 5-HT are facilitated by LSD.
6. Reuptake of 5-HT is inhibited by tricyclic antidepressants.
7. Degradation of free presynaptic 5-HT is catalysed by MAO in mitochondria and inhibited by monoamine oxidase inhibitors.

his depressive illness, Hector was in such a predicament: The demands of work were growing and his superior becoming more exacting as his company undertook a difficult administrative reorganization.

It is tempting to speculate that physical and psychological stress created an immunodeficiency, as a result of which Hector contracted influenza. Whatever its cause, the debilitating viral illness seems to have acted as a last straw; but it is impossible to determine whether Hector's depression was a concomitant or an aftermath of the influenza attack or unconnected with it.

The exhaustion accompanying Hector's viral infection evolved into a disorder of mood with agitation; insomnia; loss of interest, appetite, and libido; weight loss; demoralization; self-accusation; suicidal ideation; and impairment of concentration and memory.

Hector responded well to antidepressant medication in the hospital but returned to work prematurely. As a result, he experienced a recurrence of overwhelming anxiety, culminating in a transient dissociative episode. He subsequently responded well to a comprehensive management program involving rest, medication, family therapy, individual psychotherapy, and gradual return to work.

Assuming a connection between Hector's psychosocial stress, physical exhaustion, viral illness, and melancholia, what could the connection be? How could physical and psychosocial stressors, affecting an individual with genetic and experiential vulnerability, produce a disorder of mood with a distinctive set of neurovegetative features (insomnia, anorexia, weight loss, loss of libido, and anhedonia)?

Akiskal and McKinney (1975) proposed an integrative explanatory model for mood disorder. According to them, melancholia is one final common pathway of interlocking chemical, experiential, and behavioral processes that stem from a disorder of diencephalic functioning. A set of frustrating environmental events, for example, leads to subjective turmoil, demoralization, and a state of

Chronic hyperarousal depletes biogenic amines

Imbalance in psychomotor stress and reinforcement systems

neurophysiological arousal. Chronic hyperarousal is associated with disordered biogenic amine function, or excessive intraneuronal sodium concentration, or both. The derangement of the arousal system then unbalances other neural systems linked to it. The psychomotor system is affected, causing motor retardation or agitation. The hypothalamo-pituitary stress system reacts with hypersecretion of cortisol and intracellular sodium retention. The reinforcement system (incorporated in the mesolimbic dopaminergic pathways) is also disrupted, causing anhedonia and social withdrawal. Melancholia, thus, is a disorder of diencephalic function. It results when chronically heightened arousal has biochemical sequelae that disturb the negative feedback balance between the arousal system and the psychomotor, stress-neuroendocrine, and reinforcement systems.

Akiskal and McKinney's integrative model also suggests possible mechanisms by which genetic factors could account for a tendency of the biogenic amine system to become deranged. For example:

Hypotheses about genetic predisposition

1. A mutation in the genes that monitor the synthesis of biogenic amines in presynaptic terminals.

2. A mutation in the genes that control the active transport systems of the presynaptic neuronal membrane.
3. A mutation in the genes that code lipoproteins in postsynaptic receptor sites.

The permissive amine theory of affective disorder

The permissive amine theory of affective disorder hypothesizes that: (1) a central serotonergic deficiency is the basis of the vulnerability to react to stress with affective disorder; (2) melancholia is associated with a depletion of central serotonin and catecholamines; and (3) mania is associated with a depletion of serotonin and an increase of catecholamines. According to the third hypothesis, mania and depression are not polar opposites but on a continuum from normality through depression to mania. The switch from depression to mania, which occurs in some patients with bipolar disorder, is associated with a change from low to high catecholamine secretion.

Psychoactive drugs counteract the dysfunction of biogenic amines that perpetuates affective disorder. Tricyclic antidepressants, for example, inhibit the reuptake of serotonin and norepinephrine from synaptic junctions, thus enhancing the action of these neurotransmitters and compensating for their depletion.

This chapter ends the introductory or theoretical part of the book. Part II discusses the clinical process and the tactics and strategy of clinical reasoning.

Selected Readings

Excellent introductions to the neurobiology of behavior can be found in Carlson's (1981) *Physiology of Behavior* or Groves and Schlesinger's (1979) *Introduction to Biological Psychology.*

Two comprehensive reviews of psychoimmunology have been provided by Locke (1982) and Rogers, Dubey, and Reich (1979).

A detailed discussion of memory processes with particular reference to psychopathology may be found in a chapter by Russell (1977) in *Amnesia,* a book edited by Whitty and Zangwill (1977). The molecular basis of memory is discussed by Kandell (1979).

Provocative accounts of the neurophysiologic nature and purpose of dreaming are provided by Hobson and McCarley (1977a, b) and Crick and Mitchison (1983).

Cooper, Bloom, and Roth's (1981) *The Biochemical Basis of Neuropharmacology* is indispensible for the reader seeking a comprehensive review of the effects of drugs on neurotransmission. The reader is also referred to a series of articles in *Lancet* on "Neurotransmitters and CNS Disease" by Iversen (1982), Snyder (1982), Braestrup and Nielsen (1982), Jessell (1982), Marsden (1982), Rossor (1982), and Van Praag (1982).

Akiskal and McKinney's (1975) classic review of research in depression, although a little out of date, is cited as an exceptional attempt to integrate the physical, psychological, and social factors involved in affective disorder.

PART
II

**Tactics and strategy in
the clinical process**

6

The clinical process

A feed-forward series of steps
The clinical process is a set of steps from referral through diagnosis and treatment to termination. The sequence is illustrated in Figure 6.1 as a feed-forward series, preceding steps being organized with successive steps in mind. Diagnosis is not an end in itself but a way station en route to management.

Referral

Source of referral
The process commences with referral. Patients may be referred by physicians from ambulatory, family practice, or hospital settings. Some are referred by other professionals, and others by friends. Some come of their own accord, having sought advice about where to go and how to go about it. All bring with them, to varying degree, feelings, attitudes and coping techniques that are both conducive to and contrary to the diagnostic encounter.

Motivation for referral
Some people who seek relief from illness have clear ideas about the nature of their problems and the treatment they require; sophisticated patients know what to expect. Other people may be painfully uncertain.

Vulnerable stages in the clinical process
Referral thus represents a step of heightened vulnerability, as do the points of initial contact and negotiation (following the diagnostic encounter). An

101

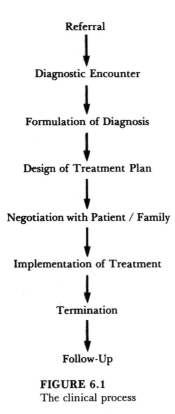

FIGURE 6.1
The clinical process

unresponsive nurse or secretary can upset a tense patient at the time of the first phone call. A poorly handled negotiation can compromise the success and even the acceptance of therapy.

The doctor-patient relationship

Patient's rights   The clinical process is an invasion of privacy, accepted by the patient in hope of a beneficial outcome. Doctor and patient are bound by an implicit contract with reciprocal obligations: the doctor to diagnose and treat appropriately, the patient to cooperate.

In the private sector, the patient has a right to choose a personal physician. He or she has the right to treatment in public institutions if he or she is involuntarily detained. While the contract operates, the patient has the right to confidentiality and the right to be fully informed about diagnosis, management plan, possible complications, and the progress of treatment. The patient has the right to decline treatment and seek help elsewhere.

Include patient in diagnosis and therapy

Although these prerogatives have been expressed in imperative, legalistic terms, they are cogent principles. They emphasize the desirability of including the patient in diagnosis and therapy and of treating the patient as an individual capable of collaborating in and contributing to the clinical process. This is the key to the negotiation stage of the clinical sequence but it should characterize the entire process.

Patients' expectations of their physicians

What do patients seek in their doctors? Mechanic (1968) surveyed a group of women in Madison, Wisconsin, who nominated the following desirable qualities, in order of emphasis: competence, personal interest and concern, readiness to make house calls, truthfulness, lack of hurry, thoroughness, availability, and willingness to explain and listen. The qualities of caring, thoroughness, lack of haste, and listening were closely associated. It is clear that these women expected competence but that technical competence alone was not enough. Davis (1968) found that a patient is less likely to comply with treatment if personal communication with the doctor is poor, if there is a struggle for control between the two of them, or if the patient feels the physician has extracted information without adequate explanation.

The rehumanization of medical care

As medicine becomes more specialized and technical, particularly in hospitals, the traditional caring function of the physician is undermined. The hospital expects the patient to submit passively to routine, impersonal procedures. It is relatively unresponsive to individual needs. The rehumanization of the hospital requires a concerted effort, an effort too readily enervated by the demands of the machine and the organization.

The effect of the physician's attitude

The physician has a powerful effect on the patient's attitude to illness. A somber or mysterious demeanor has serious implications. A positive, encouraging, open approach fosters collaboration and has a placebogenic effect, which potentiates the effect of treatment (and must be controlled in experimental studies). This effect may be dramatic if the patient is desperate for help (Schachter & Singer, 1962).

Irrational wishes and fears

Aside from reactions to the vital threat of illness, other more irrational fears and wishes hinder the development of rapport. The generic desire for mercy and cure and the inevitable fear of helplessness, invasion, and damage may be inflamed by the physician. The mysterious magician, the charismatic healer, the incisive technician, the impassive reader of others' secret thoughts, the august and learned mandarin are all familiar characters on the medical proscenium. These physicians do not allow patients to exercise or develop a sense of responsibility for their own treatment. Instead, they play on the regressive tendencies found in all people: the fantasy of being saved by a loving parent; the desire to be punished and forgiven for being bad; the need to put oneself in the hands of an omniscient elder; and the wish to find the One who understands the Mystery.

Diagnostic and therapeutic phases

Variations in the clinical process

One virtue of portraying the clinical process as a feed-forward sequence of steps is that the scheme has great adaptability. The entire process – from diagnostic encounter to implementation of treatment – can be completed in one or two interviews. On the other hand, the diagnostic phase may be prolonged in complicated cases and the implementation of treatment a lengthy business; in some cases, management never terminates – the patient needs psychosocial or pharmacological support for a lifetime. On other occasions, the direct sequence of steps must be modified, if the patient requires urgent management before diagnosis is complete, or needs referral to a more suitable facility (see Figure 6.2).

The diagnostic phase includes all stages from referral, initial contact, diagnostic encounter and formulation, through management planning. The

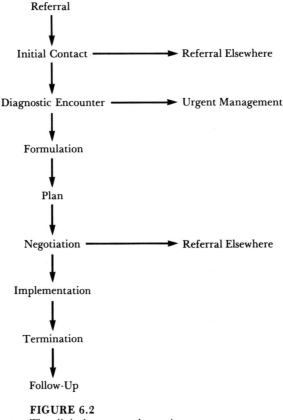

FIGURE 6.2
The clinical process: alternative routes

therapeutic or treatment phase proceeds from negotiation, through implementation of the accepted management plan, to termination (see Figure 6.3).

The interpenetration of diagnosis and therapy

Differentiating two phases, although convenient for description, is misleading. Treatment begins at the beginning; a sensitive referral and a thorough and perceptive diagnostic encounter have real significance for therapy. If the patient is confident of being understood and having personal problems accorded due weight, that patient is likely to collaborate in therapy. By the same token, one mark of a good clinician is an openness to information appearing later in the clinical process. Fresh clues may crop up during treatment and demand a revision of diagnosis.

Openness to fresh information

Case 6.1

■ Bo, an 11-year-old boy with a past history of shyness and intermittent school refusal, was often victimized by his classmates. One day, he was toppled over when one boy deliberately pushed him over another who was kneeling on all fours behind him. He complained at once of back pain and weakness of both legs and was admitted to the hospital.

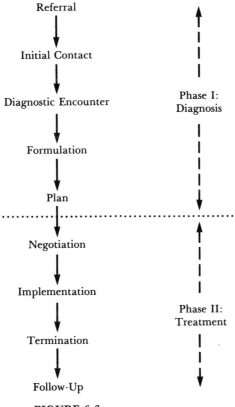

FIGURE 6.3
The clinical process: phases

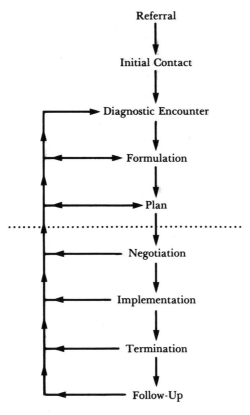

FIGURE 6.4
The clinical process: feedback

On examination, lower limb tone was normal, power reduced, tendon reflexes equivocally diminished, and plantars equivocally flexor. He had pain to jarring over L5. X-rays of the lumbar spine were normal, as were routine chest X-ray, urinalysis, and full blood count.

With strong suggestion, Bo was induced to walk briefly, but he immediately returned to bed complaining of back pain. A provisional diagnosis of conversion reaction was made, and psychotherapy begun as an urgent measure lest the symptoms become fixed. When blood chemistry results were available, hypercalcemia was apparent. A further X-ray of the lumbar spine showed a patchy demineralization of L5. Bone marrow aspiration revealed an infiltration of leukemic cells. ■

The revision of diagnosis

It might be argued that this case shows the gullibility of the diagnostic team. Another interpretation would suggest that some therapeutic measures should begin as soon as possible, before diagnosis is clarified, and that a medical team must be ready to change direction in the light of new evidence contrary to their preconceptions.

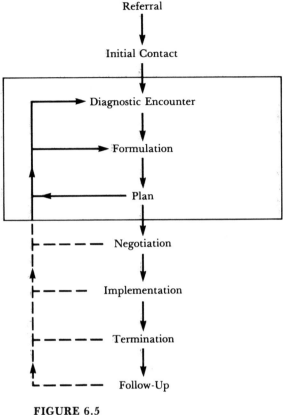

FIGURE 6.5
The diagnostic process

The feedback system

The clinical process is therefore conveniently viewed as a feedback as well as a feed-forward system. Information available later in the sequence of steps can be cycled back to the diagnostic phase for reformulation or replanning (see Figure 6.4).

Rapport

During the diagnostic encounter, the clinician must establish rapport with the patient. Patient and doctor are said to be *en rapport* when they share a sense of understanding and alliance. Subsequent enquiry will be hampered if the patient is fearful, distracted, rushed, or feels that the clinician is imperceptive, opaque, dense, or uncaring. Figure 6.5 illustrates how the pursuit of a diagnostic endeavor hinges on establishing a collaborative atmosphere.

The elements of the diagnostic encounter

The elements of the diagnostic encounter in psychiatry – history taking, mental status assessment, physical examination, and additional investigations – provide primary or secondary clues that are the grist of clinical reasoning. This point is elaborated in chapter 7, and in Figures 6.6 and 6.7.

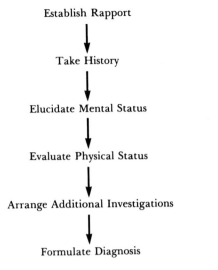

Establish Rapport

Take History

Elucidate Mental Status

Evaluate Physical Status

Arrange Additional Investigations

Formulate Diagnosis

FIGURE 6.6
Elements of the diagnostic encounter in psychiatry

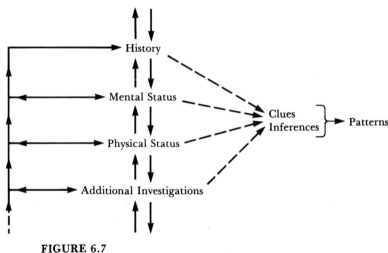

FIGURE 6.7
The eliciting of salient clues

Diagnostic formulation and management planning

Diagnostic formulation involves diagnostic categorization (see chapter 11) and an integrated formulation of the dynamic interaction of physical, psychological, and social factors operative during the predisposition, precipitation, perpetuation, and presentation of the disorder (see chapter 14). The formulation guides a plan of management organized according to feasible goals, with a prediction of time and expense, and a way of determining when the goals have been reached (see chapter 15).

Management goals guide the planners to the most suitable modes of therapy available and allow an individualization of treatment in terms of what the patient desires, what is culturally acceptable, and what is feasible. Individualization is further promoted by understanding the patient's biopsychosocial strengths and resources, which can often be exploited to compensate for, or aid the repair of, deficits and liabilities.

The triangulation of goals, strategies, and evaluation

The association between goals, therapeutic strategies, and evaluation can be seen as triangular and interactive (see Figure 6.8).

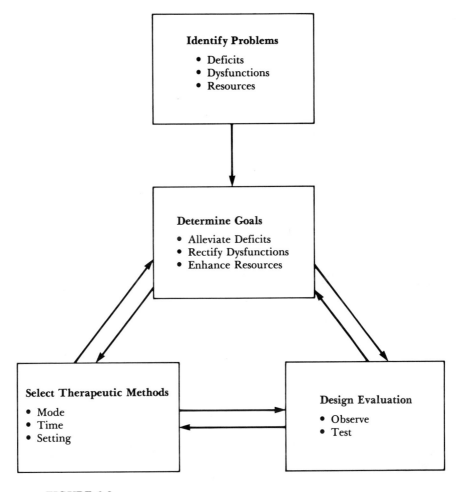

FIGURE 6.8
Management planning

Negotiation and implementation

The promotion of understanding and collaboration

Having formulated a diagnosis and designed a plan of management, the clinician must discuss conclusions and recommendations with the patient (and family, if appropriate). Even when the patient has a disorder that disrupts the capacity to interpret reality reliably, some level of understanding and cooperation is usually possible and should be solicited. The delivery of treatment against the patient's wishes is seldom necessary. It is justifiable only if the patient is suicidal, dangerous to others, or likely to endanger health and reputation by extravagant behavior.

Most patients want to discuss the therapist's conclusions and to decide whether they make sense. Most want some assurance that the conclusions are consistent with personal values and with their own views of the problem.

An active therapeutic alliance

By negotiation, the clinician enlists the patient's cooperation. Without an active therapeutic alliance, little that is enduring can be achieved; moreover, the implication that therapy is a process of active collaboration toward goals both patient and clinician have defined will counteract the fears of helplessness and victimization already described (Lazare, 1979).

Case 6.2   ■ A 10-year-old boy with severe distractibility, learning problems, and impulsiveness began to resist taking the stimulant medication prescribed for him 2 years before, despite an improvement in his ability to concentrate in school. The only rationale offered to the boy or his parents was that he had "brain damage" and was "hyper." The diagnosis and the tablets indicated to him that he was different from other children, not in control of his behavior and potentially crazy. ■

Implementation and termination

Restoration
Maintenance
Reconstruction

When patient and clinician have agreed on a plan of action, management is implemented. Depending on the radical or superficial nature of the goals, therapy can be brief or prolonged. Sometimes the clinician aims to eliminate distress and restore the patient to what he or she was before the disturbance began. Sometimes the aim is to ameliorate the most crippling symptoms and prevent deterioration. At other times, a far-reaching reconstruction is sought.

Multileveled treatment goals

Frequently, especially in more complex disturbances, the goals of treatment derive from all levels – from somatic, through psychological, to social. For the child with attention-deficit disorder (Case 6.2), for example, the following goals are conceivable:

1. Extend attention span
2. Alleviate perceptual immaturity

3. Alleviate reading disability
4. Reduce social inhibition
5. Enhance self-esteem
6. Counsel family to improve management.

Teamwork

These goals can be written more specifically and therapeutic programs designed to achieve them. Implementing such a plan will require the collaboration of pediatrician or psychiatrist, remedial teacher, psychologist, and social worker in a coordinated interdisciplinary team.

Termination

When the goals have been reached, the therapeutic alliance is terminated by mutual agreement. In some cases, the clinician or the patient may arrange a later interview to ensure the patient continues to be well.

Follow-up

Summary

The clinical process is a series of steps proceeding from referral, initial contact, diagnostic encounter, formulation, and management planning through negotiation and implementation to termination. The process operates by feed-forward, preceding steps being organized with subsequent steps in mind, and by feedback, information available later in the sequence of steps being returned for a possible revision of diagnosis and plan. Therapy therefore commences with referral, and diagnosis ceases with termination.

7

The tactics and strategy of clinical reasoning

Introduction

The clinician can be compared to a sleuth investigating a case, alert to clues, prepared to speculate about suspects and their motivation, and assiduous in the search for evidence. Conan Doyle's short story *The Speckled Band* (Doyle, 1980) illustrates the analogy well.

Sherlock Holmes and his associate Dr. Watson are awakened early in their chambers by a distressed young woman seeking their help. Her name is Helen Stoner and she lives with her stepfather, Dr. Grimesby Roylott, the last survivor of an old Surrey family. Miss Stoner tells the following story:

A succession of dissolute heirs had reduced the Roylott fortune and lands to the heavily mortgaged ancestral home and a few acres of property. Feeling the pinch, Dr. Roylott married Miss Stoner's mother in India and returned to England with his new wife, his two stepdaughters, and the former Mrs. Stoner's yearly income of 1,000 pounds. Shortly after her return, Mrs. Stoner was accidentally killed. Dr. Roylott, increasingly showing signs of an hereditary violence of temper, lived on in Surrey with his stepdaughters and with a cheetah and baboon who wandered freely on the grounds of the estate.

Two years before, Helen Stoner's sister Julia, who was planning to marry, died mysteriously in her own bedroom. On that fatal night, there was a howling storm. Helen heard Julia scream and hurried to her aid, barely in time to see her unfortunate sister die in convulsions. She remembered Julia's having been troubled that night by the odor of Roylott's cigar, which emanated from the doctor's adjoining bedroom. She also remembered hearing a low clear whistle and a clanging metallic sound shortly before her sister's demise. As Julia died, she said, "Oh, my God! Helen! It was the band! The speckled band!", a comment which Helen vaguely associated with gypsies whom Roylott allowed to camp on the manor grounds and who customarily wore spotted neckerchiefs.

The cause of Julia's death was never determined. Helen surmised she died of fright. There were no marks of violence on her body, and no signs of poisoning. The door of the room had been fastened from within, the windows were closed with iron-barred shutters, the walls and floor were sound, and the chimney was impassible.

Helen revealed that a man had recently asked her hand in marriage and that repairs to the manor wall had necessitated her moving into Julia's old bedroom, next to Dr. Roylott. The night before her journey to Holmes, she noticed the same low whistle she had heard on the fatal evening. In fear, she had dressed, left the manor, and come to London.

Miss Stoner leaves to return home. For Watson's benefit, Holmes assembles the pattern of clues: (1) the whistles in the night; (2) the presence of a band of gypsies on intimate terms with Dr. Roylott; (3) the possibility that Dr. Roylott has a pecuniary motive for getting rid of the sisters; (4) Julia's dying allusion to a band; and (5) the metallic clang (possibly caused by barred shutters falling into place). Could a gypsy have perpetrated the crime? Both Holmes and Watson discern objections to such a theory. Accordingly, the two sleuths determine to journey to the manor at once to hunt for evidence; but not before the choleric Grimesby Roylott, having followed his stepdaughter, appears at their doorstep and warns them to keep out of his affairs.

Undaunted by his threats, Holmes and Watson (who takes a revolver with him) waste no time in getting to the manor, where they are met by Miss Stoner. Holmes checks the window shutter and finds it is sound. Inside the bedroom he notes: (1) a bellrope, installed two years before (which turns out to be a dummy); (2) a nonfunctional ventilator, also installed two years before; and (3) the bed, which is clamped to the floor.

Next, the two sleuths examine Dr. Roylott's bedroom. Among other furnishings, they note (4) a large safe, (5) a saucer of milk, and (6) a small dog leash tied on itself at one end to form a loop of whipcord. Holmes apparently draws some inferences, but he keeps them to himself until clearer proofs are available, except to say that he does not think Julia died of fright (as Helen surmised) but rather of something more tangible.

Holmes arranges for Helen to retire early. As soon as Roylott returns from London and goes to bed, she is to open the shutters of her window, put the lamp there as a signal, and get out. When they see the lamp, Holmes and Watson, who will stay at a nearby inn, plan to enter the grounds, climb through the window, and spend the night in the fatal bedroom.

All this is done without mishap, save a distracting skirmish with the baboon, and the two companions settle down to a dark vigil, Holmes with a long cane, a box of matches and candle, and Watson with his revolver.

Three tense hours go by. Suddenly, there is a momentary gleam of light from the ventilator and the smell of a lamp. After another half-hour in the dark, Watson hears a gentle sound, as of steam escaping from a kettle. Holmes springs up, lights a match, dazzles Watson, and strikes furiously at the bell pull. There is a low, clear whistle. Holmes stops lashing, and a horrible cry comes from the room next door. What does it mean? "It means that it is all over," says Holmes. They enter Dr. Roylott's room, Watson with pistol in hand, and Holmes holding a lamp. There is Grimesby Roylott slumped on a chair in his dressing gown, grasping the dog leash, his eyes fixed in a rigid stare at the corner of the ceiling. Round his brow is a speckled yellow band. As Watson moves forward the strange headgear stirs and the loathesome head and puffed neck of a deadly Indian swamp adder rises from the coil. Roylott has died within ten seconds of being bitten. Holmes snatches the leash from the doctor's lap, throws the noose around the reptile's neck, draws it from its horrid perch, and throws it into the iron safe.

Holmes later retraces his reasoning. His first hunch that the crime was committed by gypsies, was generated from a misleading historical clue, the speckled band. He revised it when he realized that the fatal bedroom could not have been entered from without. Further evidence came from examining the scene of the crime. The dummy ventilator, bellrope, and fixed bed suggested the rope was a bridge from ventilator to bed. This, and the knowledge that the doctor had access to creatures from India, and a need for a rapidly acting poison, suggested a snake. But what of the whistle? Using a saucer of milk, Roylott had trained the snake to return to him when summoned. Holmes had come to this conclusion before entering Roylott's bedroom. It was supported by the finding of the noose, the milk, and the safe (which made a metallic clang when its terrible occupant was returned). Decisive proof of Holmes's hypothesis was provided in the early hours of the final morning, when Grimesby Roylott found that "violence does in truth recoil upon the violent, and the schemer falls into the pit which he digs for another."

It is pertinent that Sir Arthur Conan Doyle, who trained as a doctor, based the character of Sherlock Holmes on Dr. Joseph Bell, a physician of the Edinburgh Infirmary. Bell's brilliant deductions amazed his students, and, like Holmes, he had the rare ability to explain the steps of his reasoning. In essence, Holmes's steps in deductive reasoning were to:

The steps of deductive reasoning

1. Recognize salient clues.
2. Make cautious interpretations of the clues if indicated.
3. Assemble the clues and their interpretations to form meaningful (though possibly incomplete) patterns.

4. Generate hunches about suspects to account for the pattern of clues and interpretations.
5. Search for evidence to check the interpretation of clues and to confirm or disconfirm the hunches.
6. On the basis of the evidence, revise the salient clues, their interpretations, and the hunches, if necessary.
7. Judge the validity of the hunches by weighing positive and negative evidence.

This chapter on clinical reasoning in psychiatry deals with clues, interpretations, patterns, hunches, the search for evidence, revisions, and the weighing of evidence. In short, it describes hypothetico-deductive reasoning in the clinical process.

Recognizing salient clues

Scanning for clues

From the beginning of contact with the patient, the clinician scans the phenomenal field for clues. The referral letter, for example, provides clues about the presenting complaint, the reason for referral, and general information about sex, age, occupation, and address. It is advisable to speak directly with the

Sources of clues

referring agent (physician, school counselor, social worker, or parent, for example) to get details about the patient's background and previous history and why the patient needs attention at this time. The conversation will also help the referring agent clarify the reasons for referral.

Scanning during inception and reconnaissance

At the inception of the interview, the clinician notes physique, gait, body movement, handshake, dress, facies, eyes, eye contact, mood, affect, and attitude toward the interview and interviewer. After identificatory data have been recorded, the patient is encouraged to tell his or her own story in the reconnaisance phase of the interview. As far as possible, the patient is encouraged to talk spontaneously, the clinician acting as an attentive listener who facilitates the flow of associations (see chapter 8).

As the diagnostic encounter proceeds, questions in the clinician's mind are resolved during reconnaissance or left until the detailed inquiry: What is the main complaint? What else does the patient complain of? When did the problem begin? Was the onset associated with physical or psychosocial stress? How has the problem evolved since onset? Is it episodic, phasic, continuous, constant, intensifying, or diminishing? Has the patient ever had anything like this before? What does the patient think are the cause and nature of the illness?

Inception and reconnaissance usually take between 5 and 15 minutes. By that time, the clinician has assembled a set of clues and interpretations to form a cluster or initial pattern. Every patient presents an overwhelming number of perceptual stimuli. Color of hair, brand of jeans, belt buckle, and shine of shoes

Alertness for salient clues

all contribute to the Gestalt the individual deliberately and unwittingly projects. The experienced clinician, however, is highly vigilant for clues likely to be associated with physical or mental disorder. Many of these clues are described in chapter 9.

The definition of salient clues

Salient clues are key perceptions most likely to contribute to diagnosis. They are derived from what the clinician sees, hears, feels, smells, or has read, in, from, or about the patient. What indicates that a clue is salient? Salient clues are usually those the clinician has learned are likely to be related to disease or disorder. Blueness of the lips and nails, for example, is more likely to be part of a disease pattern than are freckles (although freckles might also be salient in some circumstances).

Other clues reach salience by virtue of their unexpected, dramatic, or discrepant qualities.

Case 7.1

■ Roger, aged 14, was referred for firesetting. A slim 6-foot, 2-inches tall, he had long arms and legs and a suggestion of webbing of the neck. He related to the interviewer as though terrified, darting glances around the room and answering questions monosyllabically. After 10 minutes, he fled the interview.

Some months later, a chromosomal analysis revealed that Roger had an XXYY/XYY mosaicism. A full investigation revealed a combination of chromosomal, physical, and psychosocial features amounting to a syndrome never before recognized. ■

Interpretations

The need to separate observation from interpretation

Some clues are stored in memory with little transformation, remaining close to the fundamental perception. Others singly or in combination are interpreted as clinical inferences. It is important to derive meaning from salient clues but no less vital to distinguish clearly between observation and inference, to be able to cite the raw data on which inferences are based, and to gauge the degree of certainty involved in each inference.

Premature inference

Inexperienced clinicians rush to inference, as though, abhorring uncertainty, they must pin down the complicated phenomena they observe. In doing so, they may close their minds to fresh clues that do not fit their premature conceptions. Consider these vaguely defined technical terms: *paranoid, hysterical,* and *schizoid.* They bias the later collection of evidence and are potentially misleading. It is better first to stick closer to the primary clues and to explore them fully before generalizing.

Case 7.2

■ An anxious adolescent girl answered positively to the examiner's question, ''Do you ever hear voices?'' On further exploration, she identified the voice as her own and located it in her own mind. The voice argued with itself about the pros and cons of interpersonal actions that had moral implications: ''Should I or shouldn't I?'' ■

*The danger of being
misled by premature
interpretation*

The voice was not a true hallucination but rather a dramatization of inner conflict. True auditory hallucinations are sensed as alien, commonly located as originating from outside the self, and (usually) less transparently related to the current emotional predicament than in this patient's case. Had the interviewer interpreted this clue as an auditory hallucination, he would have fitted a false piece to the puzzle, possibly implicating schizophrenia, for example. Later inquiry might then have gone astray, diverted by an invalid array of hypotheses.

Remember how Sherlock Holmes was temporarily beguiled by the speckled band into suspecting a band of gypsies. The clue was salient but the inference incorrect. Fortunately, he was able to go back to the words of the dying girl, which he linked to observations made in the fatal bedroom. He could then assemble a more valid pattern and revise his hunches.

Initial patterns

Categorizing clues

Keeping in mind a necessary caution about early inferences, the clinician must nevertheless attempt to categorize the perceptual clues assembled. By doing so, the clinician relates the particular phenomenon in an individual case to the general phenomena important to psychiatry (for example, hallucinations, delusions, compulsions, anxiety, etc.). Beyond these clinical signs and symptoms are more complex clues: the discrepancies, gaps, parallels and contrasts discovered in the presentation, and the clinician's intuitions—that is, rapid pattern-matching against previous experience, often with a sense of revelation.

*Molecular
discrepancies*

Discrepancies can be molecular or molar. Molecular discrepancies are minute inconsistencies detected among perceptual clues.

Case 7.3

■ In referring her obese adolescent son, a mother mentions that her main concern is his low self-esteem. Shortly afterwards, she describes how she sent him to a camp for ''fatties'' in the previous summer. ■

Case 7.4

■ A 12-year-old boy is referred for setting fire to the house next door. As she describes it, his mother smiles faintly from time to time. It becomes apparent, later, that the mother had been feuding with her neighbors. ■

Case 7.5

■ A physically mature 14-year-old girl has a dramatic, abrupt, barking vocalization for which no physical cause has been discovered. She seems unconcerned about it. When asked what she thinks is the cause, she is blandly incurious but suggests there might be something wrong with her nerves. When other children are startled by the noise and laugh at it, she laughs along with them. ''Can't do a thing with it,'' she says. ■

Molar discrepancies

Molar discrepancies are between higher-level, more inferential clues than molecular. They may be noted, for example, when the severity of symptoms and signs is disproportionate to the environmental stresses alleged to account for them. Such disproportionate disturbances may indicate that information about the environmental situation is incomplete (due to overdiscretion, obscurity, or concealment, for example) or that the problem is fueled by nonenvironmental, biologically based factors. The sophisticated clinician may also be aware of discrepant patterns of clues not matching known syndromes; in this way, new disorders may be identified.

■   In 1941, Leo Kanner noted that among the large group of children regarded as mentally defective or deaf or both were a minority who showed from birth or early childhood a unique and hitherto ill-defined pattern: a severe and pervasive inability to relate to other people, uneven developmental progress, grossly delayed and deviant language development, intolerance of environmental change, inexplicable rages or panic, and repetitive movements or object play.

Most retarded children eagerly seek human contact and their intellectual deficits are general. The combination of a striking incapacity for emotional relationships with markedly uneven abilities was a discrepant one. It led Kanner to search for associated clinical phenomena and to define an important diagnostic group.

Kanner called the disorder Inborn Autistic Disturbance of Affective Contact. The diagnosis was soon validated by clinicians from other centers and countries. This syndrome is now known as Early Infantile Autism, a pervasive developmental disorder. ■

Gaps
The clinician should also note historical gaps. Is something of importance being concealed or repressed? Why does a patient have no memory before the age of 9 years. Where was he between 1974 and 1976? Gaps are most likely to occur during the detailed inquiry, when evidence is being gathered. The clinician must decide whether to ask the patient about the gap directly or whether to leave it until later.

Parallels and contrasts
The interviewer also notes parallels and contrasts between social situations in the past, particularly in childhood, and in the present. These parallels and contrasts may give preliminary clues to interpersonal motives and attitudes that are of enduring characterological importance.

Rapid intuitions
The most complex inferences are impressive yet fallible: powerful or suggestive intuitions combining many phenomena, seemingly in a flash, yielding a fully formed impression. Sometimes the intuition has to do with a clinical diagnosis, the concept of which seems to spring fully formed into the mind.

Case 7.6
■   A tall, slim, awkward, stiffly smiling young woman enters the psychiatrist's office for the first time. She is dressed in expensive clothing, but the colors do not match. Her movements are subtly jerky and ungainly, with a hint of hesitation. She extends her hand and then withdraws it, before the psychiatrist can touch her. He has the powerful intuition that she is schizophrenic. ■

Categorical intuitions
Despite the quicksilver revelatory nature of categorical intuition, it is not magical but rooted in experience. The clinician matches features in the present

situation to the patterns of disease stored in long-term memory. As the match is made, there may be a sense of déja vù. The careful clinician, however, recognizes the danger of such spot diagnoses and develops an array of competing alternatives to keep the mind open.

Dynamic intuitions

Rapid intuitions can also deal with the dynamics of affect and motivation. The clinician learns, for example, to recognize the faltering speech pattern and eye movements of the person who is covering up or lying, the sudden conjunctival moistening when an emotional issue has been touched or approached, and the tense wrists of the patient hiding fears behind a calm exterior.

Case 7.7

■ A young woman had a very successful and socially prominent father. She was unable to sustain a close relationship with men of her own generation, whom she found superficial and unformed. On the other hand, several affairs with older married men had ended in humiliation, leaving her feeling defeated and fearful of further entanglements. Intuiting a connection between her feelings for her father and her unsuccessful relationship with men of her own generation, the psychiatrist decided to have the patient reflect on the depth and complexity of her unresolved attachment to her father. ■

Case 7.8

■ A young medical student has been referred to a psychiatrist by one of his teachers. He grins incongruously and begins at once to identify himself with Lawrence of Arabia's sadomasochistic tendencies. He speaks rapidly and intensely and smiles mirthlessly, while watching the interviewer intently. The interviewer has a sudden flash that the patient is deliberately acting crazy. He says, "It seems that you want me to think you are crazy. Why is that?" The young man deflates perceptibly and relaxes a little for the first time. He tells the interviewer how lonely he has been, how unhappy he is with the career he has chosen, and how concerned he has been that he might be going mad. ■

Cogent phrases

Experience will help the interviewer to be aware of cogent words or phrases laden with condensed meaning. What alerts the interviewer? Sometimes it is the vivid or idiosyncratic nature of the expression; sometimes it is an unusual emphasis or repetition. A gentle echoing of the phrase or an open question ("How do you mean?") may be sufficient to stimulate the patient to associate fruitfully and sometimes to recover memories of a decisive but partly repressed event.

Case 7.9

■ A disheveled young man, who has the idea that he is Jesus Christ, speaks in prophetic, biblical style. He pronounces, on several occasions, "This time, I will not be betrayed." Later in the interview, when the patient is less defensive, the clinician gently explores the connotations of betrayal. The patient recalls that when he was 7 years old, his depressed mother threatened to kill herself and all her children. ■

The interviewer's feelings

The interviewer should learn to recognize and ponder the meaning of the stray or distracting feelings patients provoke, feelings covering the entire range of emotions – from irritation, anger, contempt, disgust, boredom, and puzzlement

Empathy

to affection, caring, envy, admiration, and erotic arousal. Some of these feelings may be surprisingly powerful; indeed, the fear of their intensity and of the demands of human involvement may explain some physicians' reluctance to examine them at all. The experienced clinician learns neither to deny nor act unwisely on these emotions but to heed and understand them. Do they arise, for example, from an empathic discernment of a patient's inner state?

Case 7.10   ■ When the disturbed teenager spoke on, the interviewer began to get befuddled, as though his mind were stuffed with cotton wool. He realized he was responding to the patient's muddled thinking that meandered aimlessly around the topic without clear direction. ■

The patient's manipulation of feelings

Sometimes the patient deliberately manipulates feelings. Rebellious adolescents may intend to provoke anger, by their insulting or uncooperative behavior, to test the limits of a situation or detect an interviewer's vulnerabilities. A seductive patient may attempt to wrest control of the interview by arousing the clinician sexually. Certain sociopathic patients make a career of exploiting the fears, greed, or vanity of their dupes.

Countertransference reactions

At other times, the interviewer's emotional responses are endogenous. Something about the patient touches an inner scar and the clinician's response derives from countertransference, from attitudes left over from childhood, rather than from an empathic response to the patient's emotional state. It is remarkable how incontestable these impressions seem to those who experience them and how difficult they are to abandon without a capacity for self-exploration and openness to the help of colleagues.

Stereotyping

These endogenous impressions vary from conventional stereotypes to highly idiosyncratic reactions. You will undoubtedly recognize someone's pet belief among this list of banalities:

- An only child is always spoiled.
- Hispanics are passionate.
- Women are more intuitive than men.
- Housewives are depressed because they are oppressed.
- Mental disorder is a product of an affluent civilization and caused by too much self-absorption.
- All childhood psychopathology is caused by bad parents.
- Gifted artists are temperamental.
- Homosexuals are effeminate.
- There are no frigid women, only clumsy men.

Stereotypes often contain germs of truth. Some homosexuals are effeminate; inherited wealth may undermine achievement and be associated with boredom and destructive search for stimulation. The danger is that conventional wisdom is so convenient; it can be projected on the patient without thought or understanding. Some blacks may have a good sense of rhythm and some Englishmen may be cold-blooded, but both the patient and the interviewer can use a stereotype as a shield against closer contact, especially when a cultural gap exists between them.

Idiosyncratic reactions

More difficult to appreciate and to alter are idiosyncratic reactions derived from potent past experiences.

Case 7.11

■   A young psychiatrist became bored and irritated with older women who were depressed and self-absorbed. He wanted to give them a good shake and tell them to pull their socks up. He was responding to conflictual memories of his mother, who had been subject to periods of withdrawn melancholia during his boyhood.   ■

Hunches

The generation of hypotheses

Categorical and dynamic hypotheses

As clinicians collect and evaluate clues, make interpretations, and assemble tentative patterns, they reach a point at which they are ready to generate alternative explanations of the initial patterns delineated. These explanations are hunches or hypotheses relating either to categorical syndromes, disorders, or diseases, or to dynamic formulations about cause, precipitation, perpetuation, motivation, and meaning. The most sophisticated diagnostician approaches the problem with a coordination of both categorical and dynamic hypotheses.

Timing

Research has shown that experts start to generate hypotheses within the first minute after initial contact. By the end of the reconnaisance, an array of alternative hypotheses has been generated. These competing possibilities influence the later detailed inquiry, mental status, physical examination, and additional investigations.

Unfocused clinical inquiry: a fallacy

This view of clinical reasoning contrasts with what some medical teachers advise: the trainee should refrain from diagnostic thinking until all data have been collected and differential diagnosis should be generated only after history and examination. Experienced teachers recommend this approach for fear trainees will close on a diagnosis and ignore clues inconsistent with their premature conclusions. When their private sophisticated hypothetico-deductive reasoning is revealed, expert clinicians are often somewhat abashed since they regard it as a shortcut and are wary of exposing students to it. This leads to a regrettable inconsistency: The teacher, in effect, tells the student, "Do what I say, not what I do," (if indeed, the teacher is aware of personal reasoning). In practice, the unfocused approach to diagnosis customarily taught to medical students leads to inefficient, nonselective, mechanical, and poorly integrated data-gathering. The human mind's natural tendency to search for meaning and connection should be reinforced, systematized, and disciplined, not suppressed or denied.

The advantages of hypothesis generation

What are the virtues of an approach based on hypotheses?

1. Considering alternative hunches prevents premature closure on one diagnosis.

2. Mobilizing hypotheses spares short-term memory by separating the information derived from clues and interpretations into meaningful units.

3. An array of hypotheses that are strong conceptual competitors organizes the detailed enquiry into a systematic search for evidence for or against the diagnostic contenders.

4. The hypotheses can be framed to be open to revision in light of fresh evidence.

Like all strategies, however, hypothesis-generation has absolute and relative drawbacks:

Drawbacks to hypothetico-deductive reasoning

1. Memory is limited. Efficient though the process may be, there is a ceiling to the number of hypotheses one can juggle simultaneously. Research has demonstrated that six is maximal and four is usual. Computers have the advantage of being able to generate virtually unlimited numbers of diagnostic possibilities.

2. The human computer is overimpressed with evidence appearing early in the reasoning process and relatively less efficient at considering later information, especially if it runs counter to earlier material.

3. Clinicians seem to be better at alternative reasoning about categorical diagnosis than about diagnostic formulations involving motivation and explanation. They are more likely to close prematurely on a dynamic hypothesis than on a categorical diagnosis.

Even though the upper limit of short-term memory is fixed, the efficient use of negative evidence and of alternative dynamic hypotheses can be learned, provided they are stipulated as educational objectives.

The structure of the array of hypotheses

The pattern of clues and interpretations can be so pervasive that a particular hunch is irresistible. Nevertheless, it is advisable to marshal against a sure thing two, three, or even four outside possibilities. The clinician thus avoids premature closure, staying alert for evidence inconsistent with the spot diagnosis.

Case 7.12

■ An intense, loquacious young man has been admitted after an altercation in a bar. He demonstrates elevation of mood, irritability, psychomotor overactivity, and eccentric thinking. He claims that he plays all instruments in his rock band, arranges concerts for Fleetwood Mac, is in charge of the music department at the University, and is designing a therapeutic musical program for handicapped children. ■

This pattern of psychomotor activity, flight of ideas, and grandiosity strongly suggests mania. The condition is probably a manic episode in a bipolar affective disorder, but it could be due to a schizoaffective, schizophrenic, or schizophreniform disorder, brief reactive psychosis, or organic brain syndrome. The last of these can be divided into subclasses (cocaine and amphetamine psychosis being possible contenders).

Global hypotheses that undergo refinement

On other occasions, the pattern is less clear, and it is better to start with more general hypotheses in the form of contrasting contenders and to refine them in the direction of specificity as the evidence accrues.

The inquiry strategy

The aims of the inquiry process

The inquiry strategy is based on the array of hypotheses assembled at the end of the reconnaisance. The inquiry strategy seeks evidence in the form of secondary clues that allow revision (refinement, addition, discarding, or acceptance) of the categorical and dynamic diagnostic contenders. Inquiry pursues evidence during the detailed inquiry (past history, early development, later development, and family history), mental status, physical examination, and additional investigations.

Routine inquiry

Some sections of the inquiry are pursued *routinely* to provide a minimum data base to rule out disorders of high prevalence that mimic, contribute to, or complicate psychiatric disorder. In an inpatient setting with many severely disturbed patients, for example, alcohol and drug abuse, diabetes, neurosyphilis, epilepsy, and other organic brain disorders, must be excluded along with hematological, cardiovascular, and urological disorders.

Discretionary inquiry

Beyond routine investigation, an array of hypotheses determines which areas of the detailed inquiry, mental status, physical examination, and additional investigations will be emphasized. Detailed inquiry varies from case to case, at the interviewer's *discretion*, in accordance with the dynamic or categorical hunches guiding the inquiry plan.

When dementia is in question, for example, a history of past illnesses and recent behavior, a complete mental status (orientation, concentration, memory, language, calculation, judgment, information, abstraction), a detailed neurological examination, special neurological investigations, information from informants about recent behavior, and psychological testing may be undertaken or requested. When the pattern suggests an anxiety disorder, past illness, early development, coping techniques, current social situation, family history, mental status (especially stream, form, and content of thinking) will be stressed. Appropriate guidelines can be developed for other general patterns in different clinical contexts. Part V describes these guidelines in more detail.

Revisions: adding, refining, weighing, discarding, accepting

Revision: feed-forward and feedback

During revision, diagnostic hypotheses guide the search for evidence and may themselves be revised in the light of the evidence discovered. The process is a sophisticated mixture of feed-forward (the hypotheses direct the search) and feedback (the evidence leads to revision).

*The addition of
hypotheses*

The routine inquiry sometimes brings to light fresh clues that demand a radical revision of hypotheses. The history of past illness, for example, may reveal that the patient has epilepsy that is incompletely controlled; this fact may cause the diagnostician to conceive the initial pattern in a new way and to add a new diagnostic hypothesis to the array. The purpose of *routine inquiry* is to check for disorders with a high incidence in that clinical situation. *Discretionary inquiry*, on the other hand, pursues evidence to complete the initial pattern and enable the clinician to discard the diagnostic contenders not supported.

*The refinement
of hypotheses*

Specification

Subdivision

Before the diagnostic conclusion when the clinician weighs the evidence for or against the diagnostic contenders, the findings will often help the clinician to sharpen global or rough hypotheses and to frame them in more specific terms. For example, the hypothesis *psychotic pattern* may be expressed in more refined terms as *schizophrenic disorder*. Refining hypotheses may lead to dividing a general, inclusive hunch into two or more subordinate contenders. For example:

*General
superordinate
hypotheses*

Refinement

*Specific subordinate
hypotheses*

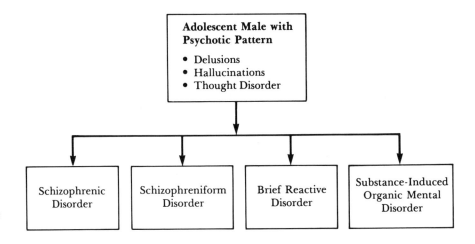

Weighing evidence

Strong evidence

Weak evidence

Evidence derived from routine or discretionary inquiry can be powerful or weak. In the case of this initial pattern: *A 17-year-old boy with 6-month history of social withdrawal, preoccupation with vague physical complaints, and a sense of alteration of facial features;* the discovery, in mental status examination of *auditory hallucinations of people commenting on his actions,* or *formal thinking disorder with difficulty in separating relevant from irrelevant ideas* and a *tendency to equate objects with a common property* would be strong evidence for schizophrenic disorder. The disclosure, in discretionary inquiry, of an uncle who had spent a long time in a mental hospital or a past personality characterized by shyness would be regarded as weak evidence for schizophrenic disorder.

Eventually, when enough evidence (weak and strong, positive and negative) has been gathered, the clinician summates and reaches a conclusion sound enough to justify a preliminary management plan. Essentially, the clinician matches the pattern of primary and secondary clues and interpretations assembled in short-term memory against the templates of abstract syndrome configurations stored in long-term memory. It is obvious that the more defined the criteria for diagnosis, the greater the likelihood that different clinicians will reach the same conclusion.

The paucity of conclusive tests

Goodness-of-fit

DSM-III attempts to foster diagnostic reliability by offering clear criteria for inclusion and exclusion. In psychiatry, however, there are few disorders for which a special investigation will provide conclusive proof (as, for example, Fölling's test does for phenylketonuria or immunological tests do for neurosyphilis), and all of these are organic brain diseases. The clinician must therefore rely on how well the patterns assembled fit the idealized disease patterns stored in memory following study and experience.

Experience involves rehearsal, practice, and direct contact with many different patients. Patients provide the clues the clinician must use as the raw material for clinical reasoning. Practice allows the clinician to sharpen and expedite thinking – namely:

Eliciting
Recognizing
Evaluating
Interpreting

} primary clues

Assembling initial patterns
Generating an array of alternative hypotheses
Developing an inquiry plan
Eliciting secondary evidence
Revising hypotheses
Weighing weak and strong, positive and negative evidence to develop a
    final pattern
Summating and matching the final pattern against idealized categorical
    and dynamic patterns
Reaching a conclusion

As with golf, practice permits the automatization of what begins in a relatively clumsy, deliberate way and facilitates the articulation of the steps to form a sequential, recycled, integrative procedure.

When is the evidence sufficient?

Since psychiatry has few clinching proofs, the clinician must decide when enough evidence has been gathered. Enough can vary from a focused 20-minute interview in an emergency room to several weeks of evaluating whether a patient is suitable for intensive psychoanalytic therapy. Sufficiency thus is relative to the kind of management appropriate to the clinical context and the gravity of the problem. Does this patient need to be admitted to the hospital? If not, what short-term measures are required until the patient is next seen? These questions are at the opposite end of a continuum from the following: Does this patient have the character structure, ego strength, degree of distress, motivation, and social resources to warrant psychoanalysis? Part V discusses how the clinical process is modified in different clinical settings.

Often, at the end of the first interview and physical examination, the clinician can make a provisional diagnosis. But a complete diagnostic formulation must usually await gathering more evidence from special investigations or informants.

A return to Baker Street

Let us now reconsider the similarity of clinician to sleuth; for the inconsistencies in this comparison are as instructive as the points of correspondence.

The analogy holds well for discerning clues and their interpretation, assembling patterns, and generating hunches. However, Sherlock tends to work with one dominant hunch at a time. Periodically, gulled by a misleading clue or a false interpretation, he reaches a brick wall and, realizing his misdirection, returns to the beginning. His investigations involve collecting evidence to support his hunch (that is, a suspect with hypothetical motive and modus operandi). The investigation culminates in a dramatic conclusion, when incontrovertible proof is produced by a brilliant maneuver, the miscreant is unmasked, and the case is closed.

The need for an array of hypotheses

Clinicians, in contrast, work from a number of hypotheses. They may have a dominant hunch, but it is pitted against alternative possibilities. Reliance on a single hunch is dangerous; the mind's eye too readily closes against evidence inconsistent with a pet hypothesis. Alternative hypotheses keep the clinician honest and are a safeguard against premature spot diagnosis. Gratifying though it may be to see Dr. Watson's face light up with admiration at one's brilliant deduction, most diagnostic work is systematic, painstaking, and fraught with seductive but false insights.

Diagnosis directs management

There are other important differences. Once Sherlock detects the culprit, the case is over; not so for the clinician. Diagnosis is a means to the next step, management planning. Holmes converges, magnifying glass in hand, on a single answer, but the clinician seeks a comprehensive evaluation. Psychiatric diagnosis converges on the problem of categorical diagnosis, and then diverges into a biopsychosocial assessment integrated by a dynamic formulation (see chapter 14).

Summary

Tactics

The sequence of tactics in the diagnostic process is as follows:

1. Elicit, recognize, and interpret salient clues.
2. Assemble initial patterns of primary clues and interpretations.
3. Generate an array of categorical and dynamic hypotheses.

4. Develop a search plan, with routine and discretionary lines of inquiry, based on the array of hypotheses.
5. Elicit evidence for or against the diagnostic contenders.
6. Revise interpretations or hypotheses if fresh evidence so demands.
7. Weigh and summate evidence.
8. Match the final pattern against abstract syndrome patterns in long-term memory.
9. Develop a comprehensive diagnostic formulation.

Strategy

The strategy is as follows:

1. Tolerate uncertainty, consider alternatives, and avoid premature closure on one possibility.
2. Give adequate weight to negative evidence and to fresh evidence appearing later in the interview.
3. Be prepared to revise interpretations, hypotheses, formulations, and plans if the secondary evidence docs not support them.
4. Try to separate observation and inference, clue and interpretation. Be prepared to cite the perceptual clues on which an interpretation is based.
5. Don't go on interminably. Reach a reasonable conclusion when enough information has been gathered. Be prepared to commit yourself to a diagnostic formulation and a therapeutic plan, but keep your eyes and ears open for fresh information suggesting the need to revise diagnosis or management.
6. Be aware of your personal reactions to the patient. Guard against stereotyping. Distinguish between genuine empathy and the projection of personal conflicts onto the patient.

Procedures

The tactics and strategy of the diagnostic process draw on technical skills and a knowledge base. The procedures are as follows:

1. Take and record history (chapter 8).
   Inception
   Reconnaisance
   Detailed inquiry
       routine
       discretionary
2. Perform mental status examination (chapter 9).
3. Perform physical examination (chapter 10).
4. Order special investigations (chapter 10).
5. Interview informants.
6. Formulate comprehensive diagnosis (chapter 14).
7. Plan goal-oriented management (chapter 15).

Knowledge   The knowledge base is as follows:

1. The clinical process as a whole (chapter 6).
2. Neurobiological systems, psychological functions, and illness behavior (chapters 3, 4 and 5).
3. Clinical syndromes (chapter 11).
4. Modes of treatment (chapter 12).

See Appendix I for the clinical reasoning of an experienced psychiatrist.

PART
III

Clinical procedures

8

The psychiatric history

Different interview settings but similar purposes

What can be achieved at the initial psychiatric interview? The outcome depends on where it is conducted and what the physician and the patient are seeking. A brisk, focused interview in an emergency room contrasts with the more extensive survey appropriate to an outpatient clinic. Both differ from what is possible at the bedside of a patient who is severely ill in a hospital ward. Despite these observations, fundamental issues can be addressed to varying degrees in any clinical situation:

1. The problem
2. Precipitation
3. Previous disorders
4. Predisposition
5. Resources, strengths, weaknesses
6. Presentation
7. Insight and desire for help

The problem

What is the problem for which the patient seeks relief? The patient may present subjective concerns for the following problems:

131

Subjective concerns

1. Physical symptoms (headache, insomnia, etc.)
2. Physical illnesses with an emotional component (asthma precipitated by tension, for example)
3. Disturbances of affect or mood (depression, explosive rage, excessive guilt, disproportionate anxiety, etc.)
4. Distressing preoccupations that seem alien (hallucinations, obsessions, etc.)
5. Scholastic or occupational problems
6. Difficulties in interpersonal relations (excessive shyness, sexual dysfunction, etc.)

Others' concerns

On the other hand, other people may be more concerned and identify the following as problems:

1. Overactivity and elevation of mood (or the reverse)
2. Increasing social withdrawal and eccentricity
3. Explosive rage
4. Substance abuse
5. Antisocial behavior
6. Forgetfulness and dilapidation of habits

Whatever the problem or problems for which the patient or associates seek help, the clinician attempts to delineate them, to understand how the patient experiences them, and to investigate their duration, onset, development, and persistence.

Precipitation

The coincidence of stress and onset

If the problems had an onset, the clinician should attempt to find whether the patient experienced physical or psychosocial stressors at that time. The mere coincidence of stress and breakdown does not substantiate a causal association; indeed, in the particular case, causation may remain speculative. It is supported, however, if the patient has had a previous breakdown when exposed to a similar stress, or if the patient's account of the stress indicates its personal significance.

Catastrophic and idiosyncratic stress

Some stressors have universal impact: the death of a beloved relative or social dislocation following a natural catastrophe, for example. Others are highly idiosyncratic, and it may require painstaking work before they are unravelled in psychotherapy. In some cases, it is a moot question whether an event was a precipitant, or the result of the disorder in its early stages, or mere coincidence.

Previous disorders

Previous similar disorders

Has the patient had any problems of a similar nature in the past? What precipitated them, if anything? Has the patient had any other emotional

Personal habits

disorders or physical symptoms related to tension? Does the patient have, or has the patient ever had, physical or neurological disease that could contribute to the present problem? Does the patient have, or has the patient had, personal habits that could cause, precipitate, or complicate the present problem (substance abuse, for example)?

Predisposition

Biopsychosocial vulnerability

What kind of person was the patient before becoming ill? What were the patient's biopsychosocial strengths. What were the weaknesses predisposing the patient to breakdown? These questions require the kind of comprehensive evaluation described in chapter 14. It is unrealistic to expect all to be elaborated in a single interview; but important pieces of the jigsaw puzzle are usually lying around, if you keep your eyes and ears open.

Resources, strengths, weaknesses

An inventory of assets and liabilities

What personal and environmental strengths, resources, and liabilities are apparent at the present time? What advantages has the patient now? What holds the patient back? What hurdles need to be faced? The clinician should take inventory of the patient's physical, intellectual, emotional, and social assets and deficiencies. This is of crucial importance to the design of an individualized plan of management (see chapters 13, 14, 15).

Presentation

The reason for seeking help

Why does the patient seek help now? Do you see the patient at the outset of a disorder or later, when a relatively defined pattern of symptoms has developed, or even later, partially recovered but still troubled by residual difficulties? Did the patient come voluntarily, or need persuasion to do so? Was the patient brought by other people? Why? This issue is considered at greater length in chapter 14.

Insight and desire for help

Unrealistic fears

Does the patient think he or she is unwell? Does the patient consider he or she has been inappropriately referred? This may be correct. If the patient recognizes personal disturbance, does he or she have any idea of its nature or cause? How realistic are these notions?

What kind of help does the patient seek, if any? Is this in line with what is advisable, appropriate, or feasible? Is the patient troubled by doubts concerning the problem and the kind of treatment to be received? Fears of craziness or of exotic psychiatric treatments are likely to be inflamed by deep-seated anxieties about helplessness and victimization and aggravated by sensational images derived from the media. It is better that such concerns be expressed as soon as possible and corrected when they are due to misinformation.

Topics covered in a psychiatric history

The following topics are the content of the psychiatric history. Do not blindly follow the order suggested below; be prepared to deal with topics in whatever sequence is natural. Some areas will be emphasized and others pursued in less detail, as different cases demand.

1. Identifying data
2. Presenting problem
3. History of present illness
4. History of past psychiatric illnesses
5. Medical history
6. History of drug or alcohol intake or of antisocial behavior
7. Early development and childhood environment
8. Educational history
9. Vocational history
10. Family history
11. Sexual history
12. Marital history
13. Characteristic coping mechanisms, values, ideals, aspirations

Stages and transitions

Inception

Clear the decks

At the opening of the interview, if you work in a clinic, go to the waiting room, introduce yourself, accompany the patient to the room, and offer a seat. After taking identifying data, it is useful to tell the patient what you already know. That way, unnecessary mysteries are avoided and the decks can be cleared for action.

> PSYCHIATRIST: Your parents came to see me yesterday. They told me they're worried because your schoolwork has fallen off – though you've always been a good student – you've dropped most of your friends, and you seem to have

become depressed. Last week, they found one of your assignments in which you
spoke about suicide. They think you may need help for an emotional problem.

PATIENT: (a 16-year-old boy) So?

PSYCHIATRIST: So they asked you to see a psychiatrist. I get the impression you're
not too happy about that.

PATIENT: No.

PSYCHIATRIST: Maybe we can start by you telling me how you feel about it.

Formality

Interviews are not always conducted in an office; they may be transacted
beside a bed, or between stacks of bottles in the side-room of an emergency clinic,
or even while driving a car. Wherever they occur, there is a pattern to the beginning, a certain formality. Introduce yourself, say why you are there, and invite
the patient to respond by telling his or her story. If the patient is reluctant to tell
you, help him or her to explain why.

Reconnaissance

Let the patient
tell the story

You must next help the patient tell his or her story as spontaneously as possible.
Listen. Do not interrupt any more than is necessary to keep the story flowing. Do
not rush the reconnaissance or try to direct it prematurely. If all you do is ask
questions, all you will get are answers. The more leading the probe, the less valid
the response, unless the issue in question is simple and unequivocal. The facilitating techniques described later in this chapter are particularly appropriate for
reconnaissance.

Detailed inquiry

After the patient has finished the story, the interviewer will want to seek further
information about the present illness, past illness, medical history, early environment, schooling, and other relevant matters from the psychiatric history. A full
detailed inquiry will take several interviews, but scanning the features most important for a provisional diagnosis can be completed within an hour.

Open-ended probes

Detailed inquiry involves questioning, but the first questions are kept as
open-ended as possible. They move from general to specific when more details
are required. Compare the following questions:

How are things in your marriage?

How are things between you and your wife?

How do you and your wife get on?

Is your marriage a happy one?

Do you love your wife?

This is not unlike the way a surgeon approaches a guarded section of a painful abdomen: from the outside in. Direct questions provoke circumscribed responses and are most appropriate to issues of fact (What year were you married?).

Some issues should be left to a later time when a therapeutic alliance has developed. Unless the patient presents it as a problem from the outset, an exploration of the details of sexual life should usually be postponed.

Transitions

When you move from one topic to another, never do so abruptly. Try to signal the change.

> THERAPIST: Okay. Well, I'd like to go on from there to something else. Could you tell me about the jobs you've had? What did you do after you left school?

Routine inquiry

Part of the detailed inquiry is routine: *minimum data base* questions obligatory for patients of that age and in that clinical situation. This routine should be defined in each clinical service. The rest of the detailed inquiry is largely

Discretionary inquiry

discretionary and involves eliciting evidence for or against the array of diagnostic hypotheses generated after reconnaissance. The detailed inquiry therefore provides evidence for the deductive reasoning described in chapter 7.

Termination

An interview may last 15 minutes or continue much longer. The usual time is about 50 minutes – long enough for a rapid survey, but not so long as to exhaust the patient. Signal the approach of the conclusion with a phrase, for example:

> Our time is almost finished, and there are a few things we need to discuss . . . .

Terminal summaries

A concluding summary of the material points of the interview can be helpful. It allows the patient to correct or modify misinterpretations and leads naturally into your plan for what happens next – a further interview, for example, or special investigations.

Facilitating the interview

Atmosphere

The need to create a favorable atmosphere

To achieve the interview's purpose – gathering information – the interviewer must develop an atmosphere favoring the expression of ideas, feelings, and attitudes (Rogers, 1951). The patient must develop a sense of trust and confidence in the interviewer in order to be as spontaneous as possible. The patient will

Spontaneity and
self-exploration

thereby see the interview as encouraging participation and collaboration toward a therapeutic end, through free expression and self-exploration.

What can you do to promote trust, spontaneity, and free expression?

Unconditional
acceptance

You must accept the patient without moral judgment. If you cannot do so, it is better to be honest with yourself and refer the patient to another physician. Anybody can help somebody, but nobody can help everybody. If a patient angers, repels, or frightens you and the feeling persists, seek help from a colleague.

Understanding

The interview is facilitated if the clinician understands the patient and conveys this by facial expression, intonation, and well-timed reflections of the content and emotion behind the patient's story. The deepest affective under-

Empathy

standing is empathy, ''feeling with,'' or sharing the patient's feelings. It contrasts with sympathy, which is a ''feeling for.''

Open-ended style

The open-ended style most appropriate to reconnaissance and detailed inquiry helps convey the spirit of collaboration, free expression, and self-exploration. An atmosphere of trust is also fostered if the interviewer is relaxed and receptive, not preoccupied, rushed, abrupt, or irritable.

A personal style

It takes time to develop a personal style. You will probably adapt to your own purposes the techniques of others who have impressed you. Some approaches you will try and discard as unsuitable. The effective interviewer is both at home with the task and aware of personal feelings throughout the task. These personal reactions can be important diagnostic clues if heeded, and serious hindrances to rapport when ignored (see chapter 7). Patients can be shrewd at perceiving when a clinician's remoteness, coldness, pomposity, abruptness, or artificiality cloak hostility or anxiety.

Setting

A skilled interviewer can be effective walking along a corridor, playing catch, or sitting by the side of a bed. Nevertheless, offices are preferable to closets and chairs an improvement on packing cases. Try to arrange your room to take advantage of its size, proportions, outlook, and design.

The size of the room

The fundamental principles are simple. The room should be large enough to fit patient, desk, chairs, other equipment, and you without crowding. It is

Seating arrangements

desirable, though not always possible, to have enough room and seating to accommodate the patient and four others, particularly if you plan to see families as well as individuals. The arrangement of desk and chairs should allow free entry and egress. Do not sit between the patient and the door. Try not to interview people across a desk, like a district attorney. Avoid harsh lighting. Make sure the patient is not blinded by glare shining directly from window or lamp. Ensure that the chairs are comfortable and that you do not tower over the patient. Do not leave the patient stranded in the middle of the room; people feel less exposed with something solid behind them. Do not sit too close (knee to knee) or too far away.

You should be near enough to make arm contact by leaning forwards. Figure 8.1 is a diagram of different seating arrangements.

One of the most popular is illustrated in Figure 8.1(a). The patient's chair is indirectly opposite the clinician's, separated by the corner of a table or desk. Patient and interviewer can make eye contact or avert gaze, at will; they are not forced to stare at each other. A swivel chair helps the interviewer vary the direction of glances. Figures 8.1(b) and 8.1(c) illustrate other useful arrangements; 8.1(c) is particularly suitable for family interviews.

Decor

Just as it is impossible not to communicate something to someone else, even if you remain silent, your office will convey something about you, even if you had nothing to do with the raddled wainscot, decrepit linoleum, and "Stag at Bay" on the wall. Pause before you hang out the "No Smoking! Lungs at Work" sign, put photographs of all the children on the desk, or allow an interior decorator to cover the walls with regency stripes and Aubrey Beardsley prints.

Professionalism

What do you want to convey? Not the panelled stolidity of a bank manager's office, the spartan bustle of a recruiting station, or the filmy ambience of a boudoir. Nor do you need to stare across a desk at your patient like a school principal. The interview is not meant to be an interrogation, a dressing down, a form of horse trading, a fireside chat, or a tête-à-tête. The therapeutic alliance connotes a certain formality, just enough for the patient to know that a professional relationship is involved and serious collaboration is planned.

Technique

During the reconnaissance and detailed enquiry, the clinician encourages free expression by the setting provided, the atmosphere created, and the interview techniques used. The interviewer should be at ease with these skills and use them naturally, without flamboyance or stiltedness. If any does not suit you, do not use it; find an alternative conveying the same spirit and with similar purpose. These are examples of useful techniques: attentive listening, subtle vocal and nonvocal encouragement, support and reassurance, the reflection of feeling, gentle indication, and judicious paraphrasing.

Attentive listening

Having invited the patient to tell the story, the interviewer waits and listens, not staring but meeting the patient's gaze from time to time to indicate he or she is following. The interviewer's intent but relaxed posture indicates involvement. If notes are taken, they are brief and unobtrusive.

Vocal and nonvocal encouragement

Oral repetition or reflection

While the flow of associations proceeds, the interviewer need do little but maintain relaxed concentration, signaling by posture, eye contact and subtle nonvocal or vocal encouragement that he or she is with the patient. A nod, an "uh-huh" or "mm-mm" at strategic points, may be all that is needed. If the flow seems to waver or pause, it is effective to repeat a significant phrase or the last word a patient has said. But do not be mechanical, and do not use this technique unless it feels natural.

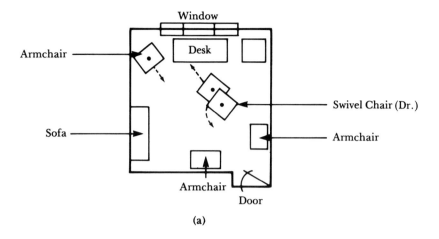

(a)

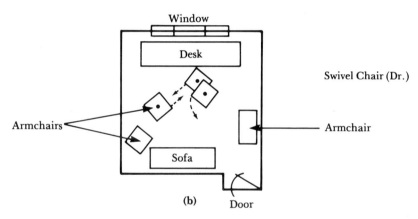

(b)

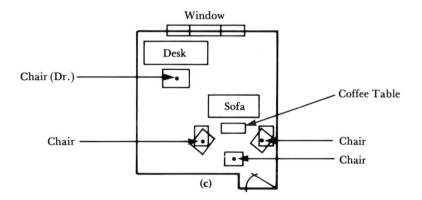

(c)

FIGURE 8.1
Three interview seating arrangements

Silences

Oral reflection

The reflection of feeling

Be alert to the patient's reactions, particularly the changes in voice intonation and speech tempo, tensing of facial muscles, alterations of skin color, and moistening of conjunctivae that herald a flush of anxiety or anger or a sudden feeling of sadness.

How does the interviewer handle silences? If the patient is thinking fruitfully, all the interviewer need do is wait. Similarly, if the patient has broken down in tears, it may be better to wait calmly until he or she can continue. If the silence occurs when the patient has lost track or has confused feelings about the topic, the interviewer can facilitate associations with a subtle oral reflection, picking up a key word, phrase, or idea from the recent conversation and repeating it gently, sometimes with a questioning intonation. Oral reflection is also useful to help circumstantial patients regain their train of thought.

The reflection of feeling is a variant of the technique of oral reflection. The clinician picks up and echoes feelings explicit or implicit in what has been said but incompletely expressed up to that point.

PATIENT: Sometimes when I get like that I can't go on. I'm in a spin . . . *(pauses)* . . .
THERAPIST: In a spin?
PATIENT: Yes . . . like "Black Magic" . . . I feel different in myself, as though I'm not really there.

The clinician could have responded in a variety of ways, picking up on the interesting phrase and asking the patient to explore its connotations:

Spin?

You're in a spin!

Tell me more about being in a spin.

How do you mean, in a spin?

What is the connection between being in a spin and "Black Magic"? Such seemingly gratuitous asides demonstrate how useful it is to share a culture (and a generation) with your patient. If you do not share it, you can always ask.

PATIENT: Yes . . . like "Black Magic" . . . I feel different in myself, as though I'm not really there.
THERAPIST: Like "Black Magic"?
PATIENT: You know, the old song about being in a spin and loving it, about Black Magic and love. *(He laughs.)*
THERAPIST: There's a connection between being in a spin and being in love?

So it goes on, the clinician listening, following, and facilitating, and the patient associating; both working towards exploration and understanding. Take this example of the reflection of feelings:

(The family – stepfather, mother, and 11-year-old daughter – have been referred because the daughter has taken an overdose. All are seated in a family interview.

They are exploring what was going on in the family at the time of the daughter's overdose.)

FATHER: . . . It was a terrible Christmas. After my mother went home, she refused to see a doctor. And I got severe flu.

MOTHER: . . . And Kerry . . .

FATHER: She's a neighbor.

MOTHER: . . . came over and dumped on me. People see me as a good listener, like a rock. I sure don't feel it, always. Kerry was having a threatened miscarriage and she wanted a baby. *(Her voice rises)* She spent all day with me!

THERAPIST: *(Quietly and slowly)* Sounds kind of overwhelming.

MOTHER: *(Weeping)* I can't do everything . . . .

Indicating inconsistencies

When the interviewer notices a discrepancy (see chapter 7) between the content of the patient's account and the feeling expressed – particularly when a strong underlying emotion is manifest in the patient's posture, face, or voice – it can be useful to indicate the inconsistency. This is a powerful technique, best left until you have had some experience. Indication is an attempt to put one's finger on something that would otherwise not be discussed, to direct the patient to something unexpressed but close to consciousness. Indication should always be based on what you see and hear, not on what you infer. Phrase indications in a neutral way and never as challenges or confronting questions.

PATIENT: *(tensely smiling)* So I wonder if she ever really cared about me, before she left, as I thought she did.

THERAPIST: *(softly)* I notice that even though you speak of sad things, you smile.

Paraphrasing

When associations flag and the ideas recently expressed have been complicated, it can be useful to offer a brief paraphrase or summary. You can thus check the validity of your understanding and help the patient to continue associating.

THERAPIST: Well, let's see. What you've been saying is that since your wife left you, you've felt confused and different, as though your mind were spinning, and that your work has lost interest for you. Does that summarize things pretty well?

The paraphrasing technique is also useful at termination to encapsulate the main points of the interview before discussing what should be done next.

Transference and countertransference

The unreasonable displacement of childhood feelings

Transference refers to the unreasonable displacement of attitudes and feelings that originated in childhood to contemporary people. This phenomenon is particularly likely to affect the doctor–patient relationship when patients are made vulnerable by fear, anxiety, guilt, despair, and hope.

Note the word *unreasonable* in the definition. The patient who is angered by overt rudeness is not displaying transference. However, if the patient is angered because you have a moustache or wear pearls, it is apparent that something is being added to an objectively neutral situation.

Different transference roles

The patient may unconsciously regard the physician as a parent or a sibling, casting you in a caring or antagonistic role. The most common roles are of nurturing mother, demanding mother, protective father, punitive father, and rivalrous sibling. Sometimes older patients will relate to the physician as though they themselves were parents, reversing the roles.

Recognizing positive and negative transference

How can you recognize transference? When the patient is exceptionally deferential, hanging on your opinions, singing your praises to others, or easily slighted by a brief or delayed appointment, you may suspect a positive transference. When the patient is unexpectedly hostile, suspicious, or competitive and there is no reasonable explanation for such antagonism, a negative transference is likely.

Crushes

It is not difficult to imagine how a positive transference can become eroticized, the patient falling in love with an idealized parental figure. Most of these infatuations are transitory, like adolescent crushes. Recognize them, respond in a professional manner, and they will go no further. Occasionally, however, unscheduled visits, notes, telephone calls, and seductive dress indicate the matter is more serious. You may need to consult a psychiatric colleague to decide how to proceed. Do not respond impulsively, out of fear or affront, lest your vulnerable patient be hurt.

Recognizing counter-transference

Transference has its counterpart in a physician's **countertransference.** Countertransference occurs when a physician irrationally transfers to a patient attitudes and feelings derived from childhood experiences. Be alert for countertransference. Suspect it whenever you have powerful feelings of affection, protectiveness, fear, frustration, irritation, hatred, or erotic excitement toward a patient; when you very much look forward to the next appointment; or when you cannot tolerate someone. If you recognize it, you will be much less likely to respond impulsively with rejection, flight, or self-indulgence. Once again, seek the help of a colleague or group of colleagues if you are unsure how to proceed in your patient's best interests.

You need not be embarrassed by transference or countertransference. Experienced clinicians know these phenomena are ubiquitous and inescapable. They are most likely to be problematic when you are overworked, preoccupied, or rendered emotionally vulnerable by vicissitudes in your personal life. Look after yourself physically and emotionally; do the best you can to ensure a fulfilling life outside of medicine itself.

Summary

The purpose of the initial interview is to obtain information from the patient about the presenting problem and its precipitation, and about previous disorders, predisposition, biopsychosocial strengths and limitations, the reason for current presentation, insight, and desire for help.

The history covers topics that range from identifying data to coping mechanisms. The four stages of the interview – inception, reconnaissance, detailed inquiry, and termination – are adapted to different topics.

In the inception, the interviewer makes introductions, gets the patient or family seated, takes identifying information, and summarizes what is known. The quality of the interview is enhanced if the clinician creates an atmosphere of trust, spontaneity, and expressiveness by acceptance, empathic understanding, open-ended style, and natural manner. The room's decor, lighting, furnishings, and arrangement can also promote (or subvert) the desired atmosphere.

During the interview, the clinician fosters free expression and association by being attentive and by using certain techniques such as vocal and nonvocal encouragement, support and reassurance, support the reflection of ideas or feelings, the indication of inconsistencies, and paraphrasing.

During the reconnaissance, the interviewer helps the patient describe the presenting problem and its precipitation and development.

During the detailed inquiry, routine and discretionary, the interviewer explores past illness; early development and environment; later educational, occupational, social, and marital history; interests, values, and aspirations; habitual coping style; family history; and mental status.

At termination, the interviewer summarizes the interview and negotiates with the patient what the next step should be.

Selected Readings

Most standard texts in psychiatry have sections on the psychiatric interview. For example, the chapters by Ripley and by Detre and Kupfer in the *Comprehensive Textbook of Psychiatry* (Freedman, Kaplan, & Sadock, Eds., 1975) are excellent. *The Harvard Guide to Modern Psychiatry* (Nicholi, 1978) also is excellent.

Enelow and Swisher (1972), Bernstein, Bernstein, and Dana (1974) and Reiser and Schroder (1980) have provided excellent monographs on interviewing for health professionals.

Colby's (1951) classic text, *A Primer for Psychotherapists*, is essential reading for the psychotherapist in training. It contains a lively account of transference and countertransference.

Siegman's chapter in *The Behavioral and Social Sciences and the Practice of Medicine* (Balis et al., Eds., 1978) is a useful summary of research in clinical interviewing.

9

The Mental Status Examination

Introduction

The context and purpose of the MSE

The **Mental Status Examination** (MSE) is a set of systematic observations and assessments undertaken by a diagnostician during the clinical interview. Properly conducted, the MSE provides a detailed and systematic description of the patient at that time, information essential for consolidating the patterns of clues and inferences required for diagnostic decision making. The MSE, guided by the hypothetico-deductive approach to diagnosis, is an essential part of the subsequent inquiry plan. This chapter deals comprehensively with the different components of the MSE. In regard to a particular patient and in accordance with the clinical context, background information, and psychiatric history, the clinician will apply the MSE tactically, pursuing brief, extensive, or discretionary lines of inquiry. These tactics are discussed in more detail at the end of this chapter.

The need for standardization

Since the MSE, like the psychiatric history, should involve routine and discretionary lines of inquiry, according to the diagnostic hypotheses being entertained, it should not be standardized as a whole; rather, the separate observations and assessments composing it should be standardized. The techniques of eliciting data should be formalized, the phenomena in question clearly defined, and the weight to be placed on each phenomenon clarified.

Reliability

The reliability of a test refers to the likelihood (usually expressed as a correlation) that similar results will be obtained on retesting **(test-retest reliability)** or that similar results will be obtained by different observers **(intertester reliability).** Test-retest reliability applies to such relatively stable characteristics as the use of language; it is not to be expected in such characteristics as mood that are changeable and often linked to the current situation. Wing, Birley, and Cooper (1967) report an attempt to train observers to reliability in the MSE.

Validity

When psychiatrists test for abstracting ability, for example, by asking subjects to explain proverbs in their own words, how certain can they be that the clinical test is a true measure of the ability in question? In other words, what is the **validity** of the test? Over the years, a number of techniques for informal mental state assessment have accumulated, but in some instances their validity is questionable. The validity of any clinical test described in this chapter is considered along with the mental faculties required for adequate performance on the test.

Sections of the Mental Status Examination

A hierarchy of functions

The sections of the MSE can be roughly graduated in a hierarchy from objective and observational to subjective and inferential. In more complex areas, such as the patient's capacity for insight, the clinician is attempting to be objective about somebody else's subjectivity. This is, at best, a relative matter.

The broad areas to be covered in the MSE are as follows:

A. APPEARANCE AND BEHAVIOR
B. RELATIONSHIP AND MOOD
C. COGNITION
D. LANGUAGE
E. THOUGHT
F. PHYSIOLOGICAL FUNCTIONS
G. INSIGHT

These areas can be further subdivided as follows:

A. Appearance and Behavior
   1. Appearance
   2. Motor Behavior
   3. Quality of speech
B. Relationship and Mood
   1. Relationship to interviewer
   2. Affect and mood

C. Cognition
1. Level of consciousness and awareness
2. Orientation, attention, and concentration
3. Memory
4. Information
5. Comprehension
6. Conceptualization and abstraction
7. Judgment
8. Combination tests of cognitive functioning
D. Language
E. Pathology of Thought
1. Abnormalities of thought processs
2. Abnormalities of thought content
F. Physiological Functions
1. Sleep
2. Appetite
3. Libido
4. Menstrual cyclc
5. Other physiological functions
G. Attitude to Illness

Each assessment area is discussed in this chapter and pertinent clinical tests described.

Appearance and behavior

Appearance

From the moment you first greet the patient, you will be aware of appearance. Try to describe it in detail before you draw inferences from it.

Physique   What is the patient's physique and habitus? Is there evidence of loss or gain of weight? Does the patient have any conspicuous marks or disfigurement?

Facies   Describe the patient's face and hair. Does the patient look ill? What is the expression of the eyes and mouth? Does the patient appear to be in touch with the surroundings?

Grooming   Is the patient clean and neat or are there deficiencies in personal hygiene revealed by poor grooming of skin, hair, and nails? How is the patient dressed? Is

Dress   the clothing neat? Is it appropriate or are there peculiarities of dress? After you have described it to yourself, can you infer what kind of statement the patient is attempting to make with this ensemble?

Motor behavior

Activity
Posture
Coordination
Movements
Stereotypies

The clinician should note general overactivity, underactivity, abnormalities of tone, gait and posture, gross incoordination, or impairment of large muscle function. Note any abnormalities of movement and posture such as tremor, chorea, tics, fidgetiness, dystonia, or torticollis.

Stereotypies are organized repetitive movements or speech or perseverative postures. They are usually associated with schizophrenia, particularly of catatonic type. A striking variant of postural stereotypy is waxy flexibility, in which the patient will remain indefinitely in a position imposed by the examiner (standing on one leg, for example). Other disorders of movement associated with catatonia include a stiff, expressionless face; facial grimacing or contortions; stiff, awkward, or stilted body movement; and unusual mannerisms of expressive movement or speech. The latter should not be confused with the gracelessness of someone who is socially anxious.

Catatonia

Rituals
Habits

Does the patient exhibit any **rituals,** such as a need to touch objects repetitively, as in obsessive-compulsive disorder, or **habits** such as nailbiting, thumbsucking, liplicking, yawning, or scratching?

Quality of speech

Pitch, tone, and tempo

The examiner will attend to the accent, pitch, tone, and tempo of speech, paying particular attention to unusually high or low pitch and abnormal tone, as in the high-pitched squawking monotone sometimes encountered in children with early infantile autism.

Production

In **mutism,** which can occur in advanced brain disorder, severe melancholia, catatonia, somatoform disorder of conversion type, or in the elective mutism of negativistic children, the patient is unable or unwilling to utter anything. In conversion disorder, mutism is less common than **aphonia,** the patient being able to speak only in a hoarse whisper.

Phonation

Fluency

The rhythm and fluency of speech is disordered in **stammering,** the patient sometimes halting and struggling tonically to get the word out, and at other times or in other cases hesitating clonically on a sound or word at the beginning of an utterance.

Relationship and mood

Relationship to interviewer

The clinician infers the quality of the patient's relationship by how he or she behaves and what is said. The relationship may be constant, it may vary with the

Inference

topic being discussed, or it may be influenced by other factors. If these factors are unexpressed (for example, when the patient is privately amused by an auditory hallucination), they may remain obscure. If such is the case, it should be noted.

Aside from matters of inconstancy and obscurity, affective states are difficult to assess. The clinician draws on a number of behavioral clues to assess the quality of the patient's relationship and mood. As a rule, the more inferential the judgment, the more unreliable the conclusion. Clinicians often differ in their inferences concerning a patient's affect, especially when it is unstable, ambiguous, complex, or shielded by interpersonal caution.

The influence of the interviewer

It is inevitable that the examiner's behavior will affect the ebb and flow of the patient's feelings. The patient may be responding appropriately to the interviewer's friendly approach (or rudeness, for that matter). The patient will also be responding to highly idiosyncratic internal predispositions, as, for example, if harboring mingled anxiety and deference for somebody perceived as a threatening authority figure who must be placated.

The fallibility of inference

Given the fallibility of inference, it is wise to stick closely to observations and be able to cite them. This skill takes training. The beginner is overimpressed by brilliant intuitive leaps; the expert heeds intuition but realizes how unreliable it is. The beginner grasps for and holds firmly to an inference, sometimes in spite of contrary evidence. The expert makes the inference, cites the clues on which it is based, can offer alternative explanations, and is prepared to discard the inference for a better one if the evidence fails to support it.

Nonverbal behavior

Eye contact

The quality of **eye contact** is important in gauging affective states. Negativistic patients, especially those with catatonia, may avert their gaze from the examiner. Children with early infantile autism characteristically demonstrate eccentricities of eye contact: staring through the examiner or averting their gaze. A delirious patient whose sensorium is impaired may stare into space; so may a melancholic or schizophrenic patient who is dominated by ruminations or preoccupations. Intermittent staring is a feature of different forms of epilepsy. Can the patient's attention be captured, albeit briefly? If not, suspect an organic brain disorder.

Some patients stare at the examiner intently. Distinguish the wide eyes of awe and fear from the narrowed slits of hypervigilant suspiciousness. Other patients make hesitant eye contact, particularly when they are embarrassed about what they are saying. Remember, however, that not all patients with shifty gaze are liars, and that some can prevaricate without batting an eyelid.

Facies

The impact of the eyes on interpersonal relations cannot be overestimated. The configuration of supraorbital, circumorbital, and facial musculature, the eyelids, palpebral fissure, gaze, depth of binocular focus, pupil size, and conjunctival moisture all combine to produce a range of social signals of great significance for (a) interpersonal dominance, competition, attraction, hostility, or avoidance, (b) the initiation and punctuation of conversation, and

(c) the feedback one requires to know how another person has responded to what one has said. Women make more eye contact than men and appear to be more likely to use eye contact to gauge when it is appropriate for them to break into a conversation. Women look at a man while speaking if they like him; men look at a woman more while listening if they are attracted to her. Same-sex pairs make more eye contact than do opposite-sex pairs (Argyle, 1967).

Posture

Eyes and face are combined with body posture and movement in a Gestalt. The face provides the clues to remoteness, bewilderment, and perplexity; the whole body is involved in tenseness (clenched fists, sweaty palms, stiff back, leaning forward, restlessness, preoccupation, boredom, and sadness).

Verbal behavior

Verbal communication

The patient may be uncommunicative or, in the extreme, quite mute. On the other hand, the patient may be friendly and communicative, even loquacious or garrulous. Patients convey antagonism by hectoring, uncooperativeness, impertinence, condescension, or even by direct threat, criticism, or abuse. In contrast, by tone of conversation and demeanor, the patient can convey respect, deference, anxiety to please, or ingratiation.

Attitudes

Note and describe the following attitudes in the patient: shyness, fear, suspiciousness, cautiousness, assertiveness, indifference, passivity, clowning, interest in the examiner, clinging, coyness, seductiveness, or invasiveness.

Affect and mood

Affect

Affect refers to a feeling or emotion usually in response to an external event or a thought. Affects are normally associated with feelings about the self or about other people who are of personal significance to the subject. Less usually, an affect is experienced without association, as though adrift from its reference point.

Affect as a monitor

Affect is the conscious component of a monitoring system signaling whether the individual is on track toward a personal goal, whether the individual is obstructed, frustrated, or prevented from achieving the goal, or whether it has already been attained. Compare, for example, the anticipatory pleasure at preparing to meet someone beloved; the anxiety and fear at seeing the beloved with a rival; the rage and despair of loss; and the exultation of reunion. Similar though more complex affects can attend mountain climbing, solving mathematical puzzles, or giving birth. Whatever the goal, its remoteness, proximity, loss, repudiation, attainment, or inaccessibility are all accompanied by self-monitoring affects.

Mood

In contrast to affect, which may be momentary, **mood** refers to an inner state persisting for some time with a disposition to exhibit a particular emotion or affect. A mood of depression, for example, may not preclude the subject's deriving momentary amusement from a joke, but gloom, sadness, and desolation prevail.

Affects and mood are inferred from the patient's demeanor and spontaneous conversation. A general query, such as

How are you feeling now?

or

How have your spirits been?

can be helpful. Try to avoid such leading questions as

Do you feel depressed?

Veiled affect

Demeanor and affect usually coincide; but sometimes they do not. For example, a stiffly smiling exterior can mask anxiety or depression. If you suspect that this is the case, an indicating or clarificatory interpretation can help the patient recover suppressed emotion.

I notice that even though you speak of sad things, you smile.

or

It's hard to smile when you feel bad inside.

Morbid affect or mood

In a mental status report, the general qualities of a patient's emotional expression should be described. Particular morbid affects or moods should be noted. Is the patient affectively **flat** – that is, emotionally dull, monotonous, and lacking in resonance? This is characteristic of chronic schizophrenia and dementia. Is the patient emotionally **constricted,** with a narrow range of affect, as in obsessional or schizoid personality? Is the patient's affect **inappropriate** or **incongruous** in that it is out of keeping with the topic of conversation?

Case 9.1

■ When she was told that her aged mother had died, the chronic schizophrenic patient began to laugh. When asked how she felt, the patient abruptly answered, "Sad," then stopped laughing and began to stare straight ahead with pursed lips, rocking in her chair. ■

Lability

Does the patient show evidence of **lability,** suddenly changing from neutral to excited, or from one emotional pole to another? Lability is often associated with emotional **intemperateness,** an abrupt, unreflective expression of heightened emotion (excited anticipation, affection, or irritation, for example).

Histrionic affect

Note **histrionic affect,** the extravagant but shallow expression of emotion found in people who exaggerate their feelings in order to avoid being ignored and who seize or fear to lose the center of the interpersonal stage. Histrionic affect is characteristic of people with histrionic, narcissistic, or borderline personality disorder.

Euphoria

Morbid **euphoria,** an exorbitant sense of well-being expressed in inexorable good spirits, is encountered in hypomania or mania, and less commonly in schizophrenia and organic brain disorder. The frontal lobe dysfunction characteristic of neurosyphilis, disseminated sclerosis, and after lobotomy, may be associated with fatuous joking and lack of foresight. **Silliness** is sometimes encountered in histrionic or immature people overwhelmed by the enormity of a difficult situation. Morbid silliness is also characteristic of some disorganized schizophrenic patients **(hebephrenia).**

Elation

As it becomes exaggerated, euphoria merges into **elation** and **excitement,** although the manic patient commonly also exhibits irritation if obstructed or thwarted. An extreme and transcendent exaltation of mood can be seen in the rare **ecstatic states** that are associated with acute schizophreniform or schizophrenic disorders and epilepsy.

Apathy

Apathy, a pervasive lack of interest and **anergia,** a lack of drive, can be found in preschizophrenic, schizophrenic, depressive, and organic brain disorders. The apathetic patient has little or no enthusiasm for work, social interaction, or recreation. Anergia is usually associated with a decrease in sexual activity. **Anhedonia,** a subjective sense that nothing is pleasurable, is commonly associated with anergia and is found in preschizophrenia, schizophrenia, and melancholia. Excessive **fatigue,** which may be manifest as hypersomnia, is found in many physical disorders, organic brain disorder, schizophrenia, anxiety disorders, depressive disorders, and abnormal illness behavior.

Fatigue

Depression

When applied to an affect or mood, **depression** refers to a pervasive sense of sadness. Depression is often, but not invariably, related to a life event involving loss, rejection, defeat, disillusionment, or disappointment. It may be associated with tearfulness and anger about the event. In more severe depression or **melancholia,** the patient feels emotionally deadened or empty, the world stale and unprofitable, and the future hopeless. The patient is preoccupied with dark forebodings and agitated by persistent self-recrimination about past failures or misdeeds. Depressed affect and gloomy ruminations are characteristically accompanied by diminished concentration and a slowing of thinking and movement **(psychomotor retardation);** in some cases, however, **agitated depression** is associated with psychomotor restlessness. Severe depression has important somatic concomitants, with characteristic posture, facies, headache, irritability, precordial heaviness, gastrointestinal slowing, anorexia, weight loss, loss of sexual interest, and insomnia. Depression typically has a diurnal variation; dysphoria, hopelessness, and agitation are worse in the morning, and the patient brightens up by evening.

Anger

Open **anger** and **irritability** are readily recognized. They may be understandable if the patient's circumstances are appreciated. **Morbid anger** however, is defined by pervasiveness, frequency, disproportion, impulsiveness, and uncontrollability. Morbid anger is associated with organic brain disorder, usually in the form of **catastrophic reactions** to frustration, especially when the patient can no longer complete a familiar or easy task. Abnormal anger is also found in some forms of epilepsy, in personality disorders of aggressive,

Controlled hostility

antisocial, borderline, or paranoid type, in the attention deficit and conduct disorders of childhood, in drunkenness, in paranoid disorders, in hypomania or mania, and in intermittent or isolated explosive disorders.

Controlled hostility may be expressed as sullenness, uncooperativeness, superiority or mockery. It can be helpful to invite the patient to express anger or resentment directly and to define its origin. This is particularly the case with adolescents:

> Whenever I ask you a question, you close up. Something about being here is making you pretty upset. Can you tell me what it is?

Anxiety and fear

Anxiety and **fear** refer to the subjective apprehension of impending danger, together with widespread manifestations of autonomic discharge (dilated pupils, cold sweaty palms, tachycardia, tachypnea, nausea, bowel hurry, urinary urgency, etc.). Fear has an object: the need to cope with uncertain odds, a charging bull or a near accident in an automobile, for example. Anxiety is associated with a threat to an essential value – being attached to someone beloved, not being a coward, being successful, or being highly regarded, for example. Fear can be eliminated by direct action – fight or flight – whereas the adaptive solution to anxiety is likely to require planning and persistence. Both affects – anxiety and fear – are biologically advantageous because they signal the need for a constructive response.

In **morbid anxiety,** affect is cast adrift from its moorings, either to float free or fasten on a substitute, phobic object, or situation (for example, on a particular animal, heights, elevators, enclosed spaces, or being fat). Morbid anxiety appears disproportionate or eccentric and is recognized as pathological by the patient and others. Many disorders of thought content (described later in this chapter) can be regarded as unconsciously determined, pathological mechanisms that detach anxiety from its object or block and divert it at origin. See also the section on ego defense mechanisms in chapter 5.

Cognition

The cognitive functions that can be assessed in a mental status examination are as follows:

1. Level of consciousness and awareness
2. Orientation, attention, and concentration
3. Memory
4. Information
5. Comprehension
6. Conceptualization and abstraction

7. Judgment
8. Combination tests of cognitive functioning

Level of consciousness and awareness

Coma

The psychiatrist may be asked to consult on a comatose or stuporous patient if a nonorganic cause is hypothesized. **Coma** is a state of nonawareness from which the patient cannot be aroused. Diminished awareness is called **semicoma** or

Stupor

stupor, the subject being temporarily rousable, by pain or noise for example, but reverting to stupor when the stimulus ceases. In stupor, eye movements become purposeful when the painful stimulus is applied and wincing or pupillary constriction may occur, but the patient remains akinetic and mute. Stupor and coma occur in primary neuronal dysfunction (as in Alzheimer's disease), secondary neuronal dysfunction (as in metabolic encephalopathy), supratentorial lesions (such as infarction, hemorrhage, and tumor), subtentorial lesions (infarction, hemorrhage, tumor, and abscess), and psychiatric disorder (dissociative disorder, depression, and catatonia).

Psychogenic coma

Psychogenic coma is suggested by normal vital and neurologic signs, resistance to opening the eyes, normal pupillary reactions, and staring (rather than wandering) eyes. Swallowing, corneal, and gag reflexes are usually intact, and electroencephalography and oculovestibular reflexes are normal. Intravenous barbiturate may increase verbalization in psychogenic stupor; it depresses awareness further in organic conditions.

Torpor

Torpor denotes a lowering of consciousness short of stupor. Awareness is narrowed and restricted; apathy, perseveration, and psychomotor retardation are found, but the more dramatic phenomena of delirium (illusions, hallucinations, agitation, etc.) are lacking. Torpor is associated with severe infection and multi-infarct dementia.

Obtundation

In **twilight** or **dreamy states,** restricted awareness (**obtundation**) is manifest as disorientation for time and place, with reduced attention and short-term memory. In addition, the subject may have the sense of being in a dream.

Case 9.2

■ A 15-year-old male jumped out of the window of a moving automobile, sustaining concussion and superficial lacerations. After admission to the hospital, he claimed to have had a vivid dream that portended his accident in every respect, except that in the dream his mother had not been in the emergency room to help him and he had felt abandoned by her.

His parents could not recall that he had spoken of a dream before the accident. The friends who drove the vehicle out of which he had jumped recalled that he had been highly excited on the way to the hospital, shouting about a dream and asking for his mother, who arrived in the emergency room shortly after he was transported there.

The most likely explanation for his 'dream' is that it never occurred but that his concussion was associated with a twilight state in which dream, false memory, and reality were interwoven. ■

Twilight states occur in dissociative disorders (especially psychogenic fugue), epilepsy and, rarely, schizophrenia.

Delirium

Delirium, a common condition in medical and surgical wards, is caused by a diffuse cerebral dysfunction of acute or subacute onset and fluctuant or reversible course. After prodromal restlessness and insomnia, delirium typically presents with obtundation, emotional lability, and visual illusions. The clinical features tend to worsen at night (''sundowning''), with insomnia, agitation, hallucinations, and delusions. It should be noted, however, that quiet deliria are common, with little more to note than **clouding of consciousness,** causing mild disorientation for time and place and reduced concentration. Restlessness, tremor, asterixis (irregular, asymmetrical jerking of the extremities), myoclonus, and disturbance of autonomic function are also common.

Clouding

Patients vary in their psychological reactions to delirium; depressive, paranoid, schizophreniform, anxious, and somatoform responses may be encountered. The patient may be fearfully or combatively hypervigilant, or torpid and apathetic.

Illusions

Visual **illusions** are characteristic of delirium, the patient misinterpreting the moving shadows, curtains, and surrounding bedroom furniture. Physical sensations may also be misperceived, the patient mistaking abdominal pain, for example, for the knives of malefactors, and tinnitus for radio waves. If poorly systemized delusional beliefs arise, the patient may act on them, seeking escape or defense. Visual **hallucinations** are more common in delirium than are auditory and vary in connotation: sometimes playful (animals romping, etc.), sometimes personal (the face of a dead relative, etc.), and sometimes horrible or threatening (dismembered bodies, accidents, etc.). Visual hallucinations are most evident at night and can be provoked when the eyes are closed, especially when the orbits are pressed on.

Hallucinosis

Confabulation

Attention and concentration wander in delirium, thinking becomes disconnected or incoherent and memory deteriorates. The patient sometimes **confabulates,** linking memories out of correct sequence (see Case 9.2).

Affect is often labile in delirium, but persistent blunting, anxiety, suspiciousness, hostility, depression, or euphoria may be encountered. The affect is usually congruent with the prevailing illusions or hallucinations.

Dissociation

Subtle restriction of consciousness often occurs during acute anxiety resulting in vagueness or amnesia for traumatic experiences. Sometimes amnesia is exaggerated, the patient wandering in a daze, to turn up in an emergency room unaware of name or address. This is known as **dissociative fugue state** and should be differentiated from epilepsy or postictal conditions.

Orientation, attention, and concentration

Disorientation

Disorders of orientation are most often found when the sensorium is clouded, as in torpor, obtundation, dreamy states, delirium, or fugue. Orientation is usually lost in the following order: time, place, person. Disorientation for time and place

TABLE 9.1
Clinical tests of orientation

1. Time
     Hour
     Day
     Date
     Month
     Year
2. Place
     Building
     City
     State
3. Person
     Name
     Address and Telephone
     Age
     Occupation
     Marital Status

usually indicates organic brain disorder. Disorientation for personal identity is actually rare and is associated with psychogenic or postictal fugue states, other dissociative disorders, and agnosia.

Orientation is assessed by asking the patient for the information in Table 9.1. The reliability of the clinical assessment of orientation is high, but its predictive validity is uncertain.

Attention and concentration

Attention is involved when a subject is alerted by a significant stimulus and sustains interest in it. **Concentration** refers to the capacity to maintain mental effort despite **distraction.** An inattentive patient ignores the clinician's questions, for example, or soon loses interest in them. The distractible patient is diverted from mental work by incidental sights, sounds, and ideas.

Simple clinical tests for attention and concentration are shown in Table 9.2. These tests have high reliability but little validity. Essentially, they test the ability to concentrate. Apart from concentration, however, arithmetical questions involve intelligence and schooling. Smith (1967) found that only 42% of 132 adults could complete the serial-sevens test without error, and only 26% of those over 45 years old could do so. Milstein, Small, and Small (1972) tested 325 hospitalized psychiatric patients and 50 age-matched nonhospitalized sibling

TABLE 9.2
Clinical tests of attention and concentration

1. Subtract sevens or threes, serially, from one hundred.
2. Reverse the days of the week or months of the year.
3. Spell simple words backward.
4. Repeat digits (two, three, four, or more) forward and backward.
5. Perform mental arithmetic:
     Number of nickles in one dollar, thirty five cents?
     Interest on two hundred dollars at four percent for eighteen months?

controls. Errors were common and were related to psychiatric disturbance, socio-economic status, intelligence, and the ability to cope with an interview situation. In summary, the procedure has little diagnostic specificity.

Memory

Short- and long-term memory

Memory has several stages. Information must first be registered and comprehended. It is then held in short-term storage. If the material is to be retained beyond immediate recall, a more durable memory trace is formed. Memory traces in long-term storage either decay, consolidate or become simplified and schematized, partly as a result of subsequent experience. Long-term memories are retrieved or recalled from storage by tagging a pattern of sensory phenomena and matching it with long-term memory schemata (see chapter 4).

In clinical practice, abnormal memory is manifest as **amnesia** (memory loss) or **dysmnesia** (distortion of memory).

Amnesia

Psychogenic amnesia occurs in several forms:

Causes of psychogenic amnesia

1. During and after severe anxiety, memory is likely to be defective.
2. Some people have the ability to repress unwelcome anxiety-laden ideas; their memory is thereby rendered patchy or selective.
3. In such dissociative disorders as psychogenic amnesia and fugue, the patient usually loses memory for a circumscribed period of time during which profoundly disturbing events took place. Less commonly, the amnesia is generalized (total) or subsequent (i.e., amnesia for everything after a particular time).
4. In psychogenic fugue, in addition to displaying generalized amnesia, the patient travels a distance from home and assumes a new identity. Not infrequently, in such cases, it is unclear whether one is dealing with unwitting self-deception or conscious imposture.

Organic amnesia

Organic amnesia occurs in acute, subacute, and chronic forms.

Retrograde and anterograde amnesia

After **acute head trauma,** there is likely to be **retrograde** amnesia, due to a disruption of short-term memory. The extent of **anterograde** amnesia following head trauma is an index of the severity of brain injury. Amnesia is also found in alcoholism (blackouts) and after acute intoxication, delirium, and epilepsy.

The amnestic syndrome

Subacute amnesia (the amnestic syndrome) occurs after Wernicke's encephalopathy, a disease caused by thiamine deficiency and encountered most commonly in alcoholics. Wernicke's encephalopathy is characterized by ophthalmoplegia, nystagmus, ataxia, and delirium. After the delirium clears, most patients have a residual **Korsakoff's syndrome,** with disorganized memory in an otherwise clear sensorium. Korsakoff patients have difficulty in recalling events from before the onset of the encephalopathy. They also have a severe impairment of the ability to lay down new memories after the encephalopathy. The retrograde amnesia affects the ability to remember the precise order in which events occurred. The anterograde amnesia, however, tends to be even more marked, the most severely affected patients, for example, being unable to store new information. As a consequence, the patient is often disoriented for place and time and may confabulate to fill the memory gaps. Thus, the characteristic pattern of Korsakoff's syndrome is of amnesia, disorientation, confabulation, a facile lack of concern, and a tendency to get stuck in the one groove of thought.

Chronic amnesia as in dementing illnesses, extends back for years. Recent memory is lost before remote.

Dysmnesia

Disorders of recognition

Disorders of recognition include **déjà vu, déjà vécu,** and **psychotic misidentification.** Déjà vu and déjà vécu are common and normal, particularly in adolescents. They involve the sudden uncanny feeling that one has experienced the present situation or heard precisely the same current conversation on a previous occasion. These phenomena are associated with anxiety and less commonly with temporal lobe epilepsy. Delusional misidentification may occur in schizophrenia, the patient describing familiar people as strangers or claiming to recognize people never met before. In the delusional syndrome named for **Capgras,** the patient regards others as doubles of whom they claim to be.

Disorders of recall

Disorders of recall include **retrospective falsification** and **confabulation.** All people indulge at times in retrospective falsification – embellishing the past to present a more appealing, tragic, or amusing impression. Histrionic people sometimes invent such an extensive and impressive past that they are drawn into imposture, while depressives find sin, failure, and occasion for self-recrimination in their unexceptional lives. After recovery from psychosis, patients often repress their memories of illness and retain only bland or vague reminiscences of the acute disorder. It is generally inadvisable to ask them to recall their experiences in detail.

Confabulation

A **confabulation** is a false memory the patient believes is true. Confabulations can be quite detailed, but they are often inconsistent and fanciful. Confabulations commonly fill memory gaps, especially in the amnestic syndrome. Some schizophrenics confabulate, spinning complicated fantasies about such topics as telekinesis, ESP, and nuclear radiation. It is difficult to draw the line between confabulation and deception in the hysterical imposter or the dramatic abnormal illness behavior of the patient with Münchausen syndrome.

Table 9.3 sets out the clinical tests for immediate, recent, and remote memory.

TABLE 9.3
Clinical tests of memory

Immediate recall
1. Repeat digits forward and backward.
   Present digits at one-second intervals.
   The average adult performance is up to six forward and four backwards.
2. Repeat unrelated words (apple, table, grass) immediately.
3. Repeat three-part phrases ("33 Park Avenue"; "brown mahogany table"; "twelve red roses").

Recent memory
4. Repeat the unrelated words after 1, 3, and 5 minutes.
5. Repeat the three-part phrases after 1, 3, and 5 minutes.
6. Recall events in the recent past.
   For example: a chronological account of the present illness; the last meal; an account of how the patient got to the office; the names of the physicians and nurses who are caring for the patient in the hospital.
7. Repeat this sentence:
   One thing a country must have to become rich and great is a large, secure supply of wood.
8. Recount the following story with as many details as possible:
   William Stern / a 63-year-old / state representative / from Walton County / Utah / was planning his reelection campaign / when he began experiencing chest pain. / He entered Logan Memorial Hospital / for three days of medical tests. / A harmless virus was diagnosed / and he, his wife / Sandra, / and their two sons, / Rick and Tommy, / hit the campaign trail again.

   The average patient should be able to reproduce 8 of the 15 separate ideas in this paragraph. Less adequate performance suggests defective recall of information requiring hierarchial analysis, short-term memory storage, and sequential recall.

Remote memory
9. Recall parents' names, date and place of birth, graduation dates, age and year of marriage, occupational history.

Reliability and validity

These tests have good test–retest and intertester reliability. Their validity is affected by intelligence and age and by such emotional states as depression and, to a lesser extent, anxiety. The most useful tests for detecting organic lesions appear to be orientation, delayed recall, sentence repetition, and general information (Hinton & Withers, 1971; Withers & Hinton, 1971).

Information

General information The patient's fund of general knowledge depends on past education and current interest in contemporary affairs. A clinical test of information is provided in Table 9.4.

TABLE 9.4
Clinical tests of information

1. Name the last four presidents starting with the current president.
2. Name the mayor, state governor, and state senators.
3. Name four large United States cities.
4. Discuss four important current events.
5. For what are these people famous?:
   George Washington, Christopher Columbus, William Shakespeare, Albert Einstein.

Organicity is suggested if the patient makes 12 (60%) mistakes or more.

Reliability and validity

If administration is standardized, reliability is high. The test is quite useful as an estimate of organicity, although it does not assess a unitary cognitive function.

Comprehension

Comprehension

Comprehension is assessed by the patient's grasp of the immediate situation. Does the patient know why he or she is at this particular location? Does the patient appreciate that he or she is ill or in need of treatment? Does the patient understand the purpose of the examination?

There are no tests for comprehension. It is assessed as the interview proceeds. Although comprehension is often disturbed in delirium and dementia, for example, there is no evidence that its assessment contributes to diagnosing organicity, beyond what is provided by other tests of the sensorium (orientation, concentration, and memory).

Conceptualization and abstraction

Similarities and differences

Simple levels of conceptualization are assessed by testing the capacity to discern the similarities and differences between sets of words. The capacity to abstract is tested by asking the subject to discern the pith of well-known metaphorical statements (see Table 9.5).

Reliability and validity

These tests have poor reliability and validity. They are affected by intelligence, educational level, culture, and age. They have little discriminating power and do not effectively detect organicity. Andreason, Tsuang, and Canter (1974) found that clinicians using these tests could not distinguish between manics,

TABLE 9.5
Clinical tests of conceptualization and abstraction

1. How are the following pairs similar or alike?
   A child and a dwarf
   A tree and a bush
   A river and a canal
   A dishwasher and a stove

2. How are the following pairs different?
   A lie and a mistake
   Idleness and laziness
   Poverty and misery
   Character and reputation

3. What is the meaning of the following proverbs? (ask if they have been heard before)
   A rolling stone gathers no moss.
   People who live in glass houses should not throw stones.
   Strike while the iron is hot.

schizophrenics, and creative writers. Such tests are most useful when they tap unmistakable formal psychotic thought disorder.

Case 9.3   ■   A young man with disorganized and accelerated thinking responds thus to the proverb, *People in glass houses should not throw stones:*
"Oh yeah. My California uncle passed the shotgun out the windows and started firing!"
To the proverb, *A rolling stone gathers no moss,* he answers:
"Put a few pebbles in your mouth when you're hiking. You'll go a few more miles." ■

Case 9.4   ■   Another young patient, who has the delusion that he is Christ, answers *Glass Houses,* thus:
"Those who know that it has been seen what they have done – and believe me it has all been seen – Let him who is without sin cast the first stone. Okay? That's what I believe it means."
The same patient responds to *Rolling Stone* in this way:
"If you can continue to move and always move and always follow yourself and no one else, you'll never have the evil one within yourself." ■

Unfortunately, the sample of thinking provoked is usually so small and its pathology so equivocal that the test is of dubious virtue.

Judgment

Judgment   Judgment is usually tested by asking the patient a question like the following:

What would you do if you found a stamped, addressed envelope in the street?

Why are there laws?

Why should promises be kept?

Good judgment requires intact orientation, concentration, and memory. There is no evidence that a finding of poor judgment adds anything to diagnosis beyond that provided by detecting deficits in the lower-order functions.

Combination tests of cognitive functions

Combination tests   A number of standardized, quantifiable clinical assessments of organic brain disorder combine different mental functions in one test. The virtues of quantification and standardization are that reliability is thereby enhanced and baseline measures are available to detect deterioration or improvement. Several combination tests are described here.

The Short Portable Mental Status Questionnaire (SPMSQ)

Kahn et al. (1960) designed the Short Portable Mental Status Questionnaire (SPMSQ). As revised and refined by Pfeiffer (1975), it consists of 10 questions concerning orientation, memory, information, and calculation (see Table 9.6). Pfeiffer (1975) provided details for scoring the SPMSQ. The categories moderate or severe impairment coincide with the diagnosis of organic brain disorder in about 90% of cases. Test-retest reliability is excellent.

TABLE 9.6
The Short Portable Mental Status Questionnaire

1. What is the date today?
2. What day of the week is it?
3. What is the name of this place?
4. What is your telephone number?
    or
4A. What is your street address?
5. How old are you?
6. When were you born?
7. Who is president of the U.S., now?
8. Who was the president just before him?
9. What was your mother's maiden name?
10. Subtract three from twenty and keep subtracting three from each new number, all the way down.

0–2 Errors: intact intellectual functioning
3–4 Errors: mild impairment
5–7 Errors: moderate impairment
8–10 Errors: severe impairment

The Set Test

Isaacs and Kennie (1973) introduced this instrument as a simple test of cognitive function. The patient is asked to name as many items as possible in each of four categories: colors, animals, fruits, and towns. One point is allotted for each correct item up to 10 in each category, to a maximum score of 40. Scores under 15 are abnormal and likely to be associated with dementia. Scores of from 15 to 24 have a low association with dementia, while over 24 there is no association. Physical illness and low social class, but not depression, may depress scores.

The Cognitive Capacity Screening Examination (CCSE)

The Cognitive Capacity Screening Examination, introduced by Kaufman et al. (1979), is a brief mental status questionnaire aiming to detect cognitive impairment. It consists of questions covering orientation, concentration, memory, and conceptualization. The total score is 30, one point for each correct answer. Scores below 20 are regarded as indicating cognitive impairment. A sample of neurological inpatients yielded relatively few false positives but a considerable number of false negatives. The CCSE is not sensitive to such specific deficits as aphasia or anosognosia. This test requires further refinement.

The Mini-Mental State (MMS)

Folstein, Folstein and McHugh (1975) proposed the MMS as a brief test of cognitive function (see Table 9.7). The first part of the test covers orientation, memory, and concentration; the second part deals with expressive and receptive language and the graphic reproduction of patterns.

    The reliability of the MMS is high with little practice effect and is useful for following the patient's progress. It satisfactorily distinguishes dementia from depression with or without cognitive impairment. Scores of from 9 to 12 out of 30 indicate a high likelihood of organic impairment. Scores of over 25 predominate in normals and functional illness of neurotic or psychotic nature.

Language

The function of language

Language is a system used both for communication and as a tool of thought. Language facilitates thinking by hierarchically organizing ideas and concepts and by syntactically indicating the relationship between them. Language and thought are not inseparable, however; psychomotor thinking, for example, does not re-

TABLE 9.7
The Mini-Mental State

Part I

1. What is the (year) (season) (date) (day) (month)?   *(5 points)*
2. Where are we: (state) (county) (town) (hospital) (floor)? *(5 points)*
3. Name 3 objects (1 second each). Ask patient to name all three after you
   have said them.   *(3 points)*
4. Serial sevens. 1 point for each correct. Stop after 5 answers. *(5 points)*
5. Ask for the 3 objects repeated above.   *(3 points)*

Part II

1. Name a pencil and a watch.   *(2 points)*
2. Repeat: No ifs, ands, or buts.   *(1 point)*
3. Follow a three-stage command:
   Take a paper in your right hand, fold it in half, and put it on the
   floor.   *(3 points)*
4. Read and obey this written instruction:
   CLOSE YOUR EYES   *(1 point)*
5. Write a sentence *(not dictated)*   *(1 point)*
6. Copy a design *(intersecting pentagons)*   *(1 point)*

quire words. Picture to yourself, for example, the way you execute a tennis backhand, or the Stars and Stripes fluttering from a flagpole.

Articulation

Language competence is assessed from the patient's speech during the interview. A history of spoken or written language difficulty or an observation of clumsy articulation, disordered rhythm, and difficulty in the understanding or choice of words should be noted and further investigated.

Syntax
Vocabulary
Comprehension

Language comprehension is tested by asking the patient to point to single objects and then to point to a number of objects in a particular sequence. The examiner may also ask the patient to perform a series of actions in an arbitrary sequence. A clinical test of language functions is provided in Table 9.8.

Expression

Expression is evaluated by asking the patient to repeat words, phrases, and sentences after you and to name correctly a number of objects. Expression and comprehension are evaluated by asking the patient to read a passage aloud and to answer questions about it. Graphic language is tested by asking the patient to take dictation. Note any errors and slowness in performance.

Aphasia

These tests are used if **aphasia** is suspected. The three most common forms of aphasia are all manifest as difficulty in repeating words or phrases. In **Broca's aphasia,** comprehension is relatively intact but expression dysfluent, sparse, telegraphic, and full of circumlocution. In **Wernicke's aphasia,** comprehension is affected. Expression, though fluent, rambles, lacks meaning, and is full of errors to which the patient seems oblivious. In **conduction aphasia,** comprehension is intact, expression fluent but full of errors and pauses, and repetition is difficult; but reading is relatively intact.

Muteness

Wells and Duncan (1980) contend that **muteness** is seldom found in neurological disease (except in the acute phase), in seizure disorder, or in advanced cerebral degeneration. The aphasic is never mute. Muteness is more

TABLE 9.8
Clinical tests of language functions

I. Comprehension
   1. Point to single objects (table, chair, book, etc).
   2. Point to objects in a specified order.
   3. Perform actions in specified sequence:
      Touch your nose with your right index finger, then point that finger at me, then put it behind your back.

II. Expression
   4. Repeat single words:
      Bird
      Calumny
      Antidisestablishmentarianism
   5. Repeat separate phrases:
      Royal British Constabulary
      No ifs, ands, or buts
   6. Repeat separate sentences:
      You can't get there from here.
      These are the times that try men's souls.
   7. Name common objects:
      Pen, matches, book, tie, dictaphone.

III. Combined and Cross Modality Functions
   8. Read a printed paragraph aloud:

   The Cowboy and His Dog

   A cowboy from Arizona went to San Francisco with his dog, which he left at a friend's, while he purchased a new set of clothes. Dressed finely, he went back to the dog, whistled to him, called him by name, and patted him. The dog would have nothing to do with him in his new hat and coat but gave a mournful howl. Coaxing was of no effect, so the cowboy went away and donned his old garments, whereon the dog immediately showed his wild joy on seeing his master as he thought he ought to be.

   9. Answer questions about it:
      What is the gist of the story?
      Where did the cowboy come from?, etc.
   10. Take dictation:
      The quick brown fox jumps over the lazy dog.

commonly a sign of melancholia, stupor, catatonic stupor, somatoform disorder, dissociation, or negativism in children (elective mutism).

Aphasia vs. schizo-phrenic language

The main diagnostic problem is to differentiate schizophrenic language from the jargon of Wernicke's aphasia. Schizophrenic patients tend to be heedlessly bizarre in thought content; aphasics are more aware of their errors and more likely to use substitutions to overcome their language defects. The confused speech of schizophrenic patients is known as **word salad** or **schizophasia**. It may be so chaotic as to be barely comprehensible.

Paralogia

Talking past the point *(Vorbeireden)* or **paralogia** occurs when the patient gives erroneous answers that reveal a knowledge of the correct response. "How many legs has a cow?" asks the interviewer. "Five," says the patient. In the same vein, for example, a centipede has 200 legs, the United States is in the

Southern Hemisphere, and 5 + 5 = 11. Talking past the point occurs in the **Ganser Syndrome** (the syndrome of approximate answers), also known as **hysterical pseudodementia.** This syndrome is most likely to be found in patients who prefer hospitalization for insanity is to incarceration for crime.

   Neologisms are new words coined by the patient. They are often condensations of ideas (portmanteau words) that attempt to capture the ineffable.

Case 9.4

■   A 20-year-old man with accelerated thinking and some loose, paranoid concerns about being photographed has grandiose ideas of climbing the world's high peaks and "dying on K2." He wants to be "the best conservation officer in the world." To him, the forest means: "pigs, pridatory, and guts." The interviewer conjectures that *pridatory* is a condensation of *pride, predatory,* and possibly, *purgatory.* ■

Word coinage

Neologisms are most typical of schizophrenia; they must be distinguished from the paraphasia and circumlocution to which the aphasic patient resorts in order to overcome expressive difficulty. A neologism sometimes reveals that the patient has been derailed by the sound or sense of an associated word or idea. At other times, neologisms are a response to hallucinations or a defense (in a private code) against the intrusion by the examiner on the patient's privacy.

Thought

Process and form

Pathology of thought can be found in the process, form, or content of thinking. The process and form of thinking may be disordered in terms of:

1. Tempo
2. Fluency
3. Continuity
4. Control
5. Logical organization
6. Intent

Normal thinking is characterized by reasonable but not excessive speed and a smooth, continuous flow from one idea to the next. Normal thinking has clear goal-direction, organization, and consensual logic in the links between and the sequence of its constituent ideas.

Problem-solving styles

   In **convergent thinking** the problem solver, being governed by a definite objective, keeps tight control over the linkage between ideas. In **divergent thinking,** the connections are more fanciful in the service of fun or creativity (lateral thinking). Nevertheless, the normal thinker perceives all thoughts as personal and is consciously in charge of how tight, loose, or logical the associations should be. Overall, if intending to communicate something, the normal thinker is concerned about whether the audience follows what is being said.

In psychological illness, particularly the turmoil associated with such psychoses as schizophrenia and mania, any or all of these characteristics may be disorganized. Pathological thinking can be sluggish, headlong, disconnected, meandering, halting, and prone to lose its track, wander off at tangents, or follow an illogical line.

The subjective experience of abnormal thought process

Abnormal thinking can be experienced by the thinker as invaded, inserted, or controlled by alien forces **(thought insertion).** It can also be sensed as leaking, stolen, lost, or broadcast from the mind into the outside world **(thought alienation** and **thought broadcasting).**

Finally, the psychotic thinker, oblivious to the need to make sense, may lose contact with the audience or use language as a mocking camouflage.

Abnormalities of thought process

Tempo

Acceleration of thought

Thinking is accelerated in **flight of ideas,** which may reach such a pitch that goal direction is lost and the connection between ideas is governed not by sense but by sound or idiosyncratic verbal or conceptual associations. Alliteration, assonance, rhyme **(clang associations),** and punning may divert the torrent of ideas. Flight of ideas is usually associated with **pressure of speech** and may be experienced by the patient as racing thoughts.

Case 9.5

■ The patient has been asked why he has been admitted to the hospital. He responds with great intensity and pressure of speech:

"What do you want to know? My birth or my death? Ha ha! Because I'm rotten, begotten, because I make my needs known to personnel, because I sit in a wheelchair and scream. I'm dizzy, busy dizzy, dizzy busy dizzy. And I'm going to college, to be the best damned conservation officer in the world, and die, when I reach 100 or 200, on Mt. Everest, or K2, or one of the 48 high peaks. . . ." ■

Flight of ideas is characteristic of mania but can also occur in excited schizophrenic patients, especially those in acute catatonia. In hypomania, the flight of ideas is less marked, the tempo being accelerated but the associations less disorganized.

Deceleration of thought

The tempo of thinking may be slowed in **retardation of thought,** especially in major depression. The patient often complains of fuzziness, woolliness, and poor concentration. Response time to questions is increased. There are long silences, during which the patient may lose the thread. In the extreme, retardation becomes mutism or even stupor.

Circumstantiality

Fluency

In **circumstantiality,** although the goal direction of thinking is retained, associations meander into fruitless, overdetailed, or barely relevant byways. The listener may feel impelled to hurry the speaker along. Circumstantiality is said to be characteristic of some epileptic patients whose peculiar combination of pedantry, perseveration, religiosity, and cliché lend their thinking a viscous quality.

Perseveration

Perseveration refers to a tendency to persist with a point or theme even after it has been exhaustively dealt with or the listener has tried to change the subject. It is also seen, for example, when a child fixedly repeats one aspect of a drawing, leaving multiple lines or dwelling on the shading interminably.

Continuity

Blocking

In **thought blocking,** the patient's speech is abruptly interrupted by silences lasting for less than a second to much longer, even a minute or more. During the pause, the eyes may flicker, particularly if the patient is listening to an auditory hallucination, although sometimes the patient becomes blank mentally. Blocking can be precipitated by questions or ideas with personal significance, particularly if their import is threatening. Blocking is an uncommon but striking sign. It tends to be identified too often, the observer mistaking the retarded thinking of a depressed or preoccupied patient for the abrupt roadblock of the true phenomenon. It is almost pathognomonic of schizophrenia but must be differentiated from the absences of petit mal epilepsy, the hesitation caused by anxiety, and the peculiar mental fixity of amphetamine intoxication.

Tangential thinking

During the period of blocking, intermediate associations may be lost by the patient recommencing on an apparently different track **(tangential thinking).** This can give rise to a phenomenon known as **the knight's move in thought:** the listener can sometimes intuit how the patient got from A to E and realize that the unspoken intermediate associations (B, C, D) were quite indirect.

The knight's move

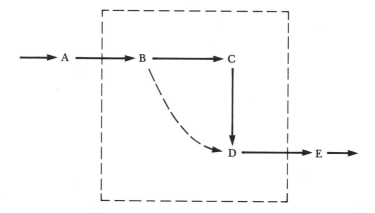

Derailing

On other occasions, thinking is subject to **derailing,** jumping the track to proceed on a different subject, particularly when a sore point has been touched on.

Patients are often aware of disturbances in the continuity of their thinking and will describe how their thoughts become paralyzed, interrupted, or jumbled.

Control

The perception of loss of control

Akin to these subjective phenomena is the patient's sense that speed, direction, form, or content of thought are out of control. Such complaints as "confused," "racing thoughts," "unable to concentrate," "scatterbrained," "jumbled," and "going crazy" often reflect the subjective perception of pathologically accelerated, dysfluent, or discontinuous thinking.

Thought alienation

Sometimes schizophrenic patients report their thinking is controlled by external forces or people, often by means of radio waves or other transmissions. Thinking may be perceived as directed by the external agency, or particular thoughts experienced as having been implanted by it. This is known as **thought insertion** or **thought alienation.**

Case 9.6

■   A former high school basketball star of 21 years who had never fulfilled his early promise as an athlete was disturbed by passers-by during pickup games. He was convinced that Linda and Paul McCartney had him under surveillance and that they interrupted his games by transmitting whispered messages that he was "a fag" and would never amount to anything.   ■

Thought deprivation

In **thought deprivation** or **broadcasting,** the patient senses that ideas are leaking out of the mind, being stolen by others, or being broadcast via radio or television. The perception that the television picks up and repeats one's thoughts may lead to a grandiose or persecutory delusional misinterpretation.

Logical organization

Pathology in the logical organization of thought

Psychotic thinking may reflect a deterioration in the capacity to think formally or logically. The schizophrenic patient commonly uses a private logic, with **overpersonalized concrete symbols.** Bleuler (1950) described the **condensation, displacement,** and **symbol-formation** of schizophrenic thought, deriving his ideas from Freud's concept of the primary process.

Private logic

Condensation equates disparate ideas that have a common property. By this means, one idea can represent another with which it has little in common. Displacement refers to an abnormal fluidity wherein one symbol can readily

Abnormal fluidity

stand for another despite its lack of similarity.

Lack of goal direction

Interpenetration of themes

Cameron (1938) refers to lack of goal direction and scattered associational flow as **asyndesis.** In **metonymic thinking,** the patient is satisfied with an erroneous, imprecise word that approximates the appropriate one. **Interpenetration of themes** is most often encountered when a rational line of discourse is interwoven with irrelevant fantasy.

Case 9.7

■ A patient could not converse with her doctor without giggling since she could not stop thinking how terrible he would look without clothes. ■

Overinclusion is another attribute of schizophrenic thought in which conceptual boundaries are blurred and conceptual thinking develops a metaphorical, overpersonal, and idiosyncratic quality.

Case 9.8

■ A 25-year-old man arrived unannounced at the door of a prominent citizen's home in order to hand the occupant a piece of paper on which he had inscribed matters of the greatest import. This document contained a number of cryptic and poorly spelled phrases alluding to cosmic problems. Among them were the following matters:

"The East is rising, 1,000,000,000."
"Z waves."
"The Dura Matter *[sic]*"
"Roman Catholic Confession"
"OPEC oil controls the West"
"Maui Waui"

He explained the connection between these phrases as follows:
China and Japan, with their teeming populations, are rising in influence. The West is in decline, controlled as it is by OPEC oil and by cosmic waves that penetrate the coverings of the human brain. The Roman Catholic Church of his parents is powerless to help. When he took a vacation in Hawaii, he enjoyed the local marijuana very much. ■

Derailment

Omission

Diffuseness

Schneider described the following features of schizophrenic thought disorder: **derailment** (see continuity), **substitution** (similar to Bleuler's concept of displacement), **omission, fusion** (the equivalent of Cameron's interpenetration), and **diffuseness.** In omission, a thought or part thereof drops out and leaves the statement puzzling or incoherent. Diffuseness refers to the blurring of a complex idea when its parts become muddled.

The following letter was received at a courthouse in Vermont. Look beyond the sense of grievance, grandiosity, and caricature of legalese to analyze closely the construction of ideas. Note the influence of alliteration on the headlong flow of associations. Note also the use of neologisms and the manner in which disparate ideas merge in a torrent of protest replete with asyndesis, metonymic thinking, overinclusion, and interpenetration of themes.

METAPHYSICAL JUSTICE OF AMERICA, INC.

The People's Ultimate Court of Metaphysical Law

Sept. 1, 1982 A.D.

Criminal Docket No. *one etc.*

President John Paul II
Metaphysical World Court
Vatican, Nation

President J. M.
Local Metaphysical Court
(Address)
Burlington, Vt.

Dear Sirs:

Matthew S. C. . . . , president of Metaphysical World and National Democratic Civil Social Justice of America, Inc., as of September 1, 1980 A.D. rules the World Court governmental officials guilty of the most heinously unconstitutional criminal world Court Cover-up Conspiracy Scandal in world court history.

Television, radio, newspaper, magazine, executive, judicial, U.S. Justice dept. officials, U.N. Justice dept. officials, civil attorneys, etc., worldwide and nationally, are immorally indebted to each other to criminally manage the social news in the interest to stonewall civil social constitutional justice and camouflage official criminal records from public knowledge. The abhorrent civil social misconduct of the civil citizen which is politically outlawed in the social interest of social order, harmony, peace and justice is doubly practiced with greater magnitude and intensity by executive and judicial officials, etc., ever scheming the distribution of their criminally social misjudgments and mispractices to all other members of the executive, judicial, etc. family gang members.

Social constitutional and general legal social justice is a criminally manipulated political and judicial, etc. social hoax in which said officials unitedly camouflage their criminal misrecords behind police, sheriff, FBI agents, etc. violence deliberately constructing a political criminal arsenal of militant political criminal misjudgements. The American taxpayers yield their tax dollars under political jail threats by judicial, attorney, police, FBI agents, IRS agents etc. militants, simultaneously governmental officials lawlessly and criminally burglarize the civil and taxpayers' treasuries to pay the cost to continue to militantly and criminally harass law abiding civil citizens.

Constitutional and social legal integrity and the so-called code of executive, judicial, attorney, etc. ethics is militantly bulldozed in the immoral interest to cover-up the executive, judicial, attorney, etc. criminal misjudgements records within the political and judicial family clan. The Richard Nixon Watergate cover-up dwarfs the present World Court and U.S. Supreme Court criminal cover-up misconduct of the James Carter, Richard Snelling [Vermont governor] and former American presidential, Vt. gubernatorial, judicial, etc. criminally, unconstitutionally, lawlessly, tyrannically, etc. political administrations. etc., etc. . . . .

Here is another letter, received by a publishing company. Try to analyze it, bearing in mind the disorders of thought process already described.

(Date)
(Address)

The (   ) Press
Poetry
(Street)
New York, NY 10022

Dear Poetry Editor,

    In the glimmer of my service to a form of servile ethics in Art, I have requested of the wife of my compilations, on the subject of my focus heart and soul of being published only on the West Coast, something more than the coy reply. My intuitions forming a coalition of tact will resound loyally, apparently where its tradition is served. Its party of one steering a course sticks to absinth *[sic]* and runs from nothing. I have mounted "a considerable press" feeling it important – not an elevator company. The children of this theory, behind a poet's place and his work, often, sadly, lurch, taking up every square inch of well-executed self-observation as if the class time were investment. Profits, their modular units, exist, to be sure, compensation for team work. When I at last know the infernal pitch by heart I will have already been scheduled with a publisher. With your patient in mind, I realize I am acting as though I owe my efforts something, which communication should yet weigh; whatever the answer it should not preclude prestigious handling, the (   ) Press the notion I have in mind.

    The cosmic force behind music and dance of poetry detonates with any 'Scorpio rising,' and maybe this unfortunate menstrual niche teaches us of famine in the hemisphere; we want it to teach us of harmonics and celestial pregnancy. This touches the hard item of campaigning with Poetry: the odious comparison the addition of weight in exercises lacking the puberty and picnic ham of the festivity. Abuse has been much the judge, when a calm focus on Work is recommended because nothing else is required.

    The philosophical parent has resisted going openface on rye because of accompanying photogenic fatality. Even as I reduce the hyperactivity, I still concern that how something is done (on whichever Coast a work is published) pursues the nimble honesty of its efforts. I think (   ) could handle the 75 poems in total, the few enclosed not so much the "naked proofs" as freedom from claustrophobic disaster. When last night I prepared the draft to this letter, the most popular of trends occurred to me – to be trends in anything; the best were queries, literal copies from *The Boston Globe,* e.g. The much-dedicated on the truth of David and John and Frank, professors or repairmen, we now have in the tight fists of the obtusely familial, with hints it is also sexual. I do not know. It sounds in Christmas allegorizing – with the few pieces I have sent along selected for the sending to represent a variant of emotional and intellectual equipment throughout, with still the best outstanding. That would be my feeling.

    To open a personal bid should not just "telephone smiling"; I am particularly tough on how I want things done and ward of no outcome, bid bagels and taste.

Cordially,

(Signature)

poet, artist

Intent of communication

Mockery and caricature in schizophrenic communication

The conventional purpose of discourse is to communicate, but the clinician may be misled by the intentions of a schizophrenic patient. The schizophrenic patient may attempt to remain private or to deride the clinician subtly by conversing in an obscure, remote, supercilious, mocking, caricatured, or farcical manner. The following passage is translated from Kraepelin's (1905) *Lectures in Clinical Psychiatry*. Kraepelin regarded this patient's talk as "only a series of disconnected sentences having no relation whatever to the general situation" (p. 80).

> The patient I will show you today has almost to be carried into the room, as he walks in a straddling fashion on the outside of his feet. On coming in, he throws off his slippers, sings a hymn loudly, and then cries twice (in English), "My father, my real father!" He is 18 years old, and a pupil of the Oberrealschule [higher-grade modern school], tall, and rather strongly built, but with a pale complexion, on which there is very often a transient flush. The patient sits with his eyes shut, and pays no attention to his surroundings. He does not look up even when he is spoken to, but he answers beginning in a low voice, and gradually screaming louder and louder. When asked where he is, he says, "You want to know that too? I tell you who is being measured and is measured and shall be measured. I know all that, and could tell you, but I do not want to." When asked his name, he screams, "What is your name? What does he shut? He shuts his eyes. What does he hear? He does not understand; he understands not. How? Who? Where? When? What does he mean? When I tell him to look, he does not look properly. You there, just look! What is it? What is the matter? Attend; he attends not. I say, what is it, then? Why do you give me no answer? Are you getting impudent again? How can you be so impudent? I'm coming! I'll show you! You don't whore for me. You mustn't be smart either; you're an impudent, lousy fellow, such an impudent, lousy fellow I've never met with. Is he beginning again? You understand nothing at all, nothing at all; nothing at all does he understand. If you follow now, he won't follow, will not follow. Are you getting still more impudent? Are you getting impudent still more? How they attend, they do attend," and so on. At the end, he scolds in quite inarticulate sounds. (pp. 79–80)

In a celebrated discourse, Laing (1960) pointed out that Kraepelin's vivid description of this patient belies his contention that the young man "has not given us a single piece of useful information." Laing suggests that the patient is carrying on a dialogue between a parody of the clinician ("What is your name? What does he shut . . . ?") and himself in an obdurate, rebellious mood ("How can you be so impudent?") He seems to resent being on show for an audience ("You don't whore for me") and being asked irrelevant, footling questions in the midst of his suffering. His communication can be evaluated in several ways: in one sense as a series of ideas too egocentrically and idiosyncratically organized to be readily comprehended (the signs of schizophrenia) and in another sense as a hostile, mocking caricature of an interrogation regarded by the patient as insensitive, authoritarian, critical, and heedless.

Abnormalities of thought content

This section classifies and defines phenomena closely aligned with severe psychopathology. These salient clues are often the key features of a psychiatric disorder; in fact, several disorders are virtually defined by their presence. In many instances, the patient will complain of these phenomena (for example, a phobia of heights); in other cases, the patient appears to have accepted an eccentric idea (for example, the delusion of being a reincarnation of Christ) and to be acting accordingly. Sometimes, however, the patient is in two minds about the phenomenon.

Case 9.9

■ Michael, a 26 year-old man who claims to be Jesus Christ in his third coming, speaks as though ex cathedra, in a manner replete with phrases from Revelations. Armageddon is imminent, he insists, but those who come unto him will be spared.

As the interview proceeds and the interviewer continues to press questions about the patient's life, he first becomes agitated, then angry, and finally bursts into bitter tears, saying: "Don't ask me, judge yourselves! Can't you see – I'm just a man, and I've always been a man. I'm just Michael." ■

Ego-syntonic and ego-alien symptoms

Abnormalities of thought content, therefore, may be accepted by the subject, that is, **ego-syntonic** (for example, a fixed delusional belief); abnormal thoughts may be resisted as **ego-alien** (for example, a recurrent obsession); or they may be intermediate between the two (for example, when the patient is still unsure of the validity of a loose delusional system). Psychosis (at best, a vague notion) is defined in part by the fidelity of reality testing; for example, by the attitude taken by the patient to his or her own aberrant mentations.

Abnormal thought can be divided into the following categories:

1. Abnormal perceptions
2. Abnormal convictions.
3. Abnormal preoccupations and impulses.
4. Abnormalities in the sense of self.

Abnormal perceptions

Abnormalities of the process of perception

Perception is physical sensation given meaning, the integration of sensory stimuli to form an image or impression in a manner or configuration influenced by past experience.

Heightened, dulled, and deviant perception

Perception can be increased or decreased in intensity. **Heightened perception** occurs in delirium, mania, after hallucinogens, and in the rare ecstatic states occurring as part of acute schizophrenia or transported hysterical trances. **Dulled perception** occurs in depression and organic delirium.

In **derealization,** the external world seems different, changed, vague, unreal, or distant. This symptom is common in normal adolescence, usually in association with depersonalization. It is also found in anxiety or dissociative disorders, depression, schizophrenia, organic brain disorder, and after hallucinogens. In **synesthesia,** the subject perceives color in response, for example, to music. This is a common psychedelic experience.

The perception of time

Abnormalities of time perception

Time may be experienced as **accelerated** under the influence of hallucinogens, in mania, or during an epileptic aura. Time may seem **slowed** or **stopped** in depression or epilepsy. In some conditions, time seems to **lack continuity** and the subject feels uninvolved in the temporal stream. This is particularly likely to be encountered in depersonalization, amnestic syndromes, depression, schizophrenia, or toxic-confusional states.

Illusions

False perception

An **illusion** is sensory stimulation given a false interpretation, that is, a false perception. Illusions are most likely when the mind is under the sway of an emotionally determined ideational set (for example, vigilance for an intruder), when sensory clarity is reduced (for example, at night), or when both sets of circumstances are operating (as when a frightened elderly patient has both eyes bandaged following ophthalmic surgery).

The modality of illusions

Illusions are common in delirium, and may be **visual** (fluttering curtains seen as intruders), **auditory** (a slamming door interpreted as the report of a pistol), **tactile** (skin sensations thought to be caused by vermin), **gustatory** (poison detected in the taste of food), **kinesthetic** (flying), or **visceral** (abdominal pain thought to be caused by ground glass). Illusions can also occur in hysteria, depression, and schizophrenia, particularly when perception is subordinated to a delusional idea (for example, of guilt or persecution) or to an emotion of great force (for example, abandonment or erotic yearning).

Hallucinations

False perception without a stimulus

A **hallucination** is a false perception occurring in the waking state in the absence of a sensory stimulus. It is not merely a sensory distortion or misinterpretation, and it carries a subjective sense of conviction. A true hallucination appears to the subject to be substantial and to occur in external objective space. In contrast, a mental image is insubstantial and experienced within internal subjective space.

Pseudohallucination

Intermediate between image and hallucination is the **pseudohallucination,** which the subject experiences as insubstantial and which seems to hover somewhere between internal and external space. Try to identify the following examples:

■ Exalted by a night of love, the young man recalled the gentle touch of his girl, inhaled again the fragrance of her hair, and remembered the very words she spoke to him as they parted. ■

■ Whenever she was tempted to shoplift, the middle-aged woman would hear an inner voice warning her to stop. The voice belonged to nobody in particular; in fact, she could not say whether it was male or female. ■

■ On his worst days, the student would hear the voices, sometimes of men, sometimes of women, commenting mockingly on everything he did. Although he got rid of his television set and discontinued the telephone, the voices persisted. ■

Circumstances conducive to hallucinosis

Fish (1967) describes five circumstances conducive to **hallucinosis:** (a) intense emotion, (b) suggestion, (c) disorder of peripheral sense organs, (d) sensory deprivation, and (e) central nervous disorder.

Melancholic patients may hear disconnected voices speaking to them in an accusatory or disparaging way (''you're rotten'') in accordance with their delusions of guilt. Hallucinations may occur in situations of great stress:

■ Cajoled, cast-down, and humiliated for a heinous crime, a young man heard a voice telling him that there was still a way out, provided he dedicated the rest of his life to Christ. ■

Hallucinations, usually visual, can spread by contagion, suggestion being very potent in situations of communal stress or privation. During World War I, many German and British troops saw an angel in the sky at Mons.

Deafness, tinnitus, or blindness, usually in association with dementia or delirium, may determine the modality of hallucinations. Sensory deprivation experiments have produced visual and auditory hallucinosis in many subjects. Hallucinosis and delirium following cataract operation probably acts by the same mechanism, especially in association with dementia.

Diencephalic and cortical disease may be associated with hallucinations (usually visual). Tumors of the olfactory or basal temporal regions may cause olfactory hallucinosis, for example as an aura. Hallucinations, especially visual (although sometimes vestibular or kinesthetic), are common in the delirium caused by toxins (drugs, hallucinogens, alcohol, toxins, and fever), cerebrovascular disease, and central degenerative disorders. Hallucinations may also be a prominent feature of the uncommon schizophrenia-like psychosis associated with epilepsy.

Aside from these circumstances, hallucinations are common and normal, especially in some people, when falling asleep **(hypnagogic)** or waking **(hypnopompic).** Severe sleep deprivation can cause a hypnagogic hallucinosis.

*The modality of
hallucinations*

Systemization

*Varieties of
hallucination*

Having defined hallucinations and described the circumstances in which they appear, let us classify them by sensory modality and relate them to the psychiatric disorders of which they are most characteristic.

Hallucinations can be (a) auditory, (b) visual, (c) olfactory or gustatory, (d) tactile, or (e) somatic. In form, they may be amorphous, elementary, or complex. They may be experienced as emanating from inner or outer space, and, if from outside, from near or far. Hallucinations may be **unsystematized,** appearing to have no link to life circumstances, or **systematized** and part of a causally interconnected delusional world.

Auditory hallucinations may be inchoate (humming, rushing water, inaudible murmurs, etc.), fragmentary (such words or phrases such as *fag, get him, beastly*), or complex. Typically, the schizophrenic patient locates complex hallucinations in inner or outer space, as a voice or voices speaking to or about him or her. The voice may be soothing, mocking, disparaging, or noncommittal. Sometimes the voice echoes the patient's thoughts or comments neutrally on actions ("Now he's getting up, . . . Now he walks to the door . . ."). Sometimes the voice orders the patient to perform actions or puts thoughts into his or her head, an experience verging on thought insertion. The voice may be perceived as coming from the radio or television, from outside the window, or even from a distant place. In alcoholic hallucinosis, usually, a conspiracy of threatening whisperers plan to injure the patient, provoking self-defense or flight.

Visual hallucinations vary from elemental flashes of light or color, as in disorders of the visual pathways and cortex, to well-formed scenes of people, animals, insects, and things. In delirium, insects or other small objects may be seen moving on the bed or in the surroundings. **Lilliputian hallucinations** (of little people on the bed, for example) occur in delirium and other organic brain syndromes. Complex audiovisual hallucinations may occur in temporal lobe epilepsy. In general, visual hallucinosis suggests acute brain disorder rather than functional psychosis and tends to occur in a setting of confusion or obtundation. Sometimes, however, a schizophrenic patient will report visual hallucinations (trips in flying saucers, for example) aligned with prevailing delusions. The visual hallucinations of hysteria or dissociative disorder have a pseudohallucinatory quality and sometimes reproduce a traumatic event, as when a war veteran relives a battle incident.

Olfactory and **gustatory hallucinations** may occur in epilepsy (burning rubber, steak and onions, etc.). Schizophrenic patients may perceive gas being pumped into their bedrooms by persecutors or taste malign substances in their food. Melancholic patients may be conscious of the stench of corruption rising from their unworthy bodies or complain of the changed metallic and tasteless quality of their meals.

Tactile hallucinations are characteristic of cocaine and amphetamine intoxication, the patient being distracted by the sensation of insects crawling on the skin **(formication).** Schizophrenic patients may detect the effect on the skin of radioactivity beamed at them from a hostile source.

Somatic hallucinations occur in schizophrenia as genital, visceral, intra-cerebral, or kinesthetic sensations, often being referred to the influence of persecutors or machines. The melancholic patient may have the sense of having no stomach, with food dropping from the throat into a void.

In schizophrenia or under the influence of hallucinogens, the patient may have the uncanny sense that somebody, a presence, is behind him or her. This can occur in states of extreme fear; it can also become a central feature of schizophrenia, in the guise of the *Doppelgänger* or *Horla*, a **hallucinatory double** of the self lurking just behind the periphery of vision.

Abnormal convictions

False belief
Overvalued idea

A **delusion** is a false belief not susceptible to argument and inconsistent with the subject's sociocultural background. Bordering on delusion is the **overvalued idea,** a notion that may be eccentric rather than false but that becomes a governing force in the patient's life. Consider the following situations:

Case 9.10   ■ A 45-year-old woman, very guilty about a sexual affair she had had several years previously, became agitated and insomniac. One day she looked into her husband's eyes, perceived that he knew everything, and realized from his expression that the marriage was finished. All this she knew without a word passing between them on the matter of her guilty secret. ■

Case 9.11   ■ A 30-year-old member of the counterculture identifies himself with the Hierophant on the tarot cards and tells the clinician that he knows he is a white wizard because he can sometimes communicate telepathically with his friends.

Case 9.12   ■ A 40-year-old man spends much of his spare time writing letters to authorities, trying to organize a grass-roots movement and attending rallies carrying a banner. He aims to combat the fluoridation of water supplies. He is convinced that water fluoridation causes sterility and that evidence to the contrary has been suppressed by profluoridation forces. ■

It is not always easy to draw the line between (a) a crank, (b) somebody holding unfamiliar views that are nevertheless consistent with a different socio-cultural system, and (c) a deluded person. Indeed, some people drift across the misty boundaries between these categories. An active delusion, however, is rigid, unshakable, and self-evident. It dominates the subject's life, subordinating all other matters. It is private, idiosyncratic, ego-centered, and inconsistent with the common experience of people from the same background. A delusion, therefore, isolates the subject from others and alienates them.

The characteristics
of a delusion

The origin of
delusional thinking

Scharfetter (1980) describes a number of situations that act as the soil in which delusions may take root and proliferate. Delusions affect people under the sway of such powerful emotion that they cannot entertain an alternative perspective of their predicament. Delusions may arise from pathology of mood, in accordance with the prevailing euphoria or dysphoria. Manic patients develop delusions of grandeur, for example; melancholics have delusions of decay, death, disease, poverty, sin, damnation, punishment, or nihilism. A person in a life situation characterized by isolation, confinement, unspoken accusation, or intolerable loss of self-esteem may be predisposed to delusional thinking. Franz Kafka described this kind of insecurity in *The Trial*. The deaf, lonely, or elderly person may be subject to ideas of persecution, as may the immigrant alone in a strange new country. The querulous litigant who has been unsuccessful in a compensation case, for example, may be consumed by the need for redress; and the impotent alcoholic may suspect his wife of infidelity. Sometimes the delusion appears to compensate for personal failure.

Case 9.13   ■ An unemployed and isolated 20-year-old man, who had never fulfilled an early promise of intellectual superiority, was convinced he would make his fortune from a complicated board game he had adapted from the floor plan of the Temple at Karnak. The game had so many rules, however, and the directions and exceptions were so complicated that nobody but the inventor could follow it. After several manufacturers of board games rejected his invention, he became convinced that there was a conspiracy to rob him of his work. ■

Severe sensory deprivation, or exhaustion and physical privation, may lead to delusional misinterpretation, often associated with wish-fulfilling hallucinations. A delusion can act as a transcendental solution to an existential wasteland.

Case 9.14   ■ His career a catalogue of failure, drug addiction, physical illness, accidents, and misery, a 25-year-old man suddenly conceives that there is a grand design behind the tortured path he has trodden. His life is a sacrifice for errant humanity; he has returned again as Christ, to receive the penitence of those who accept him. But he will not be betrayed; he will not spare those who again seek to sell him out. ■

This is the ground from which cosmic, messianic, redemptive delusions grow.

European psychiatrists have propounded the concept of the **primary**
Primary delusion   **delusion,** thought to be characteristic of schizophrenia. In this situation, the patient has a sense of something obscure but important and threatening, occurring all around. A sudden delusional revelation solves the puzzle.

Case 9.15   ■ Aware that something is amiss, the subject looks about the dining room and suddenly realizes that the layout of the cutlery has been tampered with in such a way as to indicate that the CIA has his family under surveillance. ■

It is contended that the new primary delusional interpretation of the environment cannot be understood as an extension of the patient's premorbid personality or current mood state. Primary delusions, therefore, are characterized by sudden, revelatory onset, discontinuity with previous personality or mood, and a transcendent quality.

Different kinds of delusion

The most prevalent delusions are of persecution, jealousy, love, grandeur, disease, poverty, and guilt. **Delusions of persecution** are most frequently encountered in schizophreniform disorders or schizophrenia, paranoid disorders, organic mental disorder (especially alcoholic hallucinosis, amphetamine delirium, or delusional disorder, other hallucinogenic syndromes. epilepsy, and all forms of delirium) and less commonly in melancholia or in transitory psychotic breaks in the life-course of borderline personality. The patient may perceive others as talking conspiratorially about him or her **(delusions of reference)** or spying. External agencies (communists, FBI, freemasons, etc.) are regarded as acting in concert and disconcerting the subject with radiation, poisonous gases, radio and television, intruders, or assassins. Tape recorders, cameras, and other surveillance paraphernalia are often alluded to. Delusions of poisoning, particularly by the spouse, are sometimes encountered.

Persecutory

Referential

Jealous

Delusions of jealousy occur in the same syndromes as delusions of persecution but are especially likely in association with alcoholism in men. In that case, delusions of marital infidelity (possibly related to alcoholic impotence) are characteristic, and the wife and her effects are closely scrutinized for evidence of adultery.

Grandiose

Delusions of grandeur occur in mania, schizophrenia, paranoid disorders, and organic delusional syndromes (for example, neurosyphilis). In mania and organic grandiosity, the patient's megalomania (of being God, the governor, the Virgin Mary, Napoleon, etc.) are consonant with the general high spirits. In schizophrenia and paranoid disorders, an inflated sense of importance may be reinforced by admiring auditory hallucinations and ideas of persecution may lead to grandiosity. Why else, thinks the subject, would important agencies (e.g., the FBI, Vatican, or PLO) be persecuting me?

Erotic

Erotic delusions (erotomania) are more common in female schizophrenic or paranoid patients. A lonely person develops a crush on somebody, often a celebrity or prominent citizen. Fantasies evolve into delusions, and the subject bombards his or her heart's desire with telephone calls and messages. The failure of the loved one to reciprocate is ascribed to conspiratorial forces standing in the way of destiny. In schizophrenia, the patient may receive **erotic hallucinations** (e.g., of auditory and genital type) from the beloved.

Somatic

Somatic delusions, usually of disease or ill health, occur in many psychiatric disorders. Schizophrenic patients may have bizarre complaints, possibly in an attempt to explain somatic hallucinatory experiences (e.g., of blood running backward in the head, of radiation being trained on the genitals by an outside agency, or of objects placed inside the body by malign forces). In melancholia, the patient may have delusions of being dead (no blood in the body), of internal organs rotting away, or of the brain destroyed by syphilis, in retribution for an unpardonable sin. The boundary between hypochondriasis, disease phobia, and disease conviction, on the one hand, and somatic delusions on the other may be difficult to define.

Poverty

Nihilistic

Primitive

Melancholic patients are also prone to **delusions of poverty** and **nihilism.** The future is hopeless, the present desolate, and the patient rendered destitute by a malign fate. Depressive patients may also complain of inordinate **guilt,** and that the most extreme punishments are warranted for unremarkable ancient transgressions.

Abnormal preoccupations and impulses

The following abnormal preoccupations are often associated in psychiatric disorder: phobias, obsessions, and compulsions.

The quality of phobia

A **phobia** is a morbid, irrationally exaggerated dread that focuses on a particular object, situation, or act. Phobias differ from generalized anxiety in their focused quality, although a diffuse anxiety state sometimes precedes a phobic disorder. The patient is aware of the exaggerated, irrational nature of a phobia and regards it as symptomatic. The patient often tries to avoid the phobic situation or is compelled to perform actions (such as hand washing) in order to eradicate the object of the fear or atone for tabooed action.

Many objects, situations, or acts can be foci for phobias. The custom of designating each of them with a Greek prefix is now obsolete. A few of these terms, however, are still in use: claustrophobia (fear of enclosed spaces), zoophobia (fear of animals), acrophobia (fear of heights), and agoraphobia (fear of open spaces).

Types of phobia

Agoraphobia is common and serious enough to be classified as a separate disorder in DSM–III (see chapter 10). In this condition, the patient fears being alone, incapacitated, and unaided in public places (streets, supermarkets, public transport) and, as a consequence, stays home. The childhood equivalent of agoraphobia is **school phobia,** a condition in which a fear of going to school is the superficial aspect of a fear of leaving the parent. In this condition, parental psychopathology is intricately intertwined with the child's disorder.

Social phobia involves the fear and avoidance of social groups, as in restaurants, where the patient fantasizes losing self-control in a humiliating way while under public scrutiny.

Phobias occur as a normal part of childhood development. In adults, they occur after actual trauma (the car driver who fears driving after an accident, for example) or as displaced, projected, symbolized derivatives of unconscious conflict in anxiety disorders.

Obsessions and compulsions

An **obsession** is a persistent idea, desire, image, phrase, or fragment of music cutting into the stream of conscious thinking. The patient recognizes the alien nature of the obsession and attempts to resist it, but without success. The obsession often presses the subject to perform **compulsive acts,** on pain of anxiety. The key characteristics of obsessions are their persistent, irresistible, imperative nature, ego-alien quality, and repetitiousness.

Case 9.16 ■ When scantily clad women appeared on the television screen, a very religious 13-year-old boy would become highly anxious lest impure thoughts come into his head. To ward them off, he would repeat several Hail Mary's. So often did he pester the priest at confession with dubious transgressions that the priest told his mother he had "scruples" and needed psychiatric help. ■

Case 9.17 ■ To avoid microbial contamination, the 30-year-old housewife cleaned the door-knobs and toilet daily and abraded the skin of her hands by frequent scrubbing with a hard brush. ■

Case 9.18 ■ An 18-year-old woman with a new baby began to avoid using knives. Whenever she saw one, she had a frightening impulse to stab the infant. ■

Obsessional symptoms have been reported after encephalitis. They occur in the premonitory phase of schizophrenia or as part of a major depression (for example, persistent ruminations that old tax returns were in error and ruin will result). Obsessive-compulsive symptoms are most characteristic of the anxiety disorder with the same name.

Impulsions   **Impulsions** differ from compulsions in that they are less likely to be resisted and they are episodic rather than repetitive, although the distinction may be blurred at times. Impulsions tend to occur in externalizing personalities, whereas compulsions are more typical of inhibited, constricted people. Impulsions cause difficulty for others and may lead to legal entanglements. Impulsive acts often spring from an emotional setting of anger, anxiety, frustration, rejection, sadness, or humiliation, particularly when the subject is disinhibited by alcohol.

Common impulsions include: physical assault, sexual assault, fast driving, drinking, eating, gambling, sexual exhibitionism, shoplifting, stealing, and setting fires. Sudden, episodic, if not explosive, onset is the hallmark of these phenomena. The subject does not or cannot exercise inhibition or self-control. Feeling short-circuits thought, leading to action without reflection. The subject may feel dazed, relieved or numb after the impulsive action.

Abnormalities of the sense of self

The normal person has a sense of selfhood composed of these elements: a sense of distinction between self and outside world; a sense of existing and of being involved in one's own body and activity; a sense of temporal continuity between one's past, present, and future; a sense of personal integrity.

Depersonalization   In psychiatric disorder, any or several of these phenomena may be disturbed; for example, the individual may feel uninvolved in his or her own body or actions, like a spectator looking at another person **(depersonalization)**; the

Discontinuity   sense of temporal continuity may be dislocated, past and future seeming remote, and the present but a series of disconnected scenes; the ego may feel as though it is falling apart, shedding, fragmented, or split in two; and the difference between the self and other persons or objects may have become blurred.

Derealization

The sense of depersonalization, often associated with **derealization,** the perception that the external world is unreal or remote, occurs in adolescence, epilepsy, dissociative disorders, schizophrenia, and depression. Adolescents in severe emotional turmoil **(identity diffusion)** sometimes develop a sense of **discontinuity, disintegration,** and **dedifferentiation.** These symptoms are common after ingestion of hallucinogens (in which they may be reexperienced as flashbacks), and in reactive psychosis and schizophreniform disorders.

Disintegration

Physiological functions

Sleep

Sleep disturbances are often encountered in psychiatric practice. Sleep deprivation may precipitate or accentuate psychiatric disorder. Sleep disturbance may be a prodrome, a symptom, or a sequel of psychiatric disorder. Many psychopharmacologic agents also affect sleep (see chapter 5).

Insomnia

Insomnia is a common symptom. Worry, fear, and anxiety are likely to prevent the patient from falling asleep or create restless, light sleep with frequent waking. Mania and acute schizophreniform disorders are often associated with insomnia. Early morning wakening, when the patient's mood and energy are at their lowest ebb, is associated particularly with major depression and less commonly with dementia or delirium.

Hypersomnia

Psychogenic **hypersomnia** (excessive sleep) occurs in anxiety disorders, dissociative disorder, dysthymic personality, and major depression. It should be differentiated from the sleep disturbances of encephalitis, myxedema and brain tumor, abscess, or hemorrhage. The diurnal hypersomnia of the Pickwickian syndrome is thought to be due to obstruction of the upper airways, causing nocturnal cerebral anoxia. The hypersomnia of the Pickwickian syndrome and sleep apnea tend to occur in the obese, though this is not necessarily the case with sleep apnea. Narcolepsy causes episodic attacks of hypersomnia, hypnagogic hallucinations, sleep paralysis, and cataplexy, though not all of these features need be present. The Kleine-Levin syndrome most often afflicts adolescent males, causing prolonged hypersomnia and intermittent waking with hyperphagia and apparent confusion.

Sleepwalking

Sleepwalking tends to occur in Stage III or IV sleep. The somnambulist engages in automatic activities and may even be capable of brief conversation but afterward is amnestic for the episode. Though the condition is probably a normal physiological variant, it is likely to be accentuated by waking anxiety or stress. In this, it is akin to **night terrors** in children (with which it may be associated), the child waking and screaming in fright for some time, making little sense, and eventually going back to sleep after being comforted.

Nightmares

Nightmares occur in REM sleep and are remembered on waking, at least for a time, in contrast to night terrors. They occur in normal people, anxiety disorders, early schizophrenia, delirium, and posttraumatic stress disorder. After medication suppressing REM sleep (such as tricyclic antidepressants) is withdrawn, the patient may experience transient REM rebound, with an increase of vivid dreaming.

Appetite

Increased appetite

Appetite may be increased in depression (especially dysthymic personality) and after psychotropic drug medication. Eating binges (not necessarily determined by increased appetite) may occur in **bulimia** as a condition separate from, in alternation with, or following, anorexia nervosa. Bulimia is often associated with forced vomiting.

Anorexia

Anorexia and weight loss can occur in almost any stress condition but are particularly likely in major depression, paranoid schizophrenia, somatoform disorders, alcoholism, drug addiction, and, of course, anorexia nervosa. A comprehensive physical screening is always required when anorexia and weight loss are salient.

Libido

Increase of libido

Sexual desire may be increased in mania, in some forms of acute schizophrenia, and in narcissistic or borderline personality under stress. Sexual behavior may be disinhibited after alcohol or drugs, in delirium, and in organic dementia. Nymphomania is a male fantasy about female insatiability; insofar as it exists at all, it is probably related to the sensual clinging of a dependent person.

Decrease of libido

Sexual desire is decreased by any debilitating disorder, by anxiety, worry, tiredness, age, poor nutrition, and by lack of affection for the partner. It can be reduced by depression, schizophrenia, alcoholism, substance abuse, and by neuroleptic, antihypertensive, and antidepressant medication.

Menstrual cycle

Amenorrhea

Absent, irregular, infrequent, and scanty menstrual periods (**amenorrhea** or **oligomenorrhea**) may occur in psychiatric disorder, particularly in depression, anorexia nervosa, anxiety disorders, schizophrenia, and substance abuse. Any condition reducing total body fat to below 14% in the female produces anovulation and amenorrhea.

Dysmenorrhea and pelvic pain
Dysmenorrhea, dyspareunia, vaginismus, and other pelvic complaints are common in somatoform disorders and in abnormal illness behavior generally, but a discretionary physical screen is required before a stress-related condition is diagnosed.

Other physiological functions

Hyperdynamic and hypodynamic states
Any or all body systems can be accelerated in the hyperdynamic states of anxiety, delirium, mania, and catatonic excitement or slowed in the general hypomotility of depression, organic dementia, and hypothyroidism.

Anergia
The level of energy, or fatigue, may also be affected by disorders with accelerated or sluggish mental processes. In somatoform disorders, anergia, weakness, or obscure bodily discomfort are frequently encountered.

Attitude to illness

The patient's attitude or insight into the illness has several aspects. Does the patient recognize a personal problem? Is the problem identified as personal and psychological in nature? Does the patient understand the nature and cause of the illness? Is help wanted and, if so, what kind of help?

Lack of insight
Hypomanic patients have no problems. They feel very well: high-spirited, amusing, energetic, expansive, and optimistic. The manic or schizophrenic patients may view the problem as external – other people or agencies are stupidly obstructive or malevolent. Many patients with externalizing personality disorders (borderline, antisocial and narcissistic, for example) blame others for their predicaments.

Intellectual insight
Sophisticated patients, particularly those who have undergone previous treatment, may have considerable knowledge of the formal diagnosis and the theoretical or actual causes of their disorder. This sometimes causes problems in treatment; other mental health professionals who develop psychiatric illness are notoriously difficult to manage for this reason.

Rejection of psychiatric treatment
The patient may be aware of having a problem but want no help or want help of a particular sort or from a particular kind of clinician. Whenever the latter is reasonable and feasible, it should, of course, be arranged. The patient's desires should be respected as far as possible in the negotiation phase of the clinical process.

Summary: the tactics of the Mental Status Examination

The clinician will seldom if ever need to turn over every stone and pebble in this chapter. What is required is a set of criteria to decide (1) when a brief screening

MSE is indicated; (2) when a more comprehensive screening MSE is essential; and (3) when to pursue a discretionary MSE.

The brief screening MSE

When a patient has been referred to an ambulatory clinic for a situational or personality problem and none of the indications for a comprehensive screening examination pertain, a brief, informal screen is sufficient.

The brief MSE is completed during the inception, reconnaissance, and detailed inquiry of psychiatric history-taking. In particular, note is taken of the patient's general appearance, motor behavior, quality of speech, relationship to examiner, and mood. From the patient's demeanor, conversation, and history, the clinician draws inferences about consciousness, orientation, attention, grasp, memory, fund of information, general intellectual level, language competence, and thought process. Abnormal thought content will not be investigated unless clinical clues or alerts indicate the need for such discretionary inquiry (for example, into hallucinations, obsessions, depersonalization, etc.). Physiological functions (sleep, appetite, libido, menstrual cycle, energy level) and insight should always be assessed.

The comprehensive screening MSE

The clinician should be alerted to the need for a comprehensive screen whenever there is a reasonable possibility that the patient has psychosis or has primary or secondary brain dysfunction. The settings and clues listed here mandate a comprehensive MSE:

1. The patient is seen in a hospital emergency room or crisis clinic, or is being managed on a nonpsychiatric ward and has been referred for consultation, or is being admitted to a psychiatric unit.
2. The patient is over 40 years of age.
3. The patient has a history of psychiatric disorder, substance abuse, organic brain disorder, or physical disorder that could affect brain function.
4. The patient's personal habits, memory, concentration, or grasp have recently deteriorated.
5. The patient or other informant presents clinical clues suggesting current mood disorder, psychosis, or organic brain dysfunction (for example: persistent or intermittent depression, withdrawal, elation, overactivity, bizarre ideation, hallucinations, delusions, ideas of influence and reference, headaches, loss of memory and grasp, disorientation, disordered language, seizures, motor weakness, tremor, or sensory loss).
6. The physical examination indicates or suggests brain dysfunction.
7. In forensic referrals, when mental competence or legal insanity are in question.

In summary, if you have any doubts, complete the comprehensive screen.

The comprehensive screen notes the same phenomena as in the brief screening MSE: appearance, behavior, speech, quality of relationship, and language; the physician also should ask specific questions about current or past periods of depression, sadness, irritability, alienation, withdrawal, and high spirits.

Cognitive functions should be investigated in detail. These clinical tests are recommended:

1. Observation of level of consciousness and awareness
2. Tests of orientation (see Table 9.1)
3. Tests of attention and concentration (see Table 9.2)
4. Tests of memory (see Table 9.3)
5. Tests of general information (see Table 9.4)
6. Tests of language function (see Table 9.6)

Tests for abstraction and conceptualization (Table 9.5), and judgment are of dubious validity, add little if any discriminating power, and are better avoided.

If there is any evidence or suggestion of vagueness, disorientation, lack of attention, or deterioration of memory, consider using one of the combination tests providing a composite, quantified result. For rapid assessment, the Short Portable Mental Status Questionnaire (see Table 9.6) is convenient. If there is a suggestion of disorder in central language function, the Mini-Mental State Examination (see Table 9.7) is recommended. These portmanteau tests provide a baseline score that enables the clinician to follow progress; for example, as delirium clears, as pseudodementia lifts when depression is treated, or as brain function deteriorates in the course of degenerative disease.

The tempo, fluency, continuity, control, logical organization, and communicative intent of expressed thought will become apparent during natural interchanges with the patient, although the tests for abstraction previously criticized (see Table 9.5) are sometimes useful in flushing out bizarre thoughts or disorganized thinking.

Illusions, hallucinations, delusions, phobias, obsessions, compulsions, disorders of the sense of self, and impulsions should be inquired about. It is better to ask indirectly about such matters at first and then move to more precise questions. Try not to ask the following questions in a doctrinaire, unspontaneous way. Modify them to fit your natural style and the patient's cultural background:

1. *Illusions and hallucinations*
   Have you had any unusual or strange experiences lately?
   Have you noticed or heard anything unusual or troublesome lately?
   Have you heard or seen anything out of the ordinary lately?
   Have you had any vivid imaginations lately?

Have you noticed lately any unusual:
- feelings in your head or body?
- smells or tastes?
- visions?
- voices, when you are alone?

Do you think many people have these experiences?

Why do you think they are happening to you?

2. *Delusions*

Has anyone been interfering with your life?

Does anyone or any group of people seem to be against you or want to harm you?

Have you had the sense that people are talking about you or laughing at you behind your back?

Why are these people so interested in you?

Have you noticed any other evidence that (. . .) is the case?

Has anyone been trying to influence you in anyway? How?

Have you noticed any change in the way you think? Any confusion? Any difficulty keeping to the point?

Have you had the sense that thoughts, or ideas, or pictures are put into your head? How? By whom? Why?

Have you had the sense that thoughts escape from your head? That other people can read your thoughts? That you can send messages to other people? How?

Do you think your spouse is loyal to you?

Have you ever had the sense that you were a very important person?

Do you think your face or body are changing in anyway?

Were you ever worried that there might be something wrong with your body? That your body might have some sort of disease?

Do you ever feel terribly guilty? About what?

Do you worry a lot about money?

3. *Phobias, obsessions, compulsions, impulsions*

Do you have any excessive fears?

Are there any situations, actions, things you are excessively fearful of?

Do you have any recurring thoughts, ideas, or words you cannot get out of your mind?

Are there any things you just have to do even though they seem foolish or unnecessary?

Do you ever have impulses to do unwise things?

Do you ever give in to those impulses?

What kind of impulses do you have? Violent? Gambling? Sexual? Suicidal? Risk-taking?

4. *Disturbances in the sense of time and self*

Does time seem different (changed) to you?

Does the past (the future) seem different to you?

Do you ever feel unreal?

Do you ever feel as though you were in a fog?

Does the world around you ever become remote, seem different, or appear unreal to you?

Do you ever feel as though you were a spectator of your own actions? As though you were not involved in what is going on?

Do you ever feel that things (you) are falling apart?

In a comprehensive screen, as in the brief screening MSE, physiological dysfunction and attitude to illness must be ascertained.

The discretionary MSE

The initial pattern of salient clues and clinical inferences obtained from the history and MSE is like an incomplete jigsaw puzzle. The configuration of the pieces allows the diagnostician to generate hypotheses about what the complete picture will be like. Alternative hypotheses suggest a plan of inquiry allowing the clinician to go beyond routine screens (brief or comprehensive) to investigate more deeply aspects of the MSE of particular relevance to the hypotheses in question.

Alternative hypotheses and lines of inquiry

As with the physical examination, therefore, there can be no standardized discretionary examination. Consider the following case example:

Case 9.19

■ A 20-year-old man was admitted to a psychiatric ward because his diagnosis was in doubt. He had been unemployed and at home for more than four months, cutting himself off from all outside social contact. On the evening of admission, he had become enraged while watching television, got into an altercation with his mother and sister, and damaged a door by punching and kicking it.

By the time he was interviewed, the patient was a calm, softly spoken, well built young man who gazed downward, making little eye contact with the examiner. His mood was withdrawn, subdued, and moderately depressed, but constant and never incongruous. He was capable of smiling sheepishly, but appropriately, when he spoke of how fearful he was that he might sound foolish. As the interview progressed, rapport grew between patient and interviewer.

The patient's sensorium was quite clear, he appeared to be of average intelligence, and his thought processes were normal in tempo, flow, and organization. His past health was good, he did not take drugs, and his physical examination was normal.

He told the examiner he had lost his temper because he heard noises from above, while watching television in the basement of the family home. The question of whether these noises were auditory hallucinations became the subject of a detailed discretionary inquiry. Were they of human quality? If so, how formed were they? Were the noises directed to him? Was this a recent or sudden phenomenon?

The noises were loud footsteps. They emanated from the ceiling of the basement, which was also the floor of the family kitchen above the television room. He interpreted the footsteps as those of his mother and sister, who were annoyed by his failure to seek work and his unwillingness to help with such household chores as washing up after meals.

Neither his sister nor his mother remembered deliberately making noises to upset the patient, but they freely admitted their extreme annoyance with him for not pulling his weight in the house financially, an issue that had been the subject of several family quarrels.

The clinical significance of the noises and subsequent outburst of rage in a withdrawn, depressed young man cannot be underestimated. Diagnosis moved in the direction of depression in a schizoid personality and a treatment plan was designed accordingly. ■

Selected Readings

Until the revival of concern for reliable diagnosis, as reflected in the diagnostic criteria of DSM–III, American psychiatry had lost interest in the mental status examination. In contrast, following the clinical tradition of Kraepelin and Bleuler and influenced by the phenomenological existentialism of Heidegger, Binswanger and Jaspers, European psychiatry continued to emphasize the detection, classification, and definition of psychopathological phenomena.

The term *psychopathology* reveals the essence of the European approach. Just as the great clinicians of the 19th century had identified the syndromes and morbid anatomy of physical disease, the psychopathologist proposed to define the signs of diseased mental functioning, compile syndromes of clinical features, and hunt for the underlying disorders that caused them.

The classic text on psychopathology is *Allgemeine Psychopathologie (General Psycho-pathology)* by Karl Jaspers (1913, 1962). A modern introduction to the European approach is Scharfetter's (1980) *General Psychopathology*. Volume I of the *Handbook of Psychiatry* (Shepherd & Zangwill, 1983) is a British version of the classical approach, as is a recent American text by Ludwig (1980), *The Principles of Clinical Psychiatry*. Ludwig's work relates the mental status examination to clinical reasoning.

The recently introduced scored combination tests of mental functioning can be useful for following the progress of patients with organic brain disorder. These tests are described in chapter 9.

The reader would be well advised to refer to a dictionary or glossary of psychiatric terms, as in DSM–III or Hinsie and Campbell's (1970) *Psychiatric Dictionary*.

10

The physical examination and special investigations

Neglect of the physical examination Psychiatry has neglected the physical examination. Entire books, in contrast, are devoted to the clinical interview. To comprehend this state of affairs, one must look to the historical influence of psychotherapy on American clinical practice.

Between 1950 and 1980 most psychiatrists were trained to elicit and analyze the inner psychological conflicts associated with psychiatric disorder. Many training programs were slow to accommodate new somatic interventions demanding skill in physical assessment. When their training has deemphasized medical acumen, young psychiatrists lose confidence in their ability to diagnose physical disorder. They avoid the laying-on of hands, and assume that other *Why psychiatrists avoid physical examination* physicians have greater reliability in assessing the physiologic basis of behavior. There is good evidence to the contrary (Koranyi, 1979).

Furthermore, young psychiatrists are often concerned about the unpredictable effect of physical examination on the patient's transference. In fact, the failure to detect physical disorder can have serious, even fatal, consequences outweighing the risk of distorted transference. McIntyre and Romano (1977) surveyed the views of practicing psychiatrists and psychiatric residents concerning physical examination. From their sample of 117 physicians, only one reported frequent ill effects after physical examination; half the respondents had never witnessed a complication. In fact, most considered that physical examination had a beneficial effect on the doctor-patient relationship. The authors concluded: Perhaps some of the respondents have found as we have, that after completing a physical examination and again sitting down with the patient and reviewing their situation, new ideas, fears, concerns and hopes emerge. This is often a reflection of the increased trust established as a result of the physical examination that enables the patient to speak about matters previously suppressed or repressed (McIntyre & Romano, 1977, p. 1150).

Justification for the physical examination

The physical examination is important in modern psychiatry for several reasons.

Biology affects behavior

1. Abnormal behavior does not stem exclusively from psychological conflict but rather from an interaction of biological, psychological, and social factors. Furthermore, neuroscience has determined that specific neurophysiologic systems influence behavior and contribute to the development of psychiatric disorder.

Somatic treatments

2. Somatic technologies, particularly psychopharmacology and biofeedback, have become important in treating behavioral problems and psychiatric disorder.

3. Pharmacological agents, singly or in interaction, may adversely affect normal or diseased organ systems.

Psychiatric symptoms of disease

4. Salient clues suggesting psychiatric disorder can also be manifestations of physical disorder (Hall, Popkin, & Devaul, 1978).

5. Psychiatrists encounter many patients, particularly the elderly, who are likely to have serious physical problems as well as psychiatric disorder.

Medical responsibility

6. Modern psychiatrists have more primary medical responsibility than ever before. The psychiatrist, for example, may be the only physician in a large community mental health center. The fact that a patient has been referred by another physician does not absolve the psychiatrist of the responsibility to assess physical status. It is risky to assume that the referring physician has conducted a thorough investigation. Koranyi (1979) showed that 43% of 2,000 psychiatric clinic patients had nonpsychiatric disorder. He also showed that referring physicians other than psychiatrists had missed one-third and psychiatrists one-half of serious physical disorders in patients referred to the clinic.

Consultation – liaison psychiatry

7. In recognition of the need of a multi-factorial, biopsychosocial assessment, psychiatrists today are frequently asked to collaborate diagnostically with physicians and other health workers in community and general hospital settings.

Purposes

Physical examination in diagnosis
Diagnostic phase
Treatment phase

Physical examination and laboratory investigation have both diagnostic and therapeutic utility. In the **diagnostic phase** of the clinical process, they provide data to support or refute hypotheses generated during the psychiatric interview. In the **treatment phase,** they serve two diagnostic functions:

1. They inform the physician about the function of organ systems that might be adversely affected by psychopharmacologic agents. For example, in a depressed patient, the finding of cardiac disease may influence the choice and dosage of antidepressant medication.
2. The clinician may reinstitute inquiry procedures to test new diagnostic hypotheses arising at any time in the treatment process. Sometimes the physician merely wants to establish the presence or absence of drug toxicity or side effect; but, particularly when treating patients with physical disorders, the clinician must be alert for new salient clues reflecting change in the patient's condition and be prepared to initiate appropriate diagnostic investigations.

Physical examination as therapy

The physical examination has an important, if less obvious, function in the therapeutic process. The laying-on of hands is a traditional ritual that relaxes and reassures patient, family, and doctor. Touching is an essential part of medical procedures in primitive cultures. The thoroughness, involvement, and care of a wise parent surrogate gives psychological succor to someone who is frightened or in pain.

This chapter presents:

1. A general strategy for physical diagnosis.
2. Diagnostic tactics specific to particular organs, systems, or body regions.

General strategy

How should the physician determine the scope and components of physical and laboratory investigation? Several factors impinge on this:

Factors influencing the scope of the physical examination

1. The presence or absence of suggestive physical symptoms.
2. The nature of the presenting psychiatric symptoms.
3. The clinical situation and setting.

The presence or absence of suggestive physical symptoms

Medical history as guide to physical examination

Hall et al. (1978) showed that of 650 psychiatric outpatients, 60% with four or more physical symptoms had laboratory evidence of disease, whereas only 4% with no physical symptoms had disease. Knox (1974) reviewed routine screening questionnaires and found them effective only when they were linked to a medical examination. These studies support clinical common sense – history should guide physical examination and laboratory investigation.

The nature of the presenting psychiatric symptoms

Physical disease causes psychiatric symptoms

Many medical diseases cause symptoms resembling psychiatric disorder. Common symptoms or patterns of this type are anxiety, depression, intermittent psychosis, hallucinosis, and abnormal illness behavior.

Anxiety

Somatic causes of anxiety

Hall (1980a) lists 50 somatic causes of anxiety, categorized as: neurological (15), endocrine (14), infectious (6), autonomic (4), and circulatory (5). Other causes not so readily categorized include nephritis, malignancy, malnutrition, early drug-induced Ménière's disease, and drug abuse.

    Chapter 3 discussed how emotional distress involves the interaction of several factors: social, psychological, or physical stressors; the subject's interpretation of the stressors; and the genetically and developmentally determined psychophysiologic and physiologic response to all of these. Distress can also result from faulty function of the brain centers regulating emotion. Anxiety can thus result when (a) a medical illness causes such external stressors as loss of job or severe pain; (b) illness interferes with perception and orientation, as in dementia or drug abuse; (c) illness affects the end-organs of physiologic or psychologic response, as in endocrine disorders, brain tumors, or mitral valve prolapse; or (d) the sympathetic nervous system is directly affected, as in amphetamine abuse or pheochromocytoma.

Organic anxiety

    Organic anxiety disorder has been proposed as a diagnosis meriting distinction from other anxiety disorders (Mackenzie & Popkin, 1983). Organic anxiety is usually caused by endocrine disorders (such as hyperthyroidism, pheochromocytoma, fasting hypoglycemia, and hypercortisonism) and substance use disorders (such as intoxication with stimulants or withdrawal from central nervous system depressants). Brain tumor of the third ventricle and diencephalic epilepsy are rare but established causes.

Depression

The confusion of terms associated with depression

The terms *depressed mood, depression, dysphoria, sadness, melancholia, grief, demoralization,* and *depressive episode* tend to be used interchangeably. No wonder lay people are confused by psychiatric terminology! Physical illness can provoke a temporarily depressed mood, a profound demoralization, or a major depressive episode. These distinct states can present separately, in sequence, or in combination. For example:

Physical illness and depression

1. Such disorders as Cushing's disease or such drugs as reserpine can directly affect the physiologic pathways that control mood.

2. Such debilitating diseases as cancer or disfiguring drugs as methotrexate can impair bodily function to the degree that a patient consciously experiences loss. Any disease or illness can be experienced as a loss – of vitality, of beauty, of mobility, or of potential.

3. A subliminal or suppressed awareness of a subtle loss of normal function can precipitate depression long before other symptoms of illness declare themselves.

Physical causes of depression

Hall (1980b) identified 75 nonpsychiatric disorders that can present with depression, including: infectious disease, hepatic disorder, pancreatic disorder, nutritional deficiency, electrolyte imbalance, systemic disease, and drug-induced disorder. The psychiatrist must therefore maintain a high index of suspicion when evaluating and treating patients with depressive symptomatology, a caveat that applies particularly to older patients.

Intermittent psychotic episodes

Physical causes of psychosis

Patients with recurring psychotic states usually have a psychiatric disorder such as mania, psychotic depression, schizophrenia, or borderline personality. However, Newman (1980) has described several physical illnesses that should be excluded before a psychiatric diagnosis is accepted: endocrinopathy, multiple sclerosis, alcoholism with intermittent hepatic failure or pancreatitis, systemic lupus erythematosus, acute intermittent porphyria, herpes simplex encephalitis, temporal lobe epilepsy, and the use and abuse of prescription and illicit drugs. *A physical cause must always be ruled out when psychosis presents in middle-aged patients with no previous history of psychiatric disorder.* The physician should search for other symptoms or signs of organic brain dysfunction often coexisting with psychosis.

Hallucinosis

Physical causes of hallucinations

Often regarded as a hallmark of psychological disturbance, hallucinations are actually more frequently caused by physical disorder (DeVaul & Hall, 1980). Visual and olfactory hallucinations as well as visual illusions and distortions are particularly likely to be associated with physical disorder. **Delirium,** a reversible state involving diffuse impairment of brain functioning, occurs in up to 30% of hospitalized patients (Cavanaugh, 1983) and is the most common cause of hallucinosis. Systemic causes of delirium are legion; they include metabolic, infectious, and endocrine disorders as well as states of intoxication and withdrawal. Neurological causes of delirium include vascular pathology, trauma, and infections. Hallucinosis without delirium can be caused by such central nervous pathology as temporal lobe epilepsy, migraine, tumor, and vasculitis.

Abnormal illness behavior

Disease and abnormal illness behavior

A physician may perceive that a patient's symptoms are vague or inconsistent with the typical pattern of a physical disorder. The physician may be piqued by the patient's noncompliance or doctor-shopping, puzzled by indifference to an apparently serious problem, struck by an association between symptoms and stress, or suspicious that the patient is seeking material or emotional gain by remaining sick. These impressions are clues that should alert the physician to such diagnostic hypotheses as somatoform disorder, particularly conversion disorder. Yet, as discussed in chapter 3, the physician must be cautious because other factors, including physical disorder, can account for abnormal illness behavior.

In summary, all psychiatric patients should be medically examined, but the physician must use discretionary tactics. A history of alcohol use, for example, demands an examination of the abdomen and liver function tests. A history of depressed mood and muscle weakness indicates the need for a physical and laboratory investigation of thyroid or muscle end plate function.

The clinical situation and the setting

Influences of the setting

A routine screening examination before the psychopharmacologic treatment of an outpatient contrasts with the detailed examination required in a neuropsychiatric unit. For example, the psychiatrist should screen cardiovascular, hepatic, and thyroid systems before prescribing antidepressants for a 22-year-old woman who presents to an outpatient clinic with alcohol abuse and major depression. The psychiatrist must complete a comprehensive, detailed physical examination and order a battery of laboratory tests after a 65-year-old depressed, confused man with a history of heart disease has been admitted to a neuropsychiatric ward.

Each setting is unique

Although standard diagnostic protocols have been designed for evaluating certain patient groups, the almost infinite variety of clinical situations demands that inquiry plans be tailored to each clinical problem. By the same token, although different clinical settings have common characteristics, each has particular medical and socioeconomic features that must be accommodated in clinical inquiry and management planning.

Physical examination and laboratory investigations, as hypothesis testing

Can the physician take account of these considerations to develop a rational and reliable protocol for clinical practice? Anderson (1980) suggests that if physical examination is conducted to probe hypotheses, the physician can tailor inquiry to both the clinical setting and the patient's problem. Thus, using the schema for the clinical process presented in chapter 6, physical examination becomes a dynamic part of diagnosis and management, as outlined in Figure 10.1.

Physical examination and laboratory testing, in the clinical process

Chapter 6 introduced the concept of a feed-forward series of clinical steps organized with successive clinical actions in mind. In this schema, physical and laboratory investigations are steps in a series of logical actions based on hypothesis generation and testing. As the psychiatrist takes the history and

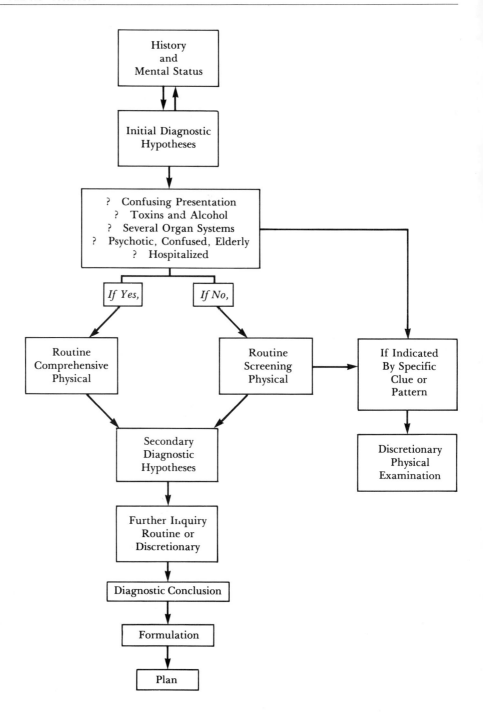

FIGURE 10.1

The physical examination in the clinical process

conducts the mental status examination, he or she may decide to extend inquiry into discretionary physical and laboratory examinations. The 65-year-old depressed man with a history of heart disease requires a comprehensive physical investigation with thorough examination of the cardiovascular system, a chest X-ray, and an electrocardiogram. The detection of a new cardiac murmur or an S-T elevation, for example, would indicate the need for further discretionary tests of cardiovascular function in consultation with an internist or cardiologist. Other systems, however, may require only routine screening. Again, a **feedback system** is emphasized: *Fresh data from interview, physical examination, and laboratory tests can indicate the need for further discretionary inquiry at any time in the clinical process.*

Physical examination and laboratory testing, as feedback

This book is not a manual on the technique of physical examination; it does not describe every discretionary inquiry. Instead, it considers the general and particular indications for undertaking:

1. The routine brief screening physical examination.
2. The comprehensive physical examination.
3. The special discretionary examination.

The routine brief screening physical examination

Rationale for screening examination

Patients are often referred to a psychiatrist after medical evaluation. However, unless referral clearly implicates an interpersonal problem such as marital disagreement or a situational difficulty such as job dissatisfaction and unless it is certain that medications will not be used, the physician should perform a screening physical examination. Referral from another physician is no guarantee that the patient has been adequately investigated.

Case 10.1

■ An internist has referred Betty, a 36-year-old housewife, to a social worker for counseling. Betty and her husband are having difficulty managing their 2-year-old son, whose temper tantrums intimidate his indecisive, insecure mother. The boy responds better to his father, who is annoyed by his wife's inability to cope.

Concerned about Betty's depression, the social worker consults a psychiatrist. The physician is impressed by Betty's sluggish speech and movement, impoverished thinking, and profoundly depressed mood. Before starting treatment, however, she undertakes a screening physical examination, during which she detects a slightly enlarged thyroid and markedly delayed patellar and Achilles tendon reflexes. Laboratory tests confirm the hypothesis of hypothyroidism. Betty responds well to thyroid replacement and her ability to cope improves dramatically. Subsequently, the couple successfully engage in couples psychotherapy with the psychiatrist and social worker. The child's temper tantrums gradually dissipate. ■

Focused examination

A screening examination should focus on organ systems and anatomical regions that (1) have a high association with psychiatric symptoms and (2) provide

Baseline examination

valuable baseline data for evaluating side effects or adverse reactions associated with psychotropic drugs. The following examination is rapidly completed in an office practice and requires little special equipment. To facilitate efficiency, it is organized by anatomical region as follows:

1. General appearance
2. Vital signs and weight
3. Skin
4. Head, neck, and cranial nerves
5. Cardiorespiratory system
6. Abdomen
7. Motor and sensory examination, reflexes, and extremities
8. Cerebellar function

General appearance

Observation

The patient's general appearance is observed during the history and mental status examination. Obvious eccentricities or abnormalities of habitus, gait, movement, coordination, posture, facies, extremities, and speech can be noted. Preliminary hypotheses can be generated. A more detailed inquiry into specific functions or anatomical regions can be left until later. These general observations are described in the previous chapter on mental status examination.

Vital signs and weight

Vital signs

These data can be obtained by trained nonmedical personnel. They yield reliable quantitative information that can be recorded on consecutive office visits.

Pulse

Blood pressure and pulse are indexes of cardiovascular function. They provide a baseline from which changes in the course of medication or physical illness can be determined. Pedal and radial pulses may reflect vascular patencies that are often reduced in degenerative disease (such as arteriosclerosis).

Abnormality in pulse regularity or rate should alert the psychiatrist to the possibility of several morbid conditions.

Tachycardia suggests:

1. Anxiety.
2. The effects on the central nervous system of drugs with stimulant, hallucinogenic, and anticholinergic properties.
3. Withdrawal from alcohol, opiates, sedative-hypnotics, and antianxiety drugs.
4. The effect on the heart of such drugs as stimulants, sympathomimetics, tricyclics, and other anticholinergics.
5. Cardiopulmonary pathology such as myocardial ischemia.

Bradycardia suggests:

1. The effect on the central nervous system of such drugs as opiates or phenothiazines.
2. The effect on the heart of such drugs as beta-blocking agents or digitalis.
3. Cardiopulmonary pathology.
4. Intracranial pathology causing increased intracranial pressure.

An irregular pulse suggests arrhythmia due to:

1. The effect on the heart of such drugs as digitalis or tricyclics.
2. Cardiopulmonary pathology.

Blood pressure

Blood pressure should be examined with the patient supine and standing for these reasons:

1. To detect orthostatic hypotension associated with withdrawal from alcohol and other central nervous system depressants or with medication (especially tricyclics and phenothiazines).
2. To establish a baseline.

Hypertension must be noted and its many causes considered.

Temperature

The temperature is a rapid nonintrusive check for several conditions:

1. Infection (fever).
2. Metabolic derangement such as hypothyroidism (hypothermia).
3. Intoxication, for example with stimulants, hallucinogens or anticholinergics (fever).
4. Drug withdrawal, for example following sedative-hypnotics, alcohol, or opiates (fever).

Weight

Weight change is easily determined, quantifiable, and, though nonspecific, a useful clue for many clinical purposes, for example:

1. To monitor the course of illness or other conditions associated with weight change. Weight gain can herald the improvement of a patient with major depression or anorexia nervosa. Weight loss can indicate a new resolve in a middle-aged man who, because of obesity, an ambitious, driving personality, and a strong family history of heart disease, needs to change his life style.
2. To check the side-effects of medication. Tricyclics and neuroleptics tend to increase weight; narcotics decrease weight.
3. To monitor compliance with treatment or health maintenance programs. Many people need to lose or gain weight in order to prevent, treat, or adjust to physical disorder. A diabetic, arthritic, or hypertensive patient may need no medication if he or she can lose fifty pounds. Patients with low back pain

due to intervertebral degeneration may avoid surgery if they reduce weight. Debilitated, hospitalized, postsurgical, or trauma patients may recover more rapidly if they can gain weight through adequate nutrition.

The second part of the screening examination assesses the function and structure of organ systems and anatomical regions. Ideally, it should be completed by a physician, although nurse practitioners can be trained to complete reliable screening physical examinations.

Skin

Abnormalities of the skin

Examining the skin begins at first contact with the handshake. Sweaty skin is associated with anxiety, thyrotoxicosis, and fever, stimulant, hallucinogen, and opiate injection, and sedative and alcohol withdrawal. Continue the examination through the history and mental status as you note the skin of exposed surfaces. Closer inspection during regional examination discloses clues about general nutrition, hydration, and disease. The psychiatrist should address the following four questions:

1. Are there any diffuse changes in color? (e.g., jaundice, cyanosis, anemia, plethora, reddening of exposed surfaces, bronzing)
2. Are there any lesions or rashes? What are their color, pattern, and location? (e.g., the erythematous, macular, malar rash associated with systemic lupus erythematosus)
3. What is the texture? (e.g., fine in hyperthyroidism) What is the turgor? (e.g., decreased in dehydration)
4. Is the skin moist? (e.g., hyperthyroidism, anxiety) Dry? (e.g., hypothyroidism)

Head, neck, and cranial nerves

General inspection

As mentioned, astute observation during history and mental status examination can yield salient clues and suggest preliminary hypotheses before function and structure are formally assessed. The psychiatrist should address the following questions:

Skin color

1. What is the skin color? (e.g., jaundice, cyanosis, anemia, plethora, reddening of exposed surfaces, bronzing)

Facies

2. Is there a facial rash? (e.g., systemic lupus erythematosus, side effects of anticonvulsants, bromism, tuberose sclerosis)

Hair

3. Is there alopecia? (e.g., hypothyroidism, hypoparathyroidism, scleroderma, alopecia areata, side effects of chemotherapy)

Breath
4. Does the breath have a particular odor? Is it foul (e.g., pyorrhea, tonsillitis, sinusitis, bronchiectasis) or musty (liver disease)? Is there an odor of acetone (e.g., diabetes mellitus, starvation), ammonia (uremia), alcohol or other toxins?

5. Is there facial asymmetry? (e.g., trauma to, or infection of, the facial nerve or a central lesion affecting the fifth cranial nerve)

Bruising
6. Is there bruising of the face or head? (e.g., domestic violence, athletic injury, accidents secondary to drugs or alcohol, skull fracture, or intracerebral hemorrhage)

7. Is there exophthalmos (hyperthyroidism)?

Eyes
8. Is blepharospasm present (tranquilizer-hypnotic withdrawal, extrapyramidal dysfunction, head injury)?

Eyelids
9. Do the eyelids droop bilaterally (myasthenia gravis) or unilaterally (Horner's syndrome, birth injury)?

Sclerae
10. Are the sclerae discolored? (jaundice, carotinemia, drugs, alcoholism)

Conjunctivae
11. What is the color of the conjunctivae? Are they red (drug use) or pale (anemia)?

Dentition
12. What is the state of dentition? Are the teeth carious, notched (congenital syphilis) or tender (abscess)? Are the gums red and swollen (periodontitis, stomatitis, dilantin side-effect) or blue (lead poisoning)?

Neck
13. Is there swelling in the neck? (e.g., thyroid disease, tumor, lymphadenopathy)

Voice
14. Is the voice hoarse? (e.g., alcohol abuse, heavy smoking, thyroid, disease, laryngeal tumor)

The psychiatrist should confirm and expand these observations during detailed inquiry into the structure and function of specific organs and body regions.

Visual system

Examining the eyes and assessing the visual system can provide salient clues about systemic disease and function.

Pupils
The size and reactivity of the pupils is influenced by the relative balance of the sympathetic and parasympathetic systems. Opiates, drugs with anticholinergic or sympathomimetic properties, and intracranial lesions can disturb autonomic balance. Normal findings are particularly valuable as a baseline for later medication. The examiner should pose the following questions. Are the pupils:

1. Unequal (intracranial tumor, multiple sclerosis)?
2. Dilated and reactive (stimulants, hallucinogens, phenothiazines)?
3. Dilated and increasingly unreactive (opiate withdrawal)?

4. Dilated and unreactive (anticholinergic drugs such as scopolamine and high doses of tricyclics)?
5. Pinpoint and unreactive (opiate intoxication)?

Fundus

During fundoscopy, the physician can directly observe the lens, humor, retinal vessels, and central nervous system (optic nerve disks and retinae) and detect manifestations of local or systemic disease. The clinician should be guided by the following questions:

1. Are cataracts present (e.g., hypoparathyroidism)?

Lens

2. Is the lens subluxated (Marfan's syndrome)?
3. Are the disk margins blurred or elevated and the disk hyperemic? When associated with visual loss, these signs indicate optic neuritis secondary to local inflammation, infectious disease, metabolic disorder or toxins. In the

Papilloedema

absence of visual loss, these signs indicate **papilloedema** which is pathognomonic of increased intracranial pressure, and a matter of immediate concern.

Retinopathy

4. Can vascular pathology be identified? In such systemic disease as hypertension, atherosclerosis, and diabetes mellitus, abnormal retinal vasculature reflects vascular pathology in other organs, and in other parts of the central nervous system. Hypertension produces uniform narrowing of the vessels ("copper or silver wiring"), "cotton wool" exudates, flower-shaped hemorrhages, and punctate pale areas of infarction. Arteriosclerosis can be associated with plaques that narrow vessels irregularly or cause "nicking" where vessels cross. Diabetes mellitus produces punctate red spots associated with retinal microaneurysms.

Nystagmus

5. Vertical, horizontal, or rotatatory nystagmus indicate many pathological conditions: the toxic effects of anticonvulsant, antianxiety and sedativehypnotic drugs, alcohol, cerebellar and vestibular dysfunction, multiple sclerosis, Wernicke's encephalopathy, encephalitis, and brain tumor.

Other cranial nerves

Extraocular movements

Vision and visual fields

Extraocular movements (Cranial Nerves III, IV, VI), visual acuity, and gross visual fields (Cranial Nerve II) are often abnormal in diseases that present with psychiatric symptoms, particularly multiple sclerosis, intracranial spaceoccupying lesions, cerebrovascular accidents, infections, Wernicke's encephalopathy, and toxic psychosis.

The corneal reflex provides a ready means of assessing the sensory integrity of Cranial Nerve V.

Cranial nerves VII, VIII, IX, XII

While examining Cranial Nerves VII, VIII, IX, and XII, the physician can scan the facial skin, evaluate the texture of the hair (thyroid, nutrition),

Mucous membranes

and check the teeth, oral mucous membranes, and tongue (for nutrition and metabolic disorders).

Thyroid
Carotid artery
Cervical lymph nodes

The thyroid gland can be palpated for size and nodules, the carotid artery palpated for patency and auscultated for the presence of bruits (arteriosclerosis), and the cervical lymph nodes checked (infection, lymphadenopathy, metastases from head or chest).

Cardiorespiratory system

Heart and lungs

Even without salient historical clues referable to this system, an examination of the heart and lungs can provide information relevant to diagnosis and treatment. The psychiatrist can palpate and auscultate for such significant abnormalities as heart murmurs or bronchospasm and refer the patient to an internist if specialized evaluation is indicated. Sometimes iatrogenic illness is exposed.

Case 10.2

■ Xavier, an 8-year-old boy, is referred to a child psychiatrist by a urologist for the evaluation of primary enuresis. Upon routine screening examination, a heart murmur is found. The anxious parents relate that their doctor told them of the murmur five years ago. Without further investigation, he had strongly recommended that they discourage Xavier from strenous activity. Consequently, he had grown up isolated from his peers and their activities.

Xavier is referred to a pediatric cardiologist, who concludes that the murmur is innocent. The psychiatrist prescribes imipramine for enuresis and counsels the parents to encourage their son to live a normal life. ■

Patients' expectations

Even though it is unusual for cardiorespiratory examination to reveal pathology, the brevity of the procedure, the potential significance of any finding, and the fact that patients expect it, support its inclusion in the screening examination.

Abdomen

Abdomen

The abdominal skin may show vascular patterns suggestive of liver disease or striae suggesting Cushing's syndrome. The prevalence of alcohol use and abuse, particularly among psychiatric patients, mandates examining the liver for tenderness and size. Other abdominal masses (renal, splenic, intestinal, retropubic) or tenderness should be noted.

Motor and sensory systems, reflexes, and extremities

The physician should observe the patient for the following abnormalities of the motor system.

Abnormal movements   1. Distinguish fine tremor (anxiety, senile tremor, thyrotoxicosis, alcohol or sedative withdrawal, lithium use) from coarse tremor (lithium toxicity, alcohol or sedative withdrawal, liver failure, anemia, cerebrovascular disease, severe pulmonary insufficiency, tabes dorsalis, parkinsonism). Note if the tremor occurs at rest (parkinsonism) or with intentional movement (multiple sclerosis, cerebellar disease).

2. Choreiform movements indicate drug toxicity (tardive dyskinesia associated with neuroleptic medication) or neurologic disease (Huntington's chorea, Sydenham's chorea).

3. Athetoid movements (disease of the basal ganglia).

4. Fasciculations, when coarse, indicate cold or fatigue, and when fine, muscle degeneration (peripheral neuritis, progressive muscular atrophy).

5. Cogwheel rigidity indicates parkinsonism.

6. Tetany or spasms may indicate metabolic disorder (hypoparathyroidism, hypocalcemia, hypomagnesemia, hypocapnia due to hyperventilation).

7. Tics (as in Gilles de la Tourette's syndrome) should be noted.

Gait   8. Gait disturbances including ataxia (cerebellar disease), steppage gait (tabes dorsalis), spastic gait (hemiplegia, paraplegia), retropulsive gait (parkinsonism), clownish gait (chorea), waddling gait (muscular dystrophy), and circumduction (hemiparesis). Bizarre gaits may be associated with somatoform disorder.

Muscle bulk and strength can be examined:

Muscle bulk and   1. Asymmetry of muscle mass and strength indicate a peripheral or central ner-
power   vous lesion.

2. Generalized weakness may indicate toxic or metabolic neuropathy, hypothyroidism, or primary muscle disorders.

Sensation   The sensory system should be checked. Test for light touch and pinprick sensation, and for graphesthesia. Particularities should be noted, such as glove or stocking anesthesia (which is more sharply demarcated in conversion disorder than in polyneuropathy).

Reflexes   The reflexes can provide information about general condition and specific lesions:

1. Hyperactive reflexes indicate central nervous arousal secondary to drug intoxication (anticholinergics, stimulants, hallucinogens), drug withdrawal (opiates, sedative-hypnotics, alcohol), hyperthyroidism, anxiety, or depression. Hyperreflexia is also characteristic of upper motor neuron disease (e.g., paraplegia, spastic hemiparesis).

2. Hyporeflexia is seen in drug intoxication (alcohol, sedative-hypnotics), electrolyte imbalance, hypothyroidism (with delayed response), Sydenham's chorea, and cerebellar disease.

3. Abnormal reflexes, such as the Hoffman or Babinski, indicate an upper motor neuron lesion.

Extremities

The extremities, particularly the hands, can be systematically inspected:

1. Are there any excoriations? These can indicate skin disease, self-inflicted lesions, stimulant overuse, an attempt to remove actual parasites or illusory vermin (as in cocainism), or pruritis of psychological or physical origin (uremia, hepatic failure, hyperthyroidism).
2. Are there needle tracks (indicating drug abuse) in the forearms, antecubital fossae, legs, or feet?
3. Do the nails and nail beds reveal clubbing (pulmonary, cardiovascular, hepatic, or thyroid disease) or other signs of systemic disorder such as brittleness or evidence of biting (indicating anxiety or stimulant overuse)?
4. Is there local or general discoloration of the skin referable to icterus, bruising, cyanosis, hemochromatosis, Addison's disease, bleeding disorder, blood dyscrasia, malnutrition, or local infection?
5. Is there edema of local, cardiovascular, hepatic, lymphatic, myxedematous, hypoproteinemic, or allergic origin?

Cerebellar function

Cerebellar function

Romberg, finger-to-nose, and heel-to-shin tests should be performed to rule out cerebellar dysfunction (drug or alcohol intoxication, cerebrovascular insufficiency, cerebellar degenerative disease, abscess, or tumor).

The comprehensive physical examination

Rationale for comprehensive physical examination

Ludwig (1980) suggests six diagnostic situations that require a comprehensive physical examination:

1. There is a pattern of symptoms suggesting diffuse pathology.
2. There is a history of alcohol or drug abuse.
3. The pattern suggests several physical disorders.
4. Psychosis, confusion, or delirium are evident.
5. The patient is over 50 years of age.
6. The patient has been admitted to hospital.

Diagnostic pattern suggestive of diffuse pathology

Does the pattern of clues and inferences suggest the diffuse effect of metabolic, autoimmune, or metastatic processes?

Case 10.3

■ A psychiatrist examines Susan, a 30-year-old woman who has been referred for the evaluation of depression and "strange thoughts." Tearful and angry during the interview, her concentration is poor.

Susan reveals a cluster of symptoms suggestive of major depression (excessive fatigue, sadness, crying spells, and sleep disturbance); but she also describes periods during which she is excessively irritable and suspicious. She has had 3 miscarriages within the previous 4 years. She also has had transient rashes and aching joints.

Puzzled by the pattern that suggests autoimmune disease, the effect of toxins, depression, and organic brain syndrome, the psychiatrist undertakes a comprehensive physical examination. This reveals slightly swollen and sore ankles and wrist joints. Laboratory investigations (LE cells, elevated sedimentation rate) implicate systemic lupus erythematosus.

The psychiatrist refers Susan to an internist. The two physicians collaborate in the design of a comprehensive management plan for systemic lupus and its behavioral and emotional complications. ■

Toxins and drugs   Has the patient been exposed to such toxins or drugs as alcohol that could damage one or more organs or alter systemic processes?

Case 10.4   ■ A psychiatrist has been treating for major depression Eve, a 38-year-old woman who is unhappily married to Adam, a liquor store clerk. Eve requests marital therapy. To begin with, she flatly denies sexual problems; but during the first joint session, while engaged in a heated argument with Adam, she blurts out derisively, ''And you can't even get it up!'' She flushes and looks down. The couple fall silent.

Inquiry into Adam's personal life reveals that he drinks heavily and eats poorly. A review of systems yields nonspecific complaints of fatigue, weakness, and nausea.

Adam is referred to an internist, who finds an enlarged tender liver and signs of peripheral neuropathy. Laboratory examination confirms the diagnosis of alcoholic hepatitis and peripheral neuropathy. Eve continues antidepressant therapy with the psychiatrist. Adam and Eve are referred to an alcohol treatment program. ■

Multiple organ systems   Does the medical review of systems reveal complaints suggesting several medical problems?

Case 10.5   ■ Quentin, a 30-year-old man, has been referred to a behavioral medicine clinic for treatment of chronic low back pain due to a herniation of the disk at L4-5, documented on myelogram. Quentin's obesity and noncompliance with treatment make surgery risky. At this point, he depends on 8 to 20 Percodan daily for the control of low-back pain.

Quentin's medical history is remarkable only for a gunshot wound to the left lower abdominal quadrant sustained in Vietnam. A review of systems reveals several complaints: burning epigastric pain, excessive fatigue, anxiety, and depressed mood.

Physical examination uncovers further salient clues. The patient is pale and sweaty. His protruding abdomen has a long, vertical midline scar, and a large ventral hernia. He has a slightly enlarged and tender liver and a tender epigastrium. He has severe bilateral spasm of the paraspinous muscles. The range of spinal motion is markedly limited, and straight leg raising bilaterally restricted.

An upper gastrointestinal series reveals ulceration and scarring of the duodenal bulb. A hemoglobin of 10.2 g/100 ml and guaiac positive stools confirm the hypothesis of bleeding peptic ulcer. Liver enzymes are elevated in a pattern consistent with alcoholic hepatitis.

Gentle, concerned inquiry eventually reveals that Quentin has been consuming 2 to 4 six-packs of beer daily. ■

Psychosis or delirium　　　　Is the patient psychotic or confused?

Case 10.6　　■ It is 2:00 A.M. on June 20, 1982. Marge, a 35-year-old housewife, is brought to the hospital by the police, who found her walking down the main street of the town, shouting obscenities. Her husband remembers that she was irritable and strange on the previous morning and that she accused him of trying to change her religious convictions after supper that night. This behavior is markedly at variance with her usual personality.

In the Emergency Room, Marge refuses to speak, except to protest that her husband, the doctors, and the police are in league and to respond that the date is January, 1980.

Her husband states that Marge has been under considerable strain in recent months due to her father's terminal illness and that she had contracted a severe upper respiratory infection five days previously. Physical examination, performed with difficulty, reveals a fever of 38° C, a pulse of 110, hyperactive deep tendon reflexes, nuchal rigidity, and an unequivocal Babinski sign on the right side. Spinal tap confirms the hypothesis of viral meningo-encephalitis. ■

Age and　　　　Is the patient over 50 years of age? Is the patient hospitalized? If so, a
hospitalization　　comprehensive physical examination is required for medical and legal reasons.

The discretionary physical examination

Discretionary physical　　The discretionary physical examination stems from either of the routine physical
examination　　examinations (screening or comprehensive) in accordance with the set of diagnostic hypotheses. It may be indicated at any point in the diagnostic or treatment phases of the clinical process. Since clinical settings, clues, inferences, and patterns are varied and diagnostic hypotheses numerous, the discretionary examination can never be standardized. On the contrary, the discretionary examination is an opportunistic inquiry designed by the astute physician to fit the resources, constraints, and epidemiological features of the clinical setting, the diagnostic hypotheses, and the individual who has the problem.

Case 10.7　　■ Joan, a 32-year-old recently divorced mother of two children, is referred to a psychiatrist by her family physician. Because of frequent severe panic attacks with hyperventilation, Joan avoids all social activities and travel and spends most of her time at home. There, she ruminates constantly about her misfortunes and contemplates suicide. If she plans to go out, she must compulsively check that her belongings have not been misplaced or stolen, sometimes to the extent that she cannot leave home. Her symptoms have worsened over the past 3 months and are now associated with neurovegetative signs.

A screening physical examination is unremarkable except for slight tachycardia and hyperreflexia consistent with anxiety. Joan is diagnosed as having a major depression in association with long-standing generalized anxiety disorder.

Initially, Joan responds to imipramine (150 mg at bedtime), oxazepam (7.5 mg every six hours as needed, for anxiety), relaxation training, and cognitive-behavioral psychotherapy (see chapter 11). Ater 8 weeks of treatment, however, she develops dizzy spells, shortness of breath, and left-sided chest pain. Her family doctor tells her not to worry, reassuring her that the symptoms are typical of anxiety and hyperventilation, and suggesting that she increase the dosage of oxazepam. Her symptoms worsen. Convinced that her treatment has failed and she is doomed to a life of despair, Joan reverts to suicidal ruminations.

The psychiatrist inquires into her new symptoms. He discovers that chest pain preceded the onset of other symptoms and is exacerbated by deep breathing or coughing, a pattern inconsistent with her long-standing anxiety state. He notices that the patient is pale and sweating. Physical examination reveals a fever of 38.2° C and fine rales in the lower left chest posteriorly. Chest X-ray confirms pneumonia. After a rapid response to appropriate antibiotics, Joan feels much better physically, is relieved of her pessimistic ruminations, and resumes psychiatric treatment with restored faith. ■

Laboratory procedures and other special investigations

Physical examination and special investigation converge on a diagnostic conclusion

Evidence elicited by appropriate physical examination allows the physician to refine or revise the diagnostic hypotheses (see Figure 10.1). The physician may then arrange appropriate special investigations in order to elicit further evidence for or against the revised array of hypotheses. The process converges progressively on a diagnostic conclusion (see Figure 10.2). The physician will then be ready to develop a diagnostic formulation and design a management plan (as outlined in detail in chapters 14 and 15).

Although psychological tests have always been important to the diagnostic process in psychiatry and are routinely ordered in some settings, laboratory tests are seldom ordered outside the hospital. However, the medical laboratory is likely to assume increasing importance in psychiatry.

Sociomedical influences

The use of laboratory and other special investigations is influenced by a number of sociomedical issues, which can be summarized as follows:

1. Cost containment versus legal security
2. Ambulatory psychiatry versus hospital psychiatry

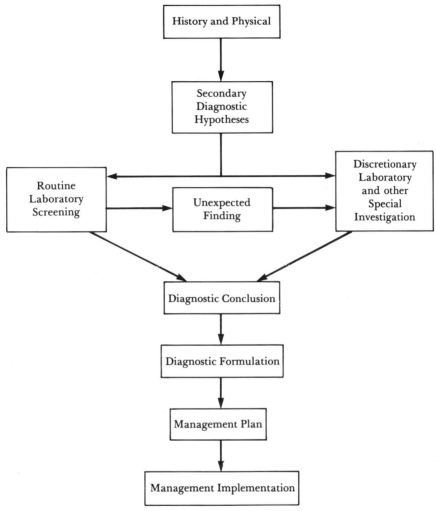

FIGURE 10.2
Special investigations in the clinical process

3. Psychological investigations versus physical investigations
4. Intrusive investigations versus benign investigations
5. Discretionary investigations versus screening investigations

Cost containment versus legal security

Medicine and psychiatry are increasingly affected by legal considerations. Physicians are no longer above suspicion; patients often question their good faith and

The cause of defensive medicine

skills. The psychiatrist is especially vulnerable because some patients, in accordance with their unconscious denial of emotional problems, would openly or secretly prefer a diagnosis of somatic disorder. Thus, the psychiatrist who overlooks such a diagnosis is vulnerable to lawsuit.

An adversarial climate fosters defensive medicine. Physicians sometimes order laboratory tests as much from fear of malpractice suits as to gather evidence about an array of diagnostic hypotheses. The cost of this aberration of the clinical process is staggering; and, ironically, many procedures themselves can lead to **iatrogenic disorder.**

Because psychiatric diagnosis relies more on the history of psychosocial patterns than on current physical phenomena, psychiatrists have not been greatly concerned about the problem of cost containment. This is no longer the case; the cost-effective use of the laboratory is becoming an issue of considerable importance.

Ambulatory versus hospital psychiatry

The convenience of the setting for physical procedures

Physicians are practical; they prefer techniques that are effective, convenient, and safe. Thus, certain features in the setting may influence a psychiatrist's preparedness to examine patients physically. Many psychiatric disorders once requiring hospitalization can now be managed in an outpatient department or office. The clinical process in a hospital lends itself to routine physical and laboratory examination, but such investigations are often inconvenient in an office arranged primarily for psychotherapy, with its comfortable chairs, couch, and desk but lack of examining table, nurse, and syringe. Chapters 16 through 21 more thoroughly discuss the effects of different settings on the diagnostic process.

Psychological versus physical investigations

Systems approach

The mind is a metaphor for self-conscious brain function, a metaphor in which physiology and psychology merge. Chapters 3, 4, and 5 illustrate how a multilevel systems perspective can help the clinician accommodate these intricate relationships. In many instances, investigations testing psychological processes relate directly to neurophysiologic function: Biofeedback, for example, uses physical parameters to define anxiety that can be treated with relaxation and psychotherapy; and tests of cognitive functioning can be used to assess brain functioning in dementia.

Psychology measures biology

Intrusive versus benign investigations

Most special investigations of psychiatric disorder are relatively benign. On the border of psychiatry and neurology, a number of **intrusive tests** (such as the

CT scan reduces morbidity

arteriogram and pneumoencephalography) carrying some risk of morbidity were often used in the past; but computerized axial tomography (discussed in detail later in this chapter) has largely superceded these procedures. In some instances, neuropsychologic testing can be psychologically intrusive, particularly if a patient is concerned about a possible loss of cognitive functioning. Ironically, the patients most likely to be referred for neuropsychological testing are those most threatened by it.

Discretionary versus screening investigations

Thoughtless batteries vs. thoughtful selection

This chapter has suggested that the psychiatrist, like all physicians, faces a dilemma – to miss nothing yet practice economical medicine. The psychiatrist may fall into the bad habit of ordering batteries of screening tests rather than thoughtfully considering which investigations are pertinent to the clinical problem. Routine batteries are indicated only if they have a reasonable possibility of yielding significant data. What is needed is a rational and economical plan for different clinical presentations. Selective routines must be established for investigating each clinical problem and the data subsequently used to generate additional hypotheses for further inquiry or to confirm preliminary diagnostic hypotheses before planning treatment.

The systematic planning of clinical inquiry

Chapter 5 outlined the steps of the clinical process; this chapter reviews how physical examination is coordinated with diagnosis and management. Laboratory procedures and other special investigations fit into the clinical process by testing the validity of superordinate and subordinate hypotheses. To review the process of hypothesis definition and redefinition, let us reconsider Betty, the 36-year-old woman referred by a social worker (see Case 10.1). Upon referral, the general superordinate hypothesis in this case was *depression*.

After history and mental status examination, specific subordinate hypotheses were generated in the following order of probability:

1. Major depressive episode
2. Hypothyroidism
3. Chronic intoxication
4. Other endocrinopathy

Screening physical examination reordered the priority of the hypotheses, as follows:

1. Hypothyroidism
2. Major depressive episode

and guided the discretionary laboratory inquiry, into thyroid dysfunction (serum T3, T4, and TSH) and chronic intoxication (serum SGOT, LDH, and protein), as well as routine CBC and urinalysis. Clearly abnormal thyroid function tests provided strong evidence in support of the provisional diagnosis of hypothyroidism, with secondary major depression. The validity of this diagnostic formulation was tested by prescribing replacement thyroxin, which by rapidly returning Betty to her premorbid personality and behavior, established the final diagnosis of hypothyroidism with major depression.

In this case, routine laboratory tests were augmented by detailed discretionary inquiry into thyroid function and liver disease.

Routine screening laboratory procedures

Every hospital seems to have its own protocols for laboratory investigation. Too often, standard practice is based on convention, hearsay or experience, rather than on the validity, specificity, sensitivity, and cost-effectiveness of the procedures in question.

Biochemical specificity is infrequent in psychiatry

Unlike detecting physical disorder, diagnosing psychiatric disorder infrequently rests on laboratory procedures. Since biochemical specificity is exceptional in psychiatry, the clinician must fit laboratory evidence into a mosaic of data from history, mental status, and physical examination. Occasionally, a test will clinch a diagnosis; for instance, when a CT scan reveals enlarged ventricles in an older patient with normal pressure hydrocephalus. Other tests may provide evidence for infective or structural or metabolic disorder of the central nervous system.

The physiologic dysfunctions of the nervous system thought to be associated with some mental disorders (such as major depression and schizophrenia) are not sufficiently defined to be diagnosable by laboratory tests. Although they may foreshadow an era of laboratory investigations in psychiatry, recent advances in neuroendocrinology have fallen short of expectations. Consider, for example, the Dexamethasone Suppression Test. Although this procedure has been widely publicized for its specificity in affective disorder (95%), its sensitivity is only 50%, it is unreliable in many medically ill patients, and it does not predict which patients will respond to medication (Gelenberg, 1983a).

Most laboratory tests are used either to rule out biomedical pathology or to provide a baseline from which to evaluate complications secondary to medication or disease processes. Other special investigations, such as neuropsychological testing, can help to identify and localize (though not define) pathology of the central nervous system.

Hospital protocols

In the hospital setting, policy determines laboratory routines. For legal protection of the hospital, most patients require a CBC, chest X-ray, and urinalysis. Other routine screening procedures are determined by such factors as age and sex; for example, over 40 years of age, men usually have an electrocardiogram and women a Papanicolaou smear. Diagnostic protocols are then developed for specific problems. For example, tests of renal, cardiac, thyroid, and liver function should be ordered in all cases of mania for whom treatment with lithium is contemplated.

There are also protocols for outpatients, depending on the particular population served. A psychopharmacology clinic may routinely order CBC, urinalysis, and EKG (the latter in patients over 40 years old); a psychotherapy clinic may order an MMPI and Rorschach; and a behavioral medicine clinic may order an electromyogram, biofeedback profile, and stress inventory.

Discretionary laboratory procedures

The use of laboratory procedures to rule out organic disorders

For certain superordinate hypotheses, discretionary laboratory procedures help the clinician rule out specific, usually biomedical, disorders. Chapter 5 presented the superordinate hypothesis of psychotic pattern needing refinement to one or other of an array of specific subordinate hypotheses, including schizophrenic disorder, brief reactive psychosis, and organic mental disorder. Although the psychotic pattern can be corroborated by mental status examination, specific organic hypotheses are usually ruled in or out by the laboratory. Other superordinate hypotheses can also be refined by use of the laboratory. Table 10.1 lists a number of common superordinate patterns with appropriate laboratory procedures.

Special procedures

This section discusses the following special diagnostic procedures:

1. The Dexamethasone Suppression Test
2. Computerized axial tomography
3. Sleep encephalography
4. Neuropsychological testing

The Dexamethasone Suppression Test

DST

Sensitivity 50%

Specificity 90%

The **Dexamethasone Suppression Test (DST)** assesses the function of the hypothalamic-pituitary-adrenal cortical axis in order to detect major depression (Carroll, Feinberg, & Greden, 1981). The sensitivity of the DST is about 50%: only about one-half of all patients with major depression have a positive test. However, the DST has a specificity of over 90% in patients with the melancholic

TABLE 10.1
Common superordinate patterns and suggested laboratory examinations

General superordinate hypothesis	*Laboratory (s = Suggestive; c = Confirmatory)*
1. Acute psychosis with confusion – delirium	Delirium can be suggested or confirmed by simple cognitive testing and general cerebral dysfunction by diffuse EEG slowing. Subtle cognitive impairment may be detected only by diffuse EEG slowing or neuropsychologic testing
Substance abuse:	urine and serum drug levels (c)
Metabolic disorders:	
porphyria	urine porphyrins (c)
Addison's disease	CBC (s); electrolytes (s); serum ACTH and cortisol (c)
Cushing's disease	CBC (s); electrolytes (s); urinary cortisol (c); DST (c)
hyper- and hypothyroid	thyroid function tests (c)
hyper- and hypoparathyroidism	X-rays (s); serum calcium and phosphorus (c)
uremia	BUN and serum creatinine (c); urinalysis (s)
hepatic failure	liver enzymes, bilirubin (c)
acid-base balance	arterial blood gases (c)
Exogenous toxins:	
anticholinergic medication	urine and serum drug levels (c)
heavy metals (lead, arsenic, mercury compounds)	tissue and serum levels (c) bone X-rays (s)
indolamines (LSD, psilocybin, DNT)	none
phenethylamines (mescaline, amphetamines, cocaine)	urine, drug screens
carbon monoxide	arterial blood gases (s) and carboxyhemoglobin (c)
Vitamin deficiency	CBC (s); serum levels (c)
Anoxia	
pneumonia	WBC (s); chest X-ray (c); blood gases (c)
congestive heart failure	chest X-ray (c); blood gases (c); EKG (s), RVG (c)
Myocardial infarct (silent)	EKG (s,c); enzymes (c)
hemorrhage	Hct/Hgb (s)
Cerebrovascular accident (frontal) lobes)	
intracranial hemorrhage	CT Scan (c); spinal tap (c); EEG (s)
intracranial thrombosis	CT Scan (c); EEG (s)
CNS Infection	
encephalitis (particularly herpes simplex virus)	CSF examination (s) and culture (c) brain biopsy (c)
meningitis	CSF examination (c) and culture (c)
syphilis	CSF and blood AL-Af (s); CSF culture (c)
abscess	CT Scan (c); CSF (c,s)

(continued)

TABLE 10.1 (continued)

General superordinate hypothesis	*Laboratory (s = Suggestive; c = Confirmatory)*
1. Acute psychosis with confusion – delirium (cont.)	
Systemic Infections	
pneumonia	WBC (s); chest X-ray (c)
septicemia	WBC (s); blood culture (c)
gastroenteritis with electrolyte disorder	serum electrolytes (c)
Functional psychoses (may appear confused)	
schizophrenia, mania, borderline	no laboratory evidence. Psychological tests: MMPI, Rorschach (s)
psychotic depressive episode	psychological tests: Beck, Zung, SCL-90 (s); DST (s)
Space occupying lesion	EEG, neuropsychologic testing, and physical exam, can suggest localization
tumor	CSF (s); CT Scan (c)
subdural hematoma	CT Scan (c); xanthochromic CSF (s)
abscess	CBC (s); CSF (s); CT Scan (c)
Degenerative disease with decompensation secondary to complication (see previously listed categories)	
Seizure disorders	EEG (c); rule out causes other than epilepsy
2. Psychosis without confusion	
Functional psychoses: (see under #1)	psychological testing (s)
Toxic psychoses: phencyclidine, LSD, amphetamine	urine and blood screen
CNS disease	neuropsychological testing (s)
vasculitis (Lupus, etc.)	sedimentation rate (s); serum ANA (s); temporal artery biopsy (c)
encephalitis	spinal tap (s); EEG (s); CT Scan (s); biopsy (c)
multiple sclerosis	spinal tap (s); CT Scan (s); cortical evoked responses (s)
temporal lobe epilepsy	EEG (c)
acute intermittent porphyria	porphyrins in urine and feces
tumor, frontal lobe	EEG (s); skull X-rays (s); CT Scan (c)
hemorrhage, frontal lobe	EEG (s); spinal tap (c); CT Scan (c)
Systemic disease	
hepatic failure	liver enzymes (s); bilirubin (c)
renal failure	urinalysis (s); serum creatinine (c) or BUN (c)

(continued)

TABLE 10.1 (continued)

General superordinate hypothesis	*Laboratory (s = Suggestive; c = Confirmatory)*
3. Chronic psychosis with cognitive deficit (dementia) (other than categories mentioned earlier in table).	
Degenerative disorders	
Senile dementia, Alzheimer's disease, Pick's Disease, Huntington's chorea, Jakob-Creutzfeldt disease, Parkinson's disease	neuropsychological testing (s); low dopamine metabolites in CSF and urine (s); CT Scan (c); biopsy (c)
Normal pressure hydrocephalus	CSF pressure (s); CT Scan (c)
Metabolic	
Wilson's disease	serum copper (c); ceruloplasmin (c)
4. Depression	
Adjustment disorder with depressed mood, dysthymic disorder	psychological testing (s)
Major depressive episode	psychological testing (s): Beck, Zung SCL-90; Dexamethasone Suppression Test (s)
Organic affective syndrome	
drug-induced: reserpine, methyldopa, hallucinogens, sedatives, alcohol	urine and serum drug screens (c)
drug withdrawal: stimulants	urine and serum drug screens (c)
Endocrine disorders: Cushing's, Addison, thyroid, parathyroid disorders	urine and serum drug screens (c)
Cancer: carcinoma of the pancreas, lung, and others	X-ray (s); CT Scan (s); biopsy (c); other tests as indicated
Viral syndromes: mononucleosis	CBC (s); monospot (c); culture (c)
5. Anxiety	
Panic disorders	
Anxiety secondary to physical disorder	
hypoglycemia	5-hour glucose tolerance test (c)
pheochromocytoma	abdominal X-ray (s); or CT Scan (s); urinary catecholamines (c)
hyperthyroidism	thyroid function tests (s); phentolamine test (c)
mitral valve prolapse	EKG (s); echocardiogram (c)
Substance intoxication	urine and serum screens (c)
caffeine	
amphetamines	
hallucinogens	
Substance withdrawal	
sedative-hypnotics (barbiturates, benzodiazepines, etc.)	urine and serum screens (s); pentobarbital tolerance tests (s)
alcohol	

subtype of depression; in other words, fewer than 10% of nondepressed psychiatric patients have positive DST tests.

Unreliable in many situations

The initial enthusiasm for the DST has waned, however. The clinical utility of the test has been challenged on statistical grounds (Modell, 1983; Shapiro, Lehman, & Greenfield, 1983; Davis et al., 1983). Moreover, several conditions or factors other than major depression have been found to cause a spurious

Spurious positives

positive test, including noncompliance with instructions, technical variations (dose, time of measurement), rapid weight loss, physical disorders such as Cushing's disease and liver disease, pregnancy, and pharmacologic agents such as dilantin, tegretol, alcohol, barbiturates and other hypnotics. In fact, it has been suggested that the DST reflects nothing more than stress (Baldessarini, 1982). The DST has not been useful in predicting response to medication (Nelson et al., 1982). At present, it cannot be regarded as reliable or cost-effective since it does not help the psychiatrist to determine which depressed patients will respond to antidepressant medication, and which patients have depression secondary to a physical disorder.

Computerized axial tomography

Nonintrusiveness

Computerized axial tomography (CT scan) was a revolutionary advance in neuropsychiatric diagnosis, but its proper use is in dispute. Because computerized axial tomography reliably and safely detects many intracranial problems that present with psychiatric symptoms (see Table 10.2), some clinicians order CT scans on all elderly or depressed patients admitted to a neuropsychiatric unit,

Dubious cost-effectiveness as a routine procedure

However, the cost of routine use is prohibitive and the yield surprisingly low. Larson et al. (1981) showed that of 105 consecutive psychiatric hospital admissions, only 6 had positive CT scans. Each of these patients had focal findings on neurologic examination, and management was altered by CT results in only 4 of the 6. In a study of 150 alcoholics with withdrawal seizures, Feussner et al. (1981) showed that neurological examination adequately indicated which patients required an initial CT scan. These studies suggest that, given the expense of the

TABLE 10.2
Conditions detectable by CT scan that are associated with psychiatric symptoms

Gross structural abnormality	
tumor	arteriovenous malformation
abcess	dementia with cortical atrophy
aneurism	hydrocephalus
subdural hematoma	
Focal edema or tissue change	
infarct	infiltrate (tumor, infection)
hemorrhage	

Selective use is preferable

procedure, computerized axial tomography should be used only in a discretionary inquiry in order to test diagnostic hypotheses based on positive findings from history, mental status, and neurologic examination.

The sleep electroencephalogram

Sleep encephalography and major depression

A standard methodology for recording and analyzing the sleep electroencephalogram (EEG) has been developed over the last two decades. It has led to an accumulation of evidence supporting a correlation between abnormalities in sleep architecture and major depressive disorder. Kupfer and Thase (1983) summarize these abnormalities as follows:

1. *Disturbance in the continuity of sleep* (nonspecific):
   a. prolonged sleep latency (time to fall asleep)
   b. increased number of awakenings
   c. early morning waking
   d. decreased sleep efficiency (time spent asleep per total recording time)
2. *Diminished slow wave sleep* (nonspecific)
3. *Increased random eye movements* (relatively specific):
   a. increased REM density $\left(\dfrac{\text{Total amount of REM activity}}{\text{Total amount of time in REM sleep}} \right)$
   b. the shifting of REM activity to the first few hours of sleep
   c. intense activity during the first period of REM sleep
   d. increased number of REM counts during the second half of each REM period
4. *Random eye movement latency shortened* (relatively specific):
   a. to less than 60 minutes in most patients, compared within normal mean value of 90 minutes

The specificity of changes in REM architecture

Increased random eye movements and ·shortened REM latency are seldom detected in physical or other (nonaffective) psychiatric disorders, in normally sad people, or in geriatric patients with dementia (as contrasted with the pseudodementia caused by primary depression). However, some patients with nonendogenous, chronic depression have a sleep EEG similar to that found in major depression. Akiskal (1983) suggests that, in the latter group of patients, the EEG distinguishes patients likely to respond to antidepressant medication.

In summary, the sleep EEG shows acceptable sensitivity (61% to 90%), specificity (80% to 100%), and diagnostic confidence (83% to 100%) for the diagnosis of major depression of primary, endogenous, or melancholic type (Kupfer & Thase, 1983). However, even though it is a promising procedure, its use is limited by the limited number of sleep laboratories, expense and inconvenience, and the difficulty in assuring the necessary 2-week drug-wash-out period.

More convenient methods of recording changes in sleep architecture (such as recording the EEG during daytime naps) are being explored (Kupfer et al., 1981; Reynolds, Coble, & Kupfer, 1982).

Neuropsychological testing

Use in neurological, neurosurgical, geriatric and physically ill patients

Neuropsychological testing (e.g., Reitan & Davison, 1974) has an important function in both diagnosis and therapy. When the patient is cooperative, psychological tests can uncover subtle deficiencies in many cerebral functions, such as perception, cognition, language and motor skills. Neuropsychiatrists in hospital psychiatric units and consultation-liaison psychiatrists in neurological, neurosurgical, and rehabilitation units are most likely to request these tests. The general psychiatrist should order them judiciously, particularly with geriatric and physically ill patients. Some indications for neuropsychological testing are as follows:

Indications for neuropsychological testing

1. To detect focal areas of dysfunction and guide further investigations.
2. To confirm the diagnosis of dementia or functional loss.
3. To identify functional deficits secondary to brain trauma, lesions, or surgery.
4. To monitor functional recovery or deterioration in association with brain pathology.

Neuropsychological tests are helpful only if the physician knows how to integrate their findings with other information in the diagnostic and therapeutic process.

Case 10.8

■ Janice, a 38-year-old ex-bookkeeper, was divorced 4 years ago and remarried 1 year ago. She has been admitted to a neurosurgery service for evaluation of chronic headaches. Her husband is exasperated because Janice will not do the housework.

Neurologic examination reveals a barely noticeable fine tremor of the hands, poor recent memory, and disorientation for time (she misses the date by one week). Blood and radiologic studies are ordered.

During the third day of her hospital stay, Janice becomes erratic. At times she is angry and irritable, at other times quiet and withdrawn. Neuropsychological testing is requested. The psychologist notes that the patient was antagonistic to testing, reports that the tests indicate generalized cerebral dysfunction, and recommends a psychiatric consultation.

The consulting psychiatrist interviews staff, patient, and husband. He notes that the husband has facial telangectasiae suggestive of liver disease. The husband admits that he and his wife have been drinking 5 to 10 beers or whiskeys daily for at least 6 months and that since her divorce, Janice has been taking Serax intermittently for bad nerves.

By this stage, the patient is patently delirious. Alcohol and benzodiazepine withdrawal syndrome is diagnosed. Three weeks after effective therapeutic withdrawal, a clinical test of cognitive function, the Mini-Mental State (see chapter 7,

Table 7.6), reveals persisting recent memory deficit. A neuropsychological battery confirms the deficit.

The psychiatrist refers Janice to an out-patient alcohol treatment team, which successfully helps her control her drinking. At 6 months, Janice is functioning well; a second neuropsychological battery reveals no residual cognitive deficit. She returns to bookkeeping and attends Alcoholics Anonymous regularly. ■

Janice's case presents five important issues related to the use of neuropsychological tests:

Integration required

1. Neuropsychological data should be incorporated with a comprehensive neuropsychiatric assessment.

Cooperation essential

2. The patient must be cooperative, otherwise the results are invalid.

Delirium invalidates

3. Psychological tests are useless in delirium.

Neuropsychological testing and rehabilitation planning

4. Neuropsychologic tests can aid the evaluation of rehabilitation from cerebral pathology due to stroke, alcohol, toxins, or encephalitis.

5. Neuropsychologic monitoring of the progression of a cerebral disease such as Alzheimer's, enables the clinician to adapt management to the patient's cognitive capacity.

Collaboration

A collaborative relationship between psychiatrist and consulting psychologist will ensure the most effective use of neuropsychological testing.

Mental status examination

As discussed in chapter 9, the astute neuropsychiatrist can adapt parts of the neuropsychological battery to the mental status examination when indicated. For example, a patient might be asked to copy geometric figures adapted from the Bender-Gestalt Visual-Motor Test to probe right parietal lobe functioning.

Projective tests

Other psychological tests can yield useful information about a patient's personality, mental processes, and mental abilities. **Projective tests,** such as the Rorschach (Exner, 1978) and Thematic Apperception Test (Murray, 1943), use ambiguous stimuli (such as inkblots or pictures) to elicit imaginative responses. They can provide insight into how a patient feels and perceives his or her personal world. Mental processes such as associative thinking, cognitive style, imagination, coping and defense mechanisms, and interpersonal style can be analyzed, enhancing psychotherapeutic planning.

Actuarial tests

Actuarial tests usually involve self-administered questionnaires, such as the Minnesota Multiphasic Personality Inventory (MMPI) (Hathaway & McKinley, 1943). They have been widely used for clinical and research purposes. However, the MMPI is of limited use. Although it has some utility as a screening instrument in nonpsychiatric settings, a clinical interview provides information that is more relevant to clinical purposes. Unfortunately, because the MMPI provides quantitated results, nonpsychiatric physicians may rely on it unduly.

Case 10.9

■ Peter, a 35-year-old college professor, is referred to an orthopedic clinic for recurrent low-back pain of 2 years' duration. Physical examination reveals bilateral lumbar muscle spasm but no other neurologic abnormality. Radiography of the spine shows spondylolisthesis.

Peter is referred to a physical therapist for an exercise and muscle-stretching regimen. Stoical by nature, he restricts none of his usual activities and splits and stacks five cords of wood. When his father suddenly falls ill, Peter is forced to do a great deal of long-distance driving to visit him. Meanwhile, the pain steadily worsens.

Angrily demanding more definitive treatment, Peter confronts his doctor, who finds no change on orthopedic examination and arranges for Peter to complete an MMPI. The MMPI reveals elevations on the scales measuring hypochondriasis (Hs) and hysteria (Hy). No further inquiry is pursued. Peter is advised to seek counseling.

Peter's wife, by now quite distraught, consults a social worker, who becomes concerned about Peter's stability and asks a psychiatrist to evaluate the problem.

The psychiatrist diagnoses major depression with agitation. As part of a routine evaluation, he asks Peter to record the factors associated with fluctuations in the pain. One week later, Peter's notes reveal that the pain worsens when his back is stressed or when he is emotionally agitated. It improves when he lies flat in a position consistent with relief from lumbar disk disease. Suspecting that Peter is exaggerating his complaints for psychological reasons but that he also has a structural problem, the psychiatrist refers the patient back to the orthopedist for further examination. CT Scan reveals a ruptured disk at the L_{4-5} level, and surgery is performed. ■

IQ testing to answer educational and vocational questions

Such **intelligence tests** as the Wechsler Adult Intelligence Scale (Wechsler, 1958) and the Wechsler Intelligence Scale for Children – Revised (Wechsler, 1974), are most useful when educational and vocational questions arise.

Case 10.10

■ Frank, a 13-year-old boy, is being considered for admission to a select, highly academic private high school. Uneven scores on a national aptitude test contrast with his consistently excellent school record. Frank is a popular and socially successful lad, but the parents and the private school are concerned he might be an overachiever who will have to struggle to keep up in a highly competitive curriculum.

The WISC-R reveals a very superior full scale IQ of 126, with particular strength in abstract-conceptual subtests. These scores give confidence to the school and parents that Frank has the ability to adapt to the private school. He eventually attends the school and prospers socially and academically. ■

The diagnostic process, management planning, and outcome evaluation

After completing laboratory and special investigations, the psychiatrist can usually proceed to a diagnostic conclusion, develop a diagnostic formulation, and design a treatment plan (see Figure 10.3). A monitoring evaluation of the effectiveness of treatment can be fed back to the system at the appropriate level and new diagnostic steps implemented as required (see chapter 15).

Summary

The physical examination is an important part of the diagnosis and treatment in psychiatry. Many nonpsychiatric medical disorders present with behavioral, emotional, or cognitive disturbances that must be diagnosed by the psychiatrist. Somatic treatments, particularly pharmacotherapy, require the evaluation and monitoring of several organ systems.

All psychiatric patients should receive at least a screening physical examination. Positive findings lead to either a comprehensive or a discretionary physical examination. Other indications for comprehensive physical examination include these situations:

1. A medical review of systems has revealed complaints suggesting dysfunction in several physical systems.
2. Diagnostic hypotheses implicate the diffuse effect of metabolic, autoimmune, or metastatic processes.
3. The patient has been exposed to toxins, drugs, or alcohol that could damage one or more organs or alter systemic processes.
4. The patient is over 50 years of age.
5. The patient has been admitted to a hospital.

The discretionary physical examination is an opportunistic inquiry designed by the astute physician to fit (a) the resources, constraints, and epidemiologic features of the clinical setting, (b) the diagnostic hypotheses, and (c) the patient.

Once the diagnostic hypotheses based on the data from history, mental status and physical examination have been revised or refined, laboratory and special investigations can be considered to support or refute the remaining hypotheses. Each clinical setting establishes its own routines for investigating particular hypotheses.

Unlike the rest of medicine, few psychiatric diagnoses rely on laboratory inquiry for confirmation. Instead, the clinician fits laboratory data into a mosaic of information from the history, mental status, and physical examination. Special procedures of importance to psychiatry include the dexamethasone suppression test, computerized axial tomography, the sleep EEG, and neuropsychological testing.

The clinician must continually reevaluate the diagnostic formulation according to the progress of the patient's disorder and the effectiveness of treatment. New physical examinations and further laboratory inquiry must be undertaken when appropriate.

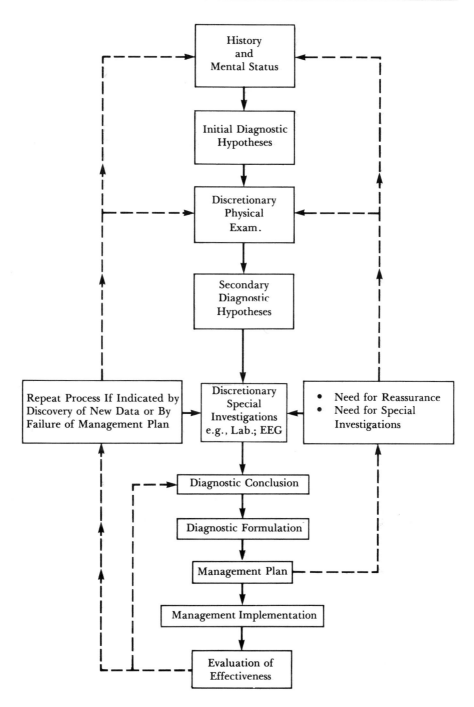

FIGURE 10.3
The diagnostic process, management planning, and outcome evaluation

Selected Readings

Ludwig's (1980) *Principles of Clinical Psychiatry* presents how the practice of clinical psychiatry integrates knowledge from general medicine, neurology, neuropsychology, and psychiatry. His text consistently and thoroughly presents how data from the physical examination assists the psychiatrist in the clinical process.

Lishman's (1978) *Organic Psychiatry* reviews the presentation and diagnosis of the organic conditions likely to be encountered in psychiatric practice.

Hall's (1980) *Psychiatric Presentation of Medical Illness* reviews the many medical disorders that can underlie psychological symptoms.

Pincus and Tucker's (1974) *Behavioral Neurology* cogently reviews the evidence for the neurological basis of psychiatric problems.

Benson and Blumer's (1975) *Psychiatric Aspects of Neurological Disease* contains useful papers about clinical problems on the border of psychiatry and neurology.

11

Patterns: categorical
diagnosis and DSM-III

The philosophic tradition in medical diagnosis

The terminology of psychiatric diagnosis embodies a checkered history and reflects a venerable philosophic debate. Cohen (1943) and Kendell (1975) have described how ancient differences between the Hippocratic and Cnidian schools of diagnosis can be traced through the subsequent evolution of medicine and psychiatry.

Hippocrates followed Aristotelian principles in emphasizing the individual patient's symptoms, signs, and prognosis. In contrast, the Cnidian school was inspired by Plato, who taught that ideas were universal and transcended sense phenomena; diseases, by the same token, had an independent existence manifest through the symptoms and signs of the patients who harbored the diseases.

The concept of disease entities

Medical taxonomy

Sydenham, who introduced the concept of **syndrome** in the 17th century, was a Platonist. Influenced by the botanical taxonomist Linnaeus, Sydenham considered that diseases were as ''real'' as botanical species and that the clinical expression of each disease must be uniform.

By the mid-19th century, however, medicine had moved in a different direction. Taking a dimensional view, Virchow described diseases as life pro-

225

cesses under altered conditions. Disease entities were therefore mental constructs, convenient fictions that summarized clinical phenomena.

The 19th century revival of disease entities

At the end of the 19th century, the great discoveries of Koch and Pasteur reversed the trend. At the heart of every disease, it seemed, was a germ; the scientist must first define the syndrome, then isolate its pathogen. The heyday of bacteriology thus revived the dormant notion of disease entities, each with its particular cause and natural history. The elucidation of the clinical features, pathology, immunology, and pathogenesis of general paralysis of the insane is a case in point. Between 1822 and 1945, Bayle defined the syndrome, Virchow and Nissl explored its morbid anatomy, Krafft-Ebing unraveled its immunology, Noguchi and Moore isolated its bacteriology, and Wagner-Jauregg described its treatment. Eventually, the antibiotic therapy of syphilis was introduced, with brilliant results.

The extreme categorical approach to psychiatry

This oft-quoted success story has sustained psychiatrists who take the following robust organic approach: The precise delineation of psychiatric syndromes is necessary because it will lead to the definition of disease entities that will then be found to have a specific etiology, pathology, prognosis, and therapy.

Categorical and dimensional approaches

Few psychiatrists today adhere fully to such a narrow model. Most have views somewhere between these extremes: (a) all psychiatric problems are true disease entities; and (b) psychiatric categories are misleading since all patients require an individual diagnostic formulation. Most would agree that medical diseases are hypothetical constructs without independent reality. Some psychiatric disorders (manic-depressive psychosis, for example) may turn out to be associated with subtle neurochemical derangements. Other disturbances, particularly those presently classified as personality disorders, will likely prove to be conceived best as loose clusters of phenomena that are themselves at the extremes of dimensional continua. Some disorders (major depression, for example) are probably categorically distinct. Others, like anxiety states, are exaggerations of, or deficiencies in, normal reactions to life stress. Few psychiatrists consider that categorical diagnosis alone is or ever will be entirely sufficient for individual management planning.

There is considerable contemporary controversy within and outside of psychiatry around these questions: Is categorical diagnosis useful at all? If so, in what way? These questions will now be addressed.

The use of categorical diagnosis

Menninger (1948) proposed the jettisoning of formal classification. He asserted that no label could convey an individual's problems, personality, relationships, and experience; the clinician needs a detailed diagnostic formulation of each patient, since few people completely fit textbook stereotypes and most fall on the borders between syndromes. Woodruff, Goodwin, and Guze (1974) take a diametrically opposite view. Like Sydenham, they compare diagnosing a psychiatric patient to identifying a botanical specimen. In their view, diagnosis has two functions: communication and prediction. They contend that psychiatric disorders should be precisely defined and will prove to have predictable causes. Their approach has had a significant influence on the planning of DSM-III.

The nomothetic and idiographic approaches to diagnosis

It is apparent that a fundamental polarity bedevils all diagnostic systems. This polarity contrasts the *nomothetic* and the *idiographic,* terms that differentiate two points of view from which an individual can be studied. On the one hand, the clinician can consider the way a subject resembles other people and is governed by universal laws. The diagnosis of schizophrenia, for example, is made by finding a similarity between the patient and a particular set or class of other patients. On the other hand, each patient can be regarded as subject to unique laws, and any evaluation ignoring uniqueness will deplete the information required for individualized management.

In practice, no clinician can function solely at either pole. However individualized the assessment, every patient has some characteristics in common with others. If not, every treatment program would have to be innovative and there would be no way of predicting when a particular kind of therapy might be effective. On the other hand, a comprehensive treatment plan demands more than a categorical label. Therapy must be more than a mere prescription for a stereotypic tag.

The balance between nomothetic and idiographic approaches

Nomothetic, categorical diagnosis is most useful for summary communication and prediction. Idiographic diagnosis is most useful for management planning. In practice, the two approaches are complementary.

The three purposes of diagnosis (communication, prediction, and planning) can now be discussed.

Diagnosis as communication

Diagnosis as summary communication

Diagnostic categories can be used to summarize the essential clinical phenomena of a case. Even though a term such as *subacute bacterial endocarditis* reveals nothing of the patient's musical ability, intelligence, marital adjustment, or alcohol intake (factors that may all be important in etiology or therapeutic management), it is a handy way of summarizing an illness's etiology, pathology, symptomatology, and likely course. It can therefore be used as a kind of verbal shorthand in discussion between practitioners, or for counting the number of cases of different illnesses diagnosed or treated each year, or for other administrative purposes.

Diagnosis for prediction

Scientific medicine began with the classification of clinical phenomena into syndromes (e.g., Bright's disease or Sydenham's chorea). In the late 19th century, this approach led to the discovery of the pathoanatomic, pathophysiologic, microbiologic, and biochemical correlates of many somatic syndromes; to the therapeutic advances of the 20th century; and to increasingly refined definitions of syndromes.

Diagnosis as a guide to research

By these criteria, psychiatry is in a phase of development akin to that of 19th century medicine; that is, it is still attempting to delineate reliable clinical syndromes. When reliability has been achieved, it may be possible in some instances to identify biological correlates (neurotransmitter anomalies, for example). In other instances, however, it is probable that temperamental variations, early experience, recent stress, or all three operating together produce broad psychopathological spectra conceptually disparate from the syndromes for which the biomedical disease model is appropriate.

Inclusiveness or exclusiveness in criteria for diagnosis

If physical correlates are sought, tight phenomenologic clusters will probably be required; for example, the RDS criteria of Feighner et al. (1972). Exclusive definitions of this type risk identifying false negatives, whereas loose definitions yield an excess of false positives. Thus, depending on its purpose, a diagnostic system may be inclusive or exclusive, loose or tight. Loose classifications are likely to be more inclusive, blanketing most or all individuals in a universe of cases; tight systems tend to exclude more cases and leave them unclassified. Since DSM-III is a mixture of tight and loose syndromes, its reliability and validity are uneven.

Categorical and multidimensional diagnosis

Biomedical diagnostic systems require the clinician to assign patients to categories: the patient either has rubella or has not. The categorical approach works better for malignant hypertension than for essential hypertension, the latter being a dimensional construct. In multidimensional categories (such as personality disorder), the cutoff points distinguishing pathology from nonpathology are blurred. Modern medicine attempts to delineate the dimensional ranges associated with normality and pathology. The application of a statistical, multidimensional approach to developmental psychopathology is illustrated by the Child Behavior Profile introduced by Achenbach and Edelbrock (1983).

Reliability and validity

A diagnostic category is **reliable** if different diagnosticians, or one diagnostician at different times, assign the same patient to that category. Diagnostic categories are also described as demonstrating more or less **validity.** Validity refers to the following:

1. The degree to which the category predicts outcome.
2. The degree to which it is associated with concurrent biological, psychological, or social factors.
3. The degree to which it is associated with antecedent factors.
4. The degree to which it embodies particular theoretical constructs as to the nature of the disorder.

Most psychiatric categories are of uncertain, unsatisfactory, or unexplored reliability and validity; indeed, until recently, the precise criteria for assigning patients were unclear. DSM-III proposes to provide such criteria as a first step to establishing the reliability and validity of its component clinical syndromes.

Diagnosis for therapeutic planning

Systemic and bio-psychosocial diagnosis

The diagnostic formulation

The diagnostic inventory

Rational therapeutic planning in psychiatry demands (1) a multilevel, cross-sectional, systemic assessment of the current pattern of symptoms, signs, and responses; (2) a longitudinal, temporal assessment of predisposition, precipitation, and perpetuation; and (3) an integrated diagnostic formulation. Planning also requires (4) an inventory of the patient's and family's biopsychosocial resources and potentials, as well as of their deficits and problems. No static taxonomy can provide the idiographic richness required to design a comprehensive, individualized plan of management. These matters are discussed in more detail in chapters 14 and 15.

The drawbacks of categorical diagnosis

Categorical diagnosis has drawbacks, many of which result from the frailties of those who diagnose rather than from the defects of diagnostic systems themselves. Nevertheless, the flaws should be squarely faced, if only to anticipate those who attack that all-purpose strawman, "the medical model."

Empty labels

People abhor a vacuum. Once a clinical problem is identified, a title tends to appear. Idiopathic megacolon, hysteria, and proctalgia fugax are good examples of these empty labels. The danger is that the clinician will be satisfied with the tag and feel that something has been achieved by pinning it on a patient. Patients, too, can be lulled or gulled by impressive but vacuous labels. Furthermore, once coined, labels acquire a life of their own. Hysteria is a case in point. Designated thus in Hellenic times because it was thought to be caused by uterine wanderlust (*hystera* means womb), hysteria was initially dropped from the lexicon of DSM-III (where it was subsumed by Somatoform Disorders) only to return, parenthetically, as hysterical neurosis: conversion type, when a lobby of influential clinicians protested its deletion.

Premature closure

Paul Valery has said, "Seeing is forgetting the name of the thing one sees." Premature diagnostic labeling may prevent the diagnostician from eliciting, perceiving, or correctly interpreting new information inconsistent with the label previously applied.

Diagnostic disparagement

Some clinicians use diagnostic epithets to disparage their patients. Such terms as *psychopath, retarded, neurotic, antisocial,* and *inadequate* are especially liable to be used in this manner. Be wary of clinicians who rely heavily on these terms when referring to people; they may be expressing dislike or fear of their patients, and using diagnosis as a pretext for keeping them at a distance.

Existential criticisms of psychiatric diagnosis

Most social critics of psychiatric diagnosis take schizophrenia as the quintessentially destructive pigeonhole. They do so because this diagnosis is likely to lead to hospitalization, and because some people, so labeled and incarcerated, have a poor prognosis.

Labeling as the cause of disturbed behavior

Scheff (1963) proposed that schizophrenic symptoms are the effect of labeling, that diagnosis excludes from society a person who is then trained to be crazy. In other words, mental illness does not occasion labeling; labeling causes mental illness.

Psychiatry and social control

Psychiatrists have been depicted as agents of a state so corrupt that it uses pseudoscientific stereotyping to control people designated socially and politically undesirable. Psychiatric institutions thus are concentration camps for labeled inmates and psychiatric treatment a thinly disguised form of political coercion.

Diagnosis as a political event

Laing (1967) described schizophrenia as a tag people pin on others who are alienated from the prevailing state of alienation. Labeling, a political event, is applied to behavior resulting from the social violence perpetrated on the patient by others, commonly within the family. The label sticks, reinforcing the very behavior that originally occasioned its ascription. Family, hospital staff, and other patients conspire to degrade and invalidate the schizophrenic who, bereft of rights and duties, is incarcerated and subjected to inhuman treatment in the name of medicine. The patient's only way out is to pretend that, if released, he or she will no longer upset the status quo of a crazy world.

Diagnosis as an obstruction to the diagnostic encounter

It is unclear whether Laing and Scheff would extend their views to all psychiatric disorders; possibly, they would take issue with the concept of diagnosis itself. Diagnostic categories, Laing might say, prevent the clinician from fully and genuinely encountering the patient and appreciating the existential situation.

Psychiatry as an obstruction to justice

Szasz (1961, 1963) described how psychiatric terminology can be used by sophistic lawyers and meretricious psychiatrists to shield miscreants from answering for their crimes. Such diagnoses as hysteria and schizophrenia represent impostures or fictions that have no place in Law, according to Szasz. In a way, therefore, Szasz's criticisms counterbalance Laing's. Szasz contends that citizens have individual rights that should not be curbed by the state until consensual limits are overstepped and the rights of others infringed on. The State, meantime, has the responsibility of ensuring that limits are observed. Psychiatry weakens the State and its citizens by interfering in this process, for lawyers have used psychiatric diagnosis to stir waters already turbid.

Can these criticisms be answered? Only partly. It is true that diagnostic categories can obscure ignorance, cause premature intellectual closure, and allow immature clinicians to disparage patients; but the fault here is in the clinician rather than diagnosis itself.

Hospitalization and dehumanization

Does diagnosis cause mental illness? Labeling may divert a patient into a dehumanized setting that provides inadequate treatment. The mental hospitals of 40 years ago were often like this. But it is the setting (rather than the label) that accentuates the patient's illness. The remedy is to provide a more therapeutic environment, not to jettison diagnosis. There is no evidence that labeling is ever the initial cause of a mental disturbance.

The political misuse of psychiatry

Is the ascription of the label schizophrenia to a patient a political event? Yes, in a way, it is. Physicians are invested by society with the authority to diagnose and treat patients. To that extent, they are agents of the State. In certain totalitarian countries, furthermore, psychiatrists are expected to diagnose and institutionalize political dissidents whom it is convenient to discredit as mentally ill. The essential question is the degree to which the clinician is acting during diagnosis in (what he or she believes are) the patient's best interests, in contrast to acting on behalf of people other than the patient. The danger of political misuse is real; but to conclude that all diagnosis is inspired by a corrupt social order is hyperbole (which is itself politically inspired).

Psychiatry and legal responsibility

Szasz's criticisms are better reasoned. They have contributed to the contemporary debate about the insanity defense in law and the use of psychiatric testimony to mitigate criminal responsibility. They have had little impact on clinical psychiatry, however, particularly as Szasz's polemics have coincided with the accumulation of research evidence that the major psychoses have genetic or biochemical correlates. The upshot is that categorical diagnosis, in the form of DSM-III, is in a more powerful position now than for many years and that the medical model, in limited form, is gaining ground.

It is appropriate at this point to analyze the concept of mental disease or disorder.

The definition of mental disease

According to Kendell (1974), there are seven different definitions of disease:

The definition of disease

1. Disease can be defined by suffering. However, many diseases produce no suffering, and not all who suffer have disease.
2. The definition of disease as what doctors treat will not do; it is too much at the mercy of contemporary vogues and private idiosyncrasies.
3. The advances of 19th century medicine suggested that the distinguishing characteristic of a disease was a lesion; that is, a divergence from standard structure or function. But what is the distinction between normal variation in, and pathological departure from, the standard pattern?
4. From another point of view, disease can be regarded as a total organism's adaptation to stress. But so is life. What bounds normality from disease? This definition leaves it quite unclear.
5. If health is an ideal state of complete normality, disease can be regarded as an imperfection in a hypothetical state of total health. This definition is too exalted to be practical.
6. More helpful, perhaps, is the statistical definition of disease as a deviation from the norm, by way of excess or defect (Cohen, 1943).

7. Scadding (1967) defines disease as the sum of the abnormal phenomena displayed by a group of living organisms in association with a specified common characteristic or set of characteristics by which they differ from the norm for their species in such a way as to place them at a biological disadvantage. How applicable is this definition to mental disorder?

The need for behavioral norms

Adapting Scadding's definition, mental disease applies to sets of abnormal mental or behavioral phenomena sufficiently deviant from the norm to place the subject at a biological disadvantage. The problem has been to define norms for psychological phenomena that are not purely social in nature. We otherwise become mired in fruitless arguments about whether criminals, homosexuals, or counterculture folk, for example, are mentally ill.

It must be concluded that there is no precise or satisfactory definition of disease and consequently none of mental disease. DSM-III (1980) essentially agrees with this but opts for the following loose definition. Mental disease is:

The definition of mental disease

- a psychological or behavioral syndrome;
- causing distress or disability;
- stemming from physical, psychological, or behavioral dysfunction;
- and not solely a reflection of disturbance between the subject and society.

The development of a standard nomenclature for psychiatric diagnosis

The standardization of psychiatric diagnosis

Until recently, the definition of psychiatric disorders was poorly standardized. As a result, there were marked apparent transatlantic differences in the prevalence of schizophrenia. Even within the same center, diagnostic reliability was often unsatisfactory. Scientific questions about the validity of formal psychiatric diagnoses could not be answered while their identification was subject to logical error, local fashion, and personal idiosyncracy.

The task force of the American Psychiatric Association, which designed DSM-III, proceeded to define each clinical category as precisely, clearly, and exclusively as possible. Field trials established the clinical acceptability of early drafts of the manual and demonstrated a diagnostic reliability generally better than that of the previous official diagnostic system.

DSM-III: the main mental disorders

DSM-III is descriptive and atheoretical. The clinical features of the various mental disorders are defined, and theoretical statements about etiology or psychopathol-

Multi-axial diagnosis

ogy are avoided. Aware that unitary pigeonholes restrict diagnostic reasoning, the authors of DSM-III recommend the following multi-axial system:

Axis I   Mental disorders
Axis II   Personality disorders
             Specific developmental disorders (children)
Axis III   Physical disorders
Axis IV   Severity of psychosocial stressors
Axis V   Highest level of adaptive functioning in the past year.

DSM-III does not aim to provide an integrated diagnostic formulation and is more useful for communication and scientific prediction than for management planning. Nevertheless, its clarity, precision, comprehensiveness, and tested reliability make it essential reading. This section touches on the system's major divisions; the reader should also refer to the *Diagnostic and Statistical Manual of Mental Disorders* (3rd ed.).

This chapter deals with the broad categories applied by DSM-III to adult mental disorder. Chapters 16 to 20 deal with the syndromes most commonly encountered in different medical settings – ambulatory, emergency, inpatient, liaison psychiatry, and family practice. Chapters 21 to 26 deal with child and adolescent psychiatry; this chapter will not discuss child and adolescent disorders.

The 12 main groups of mental disorders are:

1. Organic Mental Disorders
2. Substance Use Disorders
3. Schizophrenic Disorders
4. Paranoid Disorders
5. Affective Disorders
6. Other Psychotic Disorders
7. Anxiety Disorders
8. Somatoform Disorders
9. Dissociative Disorders
10. Psychosexual Disorders
11. Factitious Disorders
12. Personality Disorders

Each main group will be defined and the most common disorders within each group described.

Organic mental disorders

This group includes organic brain syndromes of known etiology involving reversible or permanent brain dysfunction. The clinical features of these disorders depend on site, onset, progress, and duration and on the nature of the underlying brain lesion. The symptoms and signs of organic disorders combine the behavioral effect of brain dysfunction with the patient's psychosocial reactions to it.

- **Delirium** is a clouding of the sensorium due to central neurophysiological dysfunction that is of acute or subacute onset and fluctuant course. Attention, orientation, short-term memory, and thinking are affected; perceptual illusions and hallucinations are characteristic; and nocturnal restlessness and diurnal drowsiness are common.
- **Dementia** is a loss of mental ability, due to an organic factor, that may be reversible or irreversible. It is associated with loss of recent memory, impairment of judgment and abstraction, personality change, and a gradual deterioration in habits.
- **Amnestic Syndrome** causes an impairment of recent and long-term memory; secondary to an organic factor affecting brain function.
- **Organic Delusional Syndrome** involves delusions without impairment of consciousness, memory, or intellect; secondary to an organic factor affecting brain function.
- **Organic Hallucinosis** involves hallucinations in the absence of impairment of consciousness, memory or intellect, and without disturbance of mood; secondary to an organic factor affecting brain function.
- **Organic Affective Syndrome** is an organically determined disturbance of mood without evidence of delirium, dementia, delusional syndrome, or hallucinosis.
- **Organic Personality Syndrome** is an organically determined deterioration of behavior involving loss of emotional and impulse control and indifference or suspiciousness to others, without evidence of delirium, dementia, delusional syndrome, or hallucinosis.
- **Primary Degenerative Dementia** is associated with progressive dementia, all other organic and functional causes having been excluded.
- **Multiinfarct Dementia** causes dementia progressing intermittently, with focal neurological signs; secondary to cerebrovascular disease.

The organic brain syndromes of Intoxication and Withdrawal can occur with any of the known drugs of abuse: In addition to Intoxication and Withdrawal, alcohol causes: Withdrawal Delirium, Hallucinosis, Amnestic Disorder, and Dementia. A tabular summary of the substance-induced organic mental disorders is provided in Table 11.1.

Substance use disorders

This group of disorders represents chronic maladaptive behavior associated with the persistent and pathological use of or dependence on chemical substances that alter mood and behavior.

TABLE 11.1
Substance-induced organic mental disorders

Substance	Intoxication	Withdrawal	Withdrawal delirium	Delirium	Hallucinosis	Delusional syndrome	Affective disorder	Personality disorder	Amnestic disorder	Dementia
Alcohol	+	+	+		+		+		+	+
Barbiturate	+	+	+				+		+	
Opioids	+	+								
Cocaine	+						+			
Sympathomimetics	+	+		+		+	+			
Arylcyclohexylamine	+			+	+	+				
Hallucinogens	+				+	+	+			
Cannabis	+					+				
Tobacco		+								
Caffeine	+	+								

- **Substance Abuse Disorder** involves repeated, uncontrolled, or uncontrollable use of mind-altering chemicals leading to a deterioration in social or occupational adjustment of a duration beyond 1 month.
- **Substance Dependence** causes increasing tolerance to or withdrawal symptoms after cessation of the substance in question.

Substance use disorders are usually associated with an aggravation of maladaptive personality traits. They can lead to the organic mental disorders described in the previous section. Physical complications are common in association with alcohol use.

Schizophrenic disorders

Schizophrenic disorders represent a group of serious conditions involving irrational behavior despite clear sensorium in the acute phase and a fundamental and devastating disruption of psychic and social life. The patient's irrationality stems from disturbance of perception and emotion, abnormalities in the content and process of thinking, a deterioration in will, alteration in the sense of self, abnormal psychomotor phenomena, and a retreat from social contact into a private world. The disorder usually begins in adolescence or early adulthood. DSM-III requires that the symptoms have been present continuously for 6 months in order to rule out brief, reversible psychotic reactions now categorized in Other Psychotic Disorders.

Schizophrenic disorders may present as acute psychoses, with little warning. They may be seen in a prodromal stage of weeks' or months' duration. The patient may recover completely from the disorder; or show residual impairment of social, occupational, and personal functioning after partial recovery; or have a recurrence or recurrences of active psychosis; or continue to deteriorate into chronicity.

These disorders are more likely to occur in people with personality disorder of paranoid, schizoid, schizotypal, or borderline type; but they are not restricted to people of abnormal premorbid personality. The onset of an acute or active phase of the disorder may or may not follow a physical or psychosocial stressor.

During the acute phase, the patient is likely to exhibit the following features:

1. Disturbance of mood (excitement, depression, panic, or sense of eerie foreboding).
2. Abnormal perceptual experiences, especially depersonalization, derealization, or a sense of change or strangeness.
3. Delusions of being controlled or influenced by, or of having alien thoughts inserted into the mind by, an external agent.

4. Delusions of thoughts escaping from the mind or of the mind's being read by another person.
5. Delusions of persecution, of grandiosity, of bodily change, or of exalted religious nature.
6. Auditory hallucinations that comment on the patient's behavior, speaking about or to the patient.
7. Incongruous or blunted affect. The patient's emotional expression is likely to appear inappropriate to the content of conversation or out of step with it.
8. A disturbance in the process of thought involving one or all of the following characteristics: muteness, blocking, derailing, poor goal-direction, tangential thinking, irrelevance, neologisms, verbigeration, and verbal stereotyping.
9. The use of a private logic, difficulty in generalizing, overpersonalized thinking, overinclusiveness, and blurring of conceptual boundaries.

During prodromal and residual phases, the following features are characteristic:

1. Withdrawal from social activities and impairment of occupational functioning
2. Peculiar habits
3. Deterioration in hygiene and grooming
4. Blunted or inappropriate emotions
5. Vague, woolly, tangential, metaphorical, or overdetailed thought processes
6. Magical, bizarre, or dereistic thoughts
7. Increased self-absorption, with altered perception of self and environment

The **disorganized type** of schizophrenia is characterized by abnormal affect and disorganized thinking; the **catatonic type** by stupor, excitement, extreme negativism or compliance, rigidity or strange posturing; and the **paranoid type** by persecutory or grandiose delusions and hallucinations. A **residual type** is also recognized.

Paranoid disorders

The clinical pattern of these disorders is dominated by delusions of persecution or jealousy for longer than 1 month often interwoven with grandiosity and derived from misinterpretation of environmental cues. Signs of schizophrenia or organic brain disorder are absent.

- **Paranoia** involves an elaborate and systematized delusional system lasting more than 6 months.
- In **Shared Paranoid Disorder** (or folie à deux) one paranoid person induces another to share the same delusional beliefs.
- **Acute Paranoid Disorder** has a duration of less than 6 months.

Affective disorders

Affective disorders are characterized by serious, pervasive, and enduring disturbance of mood in the form of depression, irritability, or elation.

A **Manic Episode** involves an elevation or irritability of mood lasting longer than 1 week with overactivity, flight of ideas, grandiosity, insomnia, and the tendency to get involved in reckless or extravagant adventures. Some manic patients have delusions and hallucinations consonant with their inflated views of world and self.

In a **Major Depressive Episode,** the patient has a persistent and pervasive depression of mood together with the following psychosomatic features: anorexia, weight loss, insomnia, anhedonia, anergia, fatigue, psychomotor retardation, psychomotor agitation, diurnal variation, self-reproach, and suicidal thoughts. In severe cases, the patient may develop hallucinations and delusions consonant with the prevailing dysphoria.

DSM-III adds **with Melancholia** to the main title **Major Depressive Disorder** when the following features are marked: anorexia, weight loss, morning depression, early morning waking, marked psychomotor agitation or retardation, and guilt.

In **Bipolar Disorder,** the current episode (Manic, Depressive, or Mixed) is the expression of a recurring affective disorder. **Cyclothymic Personality** is diagnosed if, over the past 2 years, there have been repeated subclinical episodes of both hypomania and depression.

Dysthymic Disorder refers to a disturbance lasting longer than 2 years that is characterized by insomnia or hypersomnia, fatigue, low self-esteem, loss of interest, social withdrawal, irritability, pessimism, tearfulness, and, sometimes, thoughts of suicide.

Other psychotic disorders

All other psychotic disorders not classified in 1 through 5 are included here.

Schizophreniform Disorder is a category applied to patients who have presented symptoms of a schizophrenic disorder for more than 2 weeks but fewer than 6 months.

Brief Reactive Psychosis involves acute disorganization of thinking and behavior with delusions and hallucinations immediately after a severe psychosocial stressor, lasting for more than a few hours and less than 2 weeks but leading to complete recovery.

Anxiety disorders

Anxiety disorders are composed of a group of disorders in which the patient experiences severe anxiety in the form of persistent or repeated phobias, panic, obsessions, or compulsions.

Phobic disorders

Anxiety is expressed as a persistent, disproportionate, irrational fear of a specific object, event, or situation.

- **Agoraphobia** is a phobia of public places, often with a panic concerning the possibility of being lost, abandoned, incapacitated, or otherwise vulnerable in unfamiliar or impersonal surroundings.
- **Social Phobia** is associated with the irrational fear of being exposed to the scrutiny of other people. Like agoraphobia, it leads to a retreat from social relations other than in the immediate family.

Other phobias are classified as Simple Phobias.

Anxiety states

- **Panic Disorder** causes repeated attacks of severe apprehension during a period of more than 1 month, together with the physical signs of anxiety (tachycardia, tachypnea, sweating, etc.).
- **Generalized Anxiety Disorder** involves persistent anxiety associated with motor tension, autonomic hyperactivity, apprehension and hyperalertness.
- **Obsessive Compulsive Disorder** is defined by repetitive, stereotyped images, thoughts, impulsions, or actions cutting across normal thinking and seeming alien to the patient. The patient usually tries to suppress or resist the obsessions or compulsions but can do so only imperfectly and with mounting anxiety.
- **Posttraumatic Stress Disorder** is a generalized Anxiety Disorder following a serious stressor. It is associated with recurrent dreams or thoughts of the traumatic event and illusions of reliving it.

Somatoform disorders

Patients with these disorders are distinguishable by their disabling physical symptoms in the absence of physical disease or conscious impersonation of illness.

- **Somatization Disorder** is a chronic disorder of several years' duration, beginning before the age of 30 and involving many physical complaints that are not the result of physical disease, injury, medication or substance use.
- **Conversion Disorder** causes involuntary loss or alteration of physical function that mimics but is inconsistent with physical disease and coincides in onset with psychosocial stress. Conversion enables the patient either to avoid an undesired activity or to receive social support or both.
- **Psychogenic Pain Disorder** is associated with involuntary severe pain that mimics but is inconsistent with physical disease, is related to stress, and enables the patient to avoid difficulty or receive support.

- **Hypochondriasis** is the persistent fear or conviction of having a disease when there is no medical evidence for its presence.

Dissociative disorders

This group of disorders is characterized by persistent or repeated impairment of consciousness, memory, or the sense of self. Patients with these disorders may exhibit thoughts and behavior that seem to be split from the self and to have a life of their own.

- **Psychogenic Amnesia** is the partial or complete loss of personally important memory.
- **Psychogenic Fugue** involves loss of memory and identity and is associated with travel to a distant place and sometimes with the assumption of a new identity.
- **Depersonalization Disorder** causes episodes of alteration in the sense of self, often in association with illusions that the external world is changing or different.

Psychosexual disorders

These disorders of sexual functioning involve disturbance of gender identity, or paraphilia, or inadequate psychosexual arousal, or disorganized sexual psychophysiology.

Factitious disorders

Factitious disorders are caused by the deliberate production of physical or psychological symptoms or of self-injury in order to impersonate illness.

Personality disorders

Personality disorders form Axis II of the DSM-III's five-tiered system. They are enduring patterns of behavior involving an excess or deficiency of traits associated with mood, the control of affect and impulse, style of thinking, attitude to self, moral development, and social relationships.

Some common personality disorders are discussed here.

- **Paranoid Personality** involves an enduring distrust and suspicion of the motives of other people.
- **Schizoid Personality** is associated with emotional coldness, lack of sociability, and an indifference to the praise and criticism of others.

- **Schizotypal Personality** adds to the schizoid traits just mentioned, the characteristics of magical thinking, bizarre ideation, ideas of reference, and recurrent bizarre illusions.
- **Histrionic Personality** leads to egocentrism, overdramatism, the constant need for attention, manipulativeness, emotional outbursts, and a deficiency in the capacity for sincerity, fidelity, and deeper human relationships.
- **Narcissistic Personality** involves a strong sense of uniqueness and entitlement, preoccupation with fantasies of success, the craving for adulation, exploitativeness, and a fundamental lack of empathy with others.
- **Antisocial Personality** demonstrates, from before age 15, three of the following characteristics: truancy, expulsion from school, delinquency, running away from home, lying, sexual promiscuity, drunkenness, thieving, and vandalism. As an adult, the patient has a poor occupational record; is unable to function as an effective spouse, parent, or friend; and exhibits recklessness, impulsiveness, aggressiveness, lying, and criminal behavior.
- **Borderline Personality** has an unstable control of affect, impulse, and mood and an unstable sense of identity; has intense but unstable personal relationships; exhibits frequent anger, depression, and feelings of emptiness or loneliness; and demonstrates suicidal, self-injurious behavior, or transient psychotic episodes, at times of stress.
- **Avoidant Personality** exhibits low self-esteem, social inhibition, and hypersensitivity to criticism.
- **Dependent Personality** has a marked passivity and subordination to those to whom the patient is attached.
- **Compulsive Personality** manifests emotional detachment, perfectionism, interpersonal control, and often a reluctance to commitment and proneness to prevarication or procrastination when beset by doubt.

Summary

Throughout the history of medicine, there has been interplay between two philosophical views. The first viewpoint regards diseases as entities with an independent existence manifest in the patient's clinical symptoms and signs. The second views diseases as intellectual constructs that have no concrete reality but are useful for communication and prediction. Despite the flurry of disease reification in the wake of the great advances of bacteriology at the end of the 19th century, the general trend has been away from entities toward medical diagnoses regarded as more or less useful theoretical constructs.

Today, most psychiatrists use versions of the limited medical model. They would predict that at least some of the major affective and schizophrenic disorders will prove to have a biochemical basis and partially genetic etiology. Other disorders, on the other hand, will probably turn out to be difficulties in living associated with variations in the interaction between temperament, early learning, and subsequent stress. In such circumstances, the traditional biomedical model seems to be both inadequate and inappropriate.

Categorical diagnosis in psychiatry is of greatest use for communication and scientific prediction. It is less helpful for management planning. Planning requires a more detailed and individualized knowledge of the patient's biopsychosocial assets and problems than a categorical label can provide. This subject is dealt with in more detail in chapters 14 and 15. Moreover, categorical diagnosis has drawbacks. Some diagnostic labels are hollow, or too broad, or lacking in reliability and validity. Labels can put a barrier between clinicians and their patients and can be used to keep them at an emotional arm's length.

Critics of psychiatry have contended that labeling causes, or at least accentuates, mental illness. Some critics have argued that diagnosis is a political act: Psychiatrists, as agents of a corrupt state, are expected to sequester those who upset the status quo. Another dispute concerns the use of psychiatric diagnosis to mitigate criminal responsibility.

Much criticism of the medical model in the mental health field has to do with the concept of disease. Disease has never been adequately defined in medicine, and the concept of mental disease is on no less shaky ground.

There is some agreement that the phenomenology that is the proper concern of clinical psychiatry ought to be psychological and behavioral in nature rather than purely social. In this view, psychiatric disorders represent clusters of mental and behavioral phenomena that deviate sufficiently from the norm to convey biological disadvantage, a disadvantage implicit in the personal distress and disability involved in psychiatric illness.

Finally, the main adult mental disorders are described under titles proposed by the third edition of the *Diagnostic and Standard Manual of Mental Disorders.* The main disorders of children are summarized in chapter 23.

Selected Readings

Kendell's (1975) *The Role of Diagnosis in Psychiatry* is a dispassionate presentation of the history, purposes, and shortcomings of categorical diagnosis in medicine generally and psychiatry in particular. It has a particularly useful comparison of dimensional with categorical approaches and a discussion of the medical model. Woodruff, Goodwin, and Guze (1974) present a hard-line medical approach to psychiatric diagnosis in *Psychiatric Diagnosis.*

For classic assaults on the psychiatric model, read Scheff (1963) for the effect of labeling, Szasz's (1961) *The Myth of Mental Illness,* Laing's (1964) *Sanity, Madness and the Family,* Rosenhan's (1973) notorious use of impostors to trick psychiatrists, "On Being Sane in Insane Places," and Spitzer's (1976) rebuttal to Rosenhan.

The *Diagnostic and Statistical Manual of Mental Disorders,* DSM-III (1980) contains the official definitions of psychiatric disorders. As a textbook of categorical diagnosis, it is essential reading.

12

Modes of treatment

The diagnostic uncertainty and theoretical complexity of psychiatry would lead one to expect controversy over treatment. A bewildering array of therapeutic methods confronts the physician designing treatment plans for psychiatric patients.

All treatments work some of the time. The problem in psychiatry is that we are often not sure which treatments are most effective in what conditions. Each method has its proponents. Persuasive anecdotes abound; scientific studies are the exception. Research has been difficult to execute in this field because of its lack of diagnostic clarity and the large samples required for statistical purposes (Spitzer, Endicott, & Robbins, 1978). The clear diagnostic criteria for psychiatric disorders provided by DSM-III will help in developing the large multicenter studies needed to compare specific treatments in homogeneous groups of patients.

The need for multicenter studies

Depression illustrates the point. Antidepressant medication works in some but not all patients who complain of depressed mood. Multicenter studies comparing outcome of treatment in subgroups of depressed patients are beginning to define more specifically which patients respond to which antidepressants (Akiskal, 1983). Patients who fit the DSM-III criteria for Major Depressive Episode respond to antidepressants in approximately 70% of cases; but few patients classified as Dysthymic Disorder respond.

The paucity of outcome studies has allowed a number of disputes to proliferate:

Unresolved
controversies

1. Purism versus eclecticism
2. Biology versus psychology
3. Dualism versus holism
4. Psychotherapy versus behavior therapy
5. Treatment versus control

Purism versus eclecticism

The limitations of
unitary doctrines

The advocates of particular theoretical schools attempt to fit patients into treatment methods based on unitary doctrines rather than choosing the treatment methods that fit the needs and personality of the patient.

Case 12.1

■ John W., a 35-year-old married professional fund raiser, is brought by friends to a community hospital emergency room in a small university town. They describe his initially charming and then intrusively insistent plans to engage them in the production of a television screen play. The psychiatric resident on duty notes the patient's rapid, colorful, wide-ranging conversation. He also notes that John will not tolerate interruption and becomes angry and threatening when confronted about his inappropriate behavior. A telephone call to his wife reveals that periodically, for several months at a time, he becomes excitable, talks rapidly, and stays up all night planning grandiose business schemes that invariably lose large amounts of money. During these periods, he also becomes sexually promiscuous; as a result, he has been named in a paternity suit. Exasperated by his erratic behavior and infidelity, Mrs. W. has recently threatened to divorce John. She also mentions that he is in psychoanalytic treatment in New York City.

The resident makes a diagnosis of manic episode. Hoping to hospitalize the patient and provide appropriate treatment to shorten this episode, the resident telephones John's psychoanalyst to enlist his support. The following conversation takes place:

ANALYST: So John is up there in the Emergency Room in a manic state?

RESIDENT: Yes. I'd like to hospitalize him and start him on lithium. He seems to have had repeated episodes of manic behavior that have caused much financial loss and suffering.

ANALYST: Well, I don't think that would be such a good idea. We are right in the middle of an important part of the analysis; he is at the point of working through some oedipal conflict around his relationship with his mother. I believe this is causing his manic episode.

RESIDENT: But he's in no condition to undergo psychotherapy. He can't sit still for 30 seconds, much less 50 minutes!

ANALYST: We've been through this before, and he usually comes out of it in time. I'd hate like hell to have him lose this important opportunity.

The resident, annoyed, hangs up after telling the analyst that he intends to persuade John to come into the hospital anyway. He tries to do so but fails. John misses a follow-up appointment next day. Three days later, the resident receives a call from John, who, still manic, tearfully complains that he has been committed to a hospital in New Jersey. He had gone to New York to see the analyst, run out of the meeting after fifteen minutes, and been arrested later that evening for drunk and disorderly behavior. His wife is mortified. Her attorney has served separation papers. John asks the resident to find a hospital bed. ■

The need for a comprehensive approach

This example of theoretical blinkers illustrates the impropriety of a narrow model in a disorder that involves a biopsychosocial dysfunction. Other examples could be cited in which narrowly biological models are inaptly applied to patients whose problems are predominantly psychosocial.

Eclectic clinicians employ treatments from a variety of theoretical perspectives. However, problems can arise if they lack the understanding and skill necessary to apply the methods they choose.

Case 12.2

■ Peter S., a 30-year-old factory worker, presents at a psychiatric clinic with panic attacks. Initial treatment includes diazepam, 5 mg 3 times daily, and supportive psychotherapy with a social worker every 2 weeks. The medication suppresses his symptoms and the counseling helps him understand some of the stressors in his life. The counselor does not explore why the anxiety symptoms began at this particular time. Within 3 months, the attacks recur. Although he had been symptom-free during the interval, Peter reports that he has not been able to stop diazepam. Supportive psychotherapy is reinstituted, and diazepam maintained at 15 mg daily. Once again he obtains temporary relief.

Two months later the symptoms recur. However, this time Peter has significant depression with suicidal ideation. He is hospitalized. Further history reveals that his first panic attack occurred when he was moving to a new home. This stressor symbolically activated repressed, unresolved resentment about the many unhappy moves he underwent as a child during his father's service career.

After a short course of focal psychodynamic psychotherapy, Peter gains insight into the symbolic significance of the domestic move in relation to his past stressful dislocations. By understanding the origin of these feelings, he gains control over them. Imipramine is used to block further panic episodes. Relaxation exercises help wean him off diazepam. Three months later, imipramine is discontinued. Peter remains symptom-free. ■

At the initial evaluation, the physician did not adequately explore Peter's past history and thus did not determine why his panic attacks began after a move at 30 years of age. Furthermore, his treatment was unfocused and merely supportive. A preferable initial plan would have included the following steps:

A comprehensive management plan

1. Block panic attacks with imipramine.
2. Control anxiety initially with diazepam, to be gradually reduced after 1 week.
3. Take a thorough psychiatric history, which would reveal:

4. The need for stress management training, including relaxation; and indicate

5. The patient's need and capacity for focal psychotherapy in order to understand the relationship between current stressors, symptoms, underlying anger, and childhood events and feelings.

Biology versus psychology

The robust biomedical model of psychiatry

The strictly biomedical model of mental disorder suggests it is caused by physical disease that should be treated by physical intervention. As discussed in chapter 3, this reductionistic doctrine often fails in general medicine, as it does in psychiatry. Although the model has had a few spectacular successes (such as the discovery of penicillin as a treatment for tertiary syphilis), it has not been possible to demonstrate an underlying biological abnormality in most psychiatric disorders.

The proliferation of psychotherapies

Following World War II, disillusionment with the strictly biomedical model led American psychiatrists to incline towards purely psychological explanations of mental disorder. This trend relied upon a model in many ways no less limited than the biomedical, and was followed by a proliferation of psychotherapies and mental health clinicians with vested interests in nonmedical treatment. There was a resistance to mounting evidence for the genetic transmission and biological mediation of such disorders as schizophrenic and manic-depressive illness, and a denial of psychotherapy's failure to change the course of these disorders (Klerman, 1983).

The return of psychiatry to medicine

As evidence for biologic causation accumulated, many psychiatrists welcomed the return of their specialty to medicine. They eagerly treated every sad patient with antidepressant agents and every tense patient with tranquilizers. Again, indiscriminate treatment led to failure. Without reliable categorical diagnosis, and without distinction between the relative influence of physical, psychological, and social factors in the generation of illness, most physicians relied on guesswork when treating psychiatric patients.

Narrow doctrines are outdated

Recent work has shown that subtypes of depression have a differential response to psychotherapy and drug therapy (Klerman, 1983; Prusoff et al., 1980). The two treatments are actually additive in acute depressive episodes (Weissman, 1979). Other work suggests that psychotherapy and psychopharmacology are complementary in treating anxiety disorders (Sheehan, 1982). Karasu (1982) presents a conceptual schema for a discriminating but diverse pharmacotherapeutic approach to psychiatric disorder. There is no longer any justification for narrow doctrines.

Dualism versus holism

Plato began the traditional Western philosophic separation of mind from body. Dualism, promoted and maintained by Judeo-Christian religion, is anachronistic

Dualism is outdated

in medicine. The arbitrary separation of mind and body has been invalidated by the same biomedical science that originally promoted dualistic reasoning. Mind is a metaphor for the influence of the brain on behavior, and the brain is very much involved in the workings of the body.

Holism is closer to the Eastern philosophical tradition. Folk healers have long exploited the body's healing processes through their emphasis on natural psychological treatments. Unfortunately, many holistic practitioners who practice in Western society have no scientific standards and little or no formal training.

The need for a scientific holism

What is needed is an integration of the sciences of mind and of body into a scientific holism. Psychosomatic medicine supports this integration; it explores the personal meaning of illness and also strives to elucidate the psychoneurologic and neurobiologic mechanisms that translate environmental events and psychological responses to physical processes (Reiser, 1975).

Although holism has some resemblance to eclecticism, the two movements are unrelated; however, the appeal of each undoubtedly stems from common practical and theoretical concerns. These concerns have found a modern expression in the theory of general systems (Von Bertalanffy, 1968) and its application to biology (Miller, 1978) and to clinical medicine in the biopsychosocial (Engel, 1977, 1980) and pluralistic (Abroms, 1983; Marmor, 1983) models of psychiatry. This book demonstrates how biopsychosocial medicine and pluralistic psychiatry can enrich the clinical process of psychiatry.

General systems theory and the biopsychosocial approach

Psychotherapy versus behavior therapy

Since the middle 1960s, the preeminence of psychoanalytic psychotherapies in the psychological treatment of psychiatric disorder has been challenged by behavioral therapies derived from the concepts of classical conditioning (Pavlov, 1941), reciprocal inhibition (Hull, 1950), and operant learning (Skinner, 1957) and applied clinically by Dollard and Miller (1950) and Wolpe (1958). The objectives of behavior therapy can usually be measured. Measurement capability appeals to people who criticize psychoanalysis because its objectives are imprecise.

The emergence of behavior therapy

Although there is some overlap, the two schools of thought stem from distinct concepts of people and behavior. Each has remained separate from, and antagonistic towards, the other (Shectman, 1975). The earlier division between physical and psychological was complicated by this new polarity, often at the expense of clinical reasoning. Recent efforts to synthesize behavioral and psychoanalytic theories often appear to be mere translations of one technique into the terminology and conceptual framework of the other (Breger & McGaugh, 1965), though some clinicians attempt to combine the two approaches (Brady, 1968; Segraves & Smith, 1976; Kaplan, 1974). This chapter contends that the two different approaches are not clinically incompatible but can be used in a complementary fashion to provide comprehensive treatment.

The antagonism between behavior therapy and psychoanalysis

The possibility of complementation

Case 12.3   ■   Marie, a 50-year-old married bank executive, visits her family physician complaining of an excessive fear of thunderstorms. Thunderstorms have worried her since adolescence but did not significantly interfere with her life until 3 years ago, when she married for the second time.

An intelligent, reflective woman, Marie seems well-suited to psychotherapy. The physician refers her to a psychologist, who commences psychodynamic psychotherapy.

After 8 months, Marie is grateful for insights that have helped her in her marriage, but to her dismay, the phobia of thunderstorms and her anxiety symptoms have increased rather than abated. Convinced her case is hopeless, she terminates treatment. During the winter months, she is symptom-free, but as the summer thunderstorm season approaches, she becomes increasingly fearful. Her doctor persuades her to see a psychiatrist, who uncovers the following information.

The symptoms increased when Marie and her second husband bought a large house on the top of a high ridge. With its panoramic view, the house provided a box seat from which to watch the thunderstorms as they moved in from the west. Moreover, due to the exposed nature of the ridge, lightning frequently strikes near the house. Marie has become so terrified that, on the approach of a thunderstorm, she will hide in a broom closet in the center of the basement. If thunderstorms are forecast, she cannot sleep.

The husband, an electrical engineer, has not yet put up lightning rods. He wants to do it himself, citing his concern about the poor quality of work by local contractors.

Marie was deserted by her first husband, who left her to raise two children alone. Marie's father had been autocratic and chauvinistic: Women were not to be heard from.

Fifteen sessions combining directive psychotherapy, behavior modification and desensitization, and insight-oriented psychotherapy clear Marie's symptoms and improve her general coping ability. The following specific tactics are used:

1. A contractor is hired to install lightning rods.
2. Marie learns relaxation techniques to modify the anxiety associated with a forecast of thunderstorms. She eventually learns to relax during them.
3. Psychodynamic psychotherapy helps her understand:
   i. how her anger at her father was warded off by subassertive behavior with men in general and her new husband in particular;
   ii. how her repressed anger escapes control under situations of stress and is expressed as anxiety.

As Marie develops conscious control of her anger, anxiety and environment, her symptoms subside. Communication with husband and children improves dramatically. She is promoted at work.   ■

Multimodal therapy   Despite early gains in insight, Marie was unable to continue psychoanalytically oriented psychotherapy because her primary symptoms were too disabling. A subsequent combination of behavioral, psychopharmacologic, and psychotherapeutic treatment was effective.

Treatment versus control

The allegedly illusory nature of psychiatric disorder

Chapter 11 presents the contentions of Szasz (1961) and others that there are no psychiatric diseases, only differences in thinking and behavior, and that psychiatry is merely a pseudoscience designed to control socially deviant behavior. However, the polemics of antipsychiatry have coincided with advances in neuroscience, genetics, and clinical phenomenology that point to the differential influence and interaction of biologic and psychosocial factors in many psychiatric disorders.

Somatic interventions

Psychopharmacology

The excessive and indiscriminate use of psychotropic drugs

In the last 30 years, the introduction of psychotropic drugs has fundamentally altered the practice of psychiatry. Psychotropics are the class of medication most frequently prescribed by primary-care physicians (Mellinger et al., 1978). They can be used as specifics for categorical diagnostic groups, as in the case of lithium for manic-depressive illness (see Case 12.1). Unfortunately, they have too often been prescribed indiscriminately for common emotional states, as with benzodiazepines for the unavoidable anxieties of daily living.

Controversies in psychopharmacology

The benefits and side effects of psychotropic drugs

The immediate benefits of pharmacotherapy must be weighed against the likelihood and severity of long-term side effects. Neuroleptics ameliorate acute psychotic episodes and prevent relapse in chronic schizophrenic patients (Goldberg et al., 1977); but they have troublesome, though usually reversible, side effects. The prolonged use of neuroleptics increases the risk of **tardive dyskinesia,** a relatively irreversible and disabling neurological disorder. Tricyclic antidepressants provide the treatment of choice for major depressive episodes, but they are lethal in overdose, and the patients who need them most have the highest risk of suicide. There are more subtle long-term side effects. Benzodiazepines are potent anxiolytics with few immediate side effects except sedation. However, the clinician who does not closely follow the patient might not discern the early signs of psychological or physiological dependency and would also miss the gradual decomposition of coping strategies that accompanies their habitual use.

Medication can suppress the normal resolution of life crises

Medication can either facilitate or impede psychotherapy. Anxiety is ubiquitous and can motivate human beings to learn more effective coping techniques. By the same token, sadness is an inevitable concomitant of grief. Drugs should not be used to suppress the feelings that punctuate and define existence and spur personal development. However, if anxiety or depression become so disabling that they impair and prevent learning, medication can be useful. Medication can reverse the neuropsychiatric disorder underlying some symptoms or suppress other symptoms sufficiently for constructive psychologic work to continue. The disruption of concentration by major depression, for example, precludes psychotherapy. In such a case, antidepressant medication restores normal brain function and enables patients to tackle the external stresses and internal distortions that predispose them to emotional disorder. On the other hand, because benzodiazepines provide immediate relief, they can prevent the patient from working out better techniques of coping with stress.

Medication can suppress disabling symptoms

The best clinical judgment can be at odds with the patient's legal rights or the prevailing social mood. In most states, patients cannot be forced to take medication unless they have a major psychiatric disorder and are a clear, present danger to themselves or others. Ironically, the patients who could benefit most are likely to be the least cooperative.

The patient's right to refuse treatment

Patients need to know the immediate effects, complications, long-term benefit, and liabilities of psychotropic drugs. Uninformed people can be influenced by prejudice, ignorance, and misplaced humanism; a little knowledge can be a dangerous thing. Some patients refer to *The Physicians' Desk Reference* to investigate the drug prescribed and note its side effects. As a consequence, they may refuse to take the drug or become hypochondriacal about it. *The Physicians' Desk Reference* lists every side effect ever reported, even if not proven to have been caused by the drug. The book is as much a legal cover for pharmaceutical companies as it is a handy reference. Physicians know this but patients do not.

The patient's right to be informed about psychotropic medication

Psychotropic medication should be used for specific purposes, not vague symptoms. Contrast the use of antidepressants in appropriate doses for major depression with the use of antidepressants in low doses in dysthymic personality; or the prescription of flurazepam to treat the insomnia associated with an undiagnosed major depression.

Prescribe psychotropic medication for specific purposes

The physician should follow the patient closely and not prescribe drugs automatically. All too often, the patient attends a clinic where the physician checks symptoms and reissues prescriptions. Because such drugs as the benzodiazepines are nontoxic, prescriptions can be refilled for years before complications develop. Mindlessness of this sort has probably contributed to the high incidence of long-term complications following anti-anxiety medication.

Never refill prescriptions without checking

Some therapeutic regimens are too complicated. Unsubstantiated claims that particular drugs or classes of drug relieve specific symptoms might account for this phenomenon. When one phenothiazine is promoted for schizophrenia with depression, and another for schizophrenia with agitation, the result can be symptom-chasing polypharmacy, no drug being given a proper trial. In pharmacotherapy, simplicity is beautiful. The patient complies better with an uncluttered therapeutic regimen, and the clinician can follow a particular medication with more assurance and fewer mistakes.

Simplicity is beautiful

Psychopharmacological regimens are sometimes standardized rather than individualized in accordance with physical status, character traits, coping styles, the severity of symptoms, the degree of dysfunction, and the specificity of the diagnosis. Obsessive patients will obediently count pills and take medication as many times a day as required. Less organized patients may be better off with once-a-day doses. Hypochondriacal patients, who focus on physical symptoms, tolerate drugs with side-effects poorly. For them, the clinician might prescribe a monoamine oxidase inhibitor or trazodone (both of which have relatively mild anticholinergic side effects) rather than some tricyclics (which have marked side effects). Hypochondriacal patients will rigorously comply with a monoamine oxidase inhibitor diet; impulsive patients are much less reliable. Other traits affecting medication use are discussed in chapter 3.

Individualize medication according to age, sex, size, and personality

Current trends in health care suggest that more nonmedical health professionals will be caring for patients with psychiatric disorder. The physician in a community mental health center may be tempted to do no more than sign pre-monoamine oxidase inhibitor or trazodone (both of which have relatively, mild anticholinergic side effects) rather than some tricyclics (which have marked side effects). Hypochondriacal patients will rigorously comply with a monoamine oxidase inhibitor diet; impulsive patients are much less reliable. Other traits affecting medication use are discussed in chapter 3.

The need for medical supervision of all patients on medication

The need for adequate medical facilities

The general principles of psychopharmacology

The following general principles should guide the physician who uses psycho-pharmacologic agents.

Interactions, side effects, and pharmacokinetics

Learn the pharmacology of the agents you use. A knowledge of drug interactions is essential, particularly when prescribing for the elderly, who are often being treated at the same time for physical disorders. Knowledge of side effects and pharmacokinetics helps the clinician decide dose frequency and magnitude. Consider the patient's coping style before determining which drug within a general class is most likely to promote compliance and symptom relief.

Case 12.4

■ Amelia, a 42-year-old bank executive, has been hospitalized recently with a diagnosis of manic-depressive illness. She is stabilized on lithium carbonate, 1200 mg daily, and discharged. For the next year, Amelia functions better both at home and at work. Then, at a routine physical examination, her physician diagnoses essential hypertension. She is placed on hydrochlorothiazide in moderate doses.

Three weeks later, Amelia notices increasing nausea and vomiting, diarrhea, and weakness. One morning, her husband finds her in bed, somnolent and confused. Amelia is rushed to the hospital, where elevated serum levels confirm the diagnosis of lithium toxicity. Fortunately, she recovers from this dangerous complication with no neurological defect. Belatedly and ruefully, her physician recalls that the sodium-depleting effect of hydrochlorothiazide tends to elevate serum lithium concentration. ■

Symptom relief is only a temporary expedient

Treat syndromes rather than symptoms.   At times, symptomatic relief facilitates crisis intervention, but this should be regarded as a temporary expedient.

Case 12.5

■   Gwen, a 33-year-old housewife, complains of sleep disturbance. She is diagnosed as having major depressive disorder. When her physician suggests antidepressant medication, Gwen protests vigorously that she does not want to be "on drugs," but she finally agrees to take amitriptyline at a starting dose of 50 mg at bedtime.

Gwen gets immediate relief of her sleep disturbance but complains bitterly of side effects, especially dry mouth. She refuses to increase the dose, saying that she feels much better. Hoping this to be true, her doctor relents.

Four days later, her insomnia returns. Gwen's mood darkens and she becomes suicidal, requiring hospitalization.   ■

Wait for the diagnosis to declare itself

Do not prescribe prematurely.   Wait for the diagnosis to declare itself. Do not confound the diagnostic process with medication unless the patient is in such danger that you have no choice.

Case 12.6

■   Steve, a 28 year old graduate student presents with neurovegetative symptoms suggesting depression. Restricted to a 10-minute office visit, the physician takes only a cursory psychiatric history and starts the patient on tricyclic antidepressants.

Steve's insomnia is relieved, but his sadness and tearfulness continue.

During a third visit 1 month later, a more detailed history reveals that the anniversary of his first wife's death fell during the previous month and that annually, for the 4 years since she died, he becomes sad. The physician ceases medication and refers Steve for psychotherapy.   ■

Prevent allergic, toxic, or interaction effects

Take a good medication history.   Minimize the chances of an allergic response, toxic side effect, or drug interaction.

Case 12.7

■   Anthea, a 45-year-old woman, has taken phenelzine for depression since late autumn. In the early summer, Anthea commences her usual hay fever medication – a combination of antihistamine and sympathomimetic. Anthea's subsequent hypertensive crisis results from the interaction of monoamine oxidase inhibitor and sympathomimetic. It could have been prevented if a more careful medication history had been taken.   ■

Use as few drugs as possible

Avoid polypharmacy.   If you are using more than one drug, it may be impossible to evaluate your management plan.

Case 12.8

■   Alicia, a 50-year-old woman diagnosed as having major depression with psychotic delusions is treated successfully as an outpatient with a combination of tranylcypromine for depression and diazepam for sleep disturbance.

At her weekly visits, Alicia is emotionally labile, complaining of frightening visual hallucinations, particularly at night. The psychiatrist adds chlorpromazine to the bedtime regimen, but her symptoms worsen and the patient starts to believe she is going crazy. The psychiatrist increases the medication.

Finally, after Alicia is hospitalized, she discloses that she was taking from 2 to 6 tablets of diazepam in order to fall asleep and avoid the painful mood. Her hallucinations were symptoms of a metabolic delirium provoked by a toxic accumulation of diazepam and the anticholinergic effects of chlorpromazine. ■

Age and somatic disease effect pharmacokinetics

Consider the effects of age and medical illness on your choice and dose of drug.   Older people and patients with liver disease often metabolize psychotropic drugs very slowly. Pay due regard, for example, to cardiovascular and renal disease.

Case 12.9

■ Grover, a 68-year-old man, complains of difficulty falling asleep. Flurazepam provides relief for 2 weeks, but at the next visit Grover seems rather sleepy and his wife says he has been confused recently. A mental status examination reveals disorientation for time and other signs of mild confusion. Remembering that flurazepam has active metabolites with long half-lives, the physician stops medication. When Grover's mental status improves, he prescribes triazolam, which has a relatively short half-life and no active metabolites. Grover sleeps better, cheers up, and becomes active once again. He uses triazolam only once or twice monthly when he cannot get to sleep because he has something on his mind. ■

Case 12.10

■ Hubert, a 50-year-old man who suffered a myocardial infarction 6 months previously, has physically recovered and returned to work. Hubert's internist refers him to a psychiatrist for the evaluation and treatment of residual major depression. The electrocardiogram shows no postatrioventricular node conduction disturbance. Nevertheless, concerned about cardiotoxic effects of tricyclic antidepressants, the psychiatrist prescribes trazodone, an antidepressant with low cardiotoxicity, in small doses spread evenly over the day to minimize the risk of a hypotensive episode. ■

Use an instruction sheet

Give explicit instructions.   Use an instruction sheet for medication if the directions are complicated or you are concerned about compliance. Many doctors use printed forms. Hospital nurses also require clear, explicit orders. Do not expect them to guess what you have in mind.

Case 12.11

■ Roger, a 38-year-old man with chronic recurrent headaches frequently appears at the emergency room asking for a shot of demerol. Often he is ataxic and slurred in speech, as though drunk. A resident gives him 2 days medication and refers him to a psychiatrist at a behavioral medicine clinic. There, it is discovered that he is taking pentazocine, diazepam, percodan, and amitriptyline.

To understand the temporal relationship between drug use and pain, mood, and environment, the psychiatrist asks Roger to record when he uses medication. Doctor and patient use this record to develop a medication protocol that successfully avoids the use of the emergency room and helps Roger stabilize his erratic life. ■

Reevaluation　　　　*Regularly reevaluate and, if necessary, adjust medication.*

Case 12.12

■ Virgil, a 26-year-old man with anxiety attacks is given a 6-month supply of diazepam with instructions to take them as needed. Medication works well, and the patient is free of anxiety for the first time in ten years. At the end of 6 months, Virgil asks for and receives a refill. This cycle is repeated thrice. Two years later, he cannot stop medication without experiencing a variety of symptoms associated with both anxiety disorder and sedative withdrawal.

After a turbulent period in the hospital, during which he is evaluated and diazepam is withdrawn, Virgil eventually learns to use the drug on an occasional basis, in close consultation with a psychiatrist. ■

Use goal-oriented outcome criteria to monitor treatment

Evaluate your treatment according to clear outcome criteria. If necessary, revise your diagnostic hypotheses, formulation or management plan. Goal-oriented evaluation is described in chapter 14.

Case 12.13

■ Beatrice, a 28-year-old schoolteacher, presents with major depressive disorder. After 3 weeks, she reports no benefit and many side effects from tricyclic antidepressant therapy. In accordance with the negotiated treatment plan, medication is stopped for 4 days and then phenelzine is prescribed. Beatrice improves rapidly. ■

Treatment requires more than medication

Never rely on medication alone. Every patient requires at least supportive psychotherapy, if only to facilitate compliance.

Case 12.14

■ Karl, a 32-year-old unemployed man with paranoid schizophrenia, will not comply with medication instructions. Karl's psychiatrist helps him recognize his anger about being ''treated like a kid.'' Karl reveals that the therapist reminded him of his father, who was always ''bossing him around.'' ■

Insure medication is for the patient

Never prescribe drugs for the benefit of someone other than the patient. The clinician may be pressed by relatives or ward staff to quiet the patient.

Case 12.15

■ Carroll, a 32-year-old patient with bipolar disorder, is calmed in the hospital with haloperidol and started on lithium. On the fifth hospital day, a Sunday, the nurses note the return of the agitated, aggressive behavior that characterized Carroll on entering the hospital. He abuses staff and threatens other patients.

The nurses call the resident on duty, who is otherwise engaged in evaluating a suicidal patient in the Emergency Room. They request an increase in the patient's antipsychotic medication. The resident, though unfamiliar with the case, complies with the nurses' request without taking a further history or examining the patient.

Later that evening, Carroll is difficult to rouse. A serum lithium level, drawn the same morning, is in the toxic range. In retrospect, the nurses recall that the patient was clumsy and confused at the time his aggressiveness recurred. ■

The classes of psychoactive drugs

Major tranquilizers

Nature

The difference between the sedative and antipsychotic effects of neuroleptics

Major tranquilizers (neuroleptics) induce a state of diminished emotional responsiveness to which patients eventually develop tolerance. This effect is to be distinguished from the therapeutic effect of neuroleptics on the symptoms of psychosis. Both effects have been ascribed to dopaminergic-blocking.

The most commonly used neuroleptics are as follows:

1. Phenothiazines: e.g., chlorpromazine, thioridazine, trifluoperazine, fluphenazine, perphenazine.
2. Butyrophenones: e.g., haloperidol.
3. Thioxanthines: e.g., chlorprothixine, thiothixene.
4. Dibenzoxazepines: e.g., loxapine.
5. Dihydroindolones: e.g., molindone

Aims

1. Reduce psychotic hyperactivity and emotional agitation.
2. Control psychotic thought disorder.
3. Counteract social withdrawal in psychosis.
4. Reduce abnormal movements (in Gilles de la Tourette's Syndrome): haloperidol.
5. Sedate: chlorpromazine and thioridazine.
6. Reduce anxiety: small doses of neuroleptic.
7. Control manic excitement.
8. Control nausea and vomiting: especially perphenazine.

Indications

1. Acute schizophreniform or schizophrenic disorder.
2. In major depressive disorder when agitation or delusions are a prominent feature of psychotic depression.
3. Acute mania.
4. Organic brain disorder with aggressive behavior.
5. Delirium (use neuroleptics in small amounts).
6. In chronic schizophrenia: to dampen thought disorder and prevent relapse.
7. Gilles de la Tourette's syndrome.

Contraindications

1. Bone marrow deficiency.
2. Central nervous system depression.
3. History of personal or family hypersensitivity.
4. Severe liver disease.

Problems and dangers

1. Anticholinergic side effects (blurred vision, urinary retention, ileus, fecal impaction, confusion): especially chlorpromazine, and thioridazine.
2. Extrapyramidal effects (bradykinesia, akathisia, dystonia, akinesia, pseudo-parkinsonism, perioral tremor): especially haloperidol, fluphenazine, trifluoperazine.
3. Orthostatic hypotension: especially chlorpromazine.
4. Photosensitivity of skin.
5. Retinitis pigmentosa: thioridazine in doses of more than 800 mg daily.
6. Pigmentation of skin, lens, and cornea.
7. Lowered seizure threshold.
8. Cholestatic jaundice.
9. Hypothalamic effects (changes in appetite; weight gain; fluid retention; breast enlargement and engorgement in both sexes; galactorrhea; change in libido; ejaculatory incompetence; and malignant neuroleptic syndrome, a rare but sometimes fatal dysregulation of hypothalamic function associated with hyperpyrexia, delirium, and hypertension).

Clinical use

Neuroleptics have revolutionized the treatment of major psychosis, controlling terror and disintegration, and thus allowing psychosocial treatment to be effective. Patients who once would have spent most of their lives in a hospital can now live in the community despite residual psychotic symptoms. Unfortunately, psychotropic agents have sometimes been used to control people rather than to treat psychiatric disorder. Too many patients have been kept on drugs without adequate review. The emergence of tardive dyskinesia underscores this danger. Consequently, the widespread overuse of these agents, particularly in institutions, has led to a public outcry obscuring their real benefit.

When and how should a physician prescribe antipsychotic drugs?

Acute schizophrenia or schizophreniform disorder
    1. A trial of neuroleptic medication is indicated for patients with acute schizophrenic or schizophreniform disorder when other causes of acute psychosis have been ruled out. If possible, drugs should be withheld for approximately

1 week to determine if the patient improves with the support of the hospital milieu alone; but if the patient is unmanageably excited or being treated at home, drugs are usually required from the outset (Simpson & May, 1982). Neuroleptics shorten hospital stay and speed rehabilitation (Davis, 1980). Select a drug according to the general principles outlined in this chapter, prescribing a small initial oral dose to test for allergic reactions and side effects.

Psychotic excitement

2. In acute psychotic excitement of schizophreniform, schizophrenic, or manic origin, rapid medication may be necessary. It can be undertaken by oral, intramuscular, or intravenous route (Donlan, Hopkin, & Tupin, 1979). The clinician should gauge the effects of each dose after 30 to 60 minutes before determining the next dose. Avoid fixed schedules lest the drug accumulate and tardive dyskinesia occur.

Manic hyperactivity

3. In manic episodes, antipsychotics help to control hyperactivity until lithium can counteract mania. To avoid uncertainty about whether the patient actually swallows the pills, liquid haloperidol or chlorpromazine can be used. If rapid onset is desired, intramuscular haloperidol is better absorbed than chlorpromazine and less likely to provoke a hypotensive episode.

Delirium or dementia

4. In delirium or dementia, because of its relatively few cardiovascular side effects, haloperidol can be used in small oral or intramuscular doses to alleviate fear and agitation (Moore, 1977; Wells, 1977).

Psychotic depression

5. Neuroleptics are useful in patients with major depressive disorder who have psychotic symptoms such as severe agitation, delusions, and hallucinations not attributable to organic brain disorder.

Prophylaxis against relapse

6. To prevent relapse, patients with chronic schizophrenic or schizoaffective disorders should be maintained on neuroleptics but in doses as low as possible. To minimize the risk of tardive dyskinesia, dosage levels should be kept as low as possible.

Tics

7. In patients with Gilles de la Tourette's Syndrome, small doses of haloperidol alleviate uncontrolled gesticulation, verbalization, and movement.

Precautions against tardive dyskinesia

Tardive dyskinesia is a constant concern. Though neuroleptics should be prescribed only when clearly indicated, they should not be underused. Once the patient's condition has stabilized, the dose of an antipsychotic drug should be gradually reduced to the minimum necessary to help the patient maintain adequate functioning. If possible, the patient should have a drug-free trial.

When should the physician consider injectable depot medication? When daily medication would be inconvenient or when cognitive disorganization or resistance impairs compliance.

When should antiparkinsonian medication be considered?

1. Not routinely. Antiparkinsonian drugs can increase the total dose of antipsychotics required, and they have troublesome anticholinergic side effects.

2. If parkinsonism occurs, or if there is a clear past history of dystonia,

*Be alert for the anti-
cholinergic synergism
of antiparkinsonian
and neuroleptic
medication*

Cholestatic jaundice

*Early signs of
agranulocytosis*

antiparkinsonian drugs should be prescribed. After several months, they can usually be gradually discontinued without a recrudescence of parkinsonism.

3. Acute dystonia should be treated with such intramuscular antiparkinsonian agents as benztropine or diphenhydramine. Be on guard against the toxicity resulting from the combined anticholinergic effects of antiparkinsonian and neuroleptic medication.

When are laboratory tests necessary? Look out for two unusual but serious complications – **jaundice** and **agranulocytosis.** Jaundice almost always occurs within the first month of treatment and is of allergic, cholestatic type. It is generally reversible following abrupt cessation of the drug. Agranulocytosis is a rare but catastrophic disorder with high mortality. It almost always occurs between the fourth and tenth week of treatment. An initial complete blood count should always be obtained. *The occurrence of infections, sores, fever, or sore throat early in the course of antipsychotic therapy should alert the physician to repeat the complete blood count.*

Antianxiety agents

Nature

Several groups of drugs are used to treat anxiety. Their exact mechanism of action is unclear, although, as discussed in chapter 5, increasing evidence indicates that each has a specific membrane receptor (Tallman et al., 1983). The following are the most commonly prescribed antianxiety agents:

1. Benzodiazepines: diazepam, chlordiazepoxide, chlorazapate, oxazepam, flurazepam, lorazepam, triazolam, alprazolam.
2. Antihistamines: particularly hydroxyzine.
3. Barbiturates: phenobarbital.
4. Tricyclics: especially imipramine.
5. Monoamine oxidase inhibitors: parnate, nardil.
6. Beta-blockers: propanolol.

Aims

1. Sedate: benzodiazepines, barbiturates, antihistamines.
2. Reduce anxiety: benzodiazepines, antihistamines.
3. Block panic attacks: tricyclics, especially imipramine; monoamine oxidase inhibitors.
4. Block peripheral autonomic sympathetic arousal in anxiety: beta blockers.
5. Induce sleep: benzodiazepines.
6. Decrease muscle tension: benzodiazepines.
7. Alleviate alcohol withdrawal symptoms: benzodiazepines.

Indications

1. Panic disorder: imipramine or monoamine oxidase inhibitors to block panic attacks; and benzodiazepines, short-term, to calm the associated anxiety state.
2. Generalized anxiety disorder: benzodiazepines, short-term, for acute episodes. If peripheral autonomic responsivity is a significant perpetuating mechanism, block with propanolol.
3. Agitation in major depressive disorder: benzodiazepines, short-term only.
4. Sleep onset insomnia: benzodiazepines, short-term, in stressful situations.
5. Muscle spasm: benzodiazepines, short-term, in musculoskeletal disorders, particularly those with a cycle of pain, anxiety, and muscle spasm.
6. Traumatic anxiety: benzodiazepines, short-term only.
7. Alcohol withdrawal: benzodiazepines.
8. Psychophysiologic disorders: benzodiazepines, short-term; tricyclics for maintenance.

Contraindications

1. A history of paradoxical excitement.
2. Because of the dangers of lethal overdose and addiction, barbiturates are rarely, if ever, indicated, except in epilepsy.
3. Acute narrow-angle glaucoma.

Problems and dangers

1. Paradoxical excitement: benzodiazepines.
2. Sedation: all, except propanolol.
3. Psychological dependence: especially barbiturates and benzodiazepines.
4. Physical dependence: especially barbiturates; also benzodiazepines with long-term use.

Clinical use

Barbiturates have little place in psychiatry

Barbiturates have little place in the therapeutic armamentarium. If a patient is hypersensitive to other sedatives, barbiturates can be used, very short-term, for sedation or hypnosis. Intravenous amobarbital has been used to facilitate the recovery of repressed memories and for the rapid sedation of dangerously violent patients.

Medication for panic disorder

Tricyclics (particularly imipramine) and monoamine oxidase inhibitors (particularly phenelzine) are effective in modifying panic disorders. Alprazolam, a newer benzodiazepine, is also effective in panic disorders. The clinician can use imipramine or phenelzine to block panic attacks that aggravate anxiety and cause anticipatory anxiety. Acute anxiety is best treated by a 1- to 6-week course of benzodiazepines in conjunction with psychotherapy (see Case 16.6).

Benzodiazepines are not a panacea

Benzodiazepines are relatively safe, so safe, in fact, that they have become drugs of overuse, though rarely of abuse. The pharmacokinetic differences between different benzodiazepines can be exploited by the astute clinician. For example, diazepam has a rapid onset of action that might be useful in sleep-onset insomnia, but it might also be abused by someone who enjoys the sudden sensation of drowsiness. A drug with more delayed absorption, such as oxazepam, could be preferable with such a patient. Because of the risk of toxicity, older patients or those with liver disease should not be given benzodiazepines such as diazepam, chlordiazepoxide, or flurazepam. These drugs either have long half-lives themselves or produce active metabolites with long half-lives. Because of its short half-life and lack of active metabolites, oxazepam might be preferable in such cases. Remember that when drugs with relatively short half-lives are abruptly stopped, blood levels will drop rapidly and acute withdrawal syndromes may occur, in some cases with seizures.

Diazepam has rapid onset of sedation

Benzodiazepines with long half-lives unsuitable in the elderly or with liver disease

Antidepressants

Nature

Antidepressants affect neurotransmitter function in the adrenergic and serotonergic systems of the nervous system. The exact mechanisms by which they counteract depression are not clear (see chapter 5), though recent evidence points to their influence on the density and sensitivity of serotonin and norepinephrine receptors. Their differential side effects and therapeutic efficacy may be attributable, in part, to differences in their effect on different bioamines. The following are examples of different classes of antidepressants:

Different side effects due to effects on different bioamines

1. Tricyclics: imipramine, amitriptyline, desiprimine, protriptyline, nortriptyline, doxepin, clomipramine.
2. Dibenzoxazepine: amoxapine.
3. Tetracyclics: maprotiline, mianserin.
4. Triazolopyridines: trazodone.
5. Tetrahydroisoquinolines: nomifensin.
6. Monoamine oxidase inhibitors: tranylcypromine, phenelzine.
7. Stimulants: dexamphetamine, methylphenidate.
8. Neuroleptics (see the previous section in this chapter).
9. Antianxiety agents (see the previous section in this chapter).

Aims

1. Counteract depressed mood in patients with major depression: tricyclics, amoxapine, tetracyclics, trazodone, monoamine oxidase inhibitors.

2. Increase energy and motor activity: stimulants.
3. Reduce panic attacks: tricyclics, monoamine oxidase inhibitors.
4. Reduce agitation and anxiety: benzodiazepines, neuroleptics.
5. Counteract depressive delusions: neuroleptics.
6. Prevent recurrence of depressive episodes: lithium, tricyclics, tetracyclics, trazodone.
7. Alleviate obsessions and compulsions: clomipramine.
8. Alleviate pain: tricyclics.
9. Reduce gastric acidity: tricyclics, especially doxepin, amitriptyline, trimipramine.
10. Increase attention span in adult attention deficit disorder: tricyclics.

Indications

1. Major depressive episode: tricyclics, triazolopyridines, tetracyclics, monoamine oxidase inhibitors.
2. Acute anxiety and agitation in major depression: benzodiazepines, short-term use.
3. Delusional melancholia: antidepressants in combination with neuroleptics.
4. Recurrent major depressive episodes: antidepressants or lithium for prophylactic purposes.
5. To energize depressed patients: stimulants, short-term.
6. To regulate sleep in major depression: amitriptyline, doxepin, trazodone.

Contraindications

1. Tricyclics: in postatrioventricular node conduction disturbance.
2. Monoamine oxidase inhibitors: if the patient is unable to avoid tyramine-containing foods, tricyclics, stimulants, and such sympathomimetic amines as L-dopa and alpha-methyldopa.
3. Regular use of stimulants.

Problems and dangers

1. Anticholinergic effects: blurred vision, constipation, urinary hesitancy, fuzzy thinking, aggravation of glaucoma, paralytic ileus. Primarily with tricyclics (though least with desipramine).
2. Insomnia: stimulants, tranylcypromine, protriptyline.
3. Sedation: amitriptyline, doxepin, trazodone, benzodiazepines.
4. Orthostatic hypotension: tricyclics.
5. Hypertension: monoamine oxidase inhibitors interacting with tyramine-containing foods or other medication (see Case 12.7).

6. Sympathomimetic effects: tachycardia, tremor, sweating, agitation, insomnia, aggravation of psychosis. Found with tricyclics and stimulants.
7. Cholestatic jaundice: tricyclics.
8. Metabolic and endocrine disturbance: weight gain, impotence, gynecomastia, amenorrhea, and hypo- or hyperglycemia in diabetics. Found with tricyclics.
9. Accentuation of depression or agitation: stimulants.
10. Lethal overdose: all, especially tricyclics, maprotilene, and monoamine oxidase inhibitors.

Clinical use

Tricyclics (and related drugs) and monoamine oxidase inhibitors are the most effective drugs for major depressive disorder. They are also sometimes helpful in dysthymic disorder. The two kinds of depression responding to medication are distinguished from other forms of depression by a short REM sleep latency, as discussed in chapter 10 (Akiskal, 1983). For many patients with mild depressive symptoms or chronic dysphoria, tricyclics and monoamine oxidase inhibitors are no more effective than benzodiazepines, placebos, or psychotherapy (Klerman, *Indiscriminate and* 1983). Unfortunately, antidepressants are often prescribed indiscriminately for *inadequate usage of* nonspecific complaints of unhappiness. Even when prescribed appropriately, *antidepressants* their dosage level too often is inadequate.

Antidepressants work slowly. Often, 2 to 4 weeks are required before a beneficial effect can be demonstrated. With this in mind, the clinician may be tempted to give several weeks' supply, a lethal dose if taken all at once. As a pre- *Need for small pre-* caution, prescribe antidepressants in small amounts and schedule frequent ap- *scriptions and frequent* pointments to check mood, suicidal ideation, and the adequacy of social support. *checks initially* If suicidal ideation becomes more serious, consider whether hospitalization is necessary to ensure safe medication.

The psychological The many troublesome anticholinergic side effects of tricyclics can reduce *response to side effects* compliance. However, properly informed patients will perceive the side effects as *of antidepressant* indications that medication is working rather than as frightening new symptoms. *medication* In depressed, hypochondriacal or somaticizing patients, side effects reinforce illness conviction and a sense of helplessness. Some clinicians therefore consider monoamine oxidase inhibitors to be the medication of choice in such cases. Trazodone, for example, has few troublesome side effects except sedation.

Dealing with patients Some patients object to "mind-altering drugs" and regard side effects as *who object to mind-* evidence for their dim view of medication. To avoid poor compliance, active *altering drugs* education is required. These patients can be instructed that antidepressants reverse abnormal brain function just as other drugs counteract the abnormal functioning of other organs. They should appreciate that side effects are an indication not of toxicity but of the effectiveness of medication, and that antidepressants will help them regain normal mind, brain, and body function.

Psychotherapy promotes compliance with medication in five ways:

Ways in which psy-
chotherapy promotes
compliance

1. By educating the patient about drugs and illness.
2. By providing emotional support.
3. By facilitating the patient's understanding of the nature of side effects and of other problems that might interfere with compliance.
4. By counteracting the pessimism that undermines compliance (see the section on psychotherapy later in this chapter).
5. By enabling the patient to identify, understand, and resolve resistance to treatment.

The delayed therapeutic action of antidepressants indicates the need to provide support in the early weeks of treatment. However, overcautious or inexperienced clinicians may increase medication too slowly, thereby further delaying therapeutic benefits and reinforcing hopelessness.

The use of blood levels
of antidepressant

Drug blood levels are of limited use (Gelenberg, 1983b). Occasionally, when side effects or poor therapeutic response confuse the picture, blood levels can help to determine if the patient has been compliant or whether the dose is within the therapeutic range. Nortriptyline, for example, has a therapeutic window: doses higher or lower than the therapeutic range are ineffective.

The therapeutic
windows

Using side effects to
counteract secondary
symptoms

Side effects can be used to the patient's advantage. The insomnia of major depression is counteracted by the sedative action of amitriptyline or doxepin. Conversely, protriptyline energizes depressed patients with hypersomnia.

Many physicians avoid monoamine oxidase inhibitors because they fear a monoamine oxidase crisis in noncompliant patients. The physician who goes beyond categorical diagnosis will appreciate the patient's coping style, predict which patients will be compliant and therefore prescribe monoamine oxidase inhibitors with confidence.

Benzodiazepines alleviate the anxiety and agitation that often accompany major depression. They can be used to provide temporary relief pending the antidepressant action of a tricyclic or monoamine oxidase inhibitor. Patients should subsequently be weaned from benzodiazepines within a few weeks.

Lithium carbonate

Nature

Possible mechanisms
for the therapeutic
action of lithium

Lithium is a monovalent cation directly exchanged for intracellular sodium. The precise mechanisms of the therapeutic action of lithium in mania are not clear; the following central effects may be involved:

1. Inhibition of the activation of postsynaptic adenyl cyclase by neurotransmitters and hormones.
2. Stabilization of neuronal membranes.

3. Down regulation of norepinephrine and dopamine function by desensitizing postsynaptic receptors, facilitating presynaptic reuptake and deactivation, and inhibiting release.
4. Increase in serotonin synthesis.

Aims

1. Counteract acute mania.
2. Prevent or dampen mood swings in bipolar depression.
3. Prevent recurrent episodes of unipolar depression.
4. Prevent recurrence of alcohol abuse; a response that may be related to the mood-stabilizing properties of lithium.
5. Prevent recurrent migraine headaches; another response that may be related to the mood-stabilizing properties of lithium.
6. Prevent ulcers.

Indications

1. Acute mania.
2. As prophylaxis against recurrent severe mood swings of depressive or manic nature in bipolar disorder.
3. As prophylaxis against recurrent major depression.
4. As prophylaxis against episodic drinking in alcoholics with primary mood disorder.
5. As prophylaxis against recurrent headaches in patients with underlying depressive disorder.
6. Peptic ulcer.

Contraindications

None.

Problems or dangers

1. Acceptable side effects.
   a. Gastrointestinal: mild nausea, anorexia, and diarrhea.
   b. Neurological: fine tremor of fingers, slight drowsiness.
   c. Metabolic/endocrinologic: weight gain, thirst and polyuria, nontoxic goiter after prolonged use.

2. Unacceptable side effects.
   a. Gastrointestinal: severe vomiting, diarrhea.
   b. Neurologic: fasciculations, coarse tremor, muscle weakness, hyperreflexia, myoclonus, ataxia, blurred vision, nystagmus, slurred speech, changes in consciousness (ranging from drowsiness and sluggishness to confusion, stupor, and coma), seizures.
   c. Renal: nephrogenic diabetes insipidus, structural damage of uncertain incidence and severity (Bernstein, 1983).
3. Hypothyroidism or goiter with normal thyroid function but elevated TSH.
4. Renal toxicity, involving polydipsia, polyuria, and decreased creatinine clearance (Gelenberg, 1981).
5. Dermatologic disorders, including psoriasis, rashes, acne, and alopecia (Gelenberg, 1982).
6. Ventricular irritability or slow atrioventricular node conduction (Mitchell & Mackenzie, 1982).
7. Respiratory depression in patients with chronic lung disease (Gelenberg, 1983c).
8. Neurotoxicity in patients on a combination of lithium and neuroleptics (Prakash, Kelwala, & Ban, 1982).
9. Seizures (rarely).

Clinical use

Small margin of safety

Lithium has a very small margin of safety. Therapeutic levels for acute mania (1 to 1.8 mEq per liter) overlap with mild toxic levels (1.5 to 2 mEq per liter). Coma and death will result from levels over 5 mEq per liter. The physician must therefore be aware of the physiologic factors influencing serum lithium levels:

1. Acid-base balance.
2. Sodium metabolism.
3. Hydration.
4. Renal function, particularly renal clearance.
5. Other drugs.

Be alert for signs and symptoms of toxicity and closely monitor serum levels for retention, especially when the patient is on a low sodium diet or losing sodium through sweating, vomiting, or diarrhea, or when the renal clearance of lithium is diminished by renal or cardiovascular disease.

Several drugs can elevate serum lithium:

Drugs that elevate serum lithium

1. Antiprostaglandins (indomethacin, phenylbutazone, piroxicam, diclophenac, ketoprophen, and oxyphenbutazone).
2. Diuretics.

Rapid loading of lithium

The usual loading dose of lithium carbonate is 300 mg t.i.d. or q.i.d. But lithium can be given in higher doses, such as 600 mg t.i.d., to bring the patient to a therapeutic level (1.0 to 1.5 mEq per liter) as rapidly as possible. Thereafter, check serum levels every 2 to 3 days and keep a close watch for signs of toxicity. Older patients who need rapid loading can be started on from 300 to 600 mg daily.

Periodic checks of serum level

Continue to check serum levels every 2 to 4 days until the desired level has been maintained for several weeks. The interval between checks can be lengthened gradually when you are confident a particular dose will maintain a serum level that is both therapeutic and nontoxic.

Teratogenicity

Because lithium is associated with fetal abnormality, a pregnancy test should be performed before a woman of reproductive age starts lithium.

Table 12.1, derived from Gelenberg (1983b), summarizes the laboratory protocols for each commonly used psychotropic agent.

Noncompliance with lithium medication

Of all psychopharmacologic agents, lithium requires the most detailed initial work-up and the most exacting supervision. Noncompliance can be problematic. Manic patients enjoy how they feel and often see no reason for medication. The effective clinician helps patients anticipate such resistances.

TABLE 12.1
Laboratory tests for patients taking psychotropic drugs (Gelenberg, 1983b)

Drug group	*Pretreatment*	*During treatment*	*Blood drug levels*
Antipsychotic	EKG? Other tests when clinically indicated	As clinically indicated	Experimental
Antidepressant	Same as for antipsychotic drugs	As clinically indicated	Compliance check; toxicity (but cautions about technique)
Antianxiety	Only when clinically indicated	As clinically indicated	Experimental
Lithium	Renal: • serum creatinine • routine urinalysis Thyroid: • T$_4$ • T$_3$RU • FT$_4$I • TSH Other: • CBC with differential • calcium? • electrolytes? • pregnancy test? • EKG?	Renal: • serum creatinine (every 3–6 months) Thyroid: • TSH (every 6 months) Other: • CBC with differential? • calcium? • EKG?	Routine, 12 hours before last dose. Order 4 days after each dosage adjustment. Blood level at least every 3 months during maintenance therapy.

Lithium is clearly indicated in acute mania: but when should maintenance lithium be prescribed? The physician must weigh the possibility of preventing disruptive mood swings against the likelihood of complications.

Electroconvulsive therapy

Issues

*Controversies about
the use of ECT*

Despite its relative safety and proven effectiveness in major depression, there is much controversy about ECT. The following issues are often raised in disputes about the legitimacy of this mode of therapy:

1. The mechanism by which ECT acts has not been clarified.
2. Many people perceive the electrically induced convulsing of a helpless patient to be torture, not treatment.
3. ECT has often been misused in the past. Although ECT is used responsibly and sparingly today, historical abuses have affected public opinion.
4. ECT can have a deleterious effect on memory (see the next "Problems and Dangers" section in this chapter).

The banning of ECT is often espoused by the advocates of patients' rights who oppose psychiatry. As a consequence, ECT has been prohibited in California by legislative action.

Nature

The patient is first anesthetized with a short-acting intravenous barbiturate and then relaxed with a neuromuscular blocking agent, such as intravenous succinylcholine. Subsequently, a 60-cycle, AC 100–170 volt stimulus is applied to bilateral or unilateral (nondominant hemisphere) temporal leads for from .1 to .7 seconds.

Aims

1. Counteract intractable melancholia.
2. Reduce life-threatening agitation and hyperactivity in schizophrenic or manic patients.

Indications

1. Severe melancholia that has not responded in 30 days to an adequate trial of antidepressant medication.

2. Suicidal emergency in a depressed patient.
3. Life-threatening agitation and hyperactivity in mania or schizophrenia.

Contraindications

Brain tumor.

Problems and dangers

1. ECT can produce confusion and recent memory loss that does not subside fully for 3 to 6 months. Confusion and memory loss are much less frequent and severe after unipolar ECT.
2. Relapse is fairly common.
3. ECT often requires hospitalization, seriously disrupting work and family relationships.
4. ECT carries the usual risks of general anesthesia.
5. The idea of ECT frightens patients.

Clinical use

The impossibility of predicting which cases will respond better to ECT than to medication

Public resistance and the risk of memory loss have relegated ECT to the second line as a treatment for major depression. Without doubt, ECT is as effective as tricyclic antidepressants and in some cases more effective. However, it is not possible to predict which cases of depression will respond better to ECT than to antidepressant medication.

Conditions in which ECT is the treatment of choice

ECT is the treatment of choice for depressed patients with postatrioventricular node cardiac arrhythmia. It is to be preferred to drugs in pregnant women. It is occasionally required to treat life-threatening manic or schizophrenic agitation and hyperactivity.

Unilateral ECT is preferable

ECT should be used only when clearly indicated and only by psychiatrists well-versed in its use. Unilateral (nondominant hemisphere) ECT should be preferred to bilateral ECT since it is no less effective and has a much lower incidence of memory loss.

Sleep interruption

Interrupting REM sleep

It has recently been shown that interrupting sleep, particularly rapid eye movement sleep, can counteract depression (Schilgen & Tolle, 1980). The mode of action is not known; but a chronobiological mechanism, involving a resetting of the circadian rhythm, has been hypothesized. Though promising, this treatment technique is still experimental.

Physical therapy and exercise

The nonspecific benefits of exercise

The evidence that physical therapy and exercise have specific therapeutic effects is more anecdotal than scientific; the psychological benefits of exercise have not been shown to exceed those conferred by such activities as transcendental meditation, biofeedback, relaxation training, and simple rest (Morgan, 1979). On the other hand, some evidence suggests that exercise enhances self-esteem and productivity (Greist et al., 1979; Morgan, 1979).

Aims

1. Provide recreation.
2. Improve physical conditioning.
3. Improve self-esteem.
4. Engage patient in socializing activity.

Indications

1. When there is a need to reduce stress and enhance self-esteem.
2. Anxiety, depression, and adjustment disorders of all types.

Contraindications

None.

Problems and dangers

Need for medical screening

1. Unsupervised physical exercise is dangerous. Patients must be medically assessed before they engage in strenuous exercise and thus incur the risk of myocardial infarction or physical injury.
2. Exercise should not replace more specific somatic and psychosocial therapy.

Clinical use

The psychological benefits of physical therapy in rehabilitation

Physical therapy, in the broad sense of the word, can benefit almost everybody; it is particularly useful during rehabilitation from physical disorder such as myocardial infarction or musculoskeletal injury. Physical therapy also has psychological benefits. Working with a sports medicine specialist and physical, occupational, and dance therapists, a psychiatrist can design programs with exercise goals graduated to reinforce and challenge the patient. Dance therapy and similar activities contribute to the therapeutic milieu of a hospital service, mobilizing and socializing withdrawn, depressed, or anxious patients.

Psychological interventions

What is psychotherapy? Despite the diverse approaches to this form of treatment, several common features can be discerned:

Features common to all psychotherapy

1. Psychotherapy involves communication between a sanctioned therapist and a person who needs help, or between several people in these roles.
2. The roles are agreed on by both patient and therapist, the patient wanting help and the therapist providing it.
3. The therapeutic technique has a theoretical basis explaining the patient's symptoms and rationalizing the technique for alleviating them. The therapist accepts the theory; the patient may or may not.
4. Therapy occurs within the context of an intense relationship between therapist and patient.

The overlap between different techniques

Although different types of psychotherapy can be distinguished on theoretical grounds, in practice there is much overlap between different techniques. All therapy is the heir to healing practices derived from prehistory. Religious conversion, faith healing, and shamanism have features in common with psychotherapy – altered cognitive states, suggestion, cognitive reorganization, and social reinforcement by a healing presence.

Many people call themselves psychotherapists. Some have had professional training in psychiatry, psychology, and social work; others have not. Although most psychiatric residency programs require systematic courses in psychotherapy, training nationally is uneven. For example, in some programs psychodynamic psychotherapy is taught, but family, group, marital, and behavioral therapies are neglected. In other programs, psychodynamic psychotherapy is ignored.

Although there is disagreement about how particular methods bring about change, the different psychotherapies have common ingredients:

The ingredients of successful psychotherapy

1. The patient must be motivated for psychotherapy.
2. Therapist and patient must agree on the rationale for therapy.
3. Therapist and patient must agree on a therapeutic plan.
4. The therapeutic alliance must be strong enough to encourage the patient to tackle the personal stresses and distortions that would otherwise be avoided.

The difficulty of evaluating the efficacy of psychotherapy

Although psychotherapy has been an integral part of medicine for millenia, its effectiveness has been difficult to demonstrate scientifically (London & Klerman, 1982). Frank (1975) suggests two reasons for this:

1. The key therapeutic agent is a human relationship that defies measurement.
2. The patient is exposed to treatment during only a small portion of waking life – at the most 5 out of more than 100 hours per week. The patient's experiences between sessions may have greater influence on outcome than does the therapy itself.

The expense of psychotherapy

Socioeconomic questions influence psychotherapy, as they do all of medicine. Psychodynamic psychotherapy, for example, is usually recommended for people who are intelligent, fluent, and psychologically minded; but intensive psychotherapy is expensive and out of reach for many patients. The advent of insurance policies that reimburse for psychotherapy has made it more available to people with lower income.

Therapy as a culturally congruent metaphor

Therapeutic methods reflect the culture. Intensive psychoanalysis evolved in turn-of-the-century Vienna and reflected the contemporary emphasis of European intelligentsia on introspection and individualism. The recent heyday of experiential and encounter therapies paralleled contemporary vogues for sensation and immediacy. Behavior therapy, on the other hand, reflects the American fondness for tinkering with malfunctioning machines. Therapy is acceptable only when it provides a culturally congruent metaphor for the nature of illness and the essence of healing.

Categorical diagnosis is of limited use to psychotherapy

Categorical diagnosis, useful in guiding the choice of somatic therapies, has limited applicability to psychotherapy. The kind of diagnosis required for psychotherapy involves exploring personal and clinical phenomena within a theoretical scheme that explains behavior, in a discourse that is at once phenomenological, dynamic, and existential.

Types of psychotherapy

Psychodynamic psychotherapies emphasize the influence of early life experiences on present thought, feelings, and behavior. **Cognitive-behavioral psychotherapies** focus more on how current events and thinking affect feeling and behavior.

Psychodynamic Psychotherapies include:

Modes of psychotherapy

1. Supportive psychotherapy.
2. Expressive symptom-relief psychotherapy.
3. Psychoanalysis.
4. Exploratory psychodynamic psychotherapy.
5. Brief focal psychotherapy.

Cognitive-behavioral psychotherapies include:

1. Behavior therapy.
2. Cognitive psychotherapy.

Psychodynamic psychotherapies

Supportive psychotherapy

Nature

Listening, reassuring, advising, and educating

Supportive psychotherapy can be used in a wide variety of settings and situations. This technique involves listening to, reassuring, advising, and educating the patient with the intent of strengthening ailing defenses and coping techniques. Like all psychotherapy, it takes place in the context of an identificatory relationship.

Aims

1. Develop a therapeutic alliance with the patient.
2. Restore patient to a previous level of functioning or prevent further deterioration.
3. Alleviate symptoms.
4. Enhance self-esteem.
5. Strengthen existing healthy defenses.

Indications

1. When a strong therapeutic alliance is required for other purposes (e.g., to facilitate difficult medical treatment, as in juvenile diabetes mellitus).
2. Temporary emotional crisis due to situational stress, particularly acute grief reactions.
3. Adolescent crises.
4. Chronic psychiatric illness, when other techniques are unlikely to be effective.
5. As an adjunct to pharmacotherapy.

Contraindications

When a more specific intervention is required.

Problems and dangers

1. If underlying conflicts are not resolved, excessive dependency on the therapist can perpetuate maladaptive behavior.

2. Neurotic or psychotic transference to the therapist can cause, perpetuate or aggravate maladaptive behavior.

Clinical use

Supportive psychotherapy requires few technical skills other than the capacity for concerned listening and giving sensitive advice. People with natural facility and a little training can provide effective supportive therapy; hence, the wide use of this treatment (e.g., the clergyman or family physician who provides grief counseling for a recently bereaved family; the physician who helps a patient accept the losses associated with a progressive or chronic illness; the school counselor who helps an adolescent with a drop in grades discuss a family problem; the psychiatrist who encourages a schizophrenic patient recovering from a psychotic illness to discuss a dislike of medication).

Expressive, symptom-relief psychotherapy

Nature

Therapist and patient meet weekly in an outpatient setting or more freqently in an inpatient setting for up to 20 to 30 sessions. The patient is encouraged to express hitherto suppressed emotion. The catharsis of feeling relieves tension; identification with the therapist's strength encourages coping; and acceptance by the therapist enhances self-esteem. This technique borrows from the concepts of client-centered therapy (Rogers, 1951) and crisis intervention (Caplan, 1964). It demands a more focused technique than supportive psychotherapy, particularly in reflecting and clarifying the patient's feelings. These clarificatory techniques have been alluded to in chapter 7.

Aims

1. Develop a relationship of acceptance, trust, and empathic concern.
2. Relieve acute tension and associated symptoms.
3. Terminate or institute more specific treatment.

Indications

1. Anxiety, tension, grief, anger, or somatic symptoms in schizophrenic, affective anxiety, somatoform and dissociative disorders, life crises, and acute grief reactions at any age.

2. Chronic characterological psychopathology when socioeconomic, geographic, and other factors make long-term psychotherapy impossible.
3. As an adjunct to the pharmacologic treatment of severe psychiatric disorder.
4. To provide urgent symptom relief during the diagnostic encounter.

Clinical use

Whatever the cause, physical, psychological, or social, patients in crisis can be helped to ventilate and assimilate their feelings about past or recent events.

Case 12.16
■ Dale, a 35-year-old single schoolteacher, is recovering from a panic disorder that required her to take medical leave from her teaching responsibilities.
As the end of summer approaches, Dale becomes troubled and insomniac. With angry tears, she admits to her physician that she expects a confrontation with her principal who, she believes, was unfair to her when she was struggling to work during the onset of her illness. The doctor listens attentively and reassures her that she will be able to cope. Convinced that she is not deteriorating, Dale begins to make preparations for returning to work rather than despairing about the future. ■

Case 12.17
■ Frederick, a 20-year-old college student arrested for drunken driving, weeps bitterly about the emptiness he has felt since his mother died 6 months previously. After several sessions of grief work, he resumes college life with renewed confidence. ■

Case 12.18
■ Earl, a 25-year-old schizophrenic man, has been admitted to the hospital for an acute episode of persecutory auditory hallucinations. He tells the hospital physician that he fears being evicted from his room by an unfriendly landlord, who has increased the rent and refused to fix an inadequate heating system. The therapist validates Earl's sense of injustice and empathizes with his feeling of helplessness. He supports the patient's determination to do something about it. Gradually, Earl's symptoms subside without an increase in medication. With the help of a social worker, he begins looking for new accommodation. ■

Psychoanalysis

Nature

The neutrality of the therapist and the development of transference

Psychoanalysis is an extensive (e.g., from 1 to 5 years) and intensive (e.g., from 3 to 5 times weekly) form of exploratory psychotherapy aiming at a fundamental change in maladaptive personality traits and coping by facilitating insight into hitherto unconscious conflicts, emotions, and attitudes. The psychoanalyst is a neutral figure on whom these unconsciously determined conflicts are projected. The ensuing intense relationship or **transference** gives the therapist an opportunity for psychological interpretation. Thus, the patient is helped to become more self-aware and to work through childhood conflicts.

Aims

1. Establish a relationship.
2. Encourage spontaneous expression of thought and emotion.
3. Aid resolution of unconscious conflict by interpreting unconscious wishes, ego defense, and transference.
4. Help the patient work through conflicts.
5. Terminate relationship.

Indications

Patients with chronic psychoneurotic symptoms, personality disorder, or maladaptive coping techniques stemming from the inadequate resolution of intrapsychic conflict.

Contraindications

1. Psychotic disorders.
2. Low intelligence.
3. Conduct disorder.
4. Severe personality disorder.

Problems and dangers

1. Expense.
2. Unresolved transference.

The need for the patient to define problems and establish goals

3. In this form of therapy patients are expected to define and explore their own problems and establish and pursue their own goals. The initial vagueness of therapy can be difficult to tolerate. The initial lack of clear goals also makes outcome difficult to evaluate.

Clinical use

Psychoanalysis is usually recommended for chronic interpersonal problems unresponsive to brief, focal psychotherapy and reflecting long-standing neurotic conflict. The patient should meet the following criteria:

1. Reasonable social functioning.
2. Adequate verbal intelligence.
3. Capable of a therapeutic alliance.
4. Capable of expressing feelings in words.

5. Capable of fantasy and introspection.
6. Reasonably tolerant of frustration, anxiety, and anger.
7. Likely to be able to terminate, at the end of therapy, without emotional trauma.

Focal or brief psychodynamic psychotherapy

Nature

This involves intense, focused, short-term (10 to 40 sessions) outpatient treatment. A specific conflict is targeted, pathological defenses confronted, and the transference actively interpreted.

Aims

1. Develop a strong therapeutic alliance.
2. Resolve a specific intrapsychic conflict underlying chronic symptoms.
3. Keep intervention brief.

Indications

A clearly delineated conflict

Patients with chronic symptoms who have the same characteristics as those for whom psychoanalysis is recommended and who have a clearly delineated unconscious conflict as the basis of their maladaptive or symptomatic behavior.

Contraindications

1. Patients who do not meet the criteria just discussed.
2. Psychotic patients.

Patients and dangers

1. The anxiety-provoking nature of the therapy can worsen symptoms and provoke regression.
2. Focal psychotherapy is dangerous in the hands of poorly trained or inexperienced therapists.

Clinical use

Prerequisites for effective focal psychotherapy

This therapy requires training and experience. The therapist must actively confront defenses, interpret transference resistance, and avoid characterological problems. Strong motivation for change, ability to trust the therapist, and the capacity to terminate without undue emotional trauma are critical to tolerating the anxiety provoked by focal psychotherapy.

Long-term exploratory psychodynamic psychotherapy

Nature

Patient and therapist meet from 1 to 3 times per week for more than 1 year, without definite time limit usually in an outpatient setting. Both interpretive and supportive techniques are used to sustain some defenses and confront others.

Aims

1. Establish therapeutic alliance.
2. Resolve intrapsychic conflict.
3. Improve self-esteem.
4. Improve interpersonal relationships.
5. Alleviate symptoms.

Indications

Patients with chronic symptoms who lack the resources for psychoanalysis, and who have more diffuse unconscious conflicts than those who are suitable for focal psychotherapy, but who can tolerate anxiety and have some introspective ability, internal resources, and life stability.

Contraindications

Inability to tolerate self-exploration.

Problems and dangers

The need for clear goals

The initial vagueness of therapeutic goals can confuse the patient and result in a lack of clear direction.

Clinical use

Many patients who begin other forms of treatment ultimately enter exploratory therapy. The constraints of the setting and the patient's initial expectations may preclude exploratory work early in treatment; but if maladaptive patterns continue despite directive therapy, the need to explore predisposing conflicts will be apparent.

Case 12.19   ■ Phil, a 35-year-old professional man, presents with alcoholism and marital problems. After detoxification, he develops a major depression, which is treated with supportive psychotherapy and tricyclic antidepressants. Marital therapy helps Phil improve his communication with his wife as the couple overcome the mutual antagonism that has resulted from years of alcohol-related strife.

Two years later, further upsets have occurred at work and home. Psychiatrist and patient decide to explore the basis of the passive-aggressive coping style that creates continual difficulties between Phil and his wife, friends and business associates. ■

Cognitive-behavioral psychotherapies

Behavior therapy

Nature

Classical and operant conditioning   Behavior is learned by two mechanisms: **classical conditioning,** in which antecedent events serve as conditioned or unconditioned stimuli to conditioned responses; and **operant conditioning,** in which the likelihood that a behavior will occur is influenced by responses that positively or negatively reinforce it. Behavior therapy is a loosely associated group of techniques concerned with learning or unlearning behavior rather than modifying personality.

Therapeutic activity   The behavior therapist is highly active, identifying the behaviors to be changed, determining the antecedent and consequent events associated with each behavior, and manipulating events to alter behavior in the desired direction. The goal of behavior therapy is symptom relief through behavior change.

Behavioral procedures that focus on antecedents include:

Procedures that focus on antecedents

1. Respondent conditioning.
2. Stimulus control.
3. Fading.
4. Therapeutic instructions.
5. Self-instructions.
6. Modeling.

Procedures that focus on consequences include:

Procedures that focus on consequences

1. Positive reinforcement.
2. Negative reinforcement.
3. Shaping.
4. Self-reinforcement.
5. Reinforcement of autonomic responses.

6. Extinction.
7. Aversion.
8. Information feedback.

Aims

1. Establish a therapeutic alliance.
2. Identify the target behavior.
3. Complete a behavioral assessment of the symptom or undesirable behavior:
   a. Analyze the events, situations, people, and physical or psychological stimuli antecedent to the behavior,
   b. Identify the aversive or rewarding reinforcement value of the consequences of each behavior.
4. Identify desirable and attainable objectives.
5. Develop plan to achieve objectives.
6. Develop an evaluation strategy.
7. Implement treatment plan.
8. Terminate, with contingency and maintenance plans.

Indications

The use of behavior therapy in combination with other treatment

Behavior therapy is most effective when combined with other approaches. It can be integrated, to some degree, in any treatment plan. Relaxation therapy, for example, has almost universal benefit. Specific indications for behavior therapy are as follows:

1. Psychophysiologic disorder.
2. Physical disorder in which stress precipitates or perpetuates symptoms or the progression of disease.
3. Anxiety disorder.
4. Somatoform disorder.
5. Organic mental disorder in which behavioral control is desirable.
6. Schizophrenic disorder in which rehabilitation is impeded by maladaptive behavior learned during prolonged institutionalization.

Cognitive psychotherapy

Nature

The theoretical basis of cognitive psychotherapy

Cognitive psychotherapists assume that psychiatric disorder is caused by distorted attitudes and thoughts. For example, a distorted interpretation of interpersonal situations can lead to irrational thoughts, unpleasant emotions, and maladaptive behavior, as in Figure 12.1.

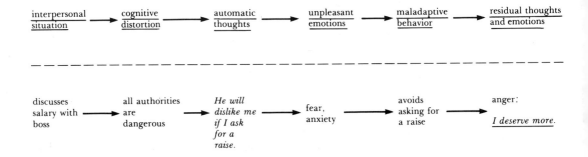

FIGURE 12.1

Assessment in cognitive psychotherapy

Cognitive psychotherapy aims to help patients focus on their cognitive responses to the stimuli that trigger maladaptive behavior. The fundamental tenet, initially proposed by Ellis (1962) and further developed by Beck (1976), is that irrational beliefs and misconceptions are at the root of emotional problems. Cognitive therapy adapts techniques from behavior therapy and psychodynamic psychotherapy while emphasizing conscious thoughts and attitudes.

Aims

1. Establish a therapeutic alliance.
2. Help the patient to:
    a. Identify the erroneous assumptions, cognitive distortions, and illogical thoughts causing and perpetuating emotional distress.
    b. Replace self-defeating, erroneous assumptions and cognitive distortions with more constructive ideas to counteract emotional distress.
    c. Develop adaptive social skills consistent with restructured cognition (e.g., self-assertiveness and effective listening).
    d. Maintain improvement change.
4. Terminate treatment.

Indications

1. Anxiety disorder.
2. Depression.
3. Somatoform disorder.
4. Habit and eating disorders.
5. Chronic schizophrenic disorder.

Contraindications

1. Acute psychosis.
2. Organic brain syndrome.
3. Severe personality disorder.

Problems and dangers

1. Cognitive therapy requires a high degree of cooperation. Some patients are so dysfunctional that they cannot concentrate on therapy and thus become further demoralized by failure.
2. The physician should not rely on this treatment exclusively when other treatments are more appropriate or complementary. For example, when unresolved conflicts impede cognitive therapy, psychoanalytic psychotherapy might be preferable to a cognitive approach.

Clinical use

The advantages of cognitive therapy

In comparison with psychodynamic psychotherapy, cognitive psychotherapy has some advantages. It is shorter, less expensive, and applicable to a wide range of patients. Patients need not be particularly introspective or verbally fluent. Some evidence indicates that cognitive therapy is as effective as medication alone in patients with unipolar depression (Kovacs et al., 1981). The technique can be used in conjunction with such other treatment as pharmacotherapy. However, unconscious conflicts may prevent the patient from working effectively. In that case, exploratory psychodynamic psychotherapy should be considered.

Social interventions

Nonspecific and specific social interventions

Social interventions aim to change a patient's self-image and coping through experience in a therapeutic setting. Social interventions range from therapeutic milieu to group, marital, and family therapy. Their widespread use has resulted from an appreciation of the influence of social factors on individual behavior (Bloch, Crouch, & Reibstein, 1981).

Two principles of group process underly therapeutic change:

The principles of group process that determine therapeutic change

1. In a group that meets regularly, individuals will display characteristic patterns of thinking, feeling, and behavior. The clinician can use the group process to elucidate these characteristic patterns.

2. Groups foster regression. As psychoanalysis provokes regression by the ambiguity of the therapeutic situation, group therapy facilitates regression by generating group tension. Early developmental conflicts regarding basic trust or autonomy, for example, are often provoked by the group. Anxiety is contagious. Characteristic defenses are mobilized. Groups can help a patient appreciate and work through unresolved conflicts.

Psychoanalytic theory
Existentialism
Learning theory

The influence of the social group on personality development is discussed in chapter 3. Psychoanalytic theory stresses the influence of early social experience on current behavior. Existential theory emphasizes the influence of the present social environment on personal experience. Learning theory deals with the influence of antecedent and subsequent social events on behavior.

Communication theory
Systems theory

Other theories explain the process of group intervention. **Communication theory** analyses the interaction of individuals in a dyad. **Systems theory** describes the way individuals affect groups and vice versa; for example, dynamic changes in individuals affect their behavior in groups. Conversely, groups influence individual dynamics. Thus, group interaction can be described in terms of individuals who respond to one another in repetitive ways (Jackson, 1957).

Structural theory

Structural theory explains how social hierarchies with culturally and dynamically prescribed roles influence social interaction (Haley, 1967).

All of these concepts should be considered when the process of a group is analyzed, whether it be 2-person, such as physician and patient, 3-person, such as physician and couple, 5-person, such as physician and family, or 25-person, such as physician and staff.

Group therapy

Therapeutic groups can be classified according to the following schemes:

The classification of different therapeutic groups

1. Theoretical orientation (e.g., psychodynamic, gestalt, transactional analysis, Tavistock).
2. Group composition (e.g., adolescent, patients with chronic pain, schizophrenic families, single mothers, disabled veterans).
3. Time (e.g., brief, extended, open-ended, etc.).
4. Size.
5. Aim (e.g., team management, group process, sensitivity, stress management, smoking cessation, etc.)

Successful group therapy requires that:

Prerequisites for successful group therapy

1. Groups be defined in terms of composition, organization, and aim.
2. Candidates be selected after diagnostic assessment.
3. Candidates be prepared for therapy.
4. The group leader be well-trained.

Aims

1. Foster group cohesion.
2. Foster trust.
3. Allow group tension to increase.
4. Identify and accomplish group tasks.
5. Terminate appropriately.

Indications

1. Patients who have neurotic conflict but cannot cope with the intimacy of individual psychotherapy.
2. Patients who have submissive, passive, or dependent traits that impede progress in individual therapy.
3. Patients who ascribe personal problems to external circumstances. In group therapy, the therapist can use other group members' observation of the patient's projective defenses.
4. Patients who are destructively competitive.
5. Patients who could benefit from other group members' feedback about socially maladaptive patterns.
6. Patients whose intellectual defenses obstruct individual psychotherapy but might yield to the regressive force of group process.
7. Patients who have unresolved sibling rivalry.
8. Patients who could benefit from group support while expressing and accepting guilt.
9. Patients who could be reassured by the realization that others have similar problems.

Contraindications

1. Egocentric, demanding patients who could disrupt the group.
2. Patients unable to tolerate assimilation by the group.
3. Eccentric patients who provoke others excessively.
4. Patients who are so impulsive that they cannot observe group rules.
5. Patients who lack the ability to confront their problems.

Problems and dangers

The dangers of ineffectual or charismatic leadership

1. Poor screening procedures may include patients whose defenses are too fragile to tolerate group tension.
2. Inadequately trained leaders may not observe interactional difficulties and facilitate their resolution. If leadership is ineffectual, group work can be

sabotaged by power struggles among participants. Autocratic, charismatic leaders can cause emotional harm to impressionable, emotionally vulnerable patients.

3. Groups are sometimes substituted for more appropriate therapies.

Clinical use

Groups fulfill several important functions:

Diagnosis

1. By providing the psychiatrist an opportunity to observe directly the patient's social actions, groups can facilitate diagnosis.

Complementation

2. Groups complement other therapies. Multiple family therapy for families with a schizophrenic member promotes compliance with medication (Laqueur, 1970). Groups can help spinal-cord-injured patients to cope with the tasks of rehabilitation (Guggenheim and O'Hara, 1976). Groups can also help patients with Type A behavior rehabilitate after myocardial infarction (Freidman et al., 1982).

Supplementation

3. Groups supplement individual psychotherapy. For example, patients with chronic anxiety disorder may not recognize their subassertive behavior until well into treatment with cognitive-behavioral psychotherapy and medication. An assertiveness training group could supplement psychotherapy.

To summarize, groups are useful for many patients and can be a cost-effective adjunct to other therapy.

Marital or couples therapy

Marital therapy has diverse origins:

The origin of marital therapy

1. The observation that the relationship between spouses could elucidate individual psychodynamics and facilitate psychotherapy.
2. The growth of marriage counseling.
3. An awareness of the influence of marriage on individual functioning, for example, an appreciation that sexual disorders are manifest within a relationship.

Nature

The therapist meets with a couple to discuss their relationship. A number of techniques can be used. Most experienced therapists use several of the following approaches in a complementary fashion:

Techniques of marital therapy

1. Individual marital therapy: Separate clinicians treat each member of the couple, but the two therapists do not communicate.

2. Collaborative therapy: The partners have different therapists who communicate about treatment.
3. Concurrent therapy: One therapist conducts the individual treatment of both partners.
4. Conjoint therapy: The couple meet in joint sessions with one or two therapists. Sometimes, individual collaborative therapy is complemented or followed by conjoint therapy, so each member of the couple meets with his or her own therapist and the four also meet on a regular basis.
5. Sometimes, couples therapy is conducted in marital groups.

Aims

1. Delineate the problems to be addressed.
2. Identify the way the couple communicate about the problems.
3. Identify maladaptive individual coping techniques and their origins.
4. Help each partner find more effective coping techniques.
5. Help the couple find alternative interpersonal tactics.
6. Monitor progress to determine whether other therapy is required.
7. Help the couple maintain their new attitudes and interpersonal skills.
8. Terminate therapy.

Indications

1. Marital discord.
2. Child-rearing difficulties.
3. Major life decisions.
4. When marital stress perpetuates individual psychopathology, or when an improvement in individual psychopathology could precipitate marital disequilibrium.
5. When the observation of marital interaction could help diagnosis.
6. In child psychiatry (see chapters 21 to 26).

Contraindications

When separation is imminent and therapy could further disturb a precarious balance.

Problems and dangers

1. The therapist must protect patients from the premature disclosure of sensitive material.
2. The introduction of a spouse may threaten the therapeutic alliance in individual psychotherapy.

3. A strong transference between marital partners may confuse both patients and therapist.

Clinical use

Couples therapy can be used to supplement other forms of treatment. It is particularly helpful when a marital problem is so stressful that an individual cannot progress in individual treatment.

Case 12.20 ■ Glenda, a 29-year-old married mother of three, is treated for obsessive-compulsive neurosis with clonidine and a combination of exploratory psychodynamic and cognitive-behavioral psychotherapy. Therapy reveals that Glenda is chronically antagonistic to her husband, a quiet, reliable man very different from her seductive, flamboyant, erratic father. These differences were initially attractive to the patient, but they now create difficulties. The more her husband gives in to her, the more resentful and guilty Glenda becomes.

The couple enter conjoint marital therapy. Glenda learns to make fewer demands on her husband and he learns to be more spontaneous and open with her. In individual therapy, Glenda explores how unresolved ambivalent feelings for her father underlie her chronic resentment. ■

Family therapy

Nature

See chapter 25.

Aims

1. Develop a therapeutic alliance with the family.
2. Identify maladaptive interaction patterns.
3. Develop and negotiate a plan to alter these patterns.
4. Facilitate family members' understanding of these patterns and their development of more effective communication.
5. Devise strategies to consolidate healthy functioning.
6. Terminate therapy.

Indications

Broad usefulness Family therapy is broadly useful when long-standing, disturbed family interaction perpetuates medical disease, abnormal illness behavior, or psychological disorder.

Contraindications

None.

Problems and dangers

As with marital and group therapy.

Clinical use

Family therapy can be used in many situations, such as:

1. For family support and education in a comprehensive medical rehabilitation program.
2. When family interaction adversely influences the course of chronic physical disorder.
3. When pathological family communication is associated with psychiatric disorder.
4. When pathological family interaction occurs in response to physical or psychiatric disorder.
5. When disturbed family interaction follows and impedes improvement in the identified patient.

As with other therapies, family therapy should be conducted with a keen eye to the need for alternative or complementary therapy.

Hospital milieu therapy

The hospital functions as a social support for seriously ill patients and for those requiring specialized diagnostic or treatment procedures. Protected in a hospital, a patient can receive diversified, individualized treatment. Psychiatric patients should be admitted to the hospital in the following circumstances:

Indications for psychiatric hospitalization

1. When the treatments required cannot be provided safely and effectively outside the hospital.
2. When there is a serious risk of suicidal or violent behavior.
3. When the patient requires an intensive, coordinated diagnostic work-up or therapeutic trial.

The relationship of marital, family, group, and milieu therapies to individual psychotherapy is represented in Figure 12.2.

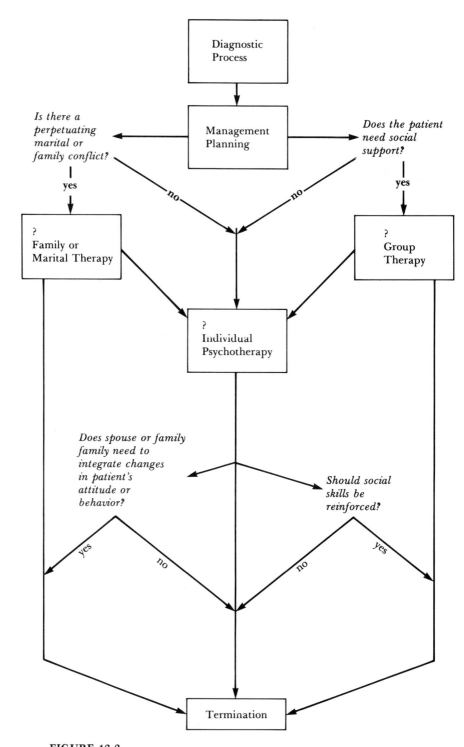

FIGURE 12.2

The relationship between psychotherapies during the clinical process

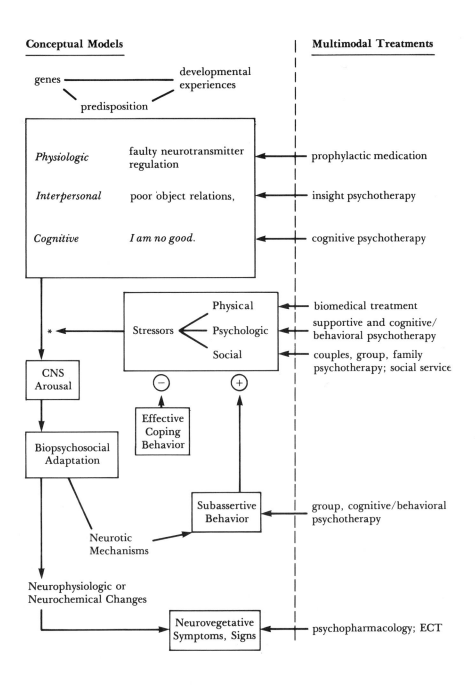

Conceptual Models

Multimodal Treatments

genes —— developmental experiences

predisposition

Physiologic   faulty neurotransmitter regulation ← prophylactic medication

Interpersonal   poor object relations, ← insight psychotherapy

Cognitive   *I am no good.* ← cognitive psychotherapy

Stressors
- Physical ← biomedical treatment
- Psychologic ← supportive and cognitive/behavioral psychotherapy
- Social ← couples, group, family psychotherapy; social service

*

CNS Arousal

⊖

Effective Coping Behavior

⊕

Biopsychosocial Adaptation

Subassertive Behavior ← group, cognitive/behavioral psychotherapy

Neurotic Mechanisms

Neurophysiologic or Neurochemical Changes

Neurovegetative Symptoms, Signs ← psychopharmacology; ECT

Key: − = inhibition
       + = augmentation

FIGURE 12.3
''Depression – A Biopsychosocial Model and Pluralistic Intervention Schema''
(from Gallagher, 1981)

Multimodal treatment

Systematic, comprehensive, diversified, individualized treatment planning

Therapeutic eclecticism and diversity were discussed in the first part of the chapter. A clinician using a comprehensive, biopsychosocial, diagnostic evaluation will be in a position to design a treatment plan that is multifaceted, individualized, and precise. Figure 12.3 illustrates the theoretical relationship between different concepts of depression and different psychiatric interventions. The left-hand column portrays the biopsychosocial formulation of a major depressive episode, incorporating many concepts related to the phenomenology of depression (see chapters 3, 4, and 5). The right-hand column lists treatment interventions directed at different levels of this formulation. The comprehensive clinician can use any of these treatments in a timely, coordinated fashion.

Chapters 14 and 15 describe in more detail the systematic assessment, biopsychosocial formulation and multimodal treatment planning required in comprehensive psychiatry. Chapters 16 through 26 will demonstrate how the comprehensive model can be applied to different clinical settings.

Selected Readings

Several books review the rapidly expanding area of psychopharmacology. Bernstein (1983) combines extensive professional experience with current scientific knowledge in a comprehensive, practical handbook. Gelenberg edits the *Massachusetts General Hospital Biological Therapies in Psychiatry*, a monthly update on recent advances in psychopharmacology.

The theoretical and practical similarities between psychodynamic and behavioral psychotherapy are discussed by Marmor and Woods (1980) in *The Interface between the Psychodynamic and Behavioral Therapies*, a collection of historical and contemporary papers on the subject. Cognitive therapy is thoroughly reviewed by Beck (1976) and Burns (1982).

In *Outpatient Psychiatry*, Lazare (1979) has compiled a balanced, thorough, and very readable book about treatment from the biological, psychological, social, and behavioral perspectives. Greist, Jefferson, and Spitzer (1982) have edited *Treatment of Mental Disorders*, a succinct overview of the contemporary physical and psychosocial treatment of each major group of psychiatric disorders.

Treatment Planning in Psychiatry (edited by Lewis & Usdin, 1982) presents a single case history. Subsequent chapters discuss the treatment of the case from different theoretical perspectives: psychodynamic, group, biological, behavioral, family and marital, child, adolescent, and geriatric.

In *Multimodal Therapy*, Lazarus (1981) describes how to integrate different theoretical treatment models.

PART IV

Diagnosis and planning

13

The problem-oriented record

Introduction

The principles of categorical diagnosis were introduced in chapter 10. There, the advantages and limitations of the categorical approach were discussed, and the administrative, investigative and managerial purposes of diagnosis defined. This chapter and the next two are concerned with the managerial purpose: How should diagnosis be framed in order to assist management planning?

Chapter 13 reviews the application to psychiatry of the problem-oriented system, a revolutionary approach to the organization, recording, storage, and use of medical information. Chapter 14 deals with comprehensive diagnostic formulation. Chapter 15 demonstrates how comprehensive diagnosis lends itself to individualized management planning.

The problem-oriented system in psychiatry

The problem-oriented medical system

The predominant contemporary influence on clinical process in medicine is the Problem-Oriented Medical Record (POMR), developed by Weed (1969).

Problem orientation has transformed record keeping, and promises to develop into a comprehensive, integrated system for diagnosis, management, record storage, data retrieval, accounting, program assessment, and research.

As we will see, the nature of psychiatric problems has made it difficult to apply the Problem-Oriented Record to psychiatry. Before discussing these difficulties, however, let us examine how the Problem-Oriented Record is currently used in psychiatry (Shaw & McKegney, 1980; Ryback, Longabaugh, & Fowler, 1981).

Data base

The Problem-Oriented System begins with the collection of a data base; for example:

    I. Identifying data
   II. Reason for admission
  III. Neuropsychiatric history
      A. History of current problems
      B. Review of psychosocial systems
      C. Patient profile
  IV. Medical history
   V. Physical examination
  VI. Mental status examination
 VII. Laboratory data
VIII. Psychological testing
  IX. Diagnostic impression

The problem list

After the data base has been collected, a problem list is prepared. The problem list includes all the patient's past and present problems – social, medical, and psychiatric. The problems are stated at a level of refinement consistent with the physician's understanding. The items included can vary in specificity from an unclarified symptom to a precise categorical diagnosis. The problem list thus generated organizes the plans and progress notes that are the body of the record.

Plans and progress notes

One advantage of starting with a master problem list is that even though problems supported by appropriate data are given specific diagnoses, more obscure problems can be recorded as symptoms (e.g., ''confusion''), signs (e.g., ''reduction of peripheral vision''), or abnormal laboratory findings (e.g., ''increased protein in cerebrospinal fluid'').

Problems as diagnosis, symptoms, signs, or abnormal laboratory findings

When sufficient data become available, problems are revised as categorical diagnoses. Whenever possible, clearly associated problems are integrated, even though a specific diagnosis is not yet possible; for example, consider the following items:

1. Auditory hallucinations of threatening voices.
2. Panic and combativeness.
3. Delusions involving the fear of pursuit and assassination.

These items could be amalgamated under the more comprehensive title, acute psychosis, etiology unknown, while precision is sought. It would be reasonable to posit alcoholic hallucinosis, among other hypotheses, as the cause and seek information on alcohol intake; but the physician should refrain from listing alcoholic hallucinosis as a problem until certain of the diagnosis.

Clarification
Resolution

As data collection proceeds, some problems are clarified and revised as etiologic diagnoses; some are resolved or become inactive; some remain active. When a symptom or sign requires separate management (for example, suicidal ideation), it is entered as a separate problem secondary to the primary problem diagnosis (e.g., major depression, unipolar type). If a new problem arises, it is added to the list.

Primary and secondary problems

Plans
Progress notes

For each active problem, a plan is designed to direct data collection (if further diagnosis is required) or to direct treatment and patient education. Progress notes are written for each problem and include any or all of the following: symptoms, objective examination, assessment, and plan.

Difficulties in the application of the problem-oriented system to psychiatry

Serious impediments have hindered the application of the Problem-Oriented System to psychiatry. These impediments relate in part to the system itself but are even more an outcome of the nature of psychiatric problems, of ambiguities in the concepts of psychiatric disease, disorder, syndrome, and illness, and of the variable reliability and validity of categorical diagnosis in this branch of medicine.

Psychiatric problems reflect all levels of functioning

A psychiatric patient presents problems reflecting every level of organismic functioning, as is the situation with all patients, whatever the branch of medicine. People are individuals within social systems, as well as vehicles for disordered chemistry and physiology. Clinical medicine dwells on biomedical problems; but psychosocial factors greatly influence the precipitation, perpetuation, presentation, and management of physical disorders.

The significance of psychosocial issues is acknowledged in the problem-oriented approach to diagnosis and management; but social, psychological, and physical problems are entered into the problem-oriented record as though they were of equivalent order. Consider the following problem list, quoted from an authoritative article on the use of the Problem-Oriented Record in psychiatry (Grant & Maletzky, 1972):

Patient B. E. 16-year-old High School Boy.
1. Sexual preoccupation, fetish-like behavior involving women's dresses and belts.
2. Educational deprivation.
3. Difficulties getting along with his aunt.
4. Difficulties following rules and restrictions.
5. Talk about imaginary friends.

     6. Inappropriate laughter.
     7. Poor eye contact.
     8. Initiated conversations with people through games or animals.
     9. Poor self-esteem.
   10. Loneliness and inability to make friends.

A lack of coherence in psychiatric problem lists

This compendium of subjective complaints, impressions, inferences, and behaviors could be readily extended by adding physical disorders and procedures; for example:

   11. Dental caries.
   12. Splenomegaly.
   13. Not immunized.
   14. Onychogryphosis.

The list lacks organization beyond the serial impact of data on the clinician's awareness. It lacks integration, and any reference to an interaction between problems. In short, it is static, piecemeal, incoherent, and unsystematic. Treatment plans directed by such a list inevitably share the same deficiencies.

What is a disease?

Feinstein (1977) defines a disease as the result of an interaction between an etiologic cause and a host. This interaction produces one or more clinical manifestations: symptoms, experienced by the patient as an illness, and signs, detected by the clinician. If the data are sufficient, the cluster of clinical manifestations may be assigned, by inference, to a disease. A disease is defined by its position in a taxonomic hierarchy of entities, a predictable course, an ideal set of clinical manifestations, and paraclinical data associated with underlying pathophysiologic or biochemical disorder.

Taxonomy

Course
Ideal manifestations
Paraclinical data

Underlying processes

Denominations

In psychiatry, however, techniques of categorical diagnosis have not been standardized, the validity of diagnostic entities is shaky, and clear criteria for selecting a particular diagnosis have only recently become available. For the most part, psychiatric diagnoses are denominations for loose clusters of clinical manifestations rather than diseases, since (aside from some organic brain disorders) they cannot be clinched by such paraclinical data as laboratory tests or radiography.

A hierarchy of psychiatric diagnoses

A rough hierarchy of psychiatric diagnoses can be traced from specific to general, and from organic to psychosocial (see Table 13.1). Upper levels take precedence in diagnosis if they can explain the clinical manifestations. Ludwig (1980) recommends that multiple diagnoses should be avoided within a particular level, that secondary diagnoses should be applied to manifestations not covered by the primary diagnosis, and that upper level diagnoses should be listed first.

The convergence of diagnosis from symptom and sign, through syndrome and psychophysiology, to disease entity is reflected in the impetus of the problem-oriented approach from general to specific. In medicine and surgery, when a categorical entity is stated in etiologic terms (for example, subacute bacterial endocarditis due to streptococcus viridans infection of an aortic valve damaged by

TABLE 13.1
Levels and syndromes

Level	Syndrome	Example
I	Structural damage to CNS	Neoplasm
II	Metabolic brain dysfunction	Delirium tremens
III	Probable metabolic dysfunction	Mania
IV	Categorical disorders based on inheritance and learned behavior, often precipitated by stress	Psychoneurosis
V	Statistical extremes in personality traits, partly inherited, partly learned	Personality disorder
VI	Maladaptive coping techniques, largely learned but related to level V	Abnormal illness behavior
VII	Expected responses to life crises, leading to normal coping	Normal grief

(Adapted from Ludwig, 1980)

A paucity of etiologic diagnoses in psychiatry reduces their usefulness as a guide

previous rheumatic fever), it provides an excellent guide to prognosis and treatment. Unfortunately, aside from structural brain lesions or known metabolic dysfunctions of the central nervous system, such precision and utility do not apply in psychiatry. Psychiatric treatment tends to be symptomatic or designed to alter feelings, attitudes, and interpersonal behavior. As it stands, the diagnosis of somatoform disorder is not much use to a clinician who is planning management. For this reason, those who have attempted to adapt the POMR to psychiatry have avoided categorical diagnoses in their problem lists.

Ryback, Longabaugh, and Fowler (1981), for example, speak of the need to develop a standardized terminology for record keeping. They define a problem as a dysfunction affecting the patient and perceived by the staff as existing or imminent in physiological, psychological, or social functioning. A problem indicator is defined as a bit of information that leads the clinician to suspect a problem in physiological, psychological, or social functioning. These authors have presented a compendium of problems which vary in nature from ICD-9 diagnoses of physical disease, through nursing observations (e.g., ''other problems involving eating/drinking, excluding alcohol and drug usage''), and social judgments (e.g., ''inadequate performance in role as member of extended family''), to environmental statements (e.g., ''no place to live''). As the items in parentheses illustrate, an all-inclusive, standard set of terms for problems can become quite strained and stilted.

Behavioral deviations in the problem list

Weed defined four classes of problem: diagnoses, psychological findings, symptoms, and physical findings. Within the class of symptoms, Grant and Maletzky (1972) include behavioral deviations, by which they refer to behavioral excesses, deficits, or inappropriateness. However, there are serious philosophical, ethical, and practical difficulties in deciding which frame of reference will be used to determine if a behavior is excessive, defective, or inappropriate. Should it be that of the patient, the physician, or the community?

Inflation of the minimum data base

Other criticisms can be directed at the way the problem-oriented system is used in contemporary psychiatry. For example, there has been a tendency to inflate the minimum data base. The minimum data base consists of (a) identifying information; (b) the historical and investigative data required to rule out other conditions likely to mimic or complicate psychiatric disorder; and (c) the data required to elicit primary clues to diagnostic hypotheses that will guide the search for secondary evidence during detailed inquiry. As it is usually used, with an overemphasis on routine data collection, the problem-oriented approach pays little heed to the sophisticated clinical reasoning required for effective problem-solving (see chapter 7). There is a danger that the clinician will be shackled by mindless data-gathering and distracted from the supple discretionary inquiry required to gather evidence in a hypothesis-directed search.

Limitations of categorical diagnosis for planning

The natural impetus of medical problem orientation – toward specific categorical diagnosis – is less appropriate to the requirements of psychiatric management planning. Only the most organic diagnoses are suitable for prescriptive treatment directed at a clear etiologic target (craniotomy for cerebral neoplasm, for example). As a consequence of the inadequacy of diagnostic categorization for psychiatric management planning, clinicians who use the problem-oriented record have been forced to revert to laundry lists of undesired behavior larded with ill-defined social deficits and physical disorders. Such gratuitous, deficit-ridden catalogues are inevitably unintegrated.

Limitations of behavioral lists

If therapy were limited to the extinction of bits of undesirable behavior, then the more molecular and behavioral the problem list, the more efficient it would be. However, behavior modification is only one of a variety of treatments. Moreover, beyond the question of utility, the following kind of problem list (Grant & Maletzky, 1972) provokes ethical, philosophical, and scientific disquiet:

> Patient G. D. 25-year-old single male:
>   1. Homosexuality.
>   a. Feminine gestures and activities.
>   2. Withdrawal from society.
>   3. Suicidal ideations.
>   4. Unemployed.
>   5. Delusions of grandeur.
>   6. Fear of people.
>   7. Possible hypertension.
>   8. Difficulty in following rules and restrictions.
>   a. Leaves ward without status.
>   b. Resists prescriptive therapy.

To whom are G. D.'s feminine gestures problematic? Why? Could his awareness that he is considered deviant be the origin of his resistance to prescriptive therapy? It is conceivable that G. D.'s lack of cooperation is a healthy reaction to a therapy governed by a problem list cramped to conform to a narrow biomedical model?

Lack of a system for deriving the problem list

These problems lack any organizing vision aside from what occurs to the recorder (or to the next person who decides to add another item to the list). When more than one person writes in the chart, the caudate jumble of disparate problems extends further and further, particularly when there is no regular mechanism of reviewing and revising it (by refinement, amalgamation, or consignment to resolved or inactive status). Inevitably, the list becomes a compilation of deficits or abnormalities, with no assurance that strengths, resources, and potentials will be taken into account.

The limitations of lists

Causal flow sequences
The flowchart

Furthermore, the listing of problems impedes considering physical, psychological, and social factors in causal interaction. There is nothing inherent in the problem-oriented system to prevent the conception of disease patterns as causal interactions; but an examination of such records suggests that this seldom occurs. Figure 13.1 presents such a pattern in the form of a conceptual flowchart.

Diagnostic flowcharts are useful in individualized management planning because they indicate points in the causal sequence at which therapy might have the greatest leverage, where the greatest gain could be achieved for the least effort, and how therapy should begin if the strategy of management demands a gradual approach with immediate, intermediate, and long-term goals. These matters are dealt with in chapters 14 and 15. Look at Figure 13.1 and try to decide which problems you would tackle first.

Multiple levels of organismic functioning

The essential obstacle to implementing the POMR in psychiatry stems from the theoretical foundations of this branch of medicine. From a narrow perspective, internal medicine can be regarded as applying the biophysical sciences to the diagnosis and management of physiological and biochemical disorders. But psychiatric diagnosis and treatment involve all levels of organismic functioning, from biochemical to social. Those who attempt to understand patients solely from a biochemical or, for that matter, a psychological or a social viewpoint, are ultimately responsible for the Lilliputian battles between those who abhor the medical model and those who defend its narrow version.

Single and multiple paradigms

The problem is even more complicated. Biological sciences have paradigms about which scientists generally agree. Even though vigorous debate about particular matters may exist at the forefront of biochemistry or physiology, for example, there is general agreement about how scientific questions should be addressed. The theoretical models that direct scientific inquiry are in contention only at times of historical crisis, when sweeping innovations are introduced and the members of a discipline struggle over whether the reigning paradigm should be superceded (Kuhn, 1970).

The lack of a dominant paradigm in the social sciences

No single paradigm governs the social sciences. In these fields, it has proven difficult to designate units of observation, to measure phenomena, and to develop an acceptable research methodology. As a consequence, social sciences abound with contending theories that use different techniques to investigate different units of behavior. The clinician seeking navigational aid must be eclectic.

Problem List: Ten-year-old boy with asthma

1. Bronchial asthma
2. Recurrent bronchitis
3. Allergies to house dust and animal danders
4. School refusal
5. Excessive dependence on mother
6. Poor peer relations
7. Low self esteem
8. Reading disability

Flowchart

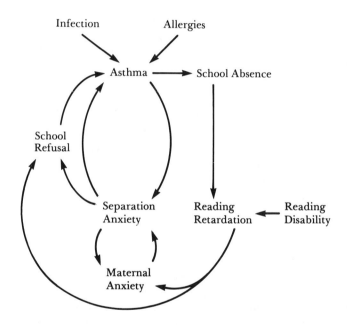

FIGURE 13.1
Diagnostic flowchart

The need for a comprehensive diagnostic formulation

Given these pragmatic and theoretical obstacles, how should we proceed? Can we exploit the thoroughness and logic of the problem-oriented system without diminishing it to a static, jumbled laundry list? Can we take account of the patient's resources and potential, as well as limitations and deficiencies? From such a vantage point, a comprehensive and individualized management plan could be provided. The next chapter introduces a system of comprehensive diagnosis designed to facilitate management planning. It does so by providing a mechanism for selecting individualized treatment goals.

Selected Readings

The classic text on the Problem-Oriented Record is Weed's (1969) *Medical Records, Medical Education and Patient Care.* The most comprehensive work on the problem-oriented record in psychiatry is by Ryback, Longabaugh, and Fowler (1981), *The Problem-Oriented Record in Psychiatry and Mental Health Care.* For a lively presentation of the problem-oriented approach in psychiatry, see the chapter by Shaw and McKegney in *Comprehensive Textbook of Psychiatry III* (Freedman, Kaplan, & Sadock, 1980).

14

The comprehensive
diagnostic formulation

The need for a comprehensive approach to diagnosis

Case 14.1 ■ Hortense, a 38-year-old married woman, is a problem patient in family practice. For more than a year, she has protested to her physician about incessant headache. Consultations with neurology, internal medicine, and psychiatry have yielded little but a medicine chest full of vials. She currently takes five capsules per day of fiorinal, 250 mg per day of amitryptaline, 120 mg per day of propanolol, up to 40 mg per day of valium, 100 mg per day of thorazine, and 100 mg of intramuscular demerol every 3 hours as required.

Hortense presses her complaints urgently and stridently, as though she anticipated being ignored, misunderstood, or rejected. Quick to criticize, importunate in her demands, and apparently impossible to help, she has exhausted all medical advisors.

Recently, additional symptoms have appeared. She feels depressed to the point of tears, has contemplated suicide, has begun to wake early in the morning, and is losing weight.

Physical examination reveals nothing of significance apart from moderate obesity. All neurological examinations have been negative, aside from brain scan findings consistent with migraine. Never before the past year have her episodes of migraine merged into a continuous headache. ■

The conventional medical approach to this patient has been exhausted. Faced with such an impasse, the physician may be tempted to prescribe more drugs, seek further consultations, or transfer the patient to someone else.

Hortense requires a more comprehensive understanding than the purely biomedical model can provide, but there are few guides for the physician who wishes to take a comprehensive view. This chapter and the next present a conceptual and practical schema for doing so.

The biopsychosocial hierarchy

Successive levels of organismic functioning

At any moment, an individual is composed of multiple systems in levels extending from biochemical to psychosocial. The individual lives in a social world and relates to others in families and groups, in a place, in a culture, in a society, in the world. It is not unlike the comprehensive addresses written by schoolchildren that begin with name and street and finish with country, hemisphere, world, solar system, and universe. In biological organisms, the levels extend from molecular to molar.

1. Physical level
   a. Biochemical systems
   b. Cell systems
   c. Organ systems
   d. Physiological systems
   e. Peripheral and central control systems
2. Psychological level
   a. Information processing
   b. Communication
   c. Attitudes and emotions
   d. Internal controls and aspirations
   e. Social competence
   f. Coping techniques
3. Social level
   a. Family
   b. Other groups
   c. Cultural institutions

The concept of emergence of each level from preceding levels

At each level in this ascending hierarchy, the individual is more than a sum of subordinate systems; each level emerges from the one before and is a unique integration of its parts. No two people, not even identical twins, share the same molecular composition, cellular structure, organ function, attitudes, feelings, family, friends, acquaintances, and enemies.

The analogy of a rope emerging from the combination of its components

We can compare the whole to a rope of many fibers combined as threads. The threads are twisted together, making strands, which are twined into strings, which are wound into cords of increasing size; and the cords in turn are coiled to form the rope. The rope is more than a collection of fibers; because of its dynamic, hierarchical organization, it transforms its components and draws strength from their combination.

The uniqueness of the individual

Although the levels and systems are common to all members of a species, the details of each are not. At the level of images and emotions, for example, nobody in the world has had the same experiences, satisfactions, hurts, frustrations, desires, and hopes as you have had or have; yet, all people are driven by the same general needs to survive, to reproduce, to love and be loved, to belong, and to be competent. It is from universal yet singular experiences that the individual constructs a unique sense of self and a distinctive outlook on the world.

Reductionism, separatism, and biomedical doctrine

The failure of reductionism

Reductionism is an important philosophical issue arising from the concept of multiple levels. Can the economics of nations be explained in terms of social interaction? Can thoughts and feelings be accounted for in terms of neurochemistry? A cautious conclusion is that the elements of one level cannot be shrunk effectively to those of another. On the whole, for example, it is more helpful to understand grief according to scientific paradigms associated with psychosocial levels of discourse. Delirium, on the other hand, is most conveniently considered in a primarily biophysical framework.

Connections between organismic levels

Nonetheless, connections between levels should be sought. Biochemistry and physiology constantly seek links between enzyme function and cell dynamics, for example. The associations between body fluid electrolytes and muscular action, between neurochemistry, behavior genetics, and mental disorder, or between individual behavior and group dynamics, for example, are scientific fields of great importance. The reductionist elucidation of bridges between levels is thus a legitimate scientific strategy, but it is more likely to be fruitful when the principles that govern adjoining levels are understood. The scientific paradigms appropriate to each level in biological, psychological, and social systems are best kept separate so that each emerges as a Gestalt from the one below.

A universal field theory

Will there ever be a set of laws comprehensive enough to apply to all levels and the bridges between them? Probably not. We lack a universal field theory for physics, the most fundamental branch of science. The notion of an even grander scheme linking all branches of science is a mirage.

So impressive are our paradigms in the biophysical domain and so tentative those at psychosocial levels, that many scientists have been influenced to concentrate on elementary biophysical explanations of complex psychological phenomena. The situation has been likened to that of a drunk looking for a lost key under a street lamp because the light is stronger there rather than under the bushes near his house where it dropped.

Adverse consequences of biomedical dogma

What is the practical importance of these philosophical considerations? Engel (1977) suggested that an exclusively biophysical approach to clinical medicine may ultimately harm the patient. But psychosocial diagnosis and treatment have not kept pace with the advances of biochemistry, physiology, pathology, and procedural medicine. The result is that as technology becomes more and more dazzling, the prestige of medicine is declining alarmingly. Rival health industries spring up, inspired by singular ideas like acupuncture, or by a reactionary holism that rejects scientific analysis.

Given the absorption of medicine in the complex gadgetry of diagnosis and treatment, is it surprising that patient and family are sometimes lost in the rush? The lack of attention to psychosocial factors is even further aggravated if the patient's illness is the result of more than one disease and treatment the responsibility of different organ specialists who do not communicate except through cryptic ward notes.

Engel submits that our contemporary predicament is the result of an inadequate and dated model of disease and medicine, linked to a set of false assumptions – namely, disease should be defined in physical terms, and other issues deemed irrelevant. Physicians are thought to be fully occupied in the task of keeping physically sick people alive and to have no time for extraneous matters.

The clinical deficiencies of the biomedical doctrine

The biomedical model is reductionist. In its strongest form, it assumes that all clinical phenomena are explicable in terms of disturbed biochemistry or physiology. Its undeniable successes have transformed it into a system dominating the behavior of physicians (Engel, 1978). Although this narrow doctrine is appropriate for understanding the cause of infectious disease, for example, it cannot cope with disorders having a substantially psychosocial predisposition, precipitation, or perpetuation. Illness always has a psychosocial component; the psychological reactions of patient and family influence and are influenced by biophysical phenomena and affect the patient's illness behavior, clinical presentation, course, and response to treatment. Moreover, the patient's psychological responses materially affect the therapeutic alliance. To ignore the psychosocial domain is to don clinical blinkers.

Reasons for resistance to the biopsychosocial approach

Beitman et al. (1982) discussed why physicians may resist the comprehensive model of diagnosis and management proposed in this book. Technicians view their responsibility as limited to diagnosing and treating physical disorder. Emotional disorders are conceived of as categorically distinct, or trivial, or irrelevant, or ultimately biophysical in origin. The physician may fear being overwhelmed by psychosocial problems and rationalize avoiding them by citing a concern that the patient will be offended by an invasion of privacy. The supposed impossibility of treating such problems may be alluded to. The physician may also have deeper fears of encountering patients with problems too like his or her own.

Countervailing arguments

On the contrary, as discussed in chapter 3, psychosocial factors are inseparable from physical disorder; indeed, many patients with physical complaints have a primary psychological disorder. Diagnosis does not obligate the clinician to provide treatment personally; some patients should be referred elsewhere, some benefit from clarification, and some will refuse psychological treatment. Some may refuse it at first but change their minds at a later date. Some patients do perceive personal questions as an invasion of privacy, but the experienced clinician learns how to ask such questions and when to withdraw gracefully. It is undeniable, however, that the physician needs training in how to explore the patient's psychosocial problems and understand his or her own reactions to them (a matter further discussed in chapter 20).

If it is accepted that the clinician must take account of all systemic levels in diagnosis, then how can they be addressed? How can such a comprehensive approach then be exploited to design an individualized plan of management? This chapter outlines a framework for comprehensive diagnosis and systematic planning. This framework integrates the systemic and temporal dimensions of illness and allows the clinician to consider the patient in detail, as a whole, and as an individual.

A model for comprehensive assessment

The axes of comprehensive assessment

A comprehensive assessment analyzes the individual by levels, in cross-section, over time. The clinician assesses the physical, psychological, and social factors operative during each of the following temporal stages of illness:

1. Predisposition.
2. Precipitation.
3. Perpetuation.
4. Current pattern.

Two axes of functioning are thus considered in comprehensive assessment (see Figure 14.1).

1. The vertical, biopsychosocial or synchronic axis.
2. The longitudinal, temporal or diachronic axis.

The next section deals with assessment in the vertical axis.

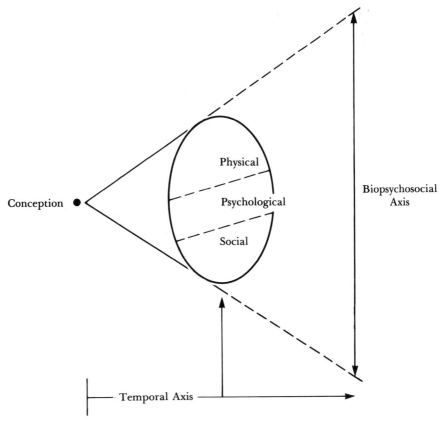

FIGURE 14.1
The two axes of functioning

The biopsychosocial axis

The vertical axis can be divided into three levels:

*Levels of the
systemic dimension*

1. Physical.
2. Psychological.
3. Social.

Physical level

The **physical level** is constituted by multiple systems in an organized peripheral and central hierarchy. The hierarchy (together with examples of abnormality in each system) is as follows:

Peripheral biosystems

1.1 Molecular (as in electrolyte disturbance due to persistent vomiting, or disturbance of enzyme function due to avitaminosis).

1.2 Cellular (as in acute poliomyelitis affecting ventral horn motoneurones in the spinal cord).

1.3 Organ System (as in malignant hypertension affecting the cardiovascular and renal systems).

These peripheral biosystems are coordinated by control biosystems operating outside conscious awareness:

Control biosystems

1.4 The autonomic nervous system (affected by diabetic neuropathy).

1.5 The neuroendocrine system (affected by thyrotoxicosis).

1.6 The subcortical homeostatic functions of the central nervous system (affected by Wernicke's encephalopathy).

Control systems are discussed in chapter 5.

Psychological level

Psychological functions

Ego processes

The **psychological level,** described in chapter 4, includes all mental functions that are conscious or have the potential for being brought to awareness. These **ego processes** have to do with mentations enabling the individual to deal with the external world, to be aware of the self and its needs, to gauge progress towards goals, and to fine-tune behavior accordingly. The principal psychological functions are manifest in the following:

Information processing

Communication

Attitudes and emotions

2.1 Information processing (disoriented in febrile delirium).

2.2 Motor control (disorganized in cerebellar disease).

2.3 Communication (disorganized in aphasia).

2.4 Attitudes and emotions (constricted, repetitive, and painful during grief).

2.5 Internal controls, rules, and aspirations (may be inadequate in antisocial personality).

2.6 Social competence (may be deficient in schizoid personality).

2.7 Coping techniques (deteriorate in dementia).

All of these psychological functions are expressed through:

Action and behavior

2.8 Behavior (accelerated and impulsive in mania).

Information processing involves orientation, attention, concentration, perception, memory, abstraction, problem solving, judgment, and insight.

Motor control regulates motility whereby the individual orientates toward, seeks, finds, and manipulates the objects required to satisfy needs.

Communication includes gesture, language, and the use of language as a tool of thought (for example, in verbal problem-solving and other symbolic operations).

Attitudes and emotions represent the subject's affectively laden impressions and ideas of the self and of significant people from the past or in the present.

Internal controls, rules, and aspirations (superego and ego ideal) involve the controls, rules, guidelines, and goals that regulate behavior and give coherence and purpose to life.

Social competence involves the capacity to discern the emotions and purposes of other people, to predict the social consequences of one's actions, and to resolve social dilemmas.

Coping techniques refer to the repertoire of coordinated cognition and activity characteristically used by the individual when subjected to stress.

Behavior is the observable manifestation of information processing, motor control, communication, attitudes, emotions, social competence, and coping (for example, blushing and aversion of gaze, etc.). The subject can report images and emotions only through the medium of language, but behavior can be observed. Images and emotions are subjective; behavior is objective. The patient's symptoms are subjective; clinical signs, in contrast, are observed.

Social level

The social environment

Each person lives in a society of more or less familiar, novel, strong, weak, friendly, neutral, and inimical relationships and interacts with others singly or in groups. Groups can be analyzed from the point of view of any member or at the higher level of the group itself. The fundamental human group (the family) has structure, a present dynamic, and an evolution through time. The capacity of the family to adapt to illness and help a sick member, for example, has a powerful effect on the outcome of that illness.

The individual belongs to extrafamilial groups at work, in recreation, and elsewhere. Their response to a sick member is of great significance. Social acceptance, support, and reentry, or rejection, abandonment, and exclusion can be important factors in the predisposition, precipitation, perpetuation, and outcome *The need to belong* of illness. Just as they need to give and receive love, people have a fundamental need to belong. The availability and adequacy of past and current social supports may be crucial to present or future physical or psychiatric disorder or illness behavior.

Social institutions

Beyond the social groups closest to the patient are such institutions as government, school, religious organization, and medicine. The medical system, for example, may overlook, reject, or accept a patient. Having been accepted by the system, the patient is involved with it briefly, episodically or chronically and is diagnosed and treated, to good or ill effect. The response of the medical system will materially affect the acute phase, course, and outcome of an illness. It can also influence subsequent illness behavior.

The **social level** can thus be divided into the following systems:

Social systems

3.1 Interpersonal system.
3.2 Family system.
3.3 Other social support systems.
3.4 Medical system.
3.5 Other institutional systems.

The temporal axis

Figure 14.1 contrasts the vertical or biopsychosocial axis and the longitudinal or temporal axis. The temporal axis is comprised of the following stages or points of time:

Stages in the temporal axis

1. Predisposition.
2. Precipitation.
3. Perpetuation.
4. Pattern of response.

All three vertical levels operate at every point or stage in the temporal dimension. Each point will now be discussed.

Predisposition

Physical and psychosocial predisposition

Predisposition refers to all factors rendering the individual vulnerable to disease or disorder. Physical predisposition could include, for example, adverse genotype, intrauterine subnutrition, birth injury, or postnatal organ damage due to infection, trauma, or toxins.

Psychological factors might include, for example, the need to succeed, anxiety over deadlines, and competitiveness that predispose some patients to coronary artery disease, together with the driving, perfectionistic lifestyle reflecting these attitudes (Type A personality).

Among the social factors predisposing to later disease or disorder are early losses and emotional deprivation (for example, when a child lives in many foster homes after family breakup); membership of an ethnic minority or subculture with values aberrant from the mainstream; and membership of a subculture promoting potentially dangerous ways of life. An example of the latter is the life-style *Dangerous life-styles* associated with hard drinking, heavy smoking, and recklessness when physically challenged.

The reinforcement of abnormal illness behavior

In addition to such social influences, the medical system may inadvertently promote attitudes that put the patient at risk of later disorder. Hypochondriasis, conversion syndromes, sedative addiction, excessive dependence on physicians, and other forms or results of abnormal illness behavior may be reinforced by clinicians who are so preoccupied with somatic disease that they are blind to the broader picture.

Precipitation

Biopsychosocial precipitation

Precipitation refers to the physical, psychological, and social stressors that tip the scales and coincide with the onset of a disease or disorder. Included in the network of precipitating factors may be a specific causative agent, such as a microorganism; but the causative agent could have no effect if it were not preceded and accompanied by a shoal of other factors. Consider these examples:

■ During a snowstorm, an aging alcoholic man falls asleep in a doorway and contracts pneumococcal pneumonia. ■

■ After a vital business luncheon, a choleric, overweight executive drops his cigarette, rises from the table clutching his chest, and passes out. ■

■ An unhappily married, hypochondriacal woman who is secretly addicted to barbiturates develops grand mal convulsions after admission to hospital for the investigation of mental confusion. ■

■ A college freshman has been drinking heavily and eating poorly after breaking up with his girlfriend. He develops a large carbuncle and is admitted to hospital in semicoma with sugar and ketone bodies in his urine. ■

■ When her mother dies, a middle-aged, unmarried woman sells the old family home but cannot get used to her new condominium. She develops anorexia, insomnia, a pervasive sense of futility, a painful red tongue, and unsteady gait. ■

Examples of precipitating stressors from each of the three domains are listed here.

Examples of stressors

1. Physical.
   a. Trauma and physiological shock.
   b. Pain.
   c. Infectious agents.
   d. Toxins, poisons.
   e. Carcinogens.
   f. Teratogens.
   g. Lack of essential nutriments.
   h. Intoxication with, or withdrawal from, addictive agents.
   i. The side effect of pharmaceutical agents.
2. Psychological.
   a. Threat to physical integrity.
   b. Loss.
   c. Rejection.

      d. Disappointment.

      e. Success.

      f. Concern for future events.

      g. Personal reactions to events described in the social domain.

3. Social.

      a. Departure or death of others who are regarded as indispensable.

      b. Rejection by significant people.

      c. Rejection by, or loss of membership in, family or supportive social groups.

      d. Forced exposure to an alien environment (for example, after migration to a foreign country).

The division of psychosocial factors into psychological and social is artificial. There is always a psychological component to social stress – a set of ideas, images, and emotions indicating fear, anxiety, grief, or unrelieved frustration about threat, loss, separation, rejection, failure, or success. Sometimes, however, the psychological component is defensively denied, repressed, or minimized and can be ascertained only indirectly (during psychotherapy, for example).

Perpetuation

Physical, psychological, and social defenses

An acute disease or disorder usually fades when the organism's defenses are mobilized. Defenses range in a hierarchy from physical (for example, immunological responses) through psychological (for example, the decision to rest, compliance with treatment, and anticipation of cure) to social (for example, the family's rallying to help and a suitable response by the medical system). But sometimes the disorder continues, becoming subacute or chronic. In that case, it must be concluded that perpetuating factors are present. Perpetuating factors

Physical, psychological, and social perpetuation

operate by subverting the patient's defenses against disease or disorder. **Physical perpetuating factors** include anything that impairs the body's front-line inflammatory or immune responses (subnutrition or antiimmune drugs, for example) or disrupts the body's reserve autonomic, neuroendocrine, and central nervous control biosystems (diabetic neuropathy, Addison's disease, or cerebral hemorrhage, for example). **Psychological perpetuating factors,** include, for example, losing hope or fearing the consequences of getting well. **Social perpetuating factors** include responses (by family, or physician, or legal system, for example) fostering continued illness behavior rather than recovery. The hope of monetary compensation for injury, for example, may prolong disability in the form of abnormal illness behavior.

Predisposition can become perpetuation

Sometimes precipitating factors (rejection by a spouse, for example) continue and become perpetuating. Precipitating and perpetuating factors may be recurrent or persistent, unitary or multiple, episodic or cumulative.

Pattern of response

This is the temporal point on which medical diagnosis traditionally dwells. A doctrinaire biomedical approach deals exclusively with current physical patterns at this stage.

The problem is partly due to the restricted viewpoint of biomedical dogma. It is associated with the fact that all diagnostic systems are bedeviled (and enlivened) by a polarity between general categories and individual descriptions. Categorical terms refer to such idealized abstractions as schizophrenia. The individual approach, in contrast, considers afresh each person's existential situation (see chapter 11). Once it is appreciated that the pattern of response is always psychosocial as well as physical, the fundamental problems of a solely categorical *The limitation* diagnosis become apparent. No label, however reliable or valid, can describe *of labels* more than a limited aspect of a person. Rational and ethical problems arise if tags block understanding and people get lost in pigeonholes.

Yet, the necessity for an individual approach to diagnosis must be balanced by an appreciation that there is always a general aspect to a unique diagnostic formulation. Otherwise, each patient would require a completely innovative diagnosis and management. The more clearly physical the dominant *The need for* pattern of response, the more likely a relatively categorical approach to diagnosis *categorization* and management will be effective. The term *subacute bacterial endocarditis* is more helpful for management planning than is *schizophrenic disorder: paranoid type*. The latter is, in turn, more useful than *personality disorder: avoidant type*.

The comprehensive approach proposed in this book combines both general categorization and individualized formulation and extends the clinician's vantage point from the narrowly biomedical to all levels of human functioning.

The comprehensive assessment of pattern of response includes the following processes:

1. Physical
   a. Peripheral biosystems: Symptoms, signs, findings, and disorder patterns referable to dysfunction of molecular, cellular, or physiological systems.
   b. Control biosystems: Symptoms, signs, findings, and disorder patterns referable to autonomic, neuroendocrine, or subcortical nervous dysfuntion.
2. Psychological: Symptoms, signs, findings, and disorder patterns referable to these functions:
   a. Information processing.
   b. Motor control.
   c. Communication.
   d. Attitudes and emotions.
   e. Internal controls, morals, and aspirations.
   f. Social competence.
   g. Coping techniques.

3. Social: Responses to the patient's illness by the patient's social support network, the medical system, and other institutions.

Variations in the temporal axis

In a complete temporal sequence, the following occurs:

1. Predisposition → Precipitation → Perpetuation → Pattern of Response → Treatment → Recovery.

There are many variations on this theme. Some disorders are precipitated by such overwhelming impact (massive vehicular trauma, for example) that the patient cannot be said to have been predisposed (unless attitudes, such as daredevil risk-taking were involved). The sequence then becomes:

No predisposition

2. Precipitation → Perpetuation → Pattern → Treatment → Recovery.

No precipitation

In other cases, there has been no precipitation, the patient harboring a disorder active since early life that has evolved into a current pattern:

3. Predisposition → Pattern → Treatment → Recovery.

In this case, treatment may become the long-term management of chronic disorder:

4. Predisposition → Pattern → Management

Other variations are possible. Treatment may produce physical or psychosocial disturbances that so complicate the pattern as to require a modification of treatment:

Patterns secondary to treatment

5. Predisposition → Precipitation → Perpetuation → Pattern 1
$$\downarrow$$
$$\begin{cases} \text{Treatment 1} \\ \text{Pattern 2} \\ \text{Treatment 2} \end{cases}$$
$$\downarrow$$
Recovery.

Patterns change with time

When treatment itself becomes a perpetuating factor, sophisticated decision-making is required. Another sequence may be encountered when an acute pattern changes over time, sometimes in response to change in perpetuation, and the current pattern is somewhat different from that of the acute phase of the disorder. Many psychiatric patients, for example, initially suffer a state of undifferentiated anxiety or tension. Later, a more defined syndrome evolves:

6. Predisposition → Precipitation → Acute Pattern → Perpetuation
   → Present Pattern.

These sequences do not exhaust the possible variations. Try to think of others.

The diagnostic net: an integration of the biopsychosocial and temporal axes

By now your knees may be buckling. How can a clinician comprehend these multileveled, interwoven, dynamically evolving processes? How can the two axes – biopsychosocial and temporal – be integrated to guide further clinical investigation and management planning? To address these questions, we propose the **diagnostic net.**

The diagnostic net

The diagnostic net or grid combines biopsychosocial and temporal axes in the one framework or matrix. Note the configuration in Table 14.1: The temporal axis is represented horizontally, from left to right; and the biopsychosocial axis, vertically. Each stage in the temporal sequence has all three vertical levels. Tables 14.2 and 14.3 demonstrate how each compartment in the diagnostic net has subcompartments, according to the schema already described. The clinician who adheres to an exclusively biophysical approach is locked into the top right corner or, at best, the uppermost horizontal level.

At this point, it is instructive to return to Hortense (Case 14.1) to demonstrate how a diagnostic net can aid diagnostic formulation, clinical inquiry, and management planning.

Case 14.1 (continued)

■ Hortense was the much-indulged, favorite daughter of a wealthy man. Though brought up to expect the best, she was never close to her mother, a woman embittered by marital strife. The divorce of her parents during her early adolescence was traumatic. Her relationship with her mother deteriorated further, becoming stormy, dramatic, and demanding, particularly after her father married his former mistress.

TABLE 14.1
The diagnostic net: biopsychosocial and temporal dimensions

		Temporal axis			
		Predisposition	Precipitation	Perpetuation	Pattern of response
Biopsychosocial	Physical				
	Psychological				
	Social				

TABLE 14.2
The diagnostic net: divisions of the axes

	Predisposition	Precipitation	Perpetuation	Pattern
Physical	*Adverse* • Genetic and physical developmental factors	• Physical stressor	*Factors that reduce:* • Immune and inflammatory response • Response of central control systems	*Disorder of:* • Peripheral systems • Central control systems
Psychological	*Maladaptive* • Attitudes • Coping techniques	• Psychological response to stressor	*Maladaptive* • Attitudes to illness	*Disorder of:* • Information processing • Motor control • Language • Emotions and attitudes • Controls • Social competence • Coping techniques
Social	*Inadequacy of:* • Previous social support network • Previous institutional responses	• Psychosocial stressor	*Inadequate or inappropriate responses by:* • Social support network • Medical system or other institution	*Response of:* • Social support network • Medical system

TABLE 14.3
The diagnostic net: examples of the factors involved

	Predisposition	Precipitation	Perpetuation	Pattern

Physical	*Adverse*
	• Genetic endowment
	• Intrauterine experience
	• Temperamental pattern
	• Postnatal experiences
	  traumatic
	  toxic
	  infectious, etc.
		• Trauma
		• Infection, etc.
			• Factors that diminish immune or inflammatory response
			• Factors that reduce response of central control systems
				Disorder of:
				• Molecular system
				• Cell system
				• Organ system
				• Autonomic system
				• Neuroendocrine system
				• Central nervous system

Psychological	*Maladaptive* • Habitual modes of thinking and feeling about self and others • Ego ideal • Superego • Habitual coping style	Sense of: • Loss • Rejection • Abandonment • Failure • Disillusion • Threat of future problem • Major life change	• Loss of hope • Reluctance to get well due to fear of more independent functioning	*Disorder of:* • Information processing • Language • Attitudes and Emotions re self and others • Ego ideal • Superego • Social competence • Coping techniques
Social	*Inadequacy of:* • Interpersonal security • Social support groups • Previous response of medical system to patient • Response of other institutions	• Departure, death, desertion, or rejection by significant others • Rejection, exclusion, or separation from social group	• Inadequate or inappropriate responses by support system that reinforce illness behavior • Inadequate or inappropriate responses by medical system or by other institutions that reinforce illness behavior	• Response of social supports • Response of medical and other institutions

Like her mother, Hortense began to experience depressive moods in adulthood, some years after her marriage. She has also suffered from migraine since adolescence, especially when she fears or experiences loss or rejection. She becomes hostile toward her family whenever she feels threatened or slighted.

Hortense's marriage was contracted on the basis of passionate mutual attraction, despite her mother's opposition. Unfortunately, her husband's business career has not been successful. Chronic marital tension arose over financial difficulties and disputes about the discipline of their only child. Their 13-year-old son, who suffers from juvenile rheumatoid arthritis, is disobedient and provocative toward his mother and openly allied with the father against her.

Hortense's present medical condition involves obesity, migraine, depression, and drug-dependency. A marked accentuation of her health problems became apparent 3 months ago, following an argument during which her son told her he hated her and her husband threatened to leave and take the boy with him. Her husband has barely spoken to her since that time.

She visits her physician frequently, demanding relief from the headache that has become constant and from insomnia and depression. Her hostile, accusatory, insistent attitude disturbs the practitioner, but he has not given up trying to help, since he is aware that she has alienated virtually everyone else. His immediate concern is how to halt the polypharmaceutical merry-go-round. He worries, also, that Hortense might become suicidal. ■

Empty compartments

Table 14.4 provides a diagnostic net of this case. Often, when an attempt is made to complete the net, the diagnostician will find certain compartments empty. In Hortense's case, for example, there appear to have been no precipitating factors in the physical domain. In some cases, however, blanks or incomplete compartments are reminders that more information should be obtained about that stage and level. If some recorded items are unclear or uncertain, the clinician should precede them with a *?*. This indicates that further information might be needed to clarify the point by additional history-taking, examination, investigations, or diagnostic procedures. The diagnostic net is thus a guide to further clinical inquiry.

Uncertain items

Memory aid

The purpose of the diagnostic net is to remind you of the interlocking complexity of the factors that must be investigated in comprehensive diagnosis. Experienced clinicians may not need such a memory aid, since they routinely consider such factors. Try the net and see if it helps you. If it cramps your thinking, think of another way to represent the matrix of systemic levels and temporal stages involved in this case. After the net or its equivalent is completed, the next step is to prepare a dynamic flowchart from the diagnostic matrix. This is described in chapter 15.

From diagnostic net to flowchart

Summary: steps to a comprehensive diagnosis

1. The clinician preparing a 4 × 3 diagnostic net or grid should start with the current pattern and enter symptoms, signs, and manifestations of potential disorder into the three vertical levels.

TABLE 14.4
The diagnostic net: Hortense

	Predisposition	Precipitation	Perpetuation	Pattern
Physical	• Migraine • Mood disorder • Obesity • Drug dependence		• Sedative intake	• Headache • Insomnia • Anorexia • Weight loss

Psychological	• Fear of abandonment
	• Low self-esteem
	• Sense of entitlement
	• Feeling of being overwhelmed by son's illness
	  • Dramatic
	  • Demanding
	  • Quarrelsome
	  • Drug-taking
		• Acute threat of being abandoned: Three months before		• Anxiety
				• Fear
				• Depression
				• Guilt
				• Futility
				• Need for attention
				  • Angry outbursts
				  • Requests medication
				  • Attention-seeking behavior

Social	• Spouse hostile to her
	• Son chronically ill and uncooperative
	  • Medical system diagnoses physical complaints and prescribes medication
		• Husband rejects her
		• Son rejects her
			• Husband rejects
			• Son rejects
			• Son's chronic illness
			  • Medical system continues to prescribe numerous drugs
				• Husband and son continue to be alienated from her
				  • Medical system is stymied

2. If the phenomena form recognizable patterns, they should be clustered. Most patterns will be located in physical or psychological levels or both.

3. If the patterns are tentative, a differential categorical diagnosis should be prepared in relation to each pattern.

4. The clinician should then go back to the three other stages: predisposition, precipitation, and perpetuation. All sections of the net can be completed with established information or speculations that may need clarification.

Inquiry planning

5. A systematic inquiry plan is now possible involving the following steps:
   a. Gathering information in order to rule in or out each element of the differential diagnosis.
   b. Gathering further information in order to clarify speculations entered with queries in the different compartments of the net.

Consolidation

6. When the inquiry plan has been completed, the diagnostic net can be consolidated by designating patterns as diseases, disorders, or dysfunctions (if justified), inserting established data, and deleting obsolete information.

7. Using the net, the clinician can now draw up a dynamic flowchart. The flowchart is a hypothetical representation of the causal interaction between the elements of the current disorder pattern and of the causal sequence involving perpetuation. From the flowchart, key problems can be selected as a guide to management planning.

15

Management planning

Systematic management planning

Goal-oriented planning

The keystone of systematic planning is the triangular relationship among problems, goals, treatments, and evaluation (see Figure 15.1).

The clinician must first identify the deficits or dysfunctions to be alleviated or rectified. These are known as problems. From the problems, therapeutic goals can be determined. Guided by the goals, the clinician chooses the treatment or combination of treatments most likely to be effective in the case in question and estimates the costs in time and people. The resources of the patient and therapeutic environment are then considered, and, if necessary, the ideal plan is pruned. Evaluation is then designed to gauge when therapeutic goals have been attained. The plan is implemented – and modified if new findings arise as treatment proceeds – until the goals are reached and the clinical process terminates.

The choice of goals

Goals are derived from the diagnostic net, in this manner:

Identify problems

1. Consider the dysfunctions, deficits, limitations, or deviations in the diagnostic net, particularly those from the pattern, precipitation, and perpetuation.

321

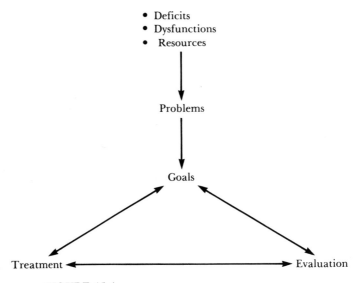

FIGURE 15.1
The key to systematic planning

Which are the most serious? Which are less so? Which could be subsumed by others? Identify the problems operating currently.

Dynamic interaction

2. How do these problems interact to produce the present disorder? What perpetuates the condition? What were the predisposing and precipitating factors? Are they still active or dormant? Draw up a flowchart indicating how the problems now interact to produce the current pattern or patterns.

Flowchart

Identify pivotal problems

3. Determine which alterable problems are pivotal. Where do the interactional vectors converge? Which centers of force have the most connections? In other words, which problems, if alleviated, should yield the greatest therapeutic benefit? Your flowchart should now include problems that are urgent, pivotal, serious, and alterable.

Remedial goals

4. Start with problems that are the most urgent, pivotal, and serious. Rewrite alterable problems as treatment goals. Use such verbs as *eliminate, alleviate, reduce, rectify,* or *ameliorate* to describe remedial goals. Remedial therapy is of several types:

Remedial therapies

a. Suppressive.
b. Substitutive.
c. Reparative.
d. Curative.

Suppressive therapy attempts to eliminate or reduce a symptom. It is appropriate when the patient needs immediate relief or to interrupt a psychosomatic vicious circle. The alleviation of pain by biofeedback, relaxation, or medication, for example, may be a crucial intermediate step towards a more curative therapy.

Substitutive therapy is often an important component of a program of behavior therapy, the extinction of an undesired behavior being facilitated by promoting a less disruptive alternative. The use of methadone to reduce a desire for narcotics is an example of substitutive pharmacotherapy.

In **reparative therapy,** the clinician helps the patient to relearn and practice skills that have become disused, damaged or disorganized following psychiatric or physical disorder. Speech therapy for aphasia after stroke is an example.

Curative therapy is aimed at an identified etiologic agent. Antibiotic therapy for neurosyphilis is an example.

Seldom, if ever, will a single approach be sufficient. Most psychiatric management plans involve combinations of suppressive, substitutive and reparative therapies.

Biopsychosocial inventory

Compensatory and substitutive goals

Urgent goals, immediate goals, and subsequent goals

5. Draw up a biopsychosocial inventory of strengths, resources, and assets. Can any of these be enhanced to compensate for the deficits? If so, write compensatory goals. Use such words as *increase, enhance, strengthen, promote* or *foster* to describe compensatory goals.

6. From your list of remedial and compensatory goals, decide which should be addressed at once (urgent and immediate goals) and which can be left until later (subsequent or eventual goals).

The choice of therapeutic methods

Having drawn up a provisional list of goals, the clinician must choose the therapeutic methods most likely to be effective. The following principles can be kept in mind:

1. Consider every goal in the provisional list.
2. Think of alternative therapeutic approaches to each goal and choose among them.

Criteria for the selection of a therapeutic method

3. When there is more than one possible method of therapy, select a method according to the following criteria:
   a. Established effectiveness.
   b. Economy of time, money, and effort.
   c. Cultural and personal acceptability.
   d. Feasibility in relation to resources available.
   e. Your own expertise in that form of therapy.

Efficiency

4. Kill several birds with one stone. When possible, choose treatments addressing more than one goal. Bracket together goals addressed by the one therapeutic method.

Evaluation

Include with each treatment a method for evaluation, and estimate the time required for the goal to be achieved. Evaluation enables the clinician to determine when therapeutic goals are attained. Some examples of evaluative methods appropriate for different biopsychosocial levels are listed here:

Methods of evaluation

1. Somatic.
    a. History (e.g., of disappearance of symptoms or restoration of function).
    b. Physical signs (e.g., apyrexia or absence of tenderness and guarding).
    c. Special investigations (e.g., normal electroencephalogram or serum amylase).
2. Psychological.
    a. History (e.g., of disappearance of symptoms or restoration of function).
    b. Mental status examination (e.g., of change in attention, orientation, memory, calculation, judgment, or abstract reasoning).
    c. Nursing reports of ward behavior.
    d. Psychological testing (e.g., of neuropsychological function).
3. Social.
    a. History (e.g., of capacity for and interest in social relationships).
    b. Mental status (e.g., of quality of relationship with interviewer).
    c. Family diagnostic interview.

Feasibility

Plan the ideal

Do not skimp on your initial plan out of fear of excessive expense. Aim for an ideal design first and then consider feasibility in terms of cost, resources, appropriateness, likelihood of successful outcome, and acceptability to the patient.

Prune later

If money, resources, or other issues of feasibility are in doubt, revise the initial plan accordingly. Why plan the ideal and revise afterwards? It is always possible to scale down, but it is more difficult to do the reverse. A skimped plan constrains imagination and impedes the consideration of alternatives. The maxim should be: *Think big; prune later.*

The case of Hortense: rational management planning

Step 1. Identify problems

From Hortense's diagnostic net (Table 14.4), it is possible to identify a number of serious and potentially alterable deficits. Note that where appropriate, the deficits have been grouped together and categorized.

1. From Pattern
   a. Insomnia, anorexia, weight loss, sense of futility, guilt, attention-seeking behavior (major depression).
   b. Anxiety, angry outbursts, demanding behavior, headache, requests for medication (anxiety reaction to threat of abandonment in a histrionic personality).
   c. Continuing estrangement of, and rejection by, husband and son (rejection by husband and son).
2. From Perpetuation
   d. Excessive intake of sedatives and other drugs for anxiety, depression, pain, migraine, and depression (polypharmacy).
   e. Chronic illness of son.
   f. Rejection by husband and son.
3. From Predisposition
   g. Migraine.
   h. Mood disorder.
   i. Obesity.
   j. Drug dependence.
   k. Fear of abandonment; sense of entitlement; dramatic, demanding, and quarrelsome behavior when frustrated (Personality Disorder).
   l. Marital disturbance.
   m. Son's chronic illness and negativism to mother.

Step 2. Draw up a flowchart

This list is a working assembly of problems. These problems can be conceived of as interacting in the manner of a vicious circle (see Figure 15.2).

Step 3. Identify the most urgent, serious, pivotal problems

The flowchart suggests that the most serious and pivotal problems are as follows:

1. Anxiety, tension, somatization.
2. Major depression.
3. Polypharmacy.
4. Rejection by husband and son.

These problems, which clearly interact, are critical to immediate management. Other problems rooted in predisposition can be tackled later. They are as follows:

5. Personality disorder.
6. Proneness to mood disorder.

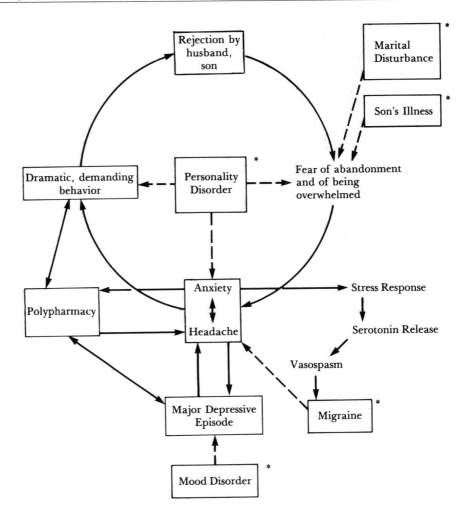

*   Influence of predisposing factors represented by dotted lines

FIGURE 15.2
Flowchart of problems: Hortense

7. Marital disorder.
8. Migraine.
9. Obesity.

Step 4. Rewrite problems as goals

Problems 1, 2, 3, and 4 should be addressed at once. They could be rewritten as immediate goals:

Immediate goals

1. Counter anxiety, tension, somatization (headache).
2. Alleviate major depressive reaction.
3. Reduce dependence on drugs.
4. Modify rejection by husband and son.

The predisposing problems could be rewritten as subsequent or eventual goals:

Subsequent goals

5. Alleviate personality disorder.
6. Reduce proneness to mood disorder.
7. Alleviate marital disorder.
8. Reduce tendency to migraine.
9. Reduce obesity.

Step 5. Take inventory of biopsychosocial resources and potentials

Let us say that after scanning Hortense's resources and potentials from all three levels of functioning, we find she once worked effectively as a bookkeeper in her husband's business and has the capacity for attending to administrative detail. A possible final compensatory goal could be, for example:

10. Enhance capacity for administrative work as a vocational choice.

We now have four immediate goals (1–4), five subsequent remedial goals (5–9), and one subsequent compensatory goal (10).

Step 6. For each goal, consider alternative treatment methods

Select an appropriate method according to effectiveness, economy, acceptability, feasibility, and efficiency.

Immediate goals

Select treatment methods

1. Alleviate depression.
   Plan: a. Admit to hospital.
   b. Change to low dose of an alternative antidepressant medication and increase cautiously.
   c. Commence individual psychotherapy.
2. Reduce anxiety, tension, and somatization.
   Plan: a. Admit to hospital.
   b. Commence individual psychotherapy.
   c. Commence relaxation training and biofeedback therapy.

3. Reduce dependence on drugs.
      Plan: a. Admit to hospital.
                b. Gradually withdraw all medication.
                c. Relaxation therapy.
                d. Individual psychotherapy.
4. Modify rejection by husband and son.
      Plan: a. Counseling of husband and son.
                b. Preparation for family therapy.

It is apparent that two (if not three) of these goals require admission to the hospital for the most effective implementation of therapy. While in the hospital, the proposed change of antidepressant medication, withdrawal from polypharmacy, relaxation training or biofeedback therapy, individual psychotherapy, and family counseling can be instituted. Hortense should be ready for discharge when her depression is relieved, when she has been withdrawn from excessive medication, and when the various psychosocial therapies are proceeding satisfactorily.

After discharge from the hospital, goals 5 and 6 (personality and mood disorder) could be addressed in individual psychotherapy of a depth and intensity determined by what the clinician decides is most appropriate for the patient. Goal 7 (marital disturbance) could be addressed through marital or family therapy, depending on which is more appropriate. Goals 8 and 9 (migraine and obesity) require a change of life-style and eating patterns and would best be served by a self-management program emphasizing relaxation, the control of tension and diet, and exercise. Goal 10 (vocational) requires vocational counseling and, perhaps, retraining.

This is an ambitious plan; but note how, in several instances, one treatment method addresses several goals (individual psychotherapy for goals 1, 2, 5, and 6, for example).

Time estimation

Step 7. Estimate how long treatment will take and how frequently it should be implemented.

Exploratory psychotherapy for personality disorder, for example, might be required at least once a week for somewhere between 6 and 12 months.

Evaluation

Step 8. Design methods of evaluation for each treatment method

These evaluation methods could vary from the patient's report of the absence of emotional disturbance and symptoms and a more productive social life (for psychotherapy) to the reduction of tension and somatic symptoms (for relaxation therapy).

Step 9. Prune the plan, if necessary

Goal 1. Depression: Alter antidepressant medication.
Goal 2. Tension: Relaxation therapy.
Goal 3. Drug dependency: Admit to hospital and withdraw from polypharmacy.
Goal 4. Rejection by family: Counseling of husband and son.
Goal 5. Personality: Reality-oriented psychotherapy.

The disadvantages of an abbreviated plan

The remaining goals could be included (rather peripherally) in the goals just listed. The danger of such an abbreviated plan would be that even if initial improvement were achieved, the lack of follow-through in regard to personality and marital disorder would probably lead to a recurrence of the problems or to their manifestation in another form. Such an undesirable outcome is also likely to occur if the plan is limited by a narrowly focused biomedical diagnosis.

The advantages of goal-oriented planning to teamwork

One virtue of this system (the goal-oriented approach) is that a management team can use it to decide who does what, when it is to be done, and how the team will know if a particular aspect of management should be modified or that treatment should terminate. Having determined goals at the outset, the team can then choose the most appropriate treatment methods. Evaluating the effect of treatment at regular intervals enables the team to revise goals or alter treatment methods when therapeutic progress has stalled. Stating the level of improvement expected enables the team to estimate how long the treatment should be implemented and how they will know when enough has been done.

The systematic organization of a plan has importance beyond the clarity it allows in a particular case. It facilitates a critical review of a clinician's or a team's general success in treatment, and it permits the evaluative comparison of different kinds of treatment.

Other advantages of goal-oriented planning

Ryback, Longabaugh, and Fowler (1981) compared goal-oriented and problem-oriented approaches to the clinical process. The proponents of goal-orientation criticize problem-orientation on a number of grounds, contending, for example, that problem-orientation stresses defects, creates pessimism, and obscures the patient's strengths. Furthermore, problems may reflect the clinician's needs rather than those of the patient. It is therefore asserted that the definition of goals by patient and physician promotes a better therapeutic alliance.

Variants of goal-oriented planning

Two goal-oriented approaches have been used in mental health settings: goal attainment scaling and goal planning. In goal attainment scaling (Kiresuk & Sherman, 1968), an expected treatment outcome is specified for up to five of the most important problems, together with a date for the evaluation of outcome. Goal planning (Houts & Scott, 1976), in contrast to goal attainment scaling, demands more attention to treatment selection. The patient's strengths and needs are specified, and the treatment team collaborate to design the management plan. The plan eventually specifies the outcome desired, the mode of treatment, the person responsible for each facet of treatment, and the target date.

The method of planning described in this chapter is essentially a form of goal planning that emphasizes the need for a multidimensional, integrated formulation of diagnosis before problems and goals are specified. It also introduces a technique of identifying pivotal problems and of determining the priority of the remedial and compensatory goals derived from those problems.

Summary

The keystone of systematic planning is the triangular relationship among goals, methods, and evaluation. In short, what is the destination, how will the patient get there, and how will you both know you have arrived?

The steps of systematic goal-directed management planning are as follows:

1. Cast the diagnostic net. Start with the current pattern and work back to precipitation, perpetuation, and predisposition. Prepare a differential diagnosis from the current pattern(s) of psychosomatic features.
2. Prepare an inquiry plan to rule in or out the hypothetical diagnoses and speculations about the causal nexus.
3. Draw up a flowchart of the dynamic interrelationships of the current patterns of response and the current perpetuating factors. Decide which problems are most pivotal. Include predisposing and precipitating factors, if they are still operative.
4. Rewrite alterable and pivotal deficits as remedial goals.
5. Define potential assets and resources from a biopsychosocial inventory and rewrite as compensatory goals those likely to foster recovery or improvement.
6. Taking each goal as a heading, decide which form of management would be most appropriate. For each goal, specify a technique of evaluation and a time estimate. Try to choose methods addressing more than one goal.
7. Review the plan according to the following criteria:
   a. The congruence of the treatment with the goal.
   b. The likelihood that the treatment could be effective.
   c. Economy in time and resources.
   d. Feasibility in time and resources.
   e. The acceptability of the treatment to the patient.
   f. The efficiency of the treatment in that it addresses more than one goal.
8. Revise the plan, if necessary, in the light of 7.
9. Negotiate the plan with the patient.

The goal-directed format provided by this scheme can be adapted to systematic record keeping. It facilitates regular, administratively efficient planning and team review. It is well suited to program evaluation and to evaluating the comparative efficiency of different therapeutic techniques.

PART V

Special situations

Thus far, we have presented a generic method of clinical reasoning involving a hypothetico-deductive diagnostic process, a comprehensive diagnostic formulation, and multifaceted, goal-oriented management planning. Part V discusses how these principles can be used in the following settings:

1. The outpatient clinic and private office.
2. The emergency room and crisis clinic.
3. The psychiatry inpatient service.
4. The general hospital.
5. The primary-care clinic.
6. The child psychiatry clinic.

Although the fundamental principles of clinical reasoning can be applied in all of these settings, each setting influences the clinical process its own way. Chapters 16 through 26 explore the following questions:

1. What are the advantages and constraints of the clinical process in each setting?

2. What kinds of clinical problems are typically referred?
3. What are the aims of clinical work?
4. What are the special features of the diagnostic process in each clinical setting?
5. What are the special features of the management process?

16

Outpatient psychiatry

The diversity and complexity of the clinical process of psychiatry find their fullest expression in the outpatient clinic and private office. This chapter summarizes the factors significantly influencing practice in these settings.

The advantages and constraints of the setting

The doctor–patient alliance

The doctor–patient relationship is voluntary and negotiated

The doctor-patient relationship is usually voluntary and negotiated in the outpatient clinic. Lazare, Eisenthal and Wasserman (1975) describe how negotiating a diagnosis and treatment plan mutually satisfactory to both parties fosters a working alliance. When the physician provides services generally akin to what the patient needs and expects, rapport is good and treatment proceeds smoothly. Otherwise, the patient may resist or terminate treatment (Borghi, 1968).

Diverse referral sources

Patients reach the outpatient clinic. from many sources. Patients may refer themselves or be referred by other physicians and mental health workers; by

Varying expectations

local, state, federal, and private agencies; and by friends and family. As mentioned, the expectations of the referring person may differ from those of the patient. If so, the physician must clarify the differences. Common reasons for referral include clinical consultation with regard to diagnosis or treatment, legal consultation, judicial referral, and self-referral.

Clinical consultation

Secondary consultation in outpatient psychiatry

Many primary-care doctors and other mental health professionals would like to treat the patient themselves but want the reassurance of a specialist's assessment. Sometimes, however, the psychiatrist is concerned that the referring clinician does not have the expertise or resources to implement the appropriate management plan. The patient also may have one of the following concerns:

1. The primary clinician is not expert enough to treat the problem.
2. If the patient communicates this concern, the clinician will be offended.
3. The cost of referral and treatment will be prohibitive.
4. The clinician thinks the patient is very ill, perhaps hopeless.
5. The patient will be labeled as *crazy* and rejected.

All parties are caught in a dilemma if the patient's expectations and concerns are not honestly and respectfully communicated by the psychiatrist to the referring agent. Negotiating the referral with primary-care physicians is discussed further in chapter 19.

Clinical referral

Reactions to referral

The patient's anticipatory concerns may become reality after referral. The psychiatrist would be wise to explore these reactions to referral lest they emerge later, overtly or covertly, and interfere with treatment.

Legal consultation

Explicit and unstated purposes for referral

The purpose of legal consultation may be explicit (for example, when a lawyer requests an expert opinion in a child custody case) or veiled (for example, when a lawyer asks for a psychiatric consultation to buy enough time to prepare the case more thoroughly).

Judicial referral

Evaluating eccentric behavior

The court may order an offender to obtain outpatient treatment for behavior that is a nuisance or danger to society or for overtly criminal behavior. Patients with psychosexual disorder (such as paraphilia), substance abuse disorder, antisocial personality, disorder of impulse control, schizophrenic disorder (especially paranoid schizophrenia), and mania are those most likely to be at odds with their community.

Self-referral

Self-referral

Lazare and Eisenthal (1977) suggest that patients seek psychiatric consultation for these reasons:

Reasons for self-referral

1. For administrative reasons e.g., about disability, draft deferment, or court testimony.
2. For advice about a personal decision.
3. To clarify the nature of, and resolve, a personal dilemma.
4. To find out where to get help.
5. To confess a guilty misdeed for which they seek absolution.
6. To ventilate burdensome feelings.
7. To control harmful impulses.
8. For the biomedical treatment of nerves or other physical problems.
9. To have the psychiatrist identify for them the psychological reasons for disturbing thoughts, feelings, and behavior.
10. To discover how psychological development has influenced current life problems.
11. To comprehend a loss of touch with reality.
12. To persuade the therapist to intervene with others who are perceived as having problems.
13. To receive succor for feelings of being empty, alone, uncared for, deprived, rejected, or abandoned.
14. For no clear reason.

The patient may not reveal the reason for seeking psychiatric consultation, and the clinician may not elicit it. This problem is discussed in the section on diagnosis in outpatient settings in this chapter.

Referral in relation to stage of the clinical process

Referral at all stages of illness and clinical process

Referral can occur at different stages of the clinical process and at any stage in the evolution of an illness, from the onset of symptoms to years afterward. The patient may be referred after unsuccessful courses of treatment and serious physical, psychological, and social complications (Cassano, Maggini, & Akiskal, 1983). Figure 16.1 relates referral to the stages of the clinical process.

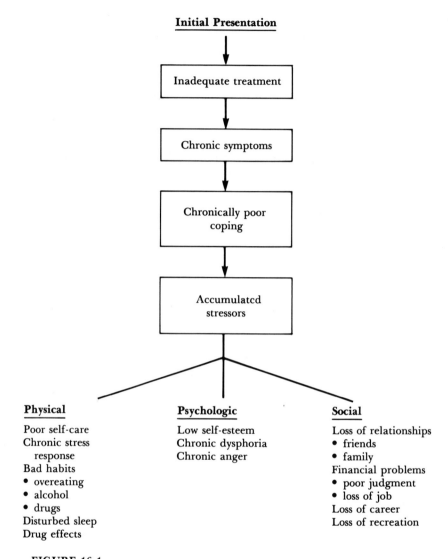

FIGURE 16.1
The consequences of inadequate treatment

Psychiatric patients are frequently referred late in the course of their illness. Most patients with psychiatric disorder are not treated by a psychiatrist. More than 50% seek help first from a primary-care physician, and many initially consult nonpsychiatric mental health professionals (Regier, Goldberg, & Taube, 1978). Some examples of late referral are provided in this chapter (see Cases 16.3 and 16.4) and in chapter 19.

Clinical problems encountered in the outpatient setting

All diagnoses

Patients can be referred to an outpatient clinic with almost any psychiatric diagnosis, although patients with acute psychosis or character disorder usually present elsewhere since they cannot tolerate waiting for an appointment.

Regardless of their diagnostic variety, most patients have the following characteristics:

Common characteristics of outpatients

1. Their symptoms are not severe enough to preclude self-care between visits.
2. They are able to negotiate a diagnosis and management plan.
3. Except in community mental health centers, they usually have the means to finance treatment.

The aims of clinical work in the outpatient setting

Outpatient clinicians and private practitioners should define their missions, aims, plans, and tactics.

Mission

Mission refers to the superordinate purpose of clinical work. For example, the mission of a general psychiatrist in a rural community might be to provide comprehensive ambulatory psychiatric care for all patients in the community.

A psychoanalyst's mission might be: to provide psychodynamically oriented psychiatric care to patients in the community.

Aims

Aims are more specific. For example, the aims of a rural psychiatrist might include the following:

1. Providing diagnostic services to the local court and schools.
2. Providing consultation for local family physicians.
3. Providing medical coverage for the staff of the community mental health center.
4. Treating patients referred for psychiatric care.

The aims of psychoanalytic practice might include:

1. Evaluating all patients referred.
2. Providing psychoanalysis or psychodynamic psychotherapy to selected patients.
3. Recommending appropriate treatment for those patients not suitable for psychoanalytic psychotherapy.

Administrative plans   Plans help clinicians achieve their aims. Plans are either administrative or clinical or both. For example, administrative plans to facilitate the rural psychiatrist's consultation to the local family physician, might include:

1. Contacting all local physicians as soon as possible.
2. Developing a reputation for competence, reliability, and efficiency.
3. Fostering the continuity of the patient's relationships with family physicians.

Clinical plans   Clinical plans might include:

1. Completing a comprehensive biopsychosocial evaluation of all new patients.
2. Developing goal-oriented, systematic management plans for all patients.
3. Conducting a systematic audit of the effectiveness of each patient's management.

Administrative tactics   Tactics represent what must be done to implement the plan. Tactics can be administrative or clinical. Specific administrative tactics to implement the plans of the rural psychiatrist might include:

1. Attending all hospital staff meetings.
2. Informing all community physicians by letter about his or her training, experience, clinical interests, and availability.
3. Telephoning all consultees immediately after seeing their patients.
4. Writing consultees a brief letter outlining assessment and recommendations.
5. Recommending follow-up with the patient's family physician.

Clinical tactics   Clinical tactics might include the following:

1. Interviewing and physically examining all patients and ordering special investigations when appropriate.
2. Formulating a comprehensive diagnosis and planning goal-oriented management for all patients (see chapters 14 and 15).
3. Designating management plans and therapeutic tactics for each clinical goal (see chapters 12, 14, and 15).

Diverse purposes   Outpatient clinical settings have diverse purposes determined by such factors as:

1. Rural or urban setting.
2. Associated institutions (e.g., hospital clinic, private solo practice, group mental health practice, community mental health center, multispecialty medical practice, primary-care practice).
3. Therapeutic approach (e.g., psychopharmacology, short-term dynamic psychotherapy, behavioral medicine).
4. Age or sex (child, geriatric, male or female).

5. Diagnostic category (e.g., anxiety disorders, pain, depression, sexual dysfunction, eating disorders).
6. Referral problem (e.g., forensic, crisis, consultation).

The name of a clinic may mislead the patient, creating incongruent expectations that impede clinical process.

Case 16.1   ■ Over a 5-year period, Henry, a 40-year-old executive, has consulted three different psychiatrists, complaining of anxiety, lack of motivation, and depression. He has never stayed in treatment longer than five sessions.

Concerned about his inadequate performance, Henry's superior at work asks the company's employee-assistance counselor to evaluate the problem. Worried about his negative attitude towards psychiatry and hoping that a medically oriented approach might foster the therapeutic alliance, the counselor refers Henry to a behavioral medicine clinic. There, an inexperienced resident takes a psychodynamically oriented psychiatric history. Expecting a more conventional medical history and examination, Henry cancels the second appointment and fails to respond to a follow-up letter. ■

Special features of the diagnostic process

Stages of diagnosis

Referral at any point in the clinical process   Referral to the outpatient setting from other clinicians can occur at any point in the clinical process. Referral occurs when the clinician or patient is concerned or dissatisfied. This may be articulated in the consultation request, though often it is not. The referring clinician may be confounded by an aspect of diagnosis or treatment, may consider the patient needs help that he or she cannot provide, or may dislike the patient. The patient, in turn, may be worried that the clinician is unhelpful or uncongenial. Sometimes, the patient or primary clinician has moved, necessitating referral.

The psychiatrist can use the time between referral and appointment to locate previous records and clarify the reasons for referral. During the diagnostic encounter, the psychiatrist must elicit a careful history of previous diagnostic work, assess its adequacy, and identify all the reasons for referral and the patients' reaction to being referred.

Since evaluation takes several weeks in most outpatient settings, the patient can assist the diagnostic process, as follows:

1. By recording the frequency and severity of a particular symptom.
2. By recording the thoughts and feelings associated with the symptom.
3. By reflecting on the initial interviews to evoke associations to be explored later.
4. By making time for additional diagnostic procedures.
5. By helping the psychiatrist locate records.

Diagnostic resources

Networks of clinicians and diagnostic services

The psychiatrist should develop a reliable network of auxiliary diagnostic services. However, there is considerable variation in the degree to which allied physicians or other mental health clinicians are available. Facilities for such special investigations as CT scanning may not be readily accessible.

Negotiated diagnosis

Since the patient is usually voluntary if not self-referred, most aspects of the diagnostic process must be negotiated. However, negotiation can founder for a number of reasons:

The reasons negotiation may founder

1. The patient's needs may not be known. The physician may have diagnostic goals in which the patient has no interest.
2. The patient may disagree with the physician's provisional diagnosis and see no point in pursuing it further.
3. The patient may be concerned about the costs of diagnostic procedures (which may not be reimbursable in ambulatory settings).
4. Diagnostic procedures may inconvenience the patient.
5. The patient may be too disturbed to negotiate.
6. The patient may be ambivalent about seeing a psychiatrist.
7. The patient may become resistant following a clash with the psychiatrist.
8. The patient may develop a negative transference to the psychiatrist (see chapter 8).
9. The patient's family may not support further diagnosis.

The need to recognize the factors influencing illness behavior

Chapter 3 presents a detailed discussion of the physical, psychological, and social factors influencing illness behavior. The psychiatrist must be attentive to all these factors during the clinical negotiation. To ignore them costs time, money, and suffering and sometimes causes the patient to defect.

The request

The patient's wishes, emphasized in this chapter, merit particular attention. The patient may expend considerable effort in consciously or unconsciously manipulating the clinician to get what he or she wants. The psychiatrist must determine what the patient fundamentally wants and accommodate it when negotiating diagnosis and treatment plans. Otherwise, frustration and resistance will confound the diagnostic process and impede treatment.

What does the patient want?

Administrative support

The need for administrative support

Administrative organization is essential for effective diagnosis in the outpatient setting. Unlike the hospital, where the diagnostic process is compressed by time and given structure by the institution's framework, outpatient psychiatry depends on other people beyond the psychiatrist's administrative domain. For example, information often arrives at the office through the mail. A system must be developed to record it and incorporate it in the clinical process.

Case 16.2

■ Maureen, a 32-year-old woman with symptoms of confusion, also reports easy fatigability and muscle weakness. Concerned about the possibility of hypothyroidism, the psychiatrist examines Maureen physically. Aside from a slight lag in deep tendon reflex return, the examination is negative. Nevertheless, the psychiatrist decides to investigate thyroid function before starting therapy.

At the subsequent visit, the psychiatrist becomes more concerned about Maureen's confusional state. He looks for the laboratory slip; it cannot be found. Pressed, he prescribes desipramine, increasing the dose when the patient returns, no better, the following week.

Another 2 weeks see no change. Urged by Maureen's husband, who is concerned about his wife's despondency, the psychiatrist hospitalizes the patient.

In the hospital, thyroid function studies confirm hypothyroidism. Chagrined, the psychiatrist searches for the laboratory slip, which he finds in a pile of junk mail. The laboratory findings indicate an abnormal thyroid profile. ■

Systematic medical records

How can such fiascos be prevented? A well-organized medical chart, with standard protocols used by all clinicians for recording information, will obviate omissions most of the time. If the recording is routine and standard, the psychiatrist need only read the chart to incorporate relevant data in the clinical process. Table 16.1 outlines a chart organization that works well in an outpatient setting.

Special features of management

The stage of illness

Check whether previous treatment was adequate

Referral can occur at any stage of an illness. Medicine and psychiatry are not standardized. A patient may have undertaken any or several of many therapies, and there is no assurance that treatment has been appropriate or sufficient. Commonly, for example, patients will have received inadequate doses of psychotropic drugs. Consequently, they will report that previous antidepressant therapy was unsuccessful. The psychiatrist thus should ask about dosage, length of treatment, and compliance before assuming a particular treatment has been ineffective.

TABLE 16.1
Chart organization: outpatient setting

A. Inside front cover

Identifying data sheet: Name; date of birth; home address and phone; business address and phone; name and address of significant other; insurance and billing information; referring person(s); primary physician and phone.

Problem list: List and number all significant medical and psychiatric diagnoses, their date of onset, their date of resolution.

Medication sheet: List all drugs: dates begun, doses, dates stopped, amounts given in each prescription.

B. Body of chart

Progress Notes section: Most recent visit on top.

Initial Assessment section: Medical history and physical examination forms; psychiatric assessment forms; biopsychosocial diagnostic net; dynamic flow chart.

Management Planning section: Prioritized problem list; goals and objectives; therapeutic techniques; evaluation.

Flow sheet section: Summary and progress data sheets for each goal.

Laboratory section: All laboratory and special investigation reports.

Communication section: Letters; other medical records; permission slips.

C. Inside back cover

Carbon copy of all prescriptions.

Case 16.3   ■   Sally, a 28-year-old divorced mother of two children, comes to the psychiatrist's office with a long history of disabling anxiety and depression. The highlights of her life include:

1. She had a middle-class upbringing.
2. At 13 years, her father, diagnosed as having cancer, became depressed.
3. At 18 years, her father died of cancer.
4. At 19 years, Sally developed anxiety attacks, requiring her to resign her job and return home.
5. At 22 years, she was married.
6. At 23 years, her first child was born.
7. At 24 years, her house burned down. Her husband blamed her because she might have forgotten to turn off the stove.
8. At 24 years, she was prescribed diazepam for anxiety at work.
9. At 24 years, she began to check things compulsively.
10. At 25 years, she gave birth to her second child (which she agreed to have only to please her husband). Her husband's infidelity precipitated a postpartum depression. She was hospitalized and treated with amitriptyline and chlorpromazine. She and her husband separated.
11. At 25 years, she returned home and began behavior therapy to diminish compulsive checking and phobic anxiety. However, she remained depressed.

12. At 26 years, she was still anxious and now had panic episodes. She began lorazepam.

13. At 26 years, she was prescribed imipramine, 25 mg t.i.d.

14. At 26 years, she was told by a psychiatrist that her compulsive checking was caused by early toilet training. Sally blamed her mother for her chronic symptoms. Her mother, who has borne the burden of her illness and helped raise the children, became angry and withdrew support.

15. At 26 years, disabled, Sally was sent to an employees' assistance program. A counselor abruptly withdrew her from all drugs saying, "We don't believe in pills here." Withdrawal symptoms, including severe anxiety and REM rebound, convinced Sally that she was "really sick." Her panic symptoms worsened. She began assertiveness training.

16. At 27 years, she returned home and recommended lorazepam, which temporarily relieved her symptoms.

17. At 28 years, severely depressed, despairing, and suicidal she is referred to a psychiatric clinic.

Sally concludes that she has tried everything without success. She is convinced she is hopeless. The psychiatrist must counteract this strong perpetuating conviction while attempting to treat the panic disorder. ∎

Sally's panic was initially precipitated by unresolved grief and subsequently aggravated by agoraphobia, compulsions, and depression. She resisted using imipramine and biofeedback because she associated them with past failure.

The need for multimodal therapy
Complex syndromes such as Sally's demand a comprehensive, biopsychosocial approach. Only after medication and biofeedback were combined with cognitive-behavioral (and subsequently exploratory, dynamic) psychotherapy did treatment prove effective.

As with medication, psychotherapy may have been inexpert or inadequately focused.

Case 16.4
∎ A family physician refers Frances, a 35-year-old unmarried teacher, for the evaluation and treatment of a depressive episode. Frances's depression has had a protracted course, beginning about 4 months after the death of her father 5 years previously. She had refused to see her father in the hospital before his death or in the funeral parlor afterwards, and she had participated in neither the funeral nor the wake.

Frances sought help from an internist, whom she met once every 2 to 6 weeks to talk over her feelings. As she became more and more dependent on her physician, a subtle pattern emerged. Physical complaints received more attention than emotions; for example, when Frances developed a new physical symptom, the physician examined her carefully and saw her more frequently. Consequently, both were frustrated: she never got the attention she wanted, and he never achieved any progress. He finally began to exhort her: "You're fine. You've just got to get yourself going." Resentfully, she sought help from another physician, only for the same pattern to recur.

On the advice of her employer, Frances sought counseling, first at a psychotherapy center, then at a community mental health clinic to which her therapist moved after 6 months. Unfortunately, the therapist's new job precluded his conducting long-term psychotherapy. Frances had to terminate rather abruptly, and she was transferred to another worker, who saw her once a month for hour-long counseling sessions.

Frances continued to have a variety of physical complaints for which she sought consultation from several physicians. As her depression deepened and she became more dysfunctional, her family doctor recommended a trial of medication. When this proved ineffective, psychiatric consultation was arranged.

Frances's job is now in jeopardy because of absenteeism, and her persistent ill-humor has alienated family and friends. Socially isolated, fearful of losing her job, and hopeless about ever recovering, she begins to harbor suicidal thoughts.

The psychiatrist negotiates a therapeutic contract for regular, weekly, hour-long psychotherapy. Initially, he offers support for her many problems, including thoughts of suicide; but once a strong alliance has developed, he helps her to address the anger at her father which has prevented her from mourning his death. After 3 weeks, he decides to increase her visits to twice weekly to provide better continuity between sessions and more support for the anxiety-provoking nature of therapy. Slowly, after she has ventilated anger and guilt and begun to grieve for her father, her chronic symptoms improve and she becomes more functional. ■

Inadequate treatment prolongs illness

Cases 16.3 and 16.4 illustrate how inadequate treatment can perpetuate illness (see Figure 16.2). Such cases also demonstrate that the clinician must not assume a particular treatment has been ineffective; a thorough history is required and sometimes only a further trial of therapy will suffice, but this time with adequate dose and clearer focus.

Negotiated responsibilities

The patient's responsibilities differ with the treatment

Outpatients must assume certain responsibilities, which are negotiated with the physician and differ with each patient and form of treatment. For example, patients have different responsibilities in the following treatment modes:

1. Behavior therapy (data-recording and data-rating; practicing behavior or relaxation exercises).
2. Pharmacotherapy (compliance with medication instructions).
3. Psychotherapy (punctuality, honesty, and reflection).

Doctor and patient negotiate a contract to fulfill these responsibilities. The doctor and patient must develop a strong therapeutic alliance to sustain the contract through the stresses that are inseparable from psychiatric illness and treatment.

Conflict

Sometimes a conflict emerges between the patient's wishes and the psychiatrist's management plan; for example:

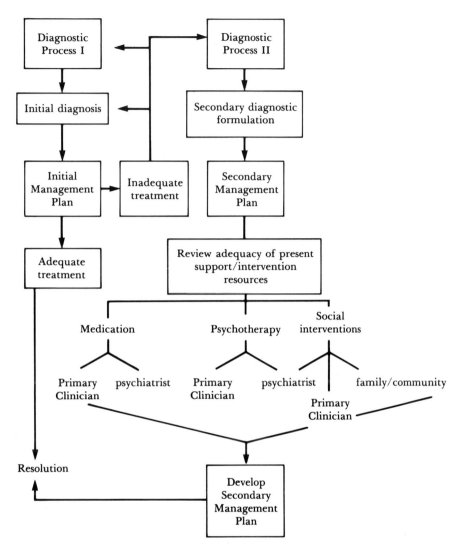

FIGURE 16.2
Review of treatment process, ambulatory setting

1. A patient with pain and major depression wants analgesics but not antidepressants.
2. A patient with panic disorder wants psychotherapy but not imipramine.
3. A patient with psychosis wants biofeedback but not antipsychotic medication.
4. A patient with unresolved grief wants pills to relieve symptoms but refuses psychotherapy.

Personal reasons for resistance to the management plan

If a comprehensive biopsychosocial assessment is completed, as outlined in chapter 14, the physician will usually understand the personal reasons for these attitudes and will develop a plan to address the conflict. Lazare (1979) classifies these conflicts according to whether they concern the problem presented by the patient, the goals, methods and conditions of treatment, or the doctor–patient relationship itself.

The conflict may be explicit or veiled (in order to avoid confrontation); direct or displaced from one area of dissatisfaction to another (again perhaps to avoid confrontation); and conscious or unconscious (on the part of either doctor or patient). The physician must strive to recognize these conflicts and develop a plan to resolve them.

Scheduling

Scheduling appointments is an important technical consideration in outpatient psychiatry. Since the schedule must be negotiated, patient and physician can use it as an arena to explore unresolved conflict.

Case 16.5

■ A busy academic psychiatrist interviews Jason, a 30-year-old man with relationship problems that jeopardize his job. Doctor and patient relate well. They decide on a short course of focal psychotherapy to explore the patient's anger at authorities. Jason requests an appointment time after work. The psychiatrist, somewhat pressed but eager to cooperate, fits him into a time that overlaps with the end of the patient's working day.

Jason is late for the first three appointments. The psychiatrist wonders about negative transference. When this is explored, Jason reveals that he really likes the doctor and is committed to therapy. However, he is caught on the horns of a dilemma: if he leaves work early enough to make the appointment, he will be fired and thus be unable to afford therapy. By being 20 minutes late, he can keep his job and get at least 30 minutes of the doctor's time.

The doctor examines his countertransference. Why had he not attended to Jason's requests? Why had he accepted the patient when he was really too busy to include him in a cramped schedule? He reflects wryly: "There I go again. Always being big brother and getting hurt because the kids are dawdling." He recognizes that he needs to make more time in his schedule for treating selected patients. ■

Consistent scheduling of appointments

Appointments and scheduling can be a source of information for the psychodynamic understanding of the therapeutic encounter. Scheduling varies with the practice and the patient. Punctuality by both parties facilitates rapport; effective psychotherapy demands consistent scheduling.

Consistent administration

Administration is a critical aspect of outpatient treatment too often overlooked by the novice clinician. Fees must be established, billing mechanisms arranged, appointment schedules planned, and staff responsibilities delineated.

Consistent data recording

An effective medical record must be developed to match the requirements of each mode of therapy. Psychopharmacology, for example, requires prescription records, symptom flowcharts and rating scales, medical history and physical forms, and laboratory data sheets; behavior therapy requires patient recording forms and biofeedback data sheets; psychotherapy necessitates goal-oriented progress notes.

All charts should have progress notes and a place for correspondence. The more standardized the chart, the less likely there will be mistakes. A sample chart is illustrated in Table 16.1 in the section on administrative support in this chapter.

Systematic management

How can the outpatient clinician use the system of diagnosis and management planning introduced in chapters 14 and 15? This chapter illustrates the problems of late intervention in two cases (16.3 and 16.4). The benefits of early intervention will be illustrated in another case example (Case 16.6), supported by a series of diagnostic nets completed at different points in the treatment process.

Case 16.6   ■   Helen, the 34-year-old mother of a 5-year-old son, experiences her first attack of panic while on a business trip with her husband. Over the previous 3 years, she has suffered anxiety episodes of increasing severity, to the extent that she has begun to avoid crowded places and outings. Diazepam has incompletely suppressed her symptoms.

Helen's panic is characteristic: a sudden upsurge of terror with pounding in the chest, profuse sweating, difficulty breathing, and numbness and tingling of the extremities. The accompanying chest pain convinces her she is having a heart attack.

Her husband drives her at once to the nearest hospital emergency room, where physical examination proves negative. After intramuscular chlorazepate partially relieves her symptoms, the trip is aborted and Helen returns home.

At a family practice clinic next day, the doctor on duty prescribes diazepam 5 mg, twice daily. Over the subsequent week, Helen's sleep and anxiety improve somewhat; but, concerned about Helen's progressive disability over the previous 2 years, the physician decides her problem requires a more comprehensive approach. He refers her to a psychiatric consultant.

The psychiatrist elicits a family history of anxiety (mother and sister) and obesity, and a strong suggestion of problems in her upbringing ("My family was messed up"). He notes several possible precipitants, including:

1. A marginal family business that leaves Helen with few funds for her personal needs.
2. Her son's beginning school.
3. The recent visit of a friend with difficult children and marital problems, who became quite dependent on Helen and did not leave for a month.
4. The recent departure of her family doctor.
5. Helen's anticipatory anxiety about the business trip, insisted on by a husband whom she cannot refuse.

The psychiatrist notes that despite her painful anxiety, Helen is unduly apologetic about taking up his valuable time. He wonders whether subassertiveness and difficulty expressing anger perpetuate her illness. His systemic and temporal assessment is summarized in Table 16.2.

To interrupt the perpetuating vicious cycle of physical symptoms and fear, he prescribes the following treatment:

1. Diazepam (1)* 5 mg h.s., to induce sleep and modify acute anxiety.
2. A thorough physical examination (2)* at the next visit.
3. Education (2)* about the nature of this frightening disorder to counteract her fearful conviction that she is about to die.

To assess the stress cycles determining the pattern of Helen's disorder, the psychiatrist asks her to keep a daily log (3)* of the sensations, events, thoughts, and feelings associated with each episode of anxiety and what she does about it. He hopes this task will give Helen something concrete to do, and a sense of control.

One week later, Helen reports a moderation of symptoms. Her sleep is improved, and she is less anxious during the day and concentrating better. The psychiatrist now prescribes:

1. Relaxation training (4)* to help Helen regulate her psychological and physiologic arousal in response to stress.
2. Low dose imipramine (5)* to block the panic attacks that perpetuate her anticipatory anxiety.

By the fourth visit, important new information has been elicited and can be included in the diagnostic net (see Table 16.3).

Powerful, long-standing stressors perpetuate Helen's stress cycle:

1. She is enmeshed in her sister's chaotic marriage in a manner that perpetuates her sister's psychopathology.
2. Her parents are chronically dependent on her for help with day-to-day household tasks they could do themselves. They make her feel guilty and obligated.
3. She lives in fear she will lose her place as responsible parent, devoted wife, and good daughter.
4. She resents the intrusion of these obligations into her family life and worries about their impact on her marriage.

Allied psychosocial factors that perpetuate the cycle include:

1. The use of denial and suppression to cope with anger. These defenses underlie maladaptive coping strategies, such as failing to confront problems and avoiding activities that might provoke an anxiety attack.

---

*Each intervention is numbered to correspond to numbers in the diagnostic cards in Tables 16.2 through 16.7.

TABLE 16.2
Diagnostic net of Helen (Case 16.6), first visit, November 1979

	Predisposition	Precipitation	Perpetuation	Pattern
Physical	• family history of anxiety, obesity	• aging • hyperventilation episode	• hyperventilation syndrome	• obesity • hyperventilation syndrome (1) — • obesity • anxiety attacks (1)
Psychological	? low self-esteem ? subassertive ? denies anger	• fear of loss of control (3) and death (2) • fear of loss of role — • unable to say "no" to trip	• fear of dying (2)	• anxiety/panic (1) • overly pleasant, minimizes her needs — • avoids places, people • hyperventilation (1)
Social	• family "messed up" • "wonderful marriage"	• child to school • failing family business • prolonged guest — • M.D. left town	• denial of marital problems — • no M.D. (2)	? strong relationship with husband — • diazepam 5 mg h.s. and p.r.n. (1) • physical examination and education (2)

Key: a. Data identified as problems to be treated at this visit are in *italic*.
b. Each problem in *italic* has a number corresponding to the numbered treatment described in the text and in the lower right box (social pattern; health care system).

349

TABLE 16.3
Diagnostic net of Helen (Case 16.6), 4th visit, January 1980

	Predisposition	Precipitation	Perpetuation	Pattern
Physical	• family history of anxiety, obesity	• aging • *hyperventilation (1, 2, 4, 5)*	• *hyperventilation syndrome (1, 2, 4, 5)*	• hyperventilation → • obesity • *anxiety attacks (1, 4, 5)*
Psychological	• anger is bad • need to be caretaker for self-esteem • chronic resentment of caretaking role • *minimizes, denies anger* • *chronic subassertive behavior; avoids conflict, resolution* • *tackles projects*	• *fear of panic attack (control, death) (6)* • *angry at guest, (6)* • *guilt (6)* • fear of loss of role (parent, wife, business) • *unable to set limits (6)*	• *fear of panic attack (2, 5, 6)* • *guilt (6)* • *fear of rejection (6)* • *subassertive coping style (6)* • *avoids conflict (6)* • *avoids driving, shopping, etc.*	• *anxiety/panic (1, 4, 5)* • *overly pleasant (6)* • *minimizes needs (6)* • *avoids conflict, people, places (6)* • *hyperventilates* • *accepts social tasks (6)*
Social	• not allowed to express anger at family • family very dependent ? "wonderful marriage"	• child to school • failing business • *prolonged guest (6)* • sister's marriage • *M.D. left town (2)*	• husband, family reinforce her subassertiveness • *society rewards "projects" (6)* • *ambivalent about behavioral approach (2)*	• family dependent on pt • strong marital relationship • social isolation • *relaxation (4)* • *therapeutic alliance with M.D. & education (2)* • *diazepam 5 mg p.r.n.* • *imipramine 50 mg h.s. (5)* • *cog behav. psychotherapy (6)*

Key: a. Data identified as problems to be treated at this visit are in *italic*.
 b. Each problem in *italic* has a number corresponding to the numbered treatment described in the text and in the lower right box (social pattern; health care system).

2. A long-standing fear of rejection.
3. The reinforcement of her self-effacement by her parents, sister, and community (she was a dedicated civic volunteer).

Factors that have predisposed her to develop these traits and be susceptible to such stressors include:

1. A family history of panic episodes, perhaps of genetic origin.
2. Her childhood experiences of being reprimanded if she directly expressed her feelings.
3. Her mother's psychiatric incapacitation. From an early age, as the oldest child, Helen assumed many parental duties. The entire family relied on her housework and emotional sustenance, and they continued to be dependent, to the extent that she could not leave home to marry until she was 29 years old. She had never had the opportunity to develop an identity distinct from that of looking after others.

Cognitive-behavioral psychotherapy (6) continues, focusing on her false assumptions and her need for greater assertiveness. By the eighth visit (March 1980), she has few symptoms. Other changes have occurred (see Table 16.4).

Free from acute anxiety, she worries less; still fearful of a panic attack, however, she continues to depend on medication. Her self-esteem has improved:

1. She has been able to refuse a request to coordinate the annual church fair. She feels some pride in her resolve instead of the guilt she anticipated.
2. Helen now perceives other subassertive patterns in her daily life and relates them to feelings of stress. But she still cannot stand up for herself with family members, and she feels guilty when she contemplates confronting her sister and parents about their burdensome demands.
3. She has learned relaxation effectively and has assumed enough control of her daily schedule to allow herself time to practice and improve her skills in this regard.

Helen and the psychiatrist develop a desensitization program (7)* for her phobic avoidance.

1. She lists all fear-provoking activities and situations and rates them on a scale of 1 (least) to 20 (most), in accordance with the amount of distress they provoke.
2. Starting with those activities rated least upsetting, she uses her new relaxation skills to avert anxiety in each activity and situation. She attempts new activities at higher anxiety levels only when she has successfully attained confidence in all activities at the previous level.

Thus, she begins driving again and is able to go shopping (in selected uncrowded situations), to church (albeit in the back row), and out to dinner (at off-peak hours).

Meanwhile, in psychotherapy, the psychiatrist helps Helen explore her difficulty recognizing anger and her self-abasing style of coping. Thirty-minute

TABLE 16.4
Diagnostic net of Helen (Case 16.6), 8th visit, March 1980

	Predisposition	Precipitation	Perpetuation	Pattern
Biological	• family history of anxiety, obesity	• aging		• obesity
Psychological	• anger is bad • need to be caretaker for self-esteem • chronic resentment of care-taking role • minimizes, denies anger • chronic sub-assertive behavior • avoids conflict resolution • tackles projects	• *fear of panic attacks without meds (4, 6, 7)* • *fear of loss of role as wife, child (6)* • *unable to set limits; refuse sister, parents, husband (6)*	• *fear of rejection (6)* • *guilt (6)* • self-esteem depends on projects, care role • *fear of panic attack without meds (6, 7)* • *avoids driving, shopping, church, restaurants (7)*	• *dependent on meds (6, 7)* • *overly pleasant (6)* • recognizes anger • reduction in anxiety • *avoids conflict with husband, parents (6)* • *sets limits on community (6)*
Social	• not allowed to express anger at family • family very dependent ? "wonderful marriage"		• *husband, family reinforce behavior (6)* • avoids psychological work • *ambivalent about behavior change (6)* • *dependency on drugs (4, 6)*	? strong relationship with husband • relaxation therapy (4) • imipramine 50 mg h.s. (5) • Cog-beh psychotherapy (6) • desensitization (7)

Key: a. Data identified as problems to be treated at this visit are in *italic.*
       b. Each problem in *italic* has a number corresponding to the numbered treatment described in the text and in the lower right box (social pattern; health

352

sessions are scheduled every 2 to 3 weeks to follow progress and help her deal with the predisposing attitudes underlying her maladaptive coping patterns (see Table 16.5):

1. Caretaking and responsibility bring approval and self-esteem.
2. Anger is unacceptable, particularly when it is directed at your parents or family or is in your self-interest.
3. Keep busy and avoid confrontations: you might lose control of your anger.

During the 10th visit, Helen glimpses the intensity of her anger and becomes more anxious for several weeks. But on the 11th visit, she reports a new confidence. She has coped by using diazepam (1) on several occasions, by relying more on her ability to control symptoms with relaxation (4), and by reducing stressors. She says that she wants to stop treatment, citing expense and her new found confidence. The psychiatrist hypothesizes that she has been frightened by a glimpse of her anger at the parents who still need her. He gently attempts to explore her resistance, but she rejects the notion. She reminds him that despite her husband's appreciation of her symptomatic improvement, he seems annoyed by what he perceives as her growing reliance on the visits. He refuses to come in to discuss the matter. The psychiatrist does not want to stress the therapeutic alliance further. He accedes to Helen's request to stop treatment but emphasizes his availability should she wish to explore further the psychological predisposition of her illness.

Two months later Helen returns to the clinic in dismay (see Table 16.5). Her anxiety has recurred. A short interview reveals a familiar pattern: Despondent about her marriage, Helen's sister has been threatening suicide. There have been numerous phone calls, often in the middle of the night, and frequent interruptions of daily business to handle emergencies. Helen's husband, who up to this point has been supportive, is becoming exasperated.

Faced with the disruption of her immediate family, Helen decides to get to the bottom of her perennial problem. ''Why do I always do this to myself?'' she asks. ''There must be something inside me that makes me do it.''

In 12 further sessions of 50 minutes each, over 4 months, Helen explores the conflicts, already outlined, in focal dynamic psychotherapy (8). Her initial task, however, is to understand that she was identifying with the psychiatrist's care-taking role to the detriment of both her sister's needs and her own. Was this not a familiar pattern? And was this behavior not alienating her husband, the one person who is receptive to her needs?

The transference interpretation strikes a chord. Helen advises her sister to seek treatment and helps her find a psychiatrist. With her husband, she works out how she can limit the sister's intrusion.

Psychotherapy continues. Helen identifies how her compliance with (what she thought was implied by) the therapist's statements was, in fact, a defense against her rage when he did not gratify her dependency needs. By January 1981, she is relatively symptom-free. More important, she understands better how to manage her emotions and personal relationships. To reinforce these gains further, patient and doctor review her progress on the diagnostic nets (9), which she takes home (see Table 16.6).

Fully active again, Helen terminates treatment except for participation in an assertiveness-training group (10), in which she functions as leader and teacher. She occasionally uses imipramine (25 mg h.s.). One year later, she reports she is seldom

TABLE 16.5
Diagnostic net of Helen (Case 16.6), 12th visit, July 1980

	Predisposition	Precipitation	Perpetuation	Pattern
Physical	• family history of anxiety, obesity	• aging		• obesity
Psychological	• anger is bad (8); • need to be caretaker for self-esteem (8); • chronic resentment of care-taking role (8); • *minimizes, denies anger (8)*; • *chronic subassertive behavior (8)*; • *avoids conflict, resolution (8)*; • *tackles projects (8)*	• *anger at guest, sister parents' dependency (6, 8)*; • *fear of panic attacks (6, 7)*; • *fear of loss of role (6, 8)*; • *unable to set limits (6, 8)*	• *guilt (6, 8)*; • *driving (7)*; • *beginning to confront family with dependency (6, 8)*	• *overt anger, anxiety, guilt (6, 8)*; • *insight = "taking time" (8)*; • *"no limits on family" (8)*
Social	• *not allowed to express anger at family (8)*; • *family very dependent (6, 8)*; ? "wonderful marriage"	• *sister's marital crisis (6, 8)*; • *patient's illness (6, 8)*; • *friend's needs (6, 8)*		• family dependent on patient; • husband supportive

Health care system (lower right box):

• M.D. p.r.n (2) • calls
• relaxation (4)
• diazepam
• "for safety" (1)
• imipramine 25 mg h.s. (5)
• Cog-beh psychotherapy (6)
• desensitization (7)
• focal, dynamic psychotherapy (8)

Key: a. Data identified as problems to be treated at this visit are in *italic*.
b. Each problem in *italic* has a number corresponding to the numbered treatment described in the text and in the lower right box (social pattern; health care system).

354

TABLE 16.6
Diagnostic net of Helen (Case 16.6), 24th visit, January 1981

	Predisposition	Precipitation	Perpetuation	Pattern
Biological	• family history of anxiety, obesity	• aging		
Psychological	• anger is acceptable (8) • self-care leads to self-esteem (8) • "I have control" (4, 8) • *driving (2)* • *awareness of anger (8, 10)* • *assertive (6, 10)* • *avoids projects in favor of self-care (6, 10)*		• guilt (6, 8) • *driving practice (7)*	• *understands and accepts NET (9)* • *more assertive with family (6, 8, 10)*
Social	• family expresses feelings (9) • family more self-reliant (9) • realistic marriage (9) • *stable M.D. relationship (2, 9)*	• sister's marriage		• *less family dependence (6, 8, 10)* • relaxation (4) • insight (8) • desensitization (7) • new coping (6) • occasional use of diazepam (1) and imipramine (5) • assertiveness group (10)

Key: a. Data identified as problems to be treated at this visit are in *italic*.
   b. Each problem in *italic* has a number corresponding to the numbered treatment described in the text and in the lower right box (social pattern; health care system).

TABLE 16.7
Treatment goals and interventions Helen (Case 16.6)

Visit	Goal (only new goals are listed)	Interventions (by number as used in text and tables 16.2–16.6)
first	modify acute anxiety modify stressors reassure about fears of heart attack develop therapeutic alliance	1. diazepam; 2. reassurance 2. prohibit further trips, with husband's support 3. physician examination and education 4. as above
fourth	block panic attack reduce helpless anticipation of panic attacks	5. imipramine; 4. relaxation training; 3. record keeping; 6. cognitive-behavioral psychotherapy; permission to avoid anxiety-provoking settings temporarily; role-playing to help set limits on obligations
eighth	reduce phobic avoidance reduce fear of losses: of role, of love and security reduce family reinforcement of subassertiveness	4. use relaxation skills in, 7. desensitization hierarchy 6. cognitive-behavioral psychotherapy: review automatic thoughts and their sources – false assumptions and cognitive distortion 6. cognitive-behavioral psychotherapy: education and role-playing at home with husband
eleventh	minimize negative consequences of premature termination	6. cognitive-behavioral psychotherapy: support, concern, statement of availability; avoid confrontational interpretation; reinforce techniques
twelfth	facilitate insight into predisposing childhood origins of perpetuating false assumptions, cognitive distortions, and maladaptive behaviors: i.e., understand cycle of dependency – anger – denial – anger – guilt – subassertiveness – unmet dependency – anger – anxiety – avoidance – more dependency – demoralization, etc.	8. focal, dynamic psychotherapy: use of transference interpretations; reinforce cognitive assessment

TABLE 16.7 (continued)

Visit	Goal (only new goals are listed)	Interventions (by number as used in text and tables 16.2–16.6)
twenty-fourth	maintain and reinforce adaptive, insightful cognitive and behavioral coping skills; diminish termination anxiety	9. biopsychosocial approach, using diagnostic net as guide. Continue to practice new skills: relaxation, desensitization, insightful thinking, assertiveness 6. cognitive-behavioral psychotherapy and follow-up health maintenance
	improve assertiveness skills	10. begin assertiveness training group
	cope with normal anxiety	4. practice relaxation skills; 6. practice new coping; 4. relaxation skills
	cope with abnormal anxiety and panic attacks	6. thought stopping, rehearsal, anger management; 1. diazepam available; 5. occasional imipramine

bothered by anxiety and then she can usually relate it to external events triggering a predictable cognitive-affective response. She continues to practice relaxation. To her surprise, she has noted the beneficial effect of her new insight and competence on other family members, particularly her chronically anxious mother, hypochondriacal father, and depressed, maritally troubled sister. ■

The interventions described in this case are summarized in Table 16.7.

In general medical practice, the treatment of panic disorder would typically involve prescribing diazepam in larger-than-needed amounts and supportive counseling. As in Case 16.3, the result might have been diazepam dependency, further deterioration in the activities and relationships sustaining Helen's self-esteem, leading to hypochondriasis, major depression, phobias, and further marital and family difficulties. To the contrary, following successful intervention it is even possible that the transmission of an ''anxiety trait'' to the patient's son will be avoided.

The results of inadequate treatment

Avoiding familial transmission

The use of serial diagnostic nets

As illustrated in this case, diagnostic nets help the physician track the effect of various interventions on the important factors influencing the illness. As benchmarks for review at nodal points in the clinical process, they are particularly useful for trainees learning the multidimensional aspects of modern psychiatric practice.

Summary

The diversity and complexity of the clinical process of psychiatry find their fullest expression in the outpatient clinic and private office. Certain features of this setting influence patient care. The doctor–patient relationship is usually voluntary and negotiated. Patients who are referred from varied sources may have different expectations from those of the referring person or the psychiatrist. The mission, aims, plans, and tactics of outpatient facilities will vary according to the patient population served. Referrals can occur at any stage of the clinical process and at any stage of the evolution of an illness. Though patients with a wide range of diagnoses are referred to this setting, patients with acute psychosis or acute organic brain syndrome are usually managed elsewhere.

Categorical diagnosis can often be established in one or two visits, but a comprehensive, biopsychosocial formulation often takes several more visits, and a psychodynamic formulation may require six or more. The psychiatrist can facilitate diagnosis by understanding what the patient wants and by negotiating a diagnostic plan with the patient. A systematic charting procedure helps organize the temporally extended, multifactorial data base.

The psychiatrist often treats patients for whom treatment elsewhere has failed and who have suffered the complications of chronic, untreated, or inadequately treated disorders. Patients must negotiate their responsibilities in treatment with the therapist. Systematic management can be helped by amplifying and revising the diagnostic net during the patient's course of treatment.

Selected Readings

In Lazare's *Outpatient Psychiatry: Diagnosis and Treatment* (1979), different specialists review the various theoretical approaches to outpatient psychiatry. They also discuss the clinical process of diagnosing and managing different clinical problems and disorders in the outpatient setting.

17

Emergency psychiatry

*Management focuses
on immediate control
and disposition*

*Serious consequences
follow clinical error*

The emergency department presents the ultimate challenge to the bio-psychosocial diagnostician. In a highly stressful environment, the psychiatrist must evaluate quickly a diversity of exacting problems. Management focuses on immediate control and disposition. Emergency patients are strangers who are often hostile, even combative, and seldom grateful. Emergency room staff vary in skill; many components of the system, such as the police, have had little or no training in handling emotionally disturbed people. Errors can have serious, if not lethal, consequences.

This chapter reviews the features of the clinical process special to this setting and presents a method of biopsychosocial assessment appropriate to this complex field.

The resources and constraints of the emergency setting

The influence of the community

Emergency psychiatric care reflects the sociocultural environment.

■ The emergency department of a large inner-city hospital provides most of the psychiatric care to a medically underserved urban ghetto. In this harsh, culturally alienated place, violence is rife and drugs are commonplace. Severely disturbed

Episodic, emergency care

patients generate an atmosphere of discord and confrontation. Unable to provide outreach or aftercare, the staff can do no more than respond to each crisis as it arises. Their mission is immediate or episodic control and disposition, not comprehensive care. An unwieldy and highly politicized bureaucracy often seems to stand in the way of change. Nevertheless, the emergency service has developed considerable expertise in the immediate handling of acutely disturbed, violent patients and in the recognition and management of drug-related disorders. ■

Contrast the urban scene to an emergency care system in an affluent community.

Coordinated care

■ It is a small, relatively wealthy city. The outreach efforts of the community's mental health center coordinate with the acute care provided by the university medical center emergency room, local emergency medical technicians, and police. All are trained. The care is individualized, interlinked, and, if required, provided in the home. The system involves the collaboration of professionals and nonprofessionals, each with clear roles according to their training and skill. Expert consultation is always available. Control is a means to care, not an end in itself. Care is systematic, individualized, and personal. Flaws in the system can be corrected because community members work together. ■

Need for community liaison

An emergency department must respond to the needs of its community, for community liaison is the cornerstone of effective planning. What is possible in a small city may be impracticable in an urban ghetto, and vice versa.

Medical and community interfaces

The emergency department relates to all elements of the health care system and the community (see Figure 17.1); for example:

Relationship to other health professionals

1. Patients may be referred for psychiatric evaluation by physicians and mental health workers, many of whom use the emergency department for night, weekend, and vacation coverage.

Walk-in patients

2. Patients often walk in. Sometimes they use the emergency department rather than establishing a therapeutic alliance. As a result, they are likely to be regarded as abusing the system.

Patients referred by other community members

3. Patients may be brought to the emergency department by family, friends, neighbors, police, or others. If they do not define themselves as sick, they are not likely to participate willingly in their own care.

Patients can be admitted to the hospital or referred to other institutions

4. The emergency department admits patients to all hospital services since emergency patients with behavioral problems often have an underlying physical disorder requiring medical treatment.

5. Patients may be sent from the emergency department to such other institutions as the state mental hospital, nursing home, detoxification center, or jail.

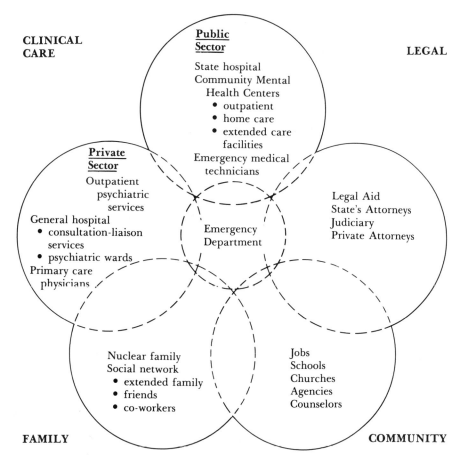

CLINICAL CARE

LEGAL

Public Sector

State hospital
Community Mental
Health Centers
- outpatient
- home care
- extended care
  facilities
Emergency medical
technicians

Private Sector

Outpatient
psychiatric
services
General hospital
- consultation-liaison
  services
- psychiatric wards
Primary care
physicians

Emergency
Department

Legal Aid
State's Attorneys
Judiciary
Private Attorneys

Nuclear family
Social network
- extended family
- friends
- co-workers

Jobs
Schools
Churches
Agencies
Counselors

FAMILY

COMMUNITY

FIGURE 17.1
Elements of the psychiatric emergency care system

Exigencies of time

Time constraints

Time affects the clinical process. In contrast to other clinical settings, the emergency service allows a psychiatrist only a short time, from minutes to a few hours, to evaluate and decide what to do about seriously disturbed, often dangerous, patients. Sometimes the need for psychiatric expertise becomes apparent to other physicians only after much of this time has expired. Other difficulties, such as the patient's inability or unwillingness to give a history, aggravate the pressure of time. Definitive treatment must often await referral to a more specialized clinical setting.

The need for special clinical tactics

The physician who works in this context must be prepared to operate within its time constraints and become adept in tactics of rapid diagnosis, management and disposition that are seldom needed elsewhere.

The effect of an atmosphere of crisis

There is no way to schedule catastrophe. The high-pitched atmosphere of the emergency room tends to exacerbate presenting problems. Fear and anxiety pervade. Clinical errors are dangerous, even fatal. Highly stressed emergency staff, distracted by other problems and perhaps untrained in psychiatry, sometimes respond to uncooperative patients with abruptness and hostility or ignore quiet, withdrawn patients.

The consequences of error

Nonlethal consequences of errors in emergency diagnosis or disposition

Mistakes can have consequences other than suicide, homicide, or major medical illness. Emergency staff seldom hear about their less dramatic errors, which can also be damaging; for example:

1. Unnecessary civil commitment, leading to humiliation, mistrust, and inappropriate management.
2. Unnecessary hospitalization, leading to regression and dependency.
3. Unnecessary medication, obscuring diagnosis and leading to morbid side-effects.
4. Missed opportunities to refer for definitive treatment, leading to a prolongation or irreversibility of the patient's disorder.

The results of variable staff training

Expertise and perspective vary greatly among the providers of emergency care. Police, paramedics, and nonspecialized personnel provide the initial care in a psychiatric emergency. The police tend to view themselves as peace keepers, not care givers. Without adequate training, they may misunderstand, or even take personally, the ravings of an angry drunk or the threats of a paranoid patient.

Need for coordination and definition of roles

Some mental health workers have had systematic clinical training; others have not. Differences in training inevitably lead to conflict. For example, there may be no leader responsible for coordination and quality assurance. The roles of different personnel may not be clearly defined and appropriate to their training and experience. Different parts of the system can develop separate and conflicting missions, aims, and plans.

Case 17.1

■ Susan, a 28-year-old woman with a 2-year history of unexplained physical symptoms diagnosed one month before as systemic lupus erythematosus, comes to the emergency department wanting to talk to someone. The nurse calls a crisis worker at the local mental health center, who talks with Susan about her marriage and family problems.

Susan is depressed about her illness and a recent therapeutic abortion, her second, following the death of a 20-week fetus. She is uncertain what to do about a deteriorating marriage and her mother's increasing dependency since Susan's father became severely ill 3 years ago. The crisis worker wishes to discuss the case with a physician, but is unable to reach Susan's doctor by phone. The on-call psychiatrist cannot be interrupted while conducting a psychotherapy session. Susan is impatient to leave, so the worker arranges an appointment for her in 1 week at the local crisis clinic.

Next day, still depressed and confused, Susan seeks help from her internist, complaining of headache. Finding that her sedimentation rate is more elevated than usual, he increases her dose of steroids. He reassures her that she will soon be feeling better about loss of her baby.

Later that week, Susan's husband, concerned about his wife's suicidal ideation, suspiciousness, and anger, brings her back to the emergency department and insists on seeing the psychiatrist on duty. His examination of her mental status reveals the following: abnormal thought process (blocking and unfinished sentences); abnormal thought content (paranoid and suicidal ideation); and impaired concentration and recent memory. Though unsure about the relationship between her abnormal mental status, the lupus erythematosus, and the medication she is taking for the disease, the psychiatrist is certain Susan is psychotic and needs hospitalization on the psychiatric service; but he cannot secure a bed. The internist agrees to admit her to a general medical unit, for a collaborative diagnostic evaluation. ■

Table 17.1 presents the potential conflicts between the roles of various personnel in a system attempting to manage sick people and control socially deviant behavior.

TABLE 17.1
Relationship of personnel in emergency psychiatric care system: potential conflicts

	Personnel				
Characteristics	*Crisis worker*	*Psychiatrist*	*Police*	*Legal aid*	*Emergency Medical Technician*
1. diagnostic training	clinical diagnosis for disposition	comprehensive diagnosis	forensic investigation	investigation	little training
2. clinical management training	crisis intervention	comprehensive treatment planning	behavior control	patient's rights	little training
3. relationship with patient	therapeutic; supportive	therapeutic; adversarial if commitment considered	supportive or adversarial (restraint)	supportive	supportive or adversarial (restraint)
4. relationship to crisis worker		colleague; supervisor	cooperative; or adversarial	little contact	cooperative
5. relationship to psychiatrist	colleague; supervisee		cooperative or adversarial	patient advocate	safe transport
6. clinical role	evaluation; care	evaluation; care	control; transport	patient advocate	safe transport

Clinical problems encountered in emergency psychiatry

The emergency psychiatrist encounters medical disorders, involuntary referrals, life-threatening emergencies, and a variety of clinical problems involving acute and chronic dysfunction.

Medical emergencies

Medical crises

The need for role definition

All medical emergency patients have emotional problems. Every patient and family with a medical emergency faces a psychological crisis fraught with pain, disability, loss, and even death. Emergency departments often have a network of personnel, including a psychiatrist, who can help in crisis situations; but their roles must be differentiated.

Case 17.2

■   Peter S., a 32-year-old carpenter, has fallen off a roof. He is brought to the emergency department, where physical and radiologic examination confirm the initial diagnosis: fracture-dislocation of the lower cervical spine with quadriplegia. Peter's wife, who accompanied him in the ambulance, insists that he should not be intubated, shouting "He won't want to live this way." The psychiatrist on duty patiently allows her to ventilate her fear that her husband will be "a vegetable." In doing so, she becomes aware of a previously undisclosed fear that she will be inadequate to care for an invalid. She finally blurts out her guilt that she might have caused the accident by demanding that her husband come off the roof and run an errand. After intubation, Peter is transferred to the intensive care unit. Meanwhile, the social worker helps Mrs. S. find lodgings and provides supportive psychotherapy for the duration of the patient's hospital stay.   ■

Involuntary referrals

Other people often bring patients, who may or may not view themselves as a psychiatric emergency. Patients with the most serious psychiatric illnesses usually have the least insight into how sick they are. How do other people determine when to bring them? The following reasons are typical:

Reasons for the referral of involuntary patients

1. The patient's behavior violates social norms (e.g., walking naked down the street).
2. The patient has no established relationship with the health care system. Patients without family physicians commonly use the emergency service for primary medical care.
3. The family, boarding home, or nursing home may have tired of the patient's behavior. Some other change, such as the illness of another family member, may have lowered tolerance for the patient.

4. Symptoms of the patient's disease or disorder may have worsened. A number of psychiatric disorders are associated with emergencies (see the section in this chapter on acute and chronic dysfunction).

Life-threatening problems

A concentration of life-threatening problems

Although the full range of psychopathology presents at the emergency department, life-threatening problems congregate there. A well-organized emergency service is the primary setting for diagnosis and disposition in the following dangerous situations:

1. Potential violence or homicide.
2. Potential suicide.
3. Occult physical disease presenting with acute or severe behavioral disturbance (e.g., delirium, dementia, organic hallucinosis).

Acute and chronic dysfunction

Other patients with the following disorders and life problems use the emergency service:

1. Acute social dysfunction.
2. Chronic social dysfunction.
3. Aggressiveness.
4. Somatoform disorder.
5. Alcohol abuse.
6. Interpersonal crises.
7. Acute loss.
8. Suicidal ideation.

The reason acute patients present

Acutely dysfunctional patients are temporarily unable to manage their lives. Such patients may be dangerous to themselves and others. They include patients with acute psychosis and delirium.

The reason chronic patients present

Chronically dysfunctional patients are unable to manage their own lives due to psychosis, dementia, or mental retardation. Such patients usually come to the emergency department periodically, in one or a combination of the following circumstances:

1. When their community support network breaks down.
2. When their psychiatric disorder relapses.
3. When they have no established physician and need care.
4. When they are troublesome, threatening, or break the law.

Some patients are threatening or actually combative. The biopsychosocial assessment of violence is discussed in more detail in the section on special features of the diagnostic process in emergency psychiatry. Disorders or situations frequently associated with violence include:

Disorders associated with violence

1. Organic mental disorders, especially those related to substance abuse (alcohol, amphetamines, phencyclidine) and temporal or frontal lobe pathology.
2. Functional psychotic disorders, especially paranoid schizophrenia and mania.
3. Paranoid disorders.
4. Explosive disorders.
5. Personality disorders, particularly conduct, paranoid, histrionic, antisocial, and borderline personality disorders.
6. Substance use disorders.
7. Adult antisocial behavior.

The misdiagnosis of somatoform disorder

Patients with somatoform disorder or other abnormal illness behavior (see chapter 3) plague emergency staff with their physical complaints. They are often not identified as emotionally disturbed but sent off with palliative drugs, only to return or go elsewhere.

The high incidence of problems associated with alcohol

People who abuse alcohol often use the emergency service. Because of the many alcoholics and the even greater number of people who drink, and because of the high association of alcohol with serious accidents and medical disorder, problems associated with alcohol are an enormous burden to emergency services. Emergency staff may evade responsibility for the care of the alcoholic.

Family strife

Some patients are in interpersonal crisis, often in association with other psychopathology. Alcohol, which disinhibits the feelings generated by family strife, is a common denominator in these situations.

Losses

People facing or responding to acute loss of self-esteem, personal resources, job, social supports, or important relationships often need emergency service.

Suicide potential

The last group includes people with suicidal ideation or behavior.

The aims of clinical work in emergency psychiatry

In contrast to inpatient or outpatient services, emergency services have a clearly defined mission: to provide rapid triage, diagnosis and management for psy-

Constituencies and aims vary with the setting

chiatric emergencies. Constituencies vary, however. Private hospitals may provide emergency care only for patients of staff physicians; whereas state- and federally funded mental health centers are mandated to care for everyone in their geographic catchment areas.

The aims of different settings and personnel vary; for example, as indicated in Table 17.1, the aims of law-enforcement agents, administrators and clinicians can sometimes be at odds.

Case 17.3

■ Paul, a 32-year-old schizophrenic patient, comes to an emergency department requesting admission to the general hospital. Acutely despondent, Paul says he hears voices telling him he must die and take others with him.

Two months before, the owner of Paul's apartment building raised the rent beyond his means, and he was evicted. He has been arrested twice in the past month for trespassing and has taken no medication for 6 weeks.

The psychiatric resident decides Paul should be admitted to the hospital for suicide prevention and urgent pharmacotherapy. The general hospital unit refuses to take him because he was admitted six months before and they consider they have nothing new to offer him. Paul refuses the offer of a bed at the state hospital, citing his fear of incarceration; nevertheless, the resident feels compelled to commit him to the state hospital because he is an imminent danger to himself and others.

In the state hospital, Paul angrily refuses drugs, keeps his bizarre thinking to himself, and is discharged within 2 weeks, following the intercession of a legal aid attorney. He has received no more than temporary shelter from the city streets. Within 3 weeks, the police will return him to the emergency department, still acutely psychotic, after he threatens a passerby. ■

Aims are achieved by planning. Administrative plans to minimize violent behavior might be to:

Administrative plans

1. Train all new staff routinely in methods of physical restraint.
2. Provide annual refresher courses for all staff in restraint skills.
3. Audit emergency management planning regularly.

Clinical plans might be to:

Clinical plans

4. Ensure the presence of a security guard in the emergency department at all times.
5. Install a panic button in the interviewing room.

Specific tactics

In every setting, special tactics must be developed to deal with different clinical problems. For example, to collect the personnel needed to subdue big, violent patients, the emergency staff in a small city must call the local police and wait for several minutes. In a large urban hospital, on the other hand, police and security personnel may be at hand.

Special features of the diagnostic process in emergency psychiatry

Time is short, the situation acute, and the stakes high.

■ Everyone looks scared. They all look mad at me. Everyone wants me to do something, something different; but I don't know what's the matter with him! What if he shoots someone? What if he shoots me? Can I take him? What's the Haldol dose? Where the hell is the attending physician? ■

These could be the thoughts of a new resident faced for the first time with a violent patient.

Settle turmoil before diagnosis possible

The physican's task is complex. Often, the physician must deal with the turmoil of patient and family before a biopsychosocial diagnosis can be completed. The priority of diagnostic questions must be ordered as follows:

The priority of diagnostic questions

Danger

1. *How dangerous is the patient?* Before proceeding, the physician must assess immediate danger. Does the patient have a weapon? How physically formidable is he or she? Is the patient irrational or confused? Is the patient out of control and angry. Is he or she physically or verbally threatening to injure others or hurt himself or herself? Is somebody or something in the environment provoking the patient? Are there enough staff available to control the patient, if it is necessary to do so? Figure 17.2 provides a schematic decision pathway for the dangerous patient.

After the patient has entered the emergency system, further diagnostic questions in order of priority include:

Psychosis
Organicity
Reversibility
Inquiry plan

2. Is the patient psychotic or delirious?
3. Is there an organic brain syndrome?
4. If so, is the cause immediately reversible?
5. What must be done to confirm an immediately treatable disease or cause?

After initial diagnosis and management, and before the patient leaves the system, other questions must be answered:

Continuing danger
Exclusion of physical disorder
Continuity of planning

6. How dangerous is the patient now personally or to others?
7. Have I completely ruled out underlying physical disorders?
8. Is my disposition consistent with the principles of comprehensive diagnosis, immediate management, and ultimate treatment?

The use of diagnostic net

These ordered clinical tasks highlight the need for systematic reasoning. Cast into shoals of data, the diagnostic net can organize facts and suggest a temporal and systemic formulation. The management of Susan (Case 17.1)

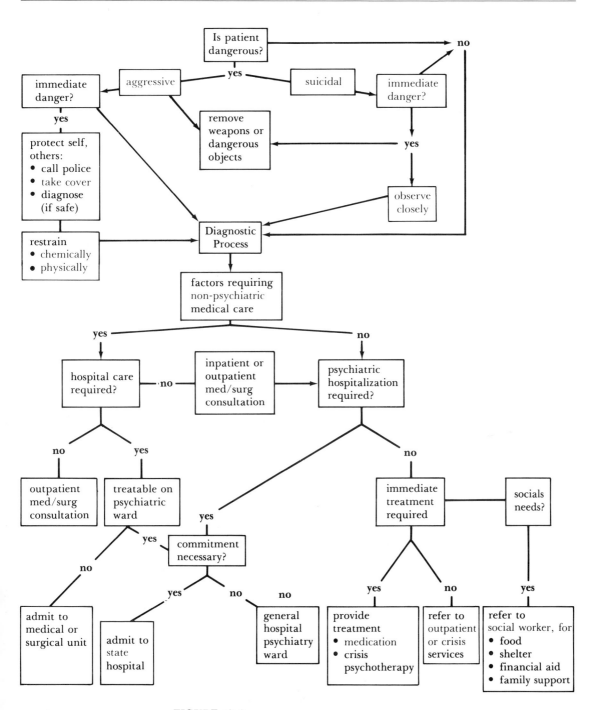

FIGURE 17.2
Dispositional algorithm, emergency psychiatry

demonstrates the utility of the net in a complex emergency case (see Table 17.2). Susan's course in the hospital is reviewed in chapter 18.

A number of features of the diagnostic process require particular comment.

Diagnosis should be related to emergency resolution

Time is of the essence. Use it wisely. When evaluating dangerousness, questions pertaining to child development, for example, have no place. Investigate only what will help you generate and test hypotheses relevant to resolving the emergency.

The use of informants

Patients may be uncooperative or unable to provide a cogent, coherent history. You must then seek data from other sources:

1. Family and friends.
2. Neighbors.
3. Employer (Be careful not to breach confidentiality. The employer may not know the patient is ill, and a job may be lost.).
4. Paramedics and police (who can be trained to observe patient and scene for diagnostic clues and ask pertinent questions of relatives, neighbors, friends, or bystanders).

Reduce fear

Fear impedes cooperation. If you can manage fear effectively, you will be more likely to enlist the patient's cooperation in the diagnostic process (see the section on management in this chapter).

Systematic clinical inquiry

Organically caused behavioral problems are prevalent. The potentially serious consequences of an overlooked physical diagnosis emphasize the significance of a thorough mental status examination, an efficient physical examination, and systematic laboratory investigations. There are several reasons why systematic clinical inquiry procedures are sometimes omitted in the very setting in which they are of greatest importance: Psychiatrists sometimes avoid physical investigations (see chapter 10); nonmedical clinicians sometimes evaluate acutely disturbed patients; and nonpsychiatric physicians, untrained in psychiatry and uncomfortable with psychiatric patients, may steer clear of evaluating and treating them.

Diagnosis should guide management

Diagnosis must be functional. It must help you make rapid and accurate decisions about management and disposition. Figure 17.2 provides an algorithm for the most important dispositional decisions in emergency psychiatry.

Ensure that appropriate laboratory facilities and medical specialty services (neurosurgeons, neurologists, and internists) are at hand to assist the diagnostic process when indicated.

As a general rule, brief screening and discretionary physical and laboratory examinations (see chapter 10) are most useful in emergencies.

Case 17.4

■ Chuck, a 25-year-old store clerk, is brought to the emergency room by his wife and brother. He tells the admitting nurse he wants help with his nerves because in recent weeks he has persistently felt irritable and been unable to concentrate. His wife blurts out, ''He's not making sense; he's gone crazy.''

TABLE 17.2
Diagnostic net, Susan, Case 17.1

	Predisposition	Precipitation	Perpetuation	Pattern
Physical	• systemic lupus erythematosus (SLE)	• SLE • pregnancy • steroids		• elevated blood sedimentation rate • headache
Psychological	? unresolved grief over previous miscarriage	? grief over impending abortion • uncertainty about marriage • fear of disease	? unresolved grief ? fear of abandonment • denial of feeling ? unable to set limits with mother	• angry and depressed mood • suicidal ideation • confused • paranoid ideation • suspiciousness
Social		? marital problems • mother's despondency • father's illness • several care providers	• unresolved marital and family issues • no psychiatric beds available	• concerned husband • physician supports her denial of grief

The nurse calls a mental health crisis worker, who interviews the patient and diagnoses "agitated depression." She asks the emergency room physician to write a prescription for a small amount of diazepam to treat the agitation and refers Chuck to a local mental health center for a follow-up appointment 4 days hence.

The next day, Chuck's wife, worried that her husband may be "sick," and not just "crazy," brings him to her family doctor, whose nurse performs a routine check on vital signs. She notes a blood pressure of 160/105, a pulse of 90, and a temperature of 100. Chuck can barely sit still during the examination.

The physician, who hypothesizes an organic cause for the patient's agitation, performs a discretionary physical examination. This reveals hyperreflexia, fine tremor of the hands, and an enlarged, tender thyroid. To confirm his secondary diagnostic hypothesis of hyperthyroidism, the physician completes a discretionary laboratory examination, which includes thyroid function studies, and hospitalizes Chuck for more definitive treatment. ■

The importance of a physical screen

This case indicates the importance of a brief screening physical examination in the emergency department, where abnormal behavior is frequently a symptom of underlying physical disorder. Ideally, a brief medical history and a routine brief screening examination (chapter 10) should be completed on all patients before formulating diagnosis and planning management.

The psychiatrist must consider the legal and administrative aspects of the case. There is no point in completing a careful biopsychosocial evaluation and negotiating an elaborate management plan that is later sabotaged by a trivial administrative oversight. The lost rapport may hinder implementing a subsequent management plan.

Case 17.5

■ A college housemaster is worried. Bill, an 18-year-old college freshman, has been behaving strangely for a month. During the last week, he has not left his room. The housemaster finds him there pacing and muttering.

Bill finally agrees to go to an emergency room, where the first-year resident diagnoses an acute psychotic episode, probably schizophrenia, and decides that hospitalization is appropriate. Bill, frightened and suspicious, is initially reluctant, but because of the good rapport he has developed with the resident, finally agrees to enter the general hospital psychiatric ward.

Once the decision has been made, Bill seems relieved. He asks to go to the ward immediately. The resident calls the unit to announce his arrival, only to find that there are no beds available. He had forgotten to check ahead.

When informed of this problem, Bill angrily declares that the resident cannot be trusted: "He is just like the rest of them." Bill becomes agitated and threatens to "break up the joint and hurt some people." Restraints are needed to contain him.

The resident tries to persuade Bill to enter the state hospital, but trust has evaporated; Bill refuses and the resident is forced to commit him on an involuntary emergency evaluation certificate. Following a court hearing 2 weeks later, Bill is discharged and lost to follow-up. ■

Special features of the management process in emergency psychiatry

Aggressive patients

Priorities in the managing of aggression

Aggressive patients present special problems in an emergency service. For effective management, you must address these key issues:

Is the patient immediately dangerous?

Urgent management

1. If so, call the police immediately. A panic button helps.
2. Warn and protect personnel and bystanders.
3. Disarm the patient without endangering yourself or others.
4. Remove all potential weapons from the immediate vicinity. Police should remove their guns, lest they be stolen in a scuffle.

Stay calm.

Calmness

1. Assure adequate security.
2. Establish clear domains of responsibility: Who does what, when?

Who is in charge? Clarify the lines of authority for staff and patient. It is essential, ahead of time, to:

Lines of authority

1. Assure that all staff have adequate training for their functions.
2. Design algorithms to facilitate decision making.
3. Develop a system of audit, feedback, and self-directed learning for the service and its personnel.

Determine cause of anger

What is the cause of the patient's anger? Determine what is precipitating or perpetuating the aggressive behavior. Can it be altered? Moyer (1971) classified several different types of mammalian aggression; Gallagher (1980) extrapolated these concepts to different clue configurations in clinical situations (see Table 17.3). The environmental interventions indicated in Table 17.3 are often quite simple and can significantly benefit the clinical process.

What is the best environment for the examination? Assess and treat the patient in the optimal surroundings:

The environment of the examination

1. Provide a quiet, secluded atmosphere. Few staff should be present, but many should be available immediately, if required.
2. Do not corner the patient by blocking the exit from the room (see Figure 17.3).

TABLE 17.3
Environmental interventions in aggressive behavior

Category of aggressive behavior (Moyer, 1971)	Clinical analogue (Gallagher, 1980)	Stimulus configurations provoking aggression	Intervention
1. Predation	drug-seeking behavior in addict; often purposeful crime	the addict sees an opportunity to steal drugs	prevention: standard, safe secure procedures for locking and dispensing drugs
2. Self-defense	the paranoid patient feels threatened and strikes out	the interviewer sits too close, stares intently, reaches out intrusively, sits between door and patient, or whispers to nurse outside of room	change these behaviors
3. Territoriality and possessiveness	the safe territory of the paranoid patient is invaded by intrusive questions or physical examination	same as 2	ask permission or warn patient that you will ask intrusive questions or complete physical examination
4. Parenthood	parents defend their child or cherished belonging	a frightened, screaming child being examined or treated	remove parents; ask parents to participate; educate parents
5. Sexuality	the angry, jealous husband; relationship problems on team	intoxicated husband angry at attempts to restrain or examine wife; may fear a doctor–wife liaison and abandonment	educate spouse about the clinical process help them participate in care and decisions as much as possible
6. Dominance	show of force in ER; leadership struggles on team	challenged male resident feels the need to control patient and puts him in his place; the chief-of-service will not change treatment plan when it is clearly indicated	do not challenge, threaten, or humiliate patient
7. Irritability	drugs; disease; pain; fatigue; frustration	any of above	identify and treat the cause of irritability

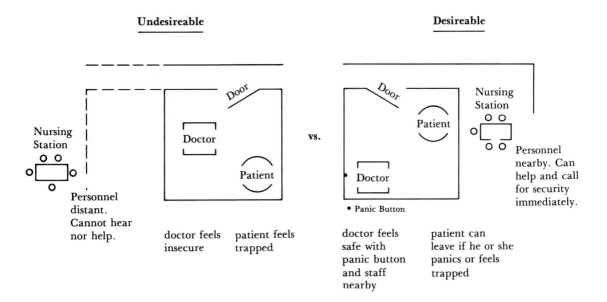

FIGURE 17.3
Interviewing the aggressive patient

What information do I need? Collate a pertinent data base, as follows:

The data base

1. Why now? What precipitated the visit to the emergency department?
2. Solicit information from accompanying friends and relatives.
3. Solicit information by telephone from other resources (physicians, therapists, record room, family, friends, etc.).

How do I relate to the patient?

Establishing a relationship

Neutral questions

1. Let the patient know who is in charge, and be reassuring that the patient will receive proper help.
2. Initiate contact with simple, neutral questions, such as ''How old are you?'' ''Where are you from?''

You may agitate the patient if you explore detailed personal matters too soon.

Gauge capacity for control

3. If the patient, without losing control, starts to talk about personal problems, gently explore them. If the patient begins to lose control, gently switch to a neutral topic. Recreational pursuits, physical health and occupation are less threatening.

Reflect feelings

4. Gently reflect the patient's feelings in order to demonstrate empathy and elicit further information: "You seem very upset by all of this, but we'll work with you to help make things better."

Realistic encouragement

5. Make reassuring (but realistic) encouraging comments, even if the patient will not communicate. "I know things seem tough right now; but I also know that we'll be able to help you, and I'm glad you decided to come here."

Restraint

How will I restrain the patient if necessary? Be prepared, if necessary, to restrain the patient physically.

1. Immediately assess the patient's potential for violence.
2. Check available resources.
3. If you think there is a possibility of violence, alert the necessary personnel, just in case.

Plan ahead

4. Plan your tactics ahead of time. Assign a leader. Do not communicate your plans to the patient in this regard.

Speedy restraint

5. Restrain the patient speedily, if necessary, without hesitation, embarrassment, or guilt. If possible, arrange for people trained in physical restraint (for example, the police) to apply it.

Physical resources

6. Do not apply physical restraint without adequate resources. You will need a minimum of one strong person for each limb.

Nonpunitiveness

7. Use restraint carefully, in a nonpunitive fashion. When patients are agitated by their fear of losing control, adequate, secure physical restraint can often be more calming than medication. The message is this: "We are in control, in your best interests. We won't let you hurt yourself or others."

Precautions

Keep in mind the following when you evaluate and manage the potentially violent patient:

Avoid threats

1. Do not threaten the patient. A show of force can be effective in calming a patient; but a threat of force only increases fear, suspicion, and agitation.

Avoid disagreement

2. Do not flatly disagree with an acutely disturbed patient. Always listen attentively.

Avoid unrealistic promises

3. Do not make promises you cannot keep. They may haunt you! Promises may relieve your anxiety and allow you to assuage demanding or angry patients temporarily, but a broken promise will spoil a hard-earned therapeutic alliance.

No levity

4. Do not joke, laugh, or discuss other problems in front of the patient and do not allow the staff to do so. This behavior will only provoke more anger and suspicion.

No staring

5. Do not stare directly at the patient.
6. Do not assume the patient is being deliberately manipulative unless there is hard evidence for it.

Avoid ridicule

Avoid unnecessary drugs

Be alert for physical disorder

7. Do not humiliate the patient. Be courteous and respectful.
8. Do not prescribe drugs rashly. Their effects may confound the diagnostic process.
9. Do not assume that disturbed behavior is psychogenic. Nonpsychiatric organic disease is frequently manifest in behavioral disturbance or psychological symptoms.

Suicidal patients

Priorities in managing suicidal patients

Assess urgency

Suicidal ideation and suicide intent must often be managed by emergency personnel. Again, effective management requires the clinician to address key issues.

Is the patient in immediate danger? If so:

1. Keep the patient under observation.
2. Remove all dangerous articles from the immediate vicinity.

Assess treatability

Does the patient have an underlying treatable disorder (e.g., major depression)? If so:

1. Refer the patient to the appropriate resources (e.g., hospital or ambulatory psychiatry).
2. Inform the patient of the nature of the problem.

Assess seriousness

Is there strong suicidal intent? If so:

1. Hospitalize the patient with appropriate precautions against suicide.
2. If the patient refuses hospitalization, consider involuntary commitment.

Assess current status of precipitating factors

Have any precipitants of the suicidal behavior or ideation changed significantly? Are they now perpetuating factors?

1. Assess the patient's insight into the situation. For example, is the patient realistic about the significance of personal losses?
2. Mobilize resources. How dependable are they?

Assess capacity for cooperation

Is the patient able to make and honor a no-suicide contract? How reliable do you think it is?

1. Assess the patient's capacity to cooperate and fulfill a minicontract during the diagnostic assessment.
2. Assess the patient's capacity for a therapeutic alliance.

Assess risks of hospitalization

What are the risks of hospitalization or commitment in terms of increased morbidity or even of eventual suicide?

1. Assess the impact of hospitalization on the therapeutic alliance.
2. Consider its impact on self-esteem.
3. Try to predict the effects of a dependency-enhancing environment.

Disposition

Handling the acute condition is only the beginning of management; the physician must also plan proper disposition. The patient may require appropriate longer-term care following the emergency visit. To accomplish this, the emergency service must liaise with a network of social, legal, and clinical services, agencies, and institutions. Successful collaboration involves:

Liaison

1. Protocols clearly delineating which patients are appropriate for referral and providing clear guidelines on how to do this.
2. Protocols for evaluating collaboration.
3. Protocols for communicating about problems during referral.
4. Personal alliances between emergency staff and allied services.

Figure 17.1 illustrates the complexity of the alliances necessary for a successful emergency service. It is important to reiterate that allied services and institutions may have different missions, aims, and strategies. These differences must be acknowledged if a coordinated and effective disposition is to be achieved.

Summary

All systems of psychiatric emergency care reflect their sociocultural milieux. Every community has its own needs and creates unique demands to which an emergency system must respond. Patients move to and from the emergency department and all elements of the health-care system and the community. Strong alliances with the community are the cornerstone of effective planning and care.

The emergency psychiatrist must often rapidly diagnose and treat crises in a setting where mistakes can be fatal for patient, family, staff, or innocent bystanders.

If the staff of psychiatric emergency services are unevenly trained, they are potentially at cross-purposes. They must diagnose and manage a full range of clinical problems, from the emotional states associated with medical and surgical emergencies, to the most severe and life-threatening psychiatric disorders. The missions of most emergency departments are similar, but the aims of different elements of the system sometimes vary or even conflict, to the patient's detriment.

When diagnosing a case, the psychiatrist must establish a priority of inquiry questions, use time efficiently, seek data from multiple sources, make functional diagnoses, modify fear, rule out organic factors, and consider the administrative and legal aspects of every case. Aggressive and suicidal patients create special management problems for the emergency psychiatrist. After immediate management, proper disposition is crucial to a favorable outcome.

Selected Readings: General References

Barton and Friedman (1982), in *Psychiatric Emergency Care: A Task Force Report of the American Psychiatric Association*, provide a comprehensive review of emergency psychiatry.

Soreff's (1981) evenly written, practical text, *Management of the Psychiatric Emergency*, cogently reviews diagnosis and management in this field. Soreff (1983) has also edited a valuable collection of up-to-date reviews of the field.

Anderson (1978) provides a succinct overview of the clinical process in the emergency room. Fauman (1983) comprehensively reviews the evaluation of the organic disorders seen in the emergency room.

Murray (1979) provides a compact review of the rapid assessment, differential diagnosis, and immediate management of violent patients. Gallagher (1980) discusses the relationship between several conceptual models of aggression and proposes a detailed method of evaluating and managing violent patients.

Gerson and Bassuck (1980) review the factors influencing the disposition of emergency patients.

18

Inpatient psychiatry

Introduction

The history of the mental hospital

The gulf between mental hospital and general hospital

The psychiatric hospital has a special place among American institutions. During the 19th century, in the heyday of moral treatment, the asylum was the embodiment of optimistic idealism. During this era, mental patients were removed from jails and workhouses and admitted to special hospitals with humane treatment programs. In the twentieth century, however, the public mental hospital has become equated with incarceration and stagnation. University medical centers have become citadels of research and technology, attracting some of the brightest minds in medicine; but the public psychiatric hospital, in contrast, has too often provided outmoded and repressive treatment administered by ill-trained staff. These historical shifts reflect a confluence of several factors (Talbott, 1978; Bachrach, 1981):

1. The procedures, staff, and patients in the hospital.
2. The authorities controlling the hospital.
3. Patterns of service delivery in the mental health system as a whole.
4. Changing attitudes to mental illness.

Another important source of change is derived from new concepts of human behavior and of psychiatric treatment. Hospital psychiatry today must be under-

TABLE 18.1
The evolution of hospital psychiatry

Era	Prevailing concepts and philosophy	Hospital practices
Confinement	The insane are immutable Rehabilitation is unlikely	Incarceration, work houses; poor houses or farms

Moral treatment	3 factors help the insane:
	• good, clean living
	• removal from stressful
	  environment
	• moral courage
		Comprehensive hospital
		  approach
		• diagnosis
		• segregation from society
		• special hospital environment
		• humanity, kindness
		• behavioral change

State hospital	State, if responsible for care
	Specialized care important; can
	  only be provided in large
	  institutions
	Mental illness is caused by de-
	  generation of the brain
		County hospitals vs. state
		hospitals
		Total environment important
		  (Meyer)

Biologic	Mental illness caused by de-
	  generation of the brain
		Bromides, convulsive therapies
		  (insulin shock, electrocon-
		  vulsive therapy)
		Custodial care

Psychoanalytic	Mental illness caused by un-
	  resolved childhood conflict
		Private psychoanalytically
		  oriented hospitals or
		  state custodial hospitals

Social Psychiatry	Interpersonal theory (Sullivan) Family theory (Lidz) Therapeutic community (Jones)	Milieu therapy ⎫ 3 settings: Psychotherapy ⎪ state hospital, Medication, ⎬ community ECT ⎭ MHC, pri- vate hospital

Biopsychosocial
Psychiatry
	Systems theory: multiple factors
	          cause psychiatric
	          disorder
	Neurosciences: dysfunction of
	          brain causes
	          psychosis
		Short-term multidisciplinary,
		  general hospital care
		
		Tertiary care in state or
		  private hospitals

stood in the context of this evolutionary history (Maxmen, Tucker, & LeBow, 1974). (See Table 18.1.)

This chapter reviews the advantages and constraints of diagnosis and treatment in the contemporary psychiatric hospital.

Fifty years ago, there were two kinds of psychiatric hospital: active treatment facilities and custodial care institutions. Today, there is a different hospital for almost every diagnostic group and mode of treatment. It would be impractical to describe each of them. Rather, this chapter describes the generic characteristics of all psychiatric hospitals with special reference to acute general hospital inpatient service.

The advantages and constraints of hospital psychiatry

The advantages of specificity

Maxmen, Tucker, & LeBow (1974) classified hospital units according to predominant treatment modality and duration of stay (see Table 18.2). Hospitals can also be categorized according to their source of funds – public or private. Some units are defined by patient age. Among the many age-related or diagnostic specialty units are the following:

Specialty units

1. Adolescent.
2. Geriatric.
3. Drug and alcohol.
4. Affective disorder.
5. Schizophrenia.
6. Eating disorders.
7. Behavioral medicine.
8. Chronic pain.
9. Sleep disorders.
10. Clinical research.

The need for mission, goals, and plans

A hospital unit should define its mission, goals, and treatment methods. Its effectiveness depends on how rigorously the staff develop and implement an admissions policy consistent with their mission and goals.

Specialization demands administrative control

Specialization requires control over admission, length of stay, and hospital environment. For example, intensive psychoanalytic psychotherapy can be conducted only in an intermediate-to-long-term hospital. Each box in Table 18.2 represents a different kind of hospital described in terms of the therapeutic approaches and ratio of staff to patients.

Admissions, missions, and community

The changing patterns of hospitalization

The flow of patients between community and hospital and among hospitals changes along with the matrix of economic, social, political, and chronological factors that determine the patterns of psychiatric care. New technologies in psychopharmacologic and psychosocial care make it possible for many severely disturbed patients, who formerly had no alternative to prolonged or frequent hospitalization, to be managed in the community. Today, these patients use hospitals infrequently and briefly, if at all.

TABLE 18.2
Typology of units

Treatment modality	Short-term (less than 3 weeks)	Intermediate-term (3 weeks to 6 months)	Long-term (longer than 6 months)
Crisis intervention	G: rapid restoration of function and discharge TS: medication; crisis psychotherapy; family therapy; mobilize community resources S/P: high		
Supportive psychotherapy	G: facilitation of psychotherapy; restoration of function outside hospital TS: doctor–patient psychotherapy; staff support S/P: medium	G: provide support restore function TS: supportive psychotherapy; organic therapy; relaxing environment S/P: medium	
Psychoanalytic		G: resolve intrapsychic conflicts TS: insight psychotherapy with one therapist administrative care by separate psychiatrist S/P: high	G: modify personality structure TS: no medication; intensive psychoanalytic psychotherapy S/P: high to very high
Therapeutic community		G: restore to optimal premorbid function TS: patient participation in planning; therapeutic groups; occupational, family, organic therapies S/P: very high	G: as intermediate term TS: as intermediate term S/P: high to medium
Token economy		G: help chronic patients learn adaptive behavior TS: systematic training using operant conditioning; adjunctive medication; occupational and recreational therapy S/P: low to medium	G: as intermediate term, but patients are more regressed
Organic therapy		G: restore to minimum function outside hospital TS: ECT; medication; adjunctive groups and supportive psychotherapy; relaxing environment S/P: low	
Custodial care			G: custodial care TS: provide biologic and medical requirements; no rehabilitation S/P: very low

Key: G = goals; TS = therapeutic strategies; S/P – staff patient ratio

Admission policies reflect these changes and, to some extent, affect the relationship between the hospital and the local community. Compare these two psychiatric hospitals in a rural state:

■ 1. A state hospital in a small rural town adopts new admission policies in response to changes in its mission and goals. Once the institution housed more than 1,000 patients, many for prolonged periods; now stringent admission criteria and a policy of brief treatment maintain the census at about 150 patients. Many patients who formerly would have been admitted from all parts of the state are managed at local hospitals and crisis services. Hospital buildings that once housed patients now provide offices for several agencies of the state government. As a result, local real estate values have risen. ■

■ 2. A large private institution continues to admit only wealthy patients who are often severely ill, from the northeastern United States. The hospital is located in a semirural environment and maintains a manicured campus. Because it is so well-staffed, the hospital directly or indirectly provides jobs for many townspeople. ■

The influence of funding

The influence of funding on admission criteria

The way a hospital is funded influences how discriminating its admission procedures can be. Public hospitals usually have broad admission criteria because they are mandated to provide services to a variety of patients. Admission to public hospitals may be determined not so much by diagnosis as by social behavior and economic considerations. A private hospital, on the other hand, may admit only patients who fit particular diagnostic and economic criteria. Publicly and privately funded hospital services are contrasted in Table 18.3.

TABLE 18.3
Differences in public and private hospital psychiatry

Factor	Public hospitals	Private hospitals
Amount of disability of patients	severe and chronic	less impaired
Typical problems encountered	schizophrenic disorders	affective disorders
Relationship with patient	adversarial (commitment)	collaborative; medical
Socioeconomic status of patients	low	middle (intermediate stay) high (long-term stay)
Social support network of patients	poor	financial and often personal and vocational resources
Nature of care provided	often custodial	specialty care multimodal care
Control of admissions	low	high

The control of time and space

The opportunity to design a responsive environment

In an ambulatory setting, the physician must rely on patient and family to implement recommended treatment. In a psychiatric hospital, the physician can provide a responsive environment (discussed in this chapter in the section on behavioral goals and management), operating 24 hours a day. The hospital can control:

1. The design of the physical space.
2. The training, experience, and character of the staff.
3. The social system of the ward.
4. Diagnostic and management procedures.
5. Admission and discharge.

Unfortunately, these factors are sometimes determined as much by economic considerations as by need.

The capacity for physical investigation and treatment

Physically and psychologically ill patients with both primary and secondary psychiatric disorders are often treated by inpatient psychiatrists. Geriatric and chronically ill patients are very likely to have complicated problems.

Case 18.1

■ Tim, an 80-year-old retired executive, has been diagnosed as having progressive senile dementia. Most of his friends have died. He can no longer drive a car or pursue his favorite hobbies. Tim drinks six highballs a day and squabbles constantly with his wife. His family requests psychiatric help. ■

The opportunity for comprehensive diagnostic investigation

This patient needs biopsychosocial evaluation. A neuropsychiatric inpatient service can best manage his irascible behavior while his dementia, coping, and social and family resources are assessed.

A hospital has the appropriate setting and facilities for the intensive diagnosis of the physical, psychological, and social dimensions of complex cases. In other settings, it could take many visits to develop a data base sufficiently comprehensive to complete the necessary diagnostic net. The hospital setting helps the physician coordinate and abbreviate the diagnostic process. Hospitals are convenient for undertaking multiple, coordinated investigations, particularly if the patient is uncooperative, or very ill, or would find it inconvenient to make several trips to complete an evaluation (see the section in this chapter on special features of the diagnostic process in hospital psychiatry).

Clinical problems encountered in hospital psychiatry

Social factors that influence hospitalization

The general characteristics of inpatients

The characteristics of the patients in an inpatient service are determined by its admission policies. What determines admission? As mentioned, each setting establishes its own criteria to achieve goals that may or may not reflect categorical diagnoses. As a general rule, however, hospital patients are likely to be more disturbed, psychotic, diagnostically complex, chronic, or treatment failures, to have severely maladaptive personality traits, to lack social supports, to be unemployed, and to have created social problems.

Public institutions must admit patients with more of these characteristics. Short-stay general hospital units tend to select patients who need a definitive assessment or who are amenable to brief treatment.

The aims of clinical work in hospital psychiatry

Missions

Each hospital unit must determine its own mission, aims, plans, and tactics. The mission of a crisis intervention unit might be:

- To provide brief hospitalization for members of the community in emotional crisis.

A crisis intervention unit might aim:

Aims

1. To admit patients appropriate for crisis intervention.
2. To provide biopsychosocial assessment.
3. To restore patients rapidly to adaptive functioning.
4. To make disposition to follow-up care that will help patients maintain adaptive functioning outside the hospital.

Plans to select admissions that are appropriate for crisis intervention, might be:

Plans

1. To admit only those who are in acute crisis.
2. To apply the following admission criteria: good premorbid functioning, well-defined precipitating stressors, and crisis pattern likely to respond to a brief hospitalization of from 2 to 5 days.

Tactics to implement the plans might include:

Tactics

1. All patients will be screened by the triage worker before they are considered as prospective patients for admission.

2. Prospective patients will be assessed by a psychiatrist.
3. Families will be interviewed by a mental health clinician.
4. If admission is deemed appropriate, the two clinicians will confer with the admissions coordinator of the crisis unit.

A generic, responsive environment

Many factors determine the mission, aims, plans, and tactics of a unit. Each is unique, although, as suggested in this chapter, hospital units with similar aims tend to resemble each other. What distinguishes the effective hospital unit?

Maxmen, Tucker, and LeBow (1974) described a generic hospital environment, the characteristics of which embody the principles of effective hospital care. They label this environment *reactive,* although *responsive* seems a more appropriate term. The responsive environment aims to provide coordinated, integrated, consistent care to patients 24 hours a day, with the ultimate purpose of returning them to productive functioning in the community as soon as possible.

Several situations obstruct or impede environmental responsiveness:

Factors that impede responsiveness

1. When treatment emanates exclusively from the doctor-patient relationship, as in a unit where psychiatrists admit their own patients as part of the psychotherapeutic process.
2. When the milieu is routine rather than individualized and rigid rather than responsive;
3. When the staff disagree about the goals of hospitalization. Should they control behavior, promote insight, treat mental disease, foster expression of feelings, or rehabilitate the patient?

The prevalence of physical problems in psychiatric inpatients

General hospital psychiatric units admit complex cases that often require both psychiatric and other medical diagnosis and intervention. Bernstein and Dreyfus (1980) studied consecutive admissions over a 3-year period to a general psychiatric unit. They found that 25% of the patients required medical or surgical consultation. 49% of these consultations were for the diagnosis, assessment, or management of physical problems unrelated to the primary psychiatric disorder. Often, the patient's primary problem was physical; but behavioral problems were so severe, or diagnosis and management so complex, that management in a psychiatric unit was warranted. The clinical course of Susan (Case 17.1), the 28-year-old woman with systemic lupus erythematosus and recent abortion, illustrates this point (see chapter 17).

Case 17.1 (continued)

■   Susan is admitted to a general medical bed with paranoid and suicidal ideation, impaired recent memory, and poor concentration. Over 1 week, her daily dose of prednisone is increased to 80 mg. Her despondency increases and her paranoid ideation begins to involve members of the hospital staff; on the 4th hospital day, a bed becomes available and she is transferred to the psychiatric inpatient service.   ■

Special features of the diagnostic process in hospital psychiatry

Monitoring the patient

The opportunity for close observation

The hospital provides a physician with the opportunity to monitor a patient around the clock. The pattern of a patient's thoughts, emotions, and behavior can be established or confirmed; social interaction can be closely observed; while through the monitoring of physiologic and biochemical indices, the relationship of behavior to pathophysiology or pathochemistry can be investigated.

Special investigations

The opportunity for complex diagnostic assessment

Several special diagnostic investigations can be completed more conveniently and reliably in a controlled setting.

1. Somatic
   a. Sleep laboratory.
   b. 24-hour urine chemistries, such as creatinine clearance.
   c. Sequential serum determinations, such as cortisol levels in the Dexamethasone Suppression Test.
   d. Radiologic studies, such as CT and PET scanning.
2. Psychologic
   a. Neuropsychological and other psychological tests can be completed and correlated with observations of mental status and physiologic profile.
   b. Close monitoring of the patient's thoughts, feelings, and behavior may reveal patterns that could never be elucidated on an outpatient basis.
3. a. Group interactions can be observed for interpersonal patterns and the appropriateness of cognitive-behavioral responses to social demands.
   b. The whole family can be interviewed to provide important clues to precipitating psychosocial or somatic stressors and long-standing interactions that might predispose patients to psychopathology.

Hospital services

The opportunity for consultation with other specialists

Chapter 8 describes the many physical diseases associated with behavioral disturbance, particularly in the elderly. Other specialty services that must be consulted during the diagnostic process are readily available in a general hospital. Geriatric patients, for example, often require the consultation of an internist while they are cared for on a psychiatry service.

Abuse of the diagnostic process

The dangers of shotgun diagnosis

Hospital services abuse the diagnostic process if they employ a shotgun approach to special investigations. Tests best ordered as part of a discretionary laboratory examination may be done routinely, significantly increasing the chances of false positive results on the basis of errors of chance (Modell, 1983). Discretionary batteries of biochemical tests, made cheap and efficient by computerized equipment, may actually be less expensive than individual tests. Hospitals should develop different specific cost-effective investigative batteries for different diagnostic hypotheses. Today's health-care costs require psychiatrists to consider the diagnostic expense of each case. A continuation of Case 17.1 illustrates this diagnostic process.

The need for specific, cost-effective test batteries

Case 17.1 (continued)

■ The admitting psychiatric resident interviews Susan after she is transferred to the psychiatric unit. She complains bitterly about her poor memory and inability to concentrate, and is convinced the doctors do not want her to have a baby. At the end of the interview, she reveals that she suspects her doctors of inducing her recent abortion with drugs. She wonders if her husband colluded with them. Without emotion, she says: "After all, he thinks that I'm no good to him anyway, now that I've got arthritis. He's the one who wants the baby." The resident suspects that Susan is denying the actual diagnosis, lupus, and her grief about the loss of the baby; but he also wonders if she might have forgotten her diagnosis as a result of impaired memory.

Cognitive examination reveals severe impairment of memory for recent events and spotty memory for events during the past 3 years.

Physical examination reveals a tall, thin woman who, despite an expensive silk nightgown and make-up, looks unkempt, ill, and older than her stated age. Other physical findings include:

1. Pale skin except over her rounded, puffy face, reddened by a diffuse malar rash.
2. Innumerable reddish papules over her entire face and neck.
3. Petechial lesions on both breasts.
4. Increased hair on her upper lip.
5. Several ulcerations of the oral mucosa.
6. Increased fatty tissue on the back of her neck, giving her a slight "buffalo hump."
7. A grade II/III ejection-type murmur loudest at the left sternal border which does not radiate.
8. Truncal obesity.
9. Purple horizontal striae over the abdomen.
10. Thin extremities.

Laboratory data from the internal medicine service reveal a mild normochromic normocytic anemia, leukopenia, lymphopenia, thrombocytopenia, elevated erythrocyte sedimentation rate, and hypergammaglobulinemia. Electrocardiogram and chest X-ray show slight cardiomegaly. Urinalysis is negative.

The resident interviews Susan's husband, Ken, a short, stocky, engaging man who readily provides additional history. Susan's wealthy mother has pressed her and Ken to return to Chicago for better medical care, but Ken is reluctant to do so. He fears that the stress created by his antipathy to his mother-in-law will aggravate Susan's insecurity and further burden their marriage. Susan opened a clothing shop 3 years ago, but because of her worsening symptoms, which were initially thought to be secondary to pregnancy not illness, she was forced to close the shop. Ken knows that if they stay in New York, he cannot support her adequately.

Ken emphasizes that the only similarity in their backgrounds is their families' protestant religion. Her family is very affluent. Susan's aloof, critical mother dominates her retired father, who is somewhat passive and who drinks too much. The mother uses money to manipulate the affection of her daughters who compete with each other. In fact, Susan was quite chagrined when her younger sister produced the first grandchild in the family. In contrast, Ken describes his own family as warm, affectionate, and supportive. ■

Table 18.4 illustrates this information on a diagnostic net. Figure 18.1 provides a flow diagram to assist in the dynamic formulation.

Special features of management process in hospital psychiatry

Problem priorities

The problems derived from Susan's diagnostic net (see Table 18.4) and dynamic formulation (see Figure 18.1) can be listed in order of priority and rewritten as goal statements addressed by diagnostic and therapeutic plans (see Table 18.5).

Behavioral goals and hospital management

Patients are admitted to a psychiatric hospital because of seriously maladaptive behavior associated with psychiatric or physical disorder. Five categories of abnormal illness behavior commonly lead to hospitalization:

Abnormal behavior that leads to hospitalization

1. Behavior intolerable to society, whatever the frequency or setting (for example, impulsive violence).
2. Behavior that becomes intolerable only if it is too frequent (for example, the repeated complaints of a melancholic patient).
3. Behavior that would be acceptable in some settings but is expressed in an inappropriate context (for example, cursing in a church).
4. The absence or deficiency of behavior appropriate to a particular situation or setting (for example, unwillingness to take appropriate medication).
5. The clearly eccentric behavioral consequences of subjective experiences (for example, shouting in public in response to hallucinations).

The need for pragmatic goals

By their ability to control the hospital environment, the staff can reinforce adaptive behavior and discourage maladaptive behavior. Behavioral goals help the staff concentrate on the pragmatic questions of rehabilitation rather than

TABLE 18.4
Diagnostic net (2), Susan (Case 17.1)

	Predisposition	Precipitation (*stressors*)	Pattern	Perpetuation
Physical	SLE	• miscarriage • steroids • exacerbation of vasculitis	• thrombocytopenia • elevated ESR • heart murmur • lymphopenia • leukopenia • exogenous Cushing syndrome • headaches	? steroids ? untreated SLE • fertility
Psychological	• family values about having children	• anticipation of move • grief over miscarriage • fear of illness • confusion ? fear of abandonment	• suicidal thoughts • paranoid thoughts • confusion • angry and depressed mood • impaired memory • suicidal behavior • self-deprecation • suspicious behavior • escape behavior	• unresolved grief • denial of illness • fear of abandonment • determination to have children
Social	• wealthy, distant family • competitive relationships with sisters • demanding, but dependent mother • passive alcoholic father	• impending move to Chicago • loss of job • conflict between husband and mother • husband anger and demoralization • several care providers	• husband reliable, concerned, but depressed and angry • overbearing mother • passive father • uncertain diagnosis • no primary physician • patient distrustful of doctors	• conflict between husband and mother • uncertain diagnosis • no primary physician

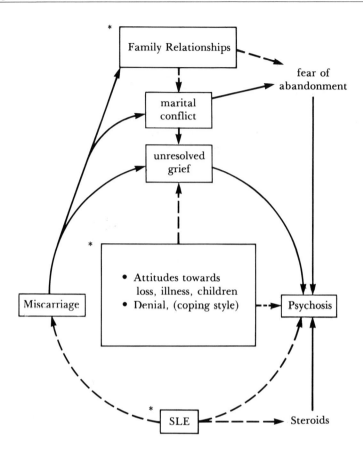

* Dotted lines represent influence of predisposing factors.

FIGURE 18.1
Dynamic flow chart: Susan (Case 17.1)

pursue an elusive "cure." This orientation does not preclude therapists from holding different theoretical positions, but it requires them to concentrate on what will help the patient adapt sufficiently to be managed out of the hospital.

Case 18.2   ■ A psychiatrist covering for a vacationing colleague is summoned from the classroom to an emergency on the psychiatric unit of a teaching hospital. As he runs to the unit with a group of orderlies and students, he reviews in his mind the principles of effective restraint.

On the unit, he is told that a patient has locked himself in his room, refused to take medication, and is threatening to hurt anybody who comes near.

The patient, John, a 25-year-old unemployed computer programmer, was admitted 5 days before with the following florid psychotic symptoms: persecutory

TABLE 18.5
Problems, goals, plans: Susan (Case 17.1) on psychiatric ward

Prioritized problems	Goal statements	Management plan
1. Abnormal mental state of uncertain etiology: • CNS vasculitis • steroid psychosis • post-partum psychosis	1. Diagnose causes and normalize mental state	1. Therapeutic trial of increased steroids to see if suppression of vasculitis produces symptomatic improvement. 2. No improvement or worsening implicates exogenous Cushing's as cause. Then taper as recommended by endocrinology consultant. 3. Daily evaluation to monitor changes in mental status with changes in steroid dose.
2. Confusion	1. Improve orientation	1. Diagnose and treat cause 2. Supportive psychotherapy 3. Haloperidol, 2 mg b.i.d.–t.i.d.
3. Low self-esteem; self-deprecating thoughts	1. Improve self-image	1. Supportive psychotherapy initially 2. Cognitive-behavioral psychotherapy eventually
4. Exogenous Cushing's	1. Modify its influence on abnormal mental status 2. Monitor disease process	1. As in problem 1 2. Screen electrolytes and cortisol
5. Suicidal behavior	1. Prevent suicide	1. Room near nurses' station 2. Frequent room checks and close observation 3. Sitter if necessary 4. Suicide pact
6. Paranoid ideation	1. Alleviate paranoid ideation	1. Neuroleptics: haloperidol 2 mg b.i.d. and q.i.h., p.r.n. 2. Explain procedures carefully and thoroughly 3. Minimize confusion
7. Family conflict	1. Assessment 2. Modify negative impact on Susan 3. Improve family support for Susan	1. Family diagnostic meeting 2. Twice weekly psychotherapy sessions with husband 3. Education of family 4. Family therapy
8. Lack of a secure relationship with primary care physician	1. Find primary physician 2. Facilitate relationship	1. Referral to local rheumatologist 2. Develop protocol for roles and responsibilities of each involved physician
9. Denial of effect of pregnancy on lupus erythematosus	1. Promote a more realistic appraisal of risks	1. Explore meaning with husband. 2. Once Susan's mental status is normal in psychotherapy, explore present and dynamic meaning of children and help Susan develop more realistic appraisal of health risks of pregnancy. 3. Help couple pursue acceptable options, such as adoption.

auditory hallucinations, paranoid delusions, ideas of reference, and fears of hurting others.

The psychiatrist assembles four orderlies but asks them to remain outside the room. He persuades the patient to let him in, and sits down on a chair beside the bed behind which John crouches, terrified.

John declares that he is angered by all the people around him and says he is afraid of hurting someone. Eventually, he admits that the staff frighten him. He agrees to be put in restraints to help him ''calm down'' and asks for more medication to ''help me get some sleep and get these voices out of my head.''

The psychiatrist reviews John's course in the hospital. A resident had prescribed low doses of phenothiazines so the patient would not be sedated too much while the dynamics thought to have precipitated the episode were explored in family therapy.

The psychiatrist and resident agree to stop family interviews, at least for the time being, move John to a less stimulating part of the ward, prohibit unstructured socialization until the patient has better control, and increase medication. ■

Treatment must be tailored to the realistic expectations of the outside world.

Case 18.3   ■ Moira, a 30-year-old woman with major depression has been encouraged in assertiveness training to vent her anger directly. Soon after discharge, she angrily confronts her boss, telling him that he is a sexual chauvinist. He fires her. Devastated, she returns to the hospital. Later, in group therapy, she learns to assert herself more effectively. ■

Abroms (1968) delimited five problems that must be ameliorated before patients are discharged from the hospital:

Problems that must be addressed before discharge

1. Destructiveness.
2. Mental disorganization of psychotic origin.
3. Rule breaking, such as drug-taking, violence, theft, or promiscuity, associated with psychiatric disorder (not antisocial personality).
4. Severe dysphoria, such as depression, mania, social withdrawal, anger, agitation, or fear.
5. Excessive dependency.

Therapeutic efforts are more efficient if directed by priorities. In most cases, for example, rule-breaking must change before the staff can help the patient change in other ways. In ideal circumstances, essential skills can be learned before discharge.

Responsibility

Skills that can be conveyed

Patients should be aware of their responsibilities in the treatment program. They should also be made aware of their important contribution to the treatment of others, a role that can help them demonstrate their progress and improve self-esteem.

Case 17.1 (continued)   ■ Since the clearing of her confusion during the 4th hospital week, Susan has participated in a therapeutic group aiming to help patients regain or acquire social skills. Susan is struck by the difficult lives of other group members. She develops particular concern for Vicki, who is about her own age. Vicki, who has been hospitalized for depression views herself as ugly and unloveable. As she tries to persuade Vicki otherwise, Susan's natural interpersonal skills as a teacher emerge. Her confidence builds and the staff encourage her leadership in the group. ■

Problem solving

The patient must learn to change or cope with the factors that precipitated the illness, to counteract the negative thinking that perpetuates symptoms, and to use reflection and introspection as means for achieving insight.

Case 17.1 (continued)   ■ Susan feels disorganized and complains bitterly of her poor memory, even though her organic brain syndrome has cleared. The staff suggest she undertake a series of memory tasks of gradually increasing difficulty with the purpose of convincing her that her memory is fundamentally intact. ■

Social skills

The patient must learn to share, to help others, and to be assertive in an appropriate manner.

Occupational skills

The patient's psychomotor skills can be restored and applied to the workplace. Vocational training may be required.

Recreational skills

The patient should be helped to rediscover the capacity for enjoyment.

Case 17.1 (continued)   ■ Susan has always enjoyed her well-developed skills as a seamstress. Her mother brings a large afghan blanket that Susan had worked on at home before her illness. It proves too complex and Susan gives up, frustrated. Ken describes this episode as "typical," referring to his mother-in-law's penchant for sabotaging her daughter's self-esteem.

The occupational therapy staff help Susan start a simple project, making a potholder, which she completes with satisfaction. They then provide her with a slightly more difficult project.   ■

Health maintenance

The patient can learn and maintain health-promoting behavior.

Case 17.1
(continued)

■   Susan enjoys swimming with the activities group and plans to return to regular swimming, which she stopped two years ago when her arthralgia began.   ■

The systems perspective of hospital management

Multimodal treatment

A hospital unit must be multimodal. Systems theory, introduced in chapter 3 and further discussed in chapters 12 and 13, is the organizational basis of biopsychosocial hospital care, which might otherwise be dismissed as pragmatic eclecticism. Group therapy, relaxation therapy, psychodrama, behavior modification, medication, electroconvulsive therapy, and psychotherapy must be coordinated in individually tailored plans in order to foster rehabilitation. Several interactional modes (group, couples, families, and individual) must be used in multiple settings (workshop, ward, expedition, etc.).

Case 17.1
(continued)

■   Susan meets daily with a psychiatric resident, who provides support while evaluating her mental status and gently exploring her concerns about pregnancy, family, and illness. He adjusts the steroid dosage according to the recommendations of her endocrinologist. He adjusts her haloperidol dose to the severity of her paranoid thinking and agitation. In group therapy, she develops assertiveness. She uses these skills during a meeting with her mother and the social worker when discharge planning is initiated.   ■

The necessity for staff cohesion

Medical autocracy impedes individualized care. Clear professional roles must be developed for all staff who maintain the responsive environment. All staff should be full-time. A physician in remote control is not enough.

The necessity for close communication between staff

Good communication is essential to coordinated, consistent work and the full use of the therapeutic potential of any ward staff. However, if the staff become preoccupied with their own group processes, they can lose sight of the primary focus – patient care. The staff must deal with the following problems:

Problems that can interrupt staff communication

1. Staff transitions: For example, patient care often suffers in teaching wards when residents change assignments at mid-year.
2. Staff dysfunction: Illness and personal or professional problems can impair the performance of key staff members.

3. Absence of leadership.
4. Lack of clarity in the unit's mission, aims, strategies, or roles.
5. Inadequate training.

Continuing education   The staff must be properly trained and provided with the opportunity for continuing education. Special expertise must be acknowledged and roles sufficiently defined to allow an appropriate division of labor in diagnosis and management. Otherwise, staff will design inappropriate management plans, as in Case 18.4.

Case 18.4   ■ During team rounds, an experienced ward nurse strongly advises a new resident to increase the dose of haloperidol for an agitated manic patient who is being treated with lithium and neuroleptics. The resident hesitates, vaguely concerned about the patient's mild confusion; but finally accedes when other staff anxiously press for better control of the patient's behavior. Next morning, the patient is difficult to rouse and markedly confused. Lithium toxicity is diagnosed. Preoccupied with medication, the team had neglected to develop an appropriate nursing plan to deal with the patient's agitation. (See Figure 18.2.) ■

This mistake in the clinical process is illustrated by algorithm in Figure 18.2.

The treatment plan must be regularly reviewed and modified if necessary in accordance with the patient's progress towards management goals.

Disruption of the unit

A number of situations are likely to impede or disrupt patient care:

Factors that impede patient care
1. When the staff are poorly trained.
2. When administrative procedures are so cumbersome that problems cannot be dealt with properly.

Case 17.1 (continued)   ■ Susan is transferred to the care of a psychiatrist in the Chicago area. One day before she leaves, the attending physician requests that the resident send a copy of a detailed discharge summary to the psychiatrist outlining the nature of the problem, the course in hospital, and the recommended management plan. Four weeks after discharge, the Chicago psychiatrist calls the attending physician, inquiring about several aspects of Susan's hospitalization. The physician is embarrassed because he does not remember essential details of the case, such as drug dosage and some of the laboratory values. He discovers that the resident has failed to dictate more than 20 discharge summaries, despite requests from the chief resident to do so. He shrugs his shoulders and spends an hour in the record room dictating a letter that provides the essential information. ■

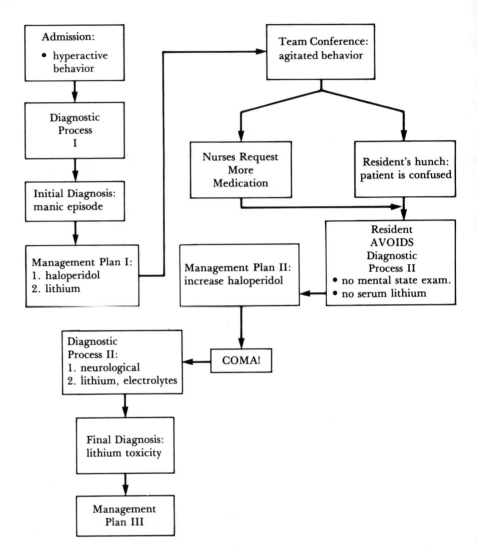

FIGURE 18.2
Clinical process on a hospital unit. Case 18.4

Patient care is also impeded in other circumstances:

3. When staff change frequently.
4. When a staff member has aims, plans, or tactics inconsistent with those of the unit.
5. When the patient's family is disgruntled.
6. When patients, such as adolescents or those with borderline or antisocial personalities, misbehave.

7. In the case of the special patient (Main, 1957) who provokes erratic behavior on the part of the referring physician, nontherapeutic reactions in the staff, and problems with discharge and outcome.

Case 18.5

■ Jane, a 25-year-old teacher, has suffered from painful posttraumatic arthritis of the left knee and hip since a car accident 7 years ago. Increasing disability and pain force her to undergo surgery for total hip replacement. Her otherwise uneventful recovery is complicated by excessive complaints of pain, for which she continues to request high doses of narcotic analgesics from both her orthopedist and primary-care physician. The former, concerned about addiction, refers her to a behavioral medicine clinic for management of pain. There, the psychiatrist diagnoses narcotic addiction and major depression. He admits her to the psychiatric unit for drug withdrawal.

Although Jane has not accepted a psychiatric diagnosis, she is willing to do something about her drug dependency. Accordingly, the psychiatrist requests the psychiatric unit to forego psychological investigation of the depression and the family situation and focus on narcotic withdrawal.

Other changes in the usual procedures soon follow. Jane refuses to let the resident perform more than a perfunctory physical examination, stating emphatically, "I've got my own doctor." However, the history reveals that she has never had a pelvic examination, although she complains about a persistent vaginal discharge. Contrary to usual ward procedure, both her internist and the psychiatrist from behavioral medicine visit her daily. Ignoring her resident, Jane calls them constantly to complain about pain and request changes in medication. Again, contrary to established procedure, the internist writes laboratory orders without consulting the resident or the ward's attending physician. Meanwhile, the nurses and activity therapists complain that the patient refuses to participate in prescribed ward activities.

The inexperienced resident, pressured by staff and unsure which physician has supervisory responsibility, delays writing medication orders for Jane's withdrawal schedule. Jane goes 12 hours without narcotics. In a typical withdrawal state, her disturbances escalate as she demands medication. The nurses respond with limit setting. They do not notify the resident, who is attending a seminar and later involved in another admission. Finally, Jane calls her orthopedist and threatens to leave the unit. The resident, aware of his oversight, orders medication and tries to persuade Jane to stay. Meanwhile, the four physicians heatedly discuss what went wrong. ■

The use of medication

Psychopharmacology is a cornerstone of hospital psychiatry. Drug treatment is discussed in chapter 11, but several features of medication specific to the hospital setting warrant emphasis:

The need for staff support

1. All staff should be able to recognize the effects and complications of medication. Responsive staff must be alert to any changes in the patient's mental or

physical status that could indicate the need for a change in medication. (See Case 18.3 and Figure 18.2.)

The need for patient education

2. If patients are educated about what to expect from medication, they will be more likely to collaborate with treatment.

Case 18.6

■ Mac, a 22-year-old unemployed man, is admitted to a psychiatric unit with an acute schizophrenic episode. Despite his distrust of physicians, he agrees to start haloperidol. Possible side-effects are not discussed. When, on the 3rd day, Mac develops a strange sensation in his mouth and neck, he is convinced that these are but a manifestation of his mental distress. He neglects to inform anyone. A full-blown dystonic reaction with painful spasm of his neck muscles emerges. Terrified, his initial suspicions about the doctors confirmed, Mac refuses further medication and leaves the hospital. ■

This patient should have been informed of the possibility of a spasm that could be easily treated. He should also have been instructed to tell a nurse immediately when he first experienced stiffness of the neck muscles.

3. The staff should have a positive attitude toward medication.

The need to identify noncompliance

4. The staff must develop ways of identifying patients who are evading medication. They then can assess why. Is it due to narcotic resistance or misinformation? If so, psychotherapy and education may help. If caused by psychotic fear, liquid or injectable medication may be required. Depot medication may be considered for patients whose compliance cannot be assured following discharge.

Psychotherapy in the hospital

The restricted utility of individual psychotherapy in hospital management

The goals of psychotherapy differ in different settings. Outpatient psychotherapy draws on the patient's account of events, thoughts, and feelings that have occurred outside the therapeutic hour. In contrast, responsive hospital psychotherapy usually aims at a change in the symptoms and signs that led to hospitalization or prolong it. Many short-stay units postpone psychotherapy by the patient's own therapist until after discharge and rehabilitation. If an outside therapist were to conduct psychotherapy in the hospital, adequate communication with ward staff would be difficult, if not impossible. However, the unit director may encourage individual psychotherapy if it can be integrated into an overall management plan.

Case 18.7

■ A psychiatric resident has spent a year between medical school and residency studying consciousness-raising therapies at a retreat in the West. Assigned to an acute psychiatric unit, he refuses to prescribe drugs for psychosis. He remains intransigent on this matter despite supervision. Instead, he proposes to use unorthodox therapeutic techniques, such as rolfing. Patients with acute psychosis get worse on this therapy and their hospitalization is significantly extended. The smooth functioning of the unit is disrupted.

Eventually, the resident must be placed on probation until he is willing to use established treatments and accept supervision. ∎

Summary

The contemporary status of hospital psychiatry cannot be understood unless the history of psychiatric theory, treatment, and institutions is appreciated. Today, there is a diversity of settings, one for almost every diagnostic group and mode of treatment. To facilitate such specialized care, the admission criteria of each hospital unit must be consistent with its stated mission and goals, and the treatment methods it adopts. Funding sources can influence the hospital's selective admission policies: public hospitals must often rely upon legal criteria, whereas private hospitals use economic and clinical criteria.

The chief advantage of the hospital setting is that it allows the physician to control more of the variables influencing treatment. Hospital patients are more likely to be psychotic, diagnostically complex, chronic cases, or treatment failures, to have severely maladaptive personality traits, to lack social support, to be unemployed, and to have created social problems.

A generic, responsive environment characterizes effective hospital care in all settings. In such an environment, patients can be closely observed during diagnosis and their response to treatment closely monitored. Special investigations and specialized hospital services can be provided more conveniently (though for the same reason they may be overused). A responsive environment concentrates on helping the patient change the maladaptive behavior that led to hospitalization rather than on seeking an elusive cure. The use of behavioral goals facilitates treatment specificity. A systems perspective helps the unit coordinate several treatment methods. The implementation of multimodal care and the prevention and management of disruptive forces require the staff to be cohesive, well-trained and full-time and to communicate effectively about all aspects of each management plan.

Selected Readings

Much literature about hospital psychiatry is contained within articles or books describing evaluative or treatment methods without specific reference to the importance of the hospital environment in the clinical process. Maxmen, Tucker, and LeBow's (1974) *Rational Hospital Psychiatry: The Reactive Environment* provides an excellent overview of the development of hospital psychiatry and the characteristics of today's successful hospital units. Talbott (1978) reviews the social forces influencing the development of the public mental hospital, and Bachrach (1981) discusses the sociology of the general hospital psychiatric unit within the context of its history. A broad overview of hospital psychiatry is found in Freedman, Kaplan, and Sadcok's *Comprehensive Textbook of Psychiatry,* Vol. 3 (1980).

Sederer's (1983) edited book, *Inpatient Psychiatry: Diagnosis and Treatment,* describes generic and problem-specific diagnostic procedures and therapeutic techniques applicable to inpatient psychiatry.

19

General hospital psychiatry

Introduction

Consultation-liaison provides psychiatric care to patients in nonpsychiatric services. The recent growth of this branch of medicine has been influenced by contemporary research and by the changing face of medical care.

Psychosocial factors influence disease

Epidemiology has implicated psychosocial factors in the pathogenesis, development, maintenance, and course of disease. Research in the neurosciences and psychosomatic medicine has explored the mediation of these effects (see chapters 3, 4, and 5). Consequently, the intellectual horizon of medicine has expanded, and the need for a psychosocial understanding of all patients has been reemphasized.

Adjustment to chronic illness

As technology improves the survival rate from acute, formerly fatal, disease more people return to their communities with chronic disorders requiring protracted treatment or management. Patients with spinal cord lesions, for example, must adjust to permanent neuromuscular disability, diminished social and occupational potential, and shattered self-esteem. Patients with such progressive diseases as cancer or diabetes, though often relatively asymptomatic at first, must eventually adapt to pain, uncertainty, progressive disability, and the likelihood of an early death. The psychiatrist working in a general hospital can contribute greatly to the care of these patients.

In the past decade, recognizing the need to promote these important activities, the National Institute of Mental Health allotted funds for the development of training programs in consultation-liaison psychiatry. The resultant advance of psychosomatic medicine greatly enriched the psychiatric understanding of medical patients, although the immediate benefits of enhanced care were less tangible (McKegney & Beckhardt, 1982). Nevertheless, despite a recent withdrawal of funding (Neill, 1983), general hospital psychiatry is firmly established (Lipowski, 1983a; Strain, 1983; Mohl, 1983). This chapter describes the clinical process of psychiatry in this setting.

Advantages and constraints of the general hospital setting

Liaison psychiatry is poorly reimbursed

Few psychiatrists rely on direct fee-for-service to compensate them for consultation-liaison. However, many psychiatrists regard consulting as a stimulating opportunity to work with other physicians and to develop sources of referral.

The consultant role can be frustrating

Consulting can be frustrating. Although consulting psychiatrists may disagree with other physicians' treatment plans, they do not have the authority to change them. The psychiatrist's role is to advise, vigorously if need be, but not take charge. It is not the psychiatrist's task to decide which patients need psychiatric consultation, unless it is hospital policy that psychiatric consultation is mandatory in such circumstances as attempted suicide.

The psychiatrist can threaten the patient's sick role

Physicians request psychiatric consultation; patients do not. The patient may view the psychiatrist as a threat, not a help, because the psychiatrist is perceived as undermining the sick role. The staff may have suggested that the patient's complaints are not real by commenting, "The pain is all in your head" or "There is too much pain for the amount of pathology". The patient thus may have already been forced to defend personal veracity, integrity, courage, and mental stability. A challenge to the legitimacy of symptoms sometimes directly threatens a sick role that is or might be financially compensated. In these unpromising circumstances, diagnosis and management planning are problematic.

Factors affecting consultation requests

Consultation work is erratic; the flow of patients is uneven. A physician's decision to request consultation can be affected by a number of factors other than the possibility that a patient has psychiatric disorder; for example:

1. *The environment of the ward and hospital.* Stressful working conditions diminish the capacity of hospital staff to tolerate difficult behavior. Consultations increase at times of tension. Some causes of stress in hospitals are discussed later in this chapter (see the section on diagnosis).

2. *The physician's training.* Specialty groups differ in their reasons for requesting consultation (Craig, 1982). Surgeons, for example, seek help in managing behavioral disturbances that impede recovery from surgery or in such conditions as burns (Billowitz, Friedson, & Schubert, 1980), spinal cord injury

(Seligson & Gallagher, 1982; Gallagher, McKegney, & Gladstone, 1982), and renal transplant surgery (Abrams, 1972). In these clinical situations, management is complicated by the patient's psychological reaction. The surgeon trained in an institution with an active psychiatric consultation service will be more likely to use one thereafter.

Case 19.1 ■ An orthopedic surgeon, trained at a renowned medical center with well-established psychiatric consultation-liaison, moves to a new hospital to develop a trauma service. He locates a psychiatrist to collaborate in establishing a program for the comprehensive care of multitrauma patients. The psychiatrist consults on every patient admitted to the trauma service, develops protocols for managing pain and psychiatric disorder, and provides education and group support programs for the staff. Before this orthopedist's arrival, the orthopedic department had rarely consulted psychiatry. ■

Internists, on the other hand, tend to consult psychiatrists because they want help in diagnosing a complex case even though they often wish to manage the case themselves.

3. *The attitude of the physician toward psychiatry.* For such private reasons as an unsatisfactory conclusion to a personal or family psychiatric illness, some physicians are antagonistic towards psychiatry; this attitude can hinder the clinical process.

Case 19.2 ■ A college chaplain refers his mother, who has rheumatoid arthritis, to an internist, who is also a friend, for evaluation and treatment in the hospital. Concerned about his mother's poor self-care, her pervasive depression over several months, and a recent deterioration in her mobility, the chaplain requests that a psychiatrist evaluate her.

The internist disagrees. Without asking for consultation, he proceeds with an exhaustive biomedical assessment. No active inflammatory disease is revealed. After two weeks in the hospital, the elderly woman continues to resist physical therapy and efforts by the internist and staff to "get her motivated." Antidepressants are prescribed, but the patient develops urinary retention.

After three weeks, under pressure from the family, the internist accedes to a consultation. Major depression and early dementia are diagnosed. The patient responds well to supportive, expressive psychotherapy focusing on her unresolved grief about the recent death of her husband and on her guilt about being a burden to her son. Angry and puzzled about the delay, the minister confronts his friend. The internist reveals that he has not had much faith in psychiatrists since the difficulty he experienced several years before trying to get help for a sister who suffered from schizophrenia. ■

A psychiatrist with a busy practice may have difficulty scheduling consultations. Yet accessibility is imperative, since advice is often urgently required.

The importance of accessibility

Compounding other time problems, the psychiatrist may find that having completed a biomedical evaluation, the physician has discharged the patient before the psychiatrist can complete the consultation. In such a case, there is a need for follow-up services, a subject discussed later in this chapter in the section on management.

On the other hand, several aspects of the general hospital facilitate the consultative process:

Factors facilitating consultation

1. Much diagnostic information, particularly of a biomedical and demographic nature, has already been acquired.
2. Family and friends are often available for interview and therapeutic planning.
3. The concentration of services that only a hospital provides can be applied to biopsychosocial diagnosis and comprehensive management.

Clinical problems in the general hospital

The consultant psychiatrist encounters a wide range of psychiatric disorders, and may also be required to cope with problems that are rarely, if ever, seen in other settings. Statistics from the Consultation-Liaison Service of the Medical Center Hospital of Vermont illustrate the problems encountered in a teaching hospital that is both a tertiary-care referral center and a community hospital (McKegney, McMahon, & King, 1983). Tables 19.1, 19.2, and 19.3 delineate the DSM-III diagnoses of 756 consultations. These consultations represent 3.3% of all 22,409 admissions to the hospital in an 18-month period. Aside from a relatively high prevalence of adjustment disorders and a deceptively low prevalence of affective disorder and psychogenic pain, this survey was similar to surveys from other centers (Wolsten & Lipowski, 1981; Taylor & Doody, 1979).

The psychiatrist deals with matters beyond immediate patient care. For example, maladaptive family responses, the reactions of staff, and the education of staff and physicians absorb much time.

The aims of clinical work in consultation-liaison

Mission

To organize clinical work within a thicket of interacting systems, each consultation-liaison service must articulate its mission, aims, plans, and tactics. These may need to vary in different circumstances. The **mission** of a consultation-liaison service in a university teaching hospital might be, for example, to improve the quality of clinical care for patients; to foster physicians' awareness of the biopsychosocial approach to medical care; and to pursue research in psychosomatic and behavioral medicine.

TABLE 19.1
Axis I diagnosis (N = 756) (percent exceeds 100 due to multiple diagnoses)

	Number	*%*
Adjustment Disorder		
depressed mood	93	
mixed emotional features	80	
anxious mood	33	
others	40	
TOTAL	246	33%
Organic Mental Disorder		
senile/presenile dementia	31	
substance induced	11	
Section 2 delirium	83	
dementia	48	
others	29	
TOTAL	202	27%
Substance Use Disorder		
alcohol	64	
other	25	
TOTAL	89	12%
Affective Disorder		
bipolar	6	
major depression	45	
other (dysthymic, cyclothymic, atypical)	29	
TOTAL	80	10%
Somatoform Disorders	47	6%
Schizophrenic, Paranoid, Other Psychotic Disorders	28	4%
Psychological Factors Affecting Physical Condition	24	3%
Anxiety Disorders	20	3%
Factitious, Psychosexual, Impulse Control, Mental Retardation, Dissociation Disorders	12	2%
V Code, or diagnosis deferred	65	9%
No Entry	70	9%

TABLE 19.2
Axis II diagnosis (N = 756)

	Number	*%*
Dependent	59	8%
Mixed/Atypical	34	5%
Passive–Aggressive	23	3%
Borderline	22	3%
Other Personality Disorders	39	5%
Personality Traits	45	6%
V Code (none) deferred	167	20%
No Entry	380	50%

TABLE 19.3
Axis III diagnosis (N = 756) (percent exceeds 100 due to multiple diagnoses)

	Number	*%*
Musculo-Skeletal/Connective (includes Spinal Cord Injuries)	163	21%
Central Nervous System (includes head injuries)	120	16%
Neoplastic	100	13%
Circulatory	89	12%
Endocrinologic, Metabolic, Nutritional	72	10%
Injury, Poisoning, Trauma (includes self-inflicted)	72	10%
Gastrointestinal	54	7%
Other	116	15%
None (specified as such)	11	1%
No Entry	108	14%

The mission of a psychiatrist who consults in a community hospital might be to provide consultation, treatment, and educational programs for the local hospital.

Aims

The **aims** of a psychiatrist in the community hospital might involve:

1. Providing consultation for hospital patients.
2. Providing advice and support to nursing staff.
3. Providing continuing education for hospital staff and physicians.

Administrative plans

General **plans** enable the psychiatrist to achieve the aims. For example, to facilitate the aim, ''To provide consultations,'' administrative plans might involve:

1. Planning a regular schedule other physicians can rely on.
2. Establishing a telephone system to enhance accessibility.
3. Developing a protocol for rapidly and efficiently communicating recommendations to consultees.

Clinical plans

Clinical plans to achieve this aim might include:

1. Undertaking biopsychosocial evaluations pertinent to the consultees' questions.
2. Designing systematic goal-oriented management plans to address the problems requiring immediate attention.
3. When appropriate, providing follow-up services.

Administrative tactics

Tactics are the specific actions required to implement plans. Administrative tactics might include:

1. Scheduling several hours for consultation, spread out over the week but at a regular time each day.
2. Designing a form to help the secretary record demographic and billing data when calling the ward secretary to schedule consultations.
3. Having the secretary notify the ward staff when your arrival is imminent so they are sure to have patient and chart available.
4. Designing a standard form to record consultation findings and recommendations and placing it in the chart.

Clinical tactics   Clinical tactics might include:

1. Reviewing the chart briefly when appropriate.
2. Generating preliminary diagnostic hypotheses before interviewing the patient.
3. If possible, arranging to interview the patient alone in a private room.
4. Introducing yourself, asking low-key questions to develop a relationship, and learning what it was about the patient's illness that brought him or her to the hospital. (See the section on diagnosis in this chapter.)

Unless the psychiatrist systematically articulates aims, plans, and tactics, the constraints mentioned in this chapter will ultimately render consultation-liaison intolerable.

Special features of the diagnostic process in general hospital psychiatry

Consultation-liaison goes well when plenty of time is available, the ward staff are helpful, and the patient, family, and consultee collaborative. In reality, consultations are often requested in less favorable circumstances.

Case 19.3   ■ Friday afternoon. The hospital calls Dr. Peters's office about a patient with low back pain. His secretary jots the information on her consultation data form: "Patient wants more pain medication. Family wants an operation. Physician wants to transfer patient to different service. The administrator wants patient discharged today. Patient without insurance. Medicaid DRG allotment has run out. Ward nurse says DSM-III diagnosis is required for the patient to get Medicaid extension."

The secretary hangs up the phone, turns, and says incredulously, "And you want to do a biopsychosocial assessment?" Dr. Peters smiles, wryly. He has been in this situation before.

The psychiatrist looks at his watch – 4:30 P.M. He is supposed to pick up his son at 5:30 to drive him to soccer. Dinner party at 7:30. He calls a friend who might be able to cover. No luck. The answering service announces that his colleague is away for the weekend.

Dr. Peters takes a breath and tells his secretary: "Call my wife. Tell her to pick up Billy after soccer. I'll meet her at dinner." Still annoyed, he finds it hard to concentrate on his last patient, but reflects: "At least I'll see Billy for a few minutes." While driving his son to soccer, he devises a plan for completing the consultation in less than an hour. Billy asks his father if he will be staying to watch the game. ■

The rest of this chapter follows Dr. Peters as he acknowledges the special features and avoids the pitfalls of diagnosis and management planning in consultation-liaison.

Initial diagnostic tactics

Strategic planning

To complete a complex consultation in a relatively brief time, the psychiatrist must carefully plan tactics and anticipate exigencies, as follows:

1. Collect as much information as possible before the interview.
2. Discuss the patient with the consultee.
3. Plan the diagnostic encounter.
4. Formulate preliminary hypotheses.
5. Read the chart.
6. Review old records.
7. Determine the purpose and goals of the interview.

Data gathering

Collect data before the examination

A secretary can acquire useful information about the consultation request from various sources – ward secretary, nurses, referring physician, and office staff. These data can be recorded on a single sheet and reviewed in order to generate preliminary diagnostic hypotheses and to consider the tactics of diagnostic inquiry.

Case 19.3 (continued)

■ Dr. Peters's secretary elicits the following information from the ward secretary:

1. The patient is on Medicaid.
2. The DRG allotment has been exhausted.
3. Discharge is contemplated.
4. The problem list includes: chronic low back pain (after having been struck by a truck), narcotic dependency, and personality disorder.

The secretary manages to catch the patient's primary nurse, who, over the phone, provides the following information:

1. The patient's wife has been complaining bitterly about her husband's care. She has tearfully confided in a nurse that she is feeling hopeless about the doctor's ability to help her husband.

2. Physician and patient seem to be annoyed with each other.
3. The patient has been admitted several times in the past year for evaluation of the same problem.
4. The staff think the patient may be ''faking'' because ''there is no organic explanation for so much pain.''
5. The patient has been taking narcotics and diazepam regularly while in the hospital and, she thinks, at home. ■

Case discussion

Talk with the consultee

Discuss the case with the consultee ahead of time whenever possible. The information gained and rapport established are invaluable.

Case 19.3 (continued)

■ Dr. Peters's secretary tries to reach the orthopedist, but he is in surgery. ■

Planning the diagnostic encounter

Organize the diagnostic encounter

Plan the diagnostic encounter ahead of time.

Case 19.3 (continued)

■ The secretary makes the following arrangements to facilitate the consultation.

1. The patient will be in his room at 6:30 P.M.
2. The patient's wife will be at the hospital at 7 P.M.
3. The patient's hospital chart and old records will be waiting at the nurses' station. ■

Hypothesis-generation

Hypotheses help diagnostic planning

Generate preliminary hypotheses. They will help you decide what should be noted or explored during the chart review and the various interviews.

Case 19.3 (continued)

■ On the way to the hospital, Dr. Peters generates several diagnostic hunches based on the fit of the available data with the clinical patterns commonly encountered in chronic pain consultations.

1. The patient has learned to behave in such a way to get attention for his pain and to legitimize his sick role.
2. The physician is frustrated by the patient's poor response to conservative treatment, by his incessant demands for medication, and by the wife's complaints.
3. The wife is annoyed with her husband for not getting better; but because it is her duty to support his sick role, she projects her anger onto the staff. She might be depressed, like the spouses of many patients with chronic pain.
4. The patient is dependent on, and perhaps physiologically addicted to, analgesics and sedative hypnotics. ■

Chart perusal

Peruse the chart for clues to diagnosis

Read the chart first. Some of your diagnostic hunches may be confirmed before you see the patient; your interview can then focus on selected or more refined hypotheses. Review the nursing notes and the physician's progress notes. Depending on their quality, thoroughness, and legibility, notes can yield valuable physiologic, cognitive, affective, and behavioral data. They can also inform the psychiatrist about staff–patient relationships and family functioning.

Case 19.3 (continued)

■ Dr. Peters notes the following:

1. Mr. S. asks for medication well ahead of his p.r.n. schedule, but he never seems to be relieved by it.
2. Mrs. S. often requests medication for Mr. S.
3. Mr. S. sometimes complains of pain even though he is apparently comfortably engaged in conversation.
4. Physical examination has revealed bilateral paravertebral muscle spasm and restricted motion of the spine, but no motor, sensory, or reflex abnormality. Diffuse tenderness has been noted along the paravertebral muscles in the lumbosacral region, with point tenderness over the lateral aspects of L5-S1. ■

Look for irrational pharmacology

Review medication.   Physicians sometimes become entangled in irrational polypharmacy, particularly when treating somatoform disorders and chronic or severe pain. In a review of hospitalized medical and surgical patients, Salzman (1981) found that nearly 50% received at least one psychotropic drug (excluding analgesics) and that the average patient was taking seven drugs.

Case 19.3 (continued)

■ Mr. S. has the following daily drug intake: percodan (oxycodone, aspirin, phenacetin and caffeine), 8 to 10 tablets; diazepam, 15 to 25 mgs.; and dioctyl sodium sulfosuccinate (a stool softener), 2 capsules. ■

Laboratory data may be overlooked

Peruse the laboratory data.   Important information sometimes is not recorded in the notes and has been overlooked by the busy physician.

Case 19.3 (continued)

■ Dr. Peters notes:

1. The lumbosacral spine X-ray films are normal.
2. The myelogram shows a slight filling defect at the L5-S1 intervertebral space, probably within normal limits.
3. CBC and sedimentation rate are normal.
4. Enzymes and blood chemistry are normal. ■

Review of previous records

Review old records

Review the old records if available. Important clues can be gleaned about disease, illness, and illness behavior and about previous doctor–patient relationships.

Case 19.3
(continued)

■ Mr. S.'s chart reveals the following:

1. There were two previous admissions, both with negative work-ups.
2. The first admission followed an accident when, as a pedestrian, Mr. S. was struck by a truck while on a construction job. Shaken up, he was taken to the hospital, where examination revealed nothing more than bruises, and he was sent home for the day. The next morning, he could barely get out of bed because of severe back pain; but he returned to work for two weeks, until the job was finished ("I have to feed the wife and kids"). He was not rehired for the next job and has been unemployed since.
3. On two previous occasions, he had adamantly refused to allow his physician to consult a psychiatrist. ■

Determining the goals of the interview

Goals help plan
the interview

Based on the consultee's questions and your preliminary hypotheses, determine the purpose and goals of the interview. For example, if the patient is about to leave the hospital against medical advice and there is a question of suicide or violence, an evaluation of dangerousness becomes paramount.

Case 19.3
(continued)

■ Dr. Peters decides on the following goals for his initial interview with Mr. S.:

1. Establish a therapeutic alliance with the patient. Very likely, Mr. S. does not wish to see him. He probably thinks that a psychiatrist will think he is crazy or imagining his pain. He must, therefore, develop rapport.
2. Engender confidence and hope. Dr. Peters anticipates that Mr. S. will question his and the orthopedist's competence to deal with the problem.
3. Analyze the pattern of the pain and its precipitation and perpetuation.
4. Rule out affective, organic, and psychotic disorders.
5. Enlist relatives and staff as collaborators in the clinical process.
6. Complete the interview in less than 45 minutes. ■

The diagnostic interview

Due to the constraints and advantages already described, the conduct of an initial interview in the general hospital may differ from the procedures described in chapter 8, even though the principles are similar. Sensitivity to the patient's needs for territorial respect, courtesy, control, safety, and comfort are critical. The physician should consider the following questions:

Privacy important

1. Can I arrange a confidential setting? Some interviews must be conducted at bedside, often with another patient in the room. When possible, move the patient to a more private setting, or ask the other patient to leave. Ask the ward staff to intercept interruptions. Draw the curtain, close the door, and hang the sign you carry in your pocket: Interview in progress – Do not disturb.

Eliminate distractions

    2. Can I eliminate distractions? Radio, television, dropped bedpans, and floor polishers impede the interview.

Promote comfort

    3. How comfortable is the patient? A patient may be emotionally distressed or physically uncomfortable. If this is so, acknowledge it and try to help the patient get comfortable. Empathy fosters confidence.

Make eye contact

    4. Can I help the patient feel less helpless, less infantilized? Do not stand over the patient. Find a comfortable position that allows good eye contact.

Case 19.4

■ Tom, a 30-year-old man with quadriplegia following a fracture-dislocation of the spine at C5-C6, refuses food and drink. He adamantly insists he wants to die and threatens to wrench himself off the Stryker frame (an immobilizing device that turns the patient to face the floor or the ceiling). When the psychiatrist arrives for the initial interview, Tom has been rotated into the prone position. At first, he rebuffs the psychiatrist's overtures, just as he has kept his distance from all the staff. Taking a gamble, the psychiatrist lies down on the floor on his back, facing up at Tom, who otherwise must talk to people behind his head. The psychiatrist accedes to Tom's request that he wipe his dribbling nose. Gradually, trust develops. Tom begins to talk about his fears of being a "vegetable." He decides, at least temporarily, to delay his plan to die so he can sort out relationships with his wife and 10-year-old son. ■

Be adaptable and resourceful

    Conducting an interview in these circumstances requires the clinician to be adaptable and resourceful. Some patients on respirators, for example, must be interviewed by means of sign language or notes. Others need the aid of a family member who is adept at reading lips. The following tactics help:

1. Introduce yourself gently in a friendly and interested manner. Confirm that the consultee has already prepared the patient for your visit. If the patient seems confused or hostile, answer questions openly but be sensitive to needs and defenses. It can be helpful if you indicate that you consult frequently at the hospital. Do not bludgeon the patient with the truth, in the manner of the medical student who told a recently injured paraplegic: "I'm here to help you adjust to your injury. How do you feel about never being able to walk again?"
2. Begin with an open-ended question about the illness. Let the patient tell the story. If the patient cannot or will not do so, shift gears and ask about the course of the illness in the hospital or about neutral topics such as sleep, pain, appetite, and energy.

Emphasize your role as physician, your interest, and your empathy

    These tactics counteract the patient's fears that you will think he or she is crazy. Moreover you indicate to the patient that you are an interested physician, sensitive to the discomfort experienced by all patients in those circumstances.

    Here is where your medical training is indispensable; the more intimate your understanding of a patient's physical disorder and its course and treatment, the more authority you will have to investigate the patient's problems.

Help patient under-stand your role

1. Be aware that patients may not understand your role; most have never heard of consultation-liaison. Many equate psychiatrists with psychoanalysts or the custodians of crazy people. Correct such misconceptions when they impede progress.

Focus on real problems

2. Focus the initial interview on immediate problems. Acknowledge and help the patient tackle such difficulties as insomnia, pain, or lack of communication with staff.

How do you broach the emotional issues involved in the case?

Emphasize that emotions are natural

3. Ask the patient about feelings in a way that indicates it is natural to have them. For example, after a patient has described a particularly difficult experience associated with the illness, you might ask: That must have been a hard time; what was it like for you? Or: These things are really tough for anyone to adjust to; what's it been like for you? Alternatively, for patients reluctant to admit what they regard as weakness: These things can be pretty tough for families. What's it been like for yours? How have you all been getting along? It's been tough, I bet.

After eliciting the pattern and the precipitating and perpetuating factors, you can inquire about predisposition, if time permits. The psychiatrist must follow the initial diagnostic plan but be adaptable enough to pursue new hypotheses suggested by the patient's story.

Case 19.3 (continued)

■ During the initial interview with Mr. S., Dr. Peters elicits a 6-month history of pain that wakes the patient several times during the night. It also wakes him early in the morning, after which he cannot get back to sleep. The sleep disturbance is consistent with a major depressive episode, a diagnosis supported by other neurovegetative symptoms.

Dr. Peters decides to foster a therapeutic alliance. He prescribes a relatively low nighttime dose of amitriptyline (50 mg) to facilitate sleep. This will also initiate antidepressant therapy, if his initial diagnostic hunch proves correct. He will complete a full psychiatric assessment over the next two or three sessions. ■

The mental status examination

Again, adaptability is the watchword. According to a standard brief examination, Cavanaugh (1983) found that 28% of medical patients admitted to a general hospital had cognitive impairment and that the house staff were usually unaware that they did. These and similar findings (Gehi et al., 1980) indicate that at least a brief cognitive screening examination should be performed on all consultations, if not all hospital admissions. Several tests for this purpose are recommended in chapter 9; for example:

Cognitive deficits are commonly overlooked

1. The Short Portable Mental Status Questionnaire (Pfeiffer, 1975).
2. The Mini-Mental Status Examination (Folstein, Folstein, & McHugh, 1975).
3. The Cognitive Capacity Screening Examination (Jacobs et al., 1977).

Be alert to emotional reactions to interview content

In addition to checking cognition as the patient tells the story, the interviewer should observe how the patient responds emotionally to each event while recalling the history of the illness. Be alert for facial blushing, moistening of the eyes, welling of tears, shifting of position, and sudden movements of the hands or feet. Does the patient attempt to show a wound or a diseased or injured part? Does the patient try to hide evidence of being unwell? What are the patient's beliefs about, attitudes towards, and understanding of, the illness? What does the patient know about personal emotional responses and the way he or she and the family are coping?

Observe motor behavior

Observe motor behavior. Are the patient's movements consistent with the disorder or disability that has been diagnosed? Does the patient tend to exaggerate, minimize, or deny illness? Does the patient do things that he or she claims to be unable to do?

**Case 19.3
(continued)**

■ Dr. Peters notes the following:

1. A grimace and stiffness as Mr. S. reaches from his bed to answer the telephone. (An appropriate response to discomfort created by shifting position.)
2. A welling of tears as, with a fixed smile, Mr. S. resentfully describes his employer's unwillingness to defray his crippling medical expenses. (A constraint of emotion consistent with the hypothesis of suppressed depression.)
3. A stiff smile as Mr. S. initially denies that he or his family have had any problems in coping with the devastating change in his life. (Also consistent with suppressed depression.)
4. Mr. S.'s conviction that the doctors will eventually find the lesion responsible for his chronic pain and cure it surgically. (Poor understanding of the nature of chronic low back pain.)
5. Mr. S.'s lack of awareness that his inflexibility impedes treatment. (He will probably have difficulty accepting the need to explore his feelings and is therefore unlikely to be receptive to insight-oriented psychotherapy.)
6. Intact cognitive functioning. ■

The physical examination

The psychiatrist may diagnose medical disorder

The consultant psychiatrist has an advantage over colleagues in other settings. Rich diagnostic data are usually already available from the admission history, physical examination, and special investigations. Yet the psychiatrist should not forego the opportunity for physical inquiry when it is appropriate. The high prevalence of undiagnosed cognitive impairment among general hospital admissions and the significant number of referrals with consultation who have organic mental disorder (28% in Vermont) or substance use disorder (12% in Vermont) mandate a keen eye for the physical causes of brain dysfunction. Moreover, a psychiatrist can detect undiagnosed disease, particularly on highly specialized services that are restricted in diagnosis and management. The consultant sometimes can identify a subtle delirium that is the first sign of deterioration or the first signs of a complication.

Case 19.5

■ Rocky, a 22-year-old man, has been hospitalized on a trauma service for multiple fractures of the extremities sustained in an automobile accident. The psychiatrist is consulted about the management of pain that has been unresponsive to the usual analgesics. During rounds on the eighth hospital day, Rocky complains that nausea prevents him from taking his drugs orally. The orthopedic resident assumes the patient is trying to hoodwink him into ordering intramuscular medication.

Next day, Rocky complains of epigastric pain in addition to his other discomforts.

At the end of the day, the psychiatrist makes her rounds. Concerned about the new symptom, and alert for stress ulcers in the trauma service, she examines the patient. Rocky's abdomen is silent to auscultation and diffusely tender with guarding, rebound, and tenderness to palpation of the epigastrium. She makes the preliminary diagnosis of acute abdomen, probably perforated peptic ulcer. Gastric lavage reveals active bleeding. Rocky is taken to the operating room and the diagnosis of peptic ulcer is confirmed at laparotomy.

Special investigations

How does the liaison psychiatrist use special investigations? Many laboratory procedures may have been completed already, but they may have been undertaken before the onset of the symptoms for which the consultation was called. Also, the laboratory investigations have seldom been directed in a discretionary way by hypotheses generated from a psychiatric interview and physical examination. The psychiatrist can assume that nonpsychiatric colleagues are not adept in assessing conditions that affect thinking, feeling, and behavior (see chapter 10).

Physicians are often inexpert in the medical assessment of emotional or behavioral problems

At this point, it would be helpful to consider the two modes of special investigation often requested in the consultation setting: psychological testing and electroencephalography.

Psychological testing

Psychological testing must be modified in several ways to fit the hospital setting (Lovitt, 1982):

Psychological testing must be modified to setting and patient

1. Most psychological tests are designed for use with physically healthy people. Almost all, in fact, were validated on healthy samples. Physically sick patients may not be able to tolerate prolonged tests which therefore should be chosen carefully, with brevity in mind.

Tests should fit an overall diagnostic plan

2. Psychological tests must be coordinated with a diagnostic inquiry plan. Too often, redundant or inappropriate tests are ordered before the psychiatric consultation. For example, psychological tests are often mistakenly ordered for delirious patients whose impaired mental function depresses test performance. In these circumstances, the test provides less information than a brief cognitive screening examination (see the previous section on the MSE).

Tests can spoil a therapeutic alliance

3. Tests that are tiring or psychologically threatening can compromise the therapeutic alliance.

4. Psychological tests should not be interpreted independently but rather within the context of a biopsychosocial evaluation.

To define the neuropsychological deficits suggested by routine history and physical examination, some psychiatrists add subtests of the Halstead-Reitan battery to the mental status examination.

The following situations call for psychological testing:

Indications for psychological testing

1. When there is a need to determine the degree of residual impairment following brain insult and to monitor recovery following brain insult.

2. When there is a need to determine how much impairment has been caused by a structural lesion of the central nervous system and to follow its progression.

3. When it is important to distinguish abnormal personality from abnormal illness behavior.

Electroencephalography

By revealing diffuse slowing, electroencephalography provides an inexpensive method of screening for metabolic delirium (Lipowski, 1983b). However, drugs that affect brain function can confound the interpretation of the electroencephalogram in suspected delirium.

A social systems assessment

The effect of social relationships on presentation

As interview proceeds, the psychiatrist will assemble and test an array of diagnostic hypotheses; but before formulating a comprehensive biopsychosocial diagnosis, the influence of all systems must be considered. How have family members (Lipsitt & Lipsitt, 1981; Waring, 1983; Waring &Russell, 1980), the primary physician (Anstett, 1980; Jensen, 1981), and the hospital milieu (Koran et al., 1983) affected the patient's psychological state and illness behavior? What factors have predisposed to or precipitated the consultation problem? What is perpetuating it? There may not be sufficient time to pursue all of these questions during the initial consultation, or even during the hospital stay, but the psychiatrist must complete a social inquiry before developing comprehensive management plans.

Case 19.3
(continued)

■ Mr. S. blurts out at the end of the initial interview that, although he is not depressed, his wife might not be "holding up." He wonders if Dr. Peters might speak with her. Peters meets briefly with Mrs. S. and arranges an appointment at his office late in the week.

At the later interview, Mrs. S. confirms his diagnostic hunch that she is, in fact, "fed up" with her husband's interminable illness. Demoralized and constantly worried, she feels guilty about her angry outbursts: "He's a good man. And he's been hurting so much since this damn back. He's just not himself anymore." Dr. Peters refers her to a trusted colleague for evaluation and treatment.

Why was the consultation called at this time? This question requires a consideration of how the staff feel about the patient and the status of the doctor–patient relationship.

Case 19.3
(continued)

■ Dr. Peters's hunch that the orthopedist is exasperated with the patient is correct. Injections, medication, and physical therapy have not helped Mr. S.'s back; and the patient continually bothers the orthopedist and his office staff for medication. The ward staff are impatient and unsure how to respond. Mr. S. thinks the staff insinuate that there is nothing wrong with him, a perception that accentuates his need to justify medication by complaining. ■

Table 19.4 and Figure 19.1 summarize Dr. Peters's assessment of Mr. S.

Factors creating stress
on medical wards

Many factors contribute to stress on a medical and surgical ward; for example, staff shortages, difficult patients, disorganized administration, poor leadership and conflicts among staff. A dysfunctional ward can be so stressful that the staff request an inordinate number of consultations, often for abnormal illness behavior of iatrogenic nature.

Case 19.6

■ A new spinal cord injury team at a tertiary care hospital becomes well known to surrounding community hospitals. As a result, the orthopedic unit, accustomed to caring at any time for only one or two patients with spinal cord injury, is deluged by ten of them. Coincidentally, there is a shortage of nursing staff.

The overburdened nurses become exhausted caring for these patients. They displace their anger onto other patients. They tolerate little frustration. They make more mistakes. An atmosphere of fear, frustration and demoralization pervades. The psychiatric consultant notes a dramatic rise in consultation requests. ■

In summary, the diagnostic process in liaison psychiatry requires the consultant to:

1. Use multiple sources of information.
2. Collaborate with different consultees in a variety of settings.
3. Enlist the cooperation of family and staff.
4. Be prepared to enter the diagnostic process at different levels.
5. Tolerate uncooperative patients.
6. Tolerate unscheduled demands for service.

TABLE 19.4
Diagnostic net: MVS. (Case 19.3)

	Predisposition	Precipitation (stressors)	Perpetuation	Pattern
Physical	• back injury	? narcotics or benzodiazepine withdrawal ? chronic noxious peripheral stimulus	• percodan dependency ? diazepam dependency ? chronic paraspinous muscle spasm • restricted spine motion	• normal L-S films, myelograms, blood work • paravertebral muscle spasm • no deficits • restricted spinal mobility • sleep disturbance • nighttime pain • neurovegetative symptoms
Psychological	? dependent personality ? passive-aggressive personality	"They don't believe me." • anger • pain behavior • passive-aggressive behavior	• major depression • "They do not believe I am in pain"	• anger • mistrust
Social	• has worked hard since age 16 • has refused to see psychiatrist • several past admissions for low back pain. Treatment failures	• wife angry, hopeless • unemployed • critical attitude of inpatient staff • wife angry at doctor • irritation between doctor and patient • hospital anxious to discharge	• reinforced by wife's attention, her asking staff for meds, and the passive-aggressive responses of staff • wife's depression • unemployable • Medicaid, disability • angry doctor • poor doctor-patient relationship	• operant pain behaviors • inappropriate affect • wife asks for pain meds • staff think patient failing • wife dislikes doctor

pain behavior

420

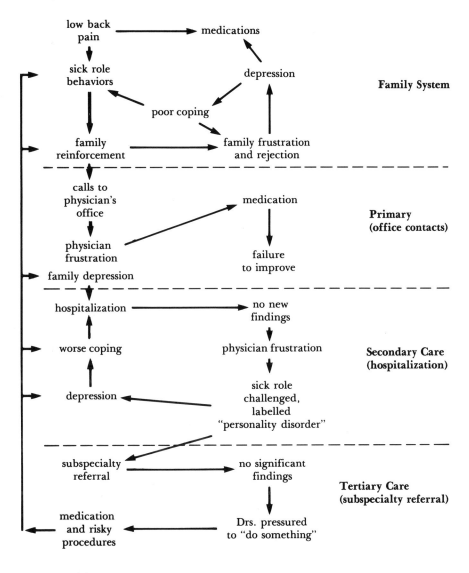

FIGURE 19.1
Dynamic flow chart: Mr. S. (Case 19.3)

Special features of management planning in the general hospital

Patients too sick for psychotherapy

Consultation-liaison psychiatry provides little opportunity for many of the treatment methods described in chapter 12. Patients are usually too sick or too briefly hospitalized to engage in dynamic psychotherapy; supportive and cognitive-behavioral approaches may be more practicable. Medication can be used, but the psychiatrist seldom observes its eventual effect. The success of an intervention may be measured by its beneficial impact on the clinical process rather than its effect on the outcome of a disorder; for example:

Success measured by impact on the clinical process

1. A patient agrees to an important diagnostic test that was initially refused because of distrust of the physician or a previous traumatic experience.
2. A nursing home is persuaded to take back a cantankerous 70-year-old man now that his depression has been diagnosed and a management plan successfully implemented in the hospital.
3. A patient with recent myocardial infarction remains in bed rest in the hospital rather than precipitously discharging himself against medical advice.
4. The ward staff alter their schedule to allow primary nursing of spinal cord injury patients.
5. The consultee is able to share with a patient's family, an unavoidable uncertainty about a particular treatment plan.

Lead informally

Use multimodal skills

The consultation-liaison psychiatrist operates in someone else's territory. Some interventions are directed not at the patient but at staff, consultee, or family. The psychiatrist may provide leadership in the clinical team yet not be the formal clinical leader. Since interventions must be practical and opportunistic, the psychiatrist must have multimodal skills (see chapter 12). This is illustrated by the clinical interventions typically required of a liaison psychiatrist, for example:

1. The management of grief.
2. Family counseling.
3. The treatment of complex pain.
4. The management of delirium.
5. The exploitation of the ward as a system.

The management of grief

Grief work

Patients in the hospital often face loss. Some people prefer death to a prolonged, painful, or debilitating illness that robs them of dignity, humanity, and savings. The loss may involve no more than a few days work, but even a brief, curable illness can have catastrophic meaning for some patients.

Case 19.3 (continued)

■ Dr. Peters completes his initial biopsychosocial evaluation of Mr. S., with:

1. A diagnostic net (Table 19.4).
2. A dynamic flowchart (Figure 19.1).
3. A list of pivotal problems (Table 19.5).

His comprehensive management plan incorporates:

1. A statement of goals (Table 19.5).
2. A set of treatment interventions (Table 19.5).

TABLE 19.5
Pivotal problem, goals, and plans: Mr. S (Case 19.3) in general hospital

Pivotal problems	Relevant goals	Relevant treatment
1. Sleep disturbance	1. sedate; treat causes	1. prescribe amitriptyline (see treatment for depression)
2. Muscle spasm	1. modify	2. physical therapy and relaxation
3. No insurance; DRG's ran out	1. obtain DRG extension; 2. minimize expenses	1. provide psychiatric diagnosis 2. facilitate discharge
3. Wife's demoralization	1. engage her in treatment	1. education and psychotherapy
3. Poor relationship with doctor	1. improve trust, compliance	1. educate patient and physician 2. assume some therapeutic responsibility
4. Major depression	1. alleviate symptoms; 2. treat causes	1. prescribe amitriptyline 2. promote grief work 3. educate re back
4. Poor understanding of low back pain	1. improve understanding and compliance	1. educate patient about back disorders 2. stop reinforcement of mind-body dichotomy by family, hospital, and doctor by educating them re their appropriate roles
4. Pain behaviors	1. minimize	1. change family and health care system reinforcement – no more ''attention'' for pain (either positive or negative) 2. avoid p.r.n. analgesics (see below)
4. Wife's depression	1. alleviate	1. refer to psychiatric colleague
5. Percodan addiction and dependency	1. eliminate chronic regular use	1. plan withdrawal schedule using regular, not p.r.n., medication (see text)
6. Unresolved grief over loss of function	1. explore grief; 2. improve function	1. regular psychotherapeutic visits 2. educate re back function
6. Chronic disability	1. improve vocational outcome	1. voc. rehab. referral 2. psychotherapy (grief work)
7. Diazepam dependency (? addiction)	1. avoid regular use	1. train in psychophysiologic relaxation 2. gradually withdraw from diazepam

Allowing the patient to ventilate anger about losing his masculinity helps him develop a plan for activities that will restore a sense of mastery, control, and self-respect. ■

Some patients experience concrete losses. Injury and illness can threaten not only recreation but also relationships fundamental to well-being. Loss is the common denominator.

Distinguish grief from depression

The psychiatrist must distinguish grief from clinical depression and plan appropriate management. Antidepressants should be prescribed cautiously for patients who are at high risk for anticholinergic side-effects. Expressive psychotherapy and cognitive therapy (see chapter 12) can help the patient work through the denial, anger, and sadness inseparable from loss.

Helping the family

Family coping

Families must cope with loss, accommodate to new roles, and bear the emotional and financial burdens associated with the illness of a relative. Psychiatrists can help the family adapt to the hospital environment, their relative's illness, and real or anticipated losses. A social worker may also be available to help the family.

The treatment of complex pain

Pain ubiquitous

Pain is ubiquitous in medical and surgical settings. Unfortunately, when treating patients in pain, physicians tend to be preoccupied with the peripheral stimulus. Pain is a multidimensional biopsychosocial experience subserved by several neurophysiologic process (see chapter 5). Somatic considerations are as follows:

Somatic influence on pain

1. The nature and intensity of the peripheral stimulus.
2. The integrity of the neural structures subserving reception, transmission, processing, modulation, and perception.
3. The influence of the neurotransmitters and neuromodulators associated with these structures.

The following psychosocial factors also should be considered:

Psychological factors

1. The degree to which the complaint of pain is reinforced by financial gain or the hope of it (e.g., compensation, litigation), interpersonal advantage (e.g., dependency, affection, power), or escape from irksome obligations (e.g., school, work, marrriage).
2. The presence and influence of anxiety and depression.
3. The extent to which the patient interprets the situation as dangerous.
4. The patient's attitudes toward the sick role.
5. Personality and coping techniques.
6. The patient's cultural attitudes towards pain and illness behavior.

At the Medical Center Hospital of Vermont, the Behavioral Medicine Service uses a clinical algorithm to assist the evaluation of patients with chronic pain (see Figure 19.2).

When dealing with self-limiting illness, acute injury, or surgery, it is appropriate for the physician to take an unidimensional approach to pain management. The standard treatment for pain, for example, includes immobilization and medication. But when the peripheral painful stimulus persists, or when much is to be gained from the sick role, psychosocial factors begin to dominate the clinical picture. In those circumstances, the biopsychosocial approach to diagnosis and management is indispensable.

1. WHAT IS THE PERIPHERAL STIMULUS NOW? IN THE PAST?
   a. Obtain old records.
   b. Interview family members.
   c. Determine what the past stimulus has been.

2. WHAT MAKES IT BETTER OR WORSE?
   a. Record patient's amount of personal behavior, thoughts, and feelings
   b. Record patient's and family's account of family member's behavior
   c. Examine environment for physical stressors
   d. Explore patient's life situation
   e. Identify reinforcers

3. IS THE PAIN CONSISTENT WITH THE PERIPHERAL STIMULUS?
   (If yes, go to #4; if no, go to #4 and #5.)

4. DOES THE PATIENT DO EVERYTHING POSSIBLE TO MAKE IT BETTER?
   (If yes, go to #6; if no, go to #5, then #6.)

5. WHAT ARE THE POSSIBLE CAUSES?
   a. Psychiatric disorder
      • depression
      • anxiety
      • somatoform disorder
      • drug addiction
   b. Personality type and psychological factors
   c. Psychological factors
      • dependency
      • security
      • revenge
   d. Social factors
      • job
      • income
      • family

6. HAVE ALL TREATMENT STRATEGIES BEEN REVIEWED?
   a. Peripheral stimulus
      • physical therapy
      • surgery, anesthesia, transcutaneous nerve stimulation
   b. Perception and coping
      • analgesics, antidepressants, sedative-hypnotics
      • psychophysiologic treatment: relaxation hypnosis, biofeedback
      • coping and adaptation: psychotherapy

FIGURE 19.2
Chronic pain evaluation

Peter, the 24-year-old maintenance man with multiple fractures (Case 3.23), illustrates this point. When narcotics are given on request for a period of time, the patient is likely to complain more frequently. If, as in this case, getting and giving drugs becomes entangled in a struggle for control and autonomy and the struggle arouses latent hostility and mistrust toward authority, then it is likely that pain will be exacerbated. In these circumstances, the psychiatrist can be an invaluable collaborator in planning immediate and long-range management.

Immediate management

What are the principles of immediate management planning for pain?

Principles for managing acute pain

1. Identify the peripheral stimulus. Alleviate it as much as possible, for example by immobilization, heat and cold, anti-inflammatory agents, elevation, local analgesia, or peripheral nerve block.
2. Review medication and develop a rational plan for adequate analgesia. For example, the following plan is useful for patients in chronic pain who are dependent on narcotics. Over a 24-hour period, prescribe the amount of analgesic the patient requests for relief of pain; but take the total dose required and divide it into equal doses to be given at intervals that approximate the duration of effective action of the particular medication. Thus, if 80 mg of morphine sulfate is required, the clinician might prescribe 15 mg every four hours. Do not wake the patient during the night to give medication. Gradually reduce the dose by 10% a day, or more rapidly, if appropriate.
3. Identify and modify anxiety-provoking stimuli: relatives, difficult staff relationships, problematic roommates, financial worries, and so on.
4. Treat anxiety: use medication initially, then train the patient to relax. Relaxation will also reduce muscle tension.
5. Consider using hypnosis to modify pain and facilitate relaxation.
6. Use cognitive therapy (see chapter 12) to modify misconceptions about the illness and to encourage the patient to develop more optimistic and collaborative attitudes to treatment.
7. Enlist support from consultee, staff, and family.
8. Without compromising therapeutic goals, give the patient as much control as possible over decisions; but be sure the decisions are in the patient's best interest.
9. Avoid sedative-hypnotics. Use low doses of sedating antidepressants instead. Sedatives accumulate causing side-effects that confuse the clinical presentation, make the patient drunk and difficult, and prevent the patient from cooperating in rehabilitation.

Long-term management

What are the principles of planning for chronic pain?

Psychosocial approaches to the alleviation of chronic pain

1. Narcotics are a problematic treatment for patients with chronic pain. Tolerance is predictable, the drugs becoming increasingly ineffective, forcing the patient to request more and more for less and less relief. Operant conditioning is almost inevitable; patients soon learn they must clamor to justify relief. Narcotics should be used only temporarily for the alleviation of acute exacerbations of pain.
2. Psychophysiologic techniques such as relaxation can counteract the augmentation of pain by anxiety and muscle spasm.
3. Hypnosis can facilitate relaxation, dispel anxiety, and modify the patient's emotional reaction to pain.
4. Distraction, the pacing of activities, and a carefully designed exercise plan can be helpful.
5. The cooperation of the family and place of employment are critical in managing the inevitable social consequences of chronic pain. The consultation psychiatrist, while often not directly involved in long-term management, can facilitate matters by contributing to the plan before discharge. A vicious cycle thus can be broken. (See Case 14.1 in chapters 14 and 15.) The psychiatrist should be aware of the local behavioral medicine or pain centers specializing in management of difficult cases.
6. Close monitoring for depression is required. Depression is a common complication as well as a precipitating or perpetuating factor in chronic pain.

The management of delirium

The psychiatrist frequently encounters delirium in hospital patients. After evaluation, the following strategic plan should be considered:

The strategic management of delirium

1. Remedy the underlying causes of the delirium.
2. Control agitation and its common sequelae. Begin with low doses of a neuroleptic. In an older person, prescribe haloperidol 0.5 mg at noon and 6 P.M., with 0.5 mg every 30 minutes for agitation as needed. Be prepared to change medication if a regimen fails or its side effects become troublesome.
3. Keep the environment well-lighted and free of confusing stimuli.
4. Have orienting calendars and familiar and friendly objects at hand.
5. Maintain continuity of staff.
6. Explain things simply; repeat your explanations.
7. Do not shout; the patient can usually hear quite well.

8. If the patient is easily distracted, retain the patient's attention by holding and pressing the hand, while keeping close eye contact.

Systems management

The psychiatrist must evaluate how the medical system influences illness behavior, a subject discussed at length in chapter 3. Sometimes, the psychiatrist must intervene to modify a nontherapeutic (or even dangerous) milieu in a hospital ward. Group meetings with the staff and individual discussions with head nurse, chief physician, or administrator can improve ward communication and initiate planning to ameliorate problems.

Case 19.7

■ On an intensive care unit, Leah, a 23-year-old woman with severe burns, screams most of the time she receives treatment in Hubbard tanks. Despite kindly, meticulous nursing, Leah is sour and hypercritical toward the staff. Their reactions vary; some are angry, others hurt. Some frankly refuse to care for Leah, placing a greater burden on those who do. Eventually, the staff become demoralized. Sick days increase.

The consultant psychiatrist helps the staff develop a protocol for managing medication and providing care in short shifts. He establishes a weekly meeting with the nurses to help them understand and cope with the hostility Leah engenders in them. ■

Case 19.8

■ Nan, a 42-year-old woman, has just been admitted after an apparently accidental overdose of methotrexate, which she has been taking for psoriasis. Nan is antagonistic to the staff and her physician, who requests psychiatric consultation. The nurse tells the psychiatrist there is rumor of a lawsuit: it is said there was a "mix up" in the instructions on the label of the bottle of methotrexate prescribed for the patient.

Nan reveals to the psychiatrist that she was enraged when her doctor, whom she had always trusted, would accept no responsibility for the error. A further interview reveals a history of similar "rifts" with other physicians. Nan alludes in passing to an alcoholic father who was lovable but totally unreliable.

The psychiatrist calls the consultee and advises him to spend time with Nan to review matters and reestablish a therapeutic alliance. Though hesitant to do so, on the advice of legal counsel, the physician decides he will discuss the situation with the patient. He acknowledges to her that he might have contributed to the mix up. At first, Nan expresses annoyance at the psychiatrist for breaching confidentiality; but she has begun to regain confidence that her doctor is truly concerned for her. She leaves the hospital, recovers uneventfully, and does not pursue legal action. ■

Case 19.9

■ A psychiatrist is called to consult on Mort, a 35-year-old man with chronic low back pain, who has already had two surgical operations for ruptured lumbar discs. Mort is addicted to methadone, has lost 40 pounds weight, and has suffered a recent bout of pneumonia. As part of the management plan, the psychiatrist collaborates with the patient and company management to develop a schedule that allows Mort to lie flat for three 30-minute periods every day. He also orders for Mort a special chair that provides lumbar support. ■

Summary

Epidemiologic research has established that psychosocial factors influence disease, illness, and illness behavior. Psychosomatic medicine and behavioral medicine have each contributed to our understanding of the nature of this influence, and the neurosciences have begun to elucidate the underlying biological mechanisms. Meanwhile, technology has improved the survival rate of many formerly fatal illnesses, only to leave patients in the hospital for prolonged periods or return them to the community with chronic disability. These social trends have created the need for a psychiatrist who can synthesize biopsychosocial knowledge and apply it to the clinical practice of medicine. Modern consultation-liaison psychiatry has emerged in response.

Consultation-liaison is arduous. The consultant may be frustrated by erratic referral and by some consultees' poor acceptance of psychiatric recommendations (Billowitz and Friedson, 1978–79). The psychiatrist must also cope with patients' misconceptions of and resistance to psychiatry.

On the other hand, consultation-liaison is facilitated because the hospital concentrates many diagnostic services and provides to the discerning clinician a wealth of information from chart, staff and family.

The consultant psychiatrist encounters a wide range of psychiatric diagnoses in the hospital and deals with problems related to family, physician, staff, and institutional systems. Clinical work requires clear aims, goals, strategy and tactics.

The psychiatrist who acquires diagnostic data from consultee, staff, chart, and past records can develop preliminary hypotheses and plan tactics to focus subsequent interviews and examinations. Interviews must be conducted in a variety of clinical settings with patients who have different medical illnesses and levels of pain, distress, and awareness. Special diagnostic procedures are required. The psychiatrist must also be able to assess the effect of the ward milieu on the patient and modify it when necessary.

Selected Readings

For a thorough review by experienced clinicians of the problems encountered by psychiatrists in the general hospital, the reader is referred to Hackett and Cassem (1978), *Handbook of General Hospital Psychiatry*. Lipowski, Lipsitt, and Whybrow's (1977) *Psychosomatic Medicine* comprehensively reviews the origins and status of the key concepts in psychosomatic medicine.

Kimball's (1981) *The Biopsychosocial Approach to the Patient* reviews psychosomatic medicine, illustrating its points with excellent clinical examples.

Theoretical and practical papers in Strain's (1981) *The Medically Ill Patient* review the application of current knowledge in psychosomatic medicine and neuroscience to medically ill patients. The papers in Kimball's (1979) *Liaison Psychiatry* cover much the same ground, while tracing some of the important ideas that have influenced the development of liaison psychiatry. Lipowski (1979, 1983) hails the historical development of the present practice of consultation-liaison psychiatry.

McKegney and Beckhardt (1982) comprehensively review research in consultation-liaison psychiatry.

Keefe and Blumenthal's (1982) *Assessment Strategies in Behavioral Medicine* reviews the techniques of assessing many clinical problems a consultation-liaison psychiatrist confronts in the general hospital setting.

20

Primary care

Introduction

The high incidence of psychosocial problems in primary care

The family practitioner provides initial care to more than half of all patients who seek help for psychiatric disorder and emotional problems (Regier, Goldberg, & Taube, 1978). About half of all primary-care patients have psychiatric disorder or disability (Rosen et al., 1972). A disproportionate amount of a physician's time is spent in the care of these problems (Gardner, 1970). A recent survey of family practice indicates that 33% of all diagnoses are of psychosocial nature (Cassata & Kirkman-Liff, 1981).

This chapter reviews how the nature, setting, and personnel of primary care medicine influence the clinical enterprise when psychological problems are at stake.

The advantages and constraints of the setting

The following characteristics apply to primary care, particularly family practice:

The characteristics of primary care

1. The physician deals with patients in all stages of the life cycle.
2. The physician is involved in a continuum from health, through illness and disease, to death.

431

3. The relationship between patient and physician is multidimensional.

4. Primary care demands an appreciation of the patient's family and community.

Life-span care

The opportunity for preventive intervention

Family physicians and pediatricians have a unique opportunity to influence psychiatric disorder and psychosocial problems. The enlightened physician might ask, when treating a child: "What advice can I give now or what intervention could I undertake to prevent disorder in the future?"

Opportunities for timely intervention

There are milestones in the development of psychiatric disorder. The identification of excessive drinking in a young adult, for example, may lead to treatment that averts the marital discord and erratic parental care resulting from this disorder, that in turn predispose a child reared in such circumstances to later psychiatric disorder (see Case 20.7). The effective management of a dying patient, for example, can ease the distress of those who are bereaved and prevent permanent psychological damage due to unresolved grief.

Early points in the natural history of psychiatric disorder

As the understanding of different psychiatric disorders improves, the manner of their development will be clarified. Consider, for example, current perspectives regarding panic disorder with agoraphobia (Sheehan, 1982a). Panic disorder typically begins with an episode of acute anxiety and evolves into a web of psychophysiologic symptoms, maladaptive coping, and social complications. Many patients with panic present first to a family practitioner, who commonly prescribes benzodiazepines and offers supportive psychotherapy. Though this treatment regimen generally produces temporary relief, the syndrome progresses inexorably, and the treatment, itself, can have serious complications such as benzodiazepine dependency. Fearful of panic attacks, patients begin to avoid the situations they fear might provoke them. Eventually, patients become too afraid to leave the house. The ineffectiveness of treatment and the inevitable losses (jobs, relationships, self-esteem) can lead to depression and suicide, or chronically maladaptive behavior. Helen, the 35-year-old woman with panic disorder discussed in chapter 16 (Case 16.6), illustrates the natural history of this syndrome. The appropriate treatment of these patients is necessarily comprehensive, combining pharmacotherapy, relaxation therapy, cognitive-behavioral psychotherapy, and dynamic psychotherapy.

The continuum of health states

Changing risky lifestyle and habits

Primary-care physicians are concerned with health, illness, disease, and death. They promote good health by advising their patients about health and persuading them to change risky or maladaptive behavior. For example, they may help or advise their patients to:

1. Stop smoking.
2. Reduce cholesterol intake.
3. Exercise more.
4. Avoid stress.
5. Plan pregnancies.
6. Plan nutrition.
7. Breast feed their babies.
8. Learn the mechanics of the back.

The primary-care physician as an educator

In these and other circumstances, knowledge about the patient's personality and coping style helps the physician implement brief interventions to correct distorted thinking and obviate noncompliance.

Physicians assume they will care for illness and disease, but many do not appreciate that death is a biopsychosocial event requiring comprehensive management. The family of dying or deceased patients needs help, as does the

Bereavement counseling

primary patient. Bereavement counseling can avert psychosocial disorder and physical disease in survivors (see chapters 3 and 5).

The multidimensional nature of the doctor–patient relationship

Physicians caring for critically ill, hospitalized patients can treat them as a captive audience. Not so the primary-care physician who must balance a complex set of coincidental relationship models. Freeman and Sack (1979) have described several different relationship models relevant to primary care, including the following:

Relationship models that operate in the doctor–patient relationship

1. The biomedical model, in which the physician provides care based on medical science. This model alone is inadequate in primary-care settings because it ignores other dimensions of human functioning critical to medical care.
2. The psychoanalytic model, in which the relationship between patient and physician is affected by reciprocal transference reactions that originate in the protagonists' early relationships with parental figures.
3. The fiduciary model, in which the physician, as an expert, acts on the patient's behalf, while the patient is expected to defer to a superior authority.
4. The market model, in which patient and doctor are free to choose each other and contract for care on a fee-for-service basis.
5. The professional model, in which the doctor defers to a code of ethics which guides professional relationships.
6. The institutional model, in which the doctor has an allegiance to an institution, such as the Veterans' Administration or a Health Maintenance Organization.
7. The social control model, in which the doctor assumes responsibility for the

public good, if necessary against the wishes of the patient, as in reporting infectious disease or detaining dangerous patients.

8. The ritualistic model, in which the physician provides care based on rituals or vogue rather than science, as when all babies are delivered in hospital delivery rooms or when psychiatrists avoid physically examining their patients.

Every doctor–patient relationship reflects one or more of these models. Primary-care physicians should understand the relevance of these models to clinical planning. Consider for example, the predicament of a family physician who is required by law to report the venereal disease of a long-standing patient who is also a friend.

The family and community context

The physician who cares for all members of a family and knows the local community has four advantages:

The advantages of knowing the family and community

1. By virtue of a physician's special authority, he or she has access to information about private matters or community forces that could influence the predisposition, precipitation, perpetuation or prognosis of biopsychosocial disorder.
2. The physician may already have the trust of the patient and family.
3. The physician may know the patient's characteristic coping style, illness behavior, and life history.
4. The physician can follow a patient's psychological problems while ostensibly treating a physical disorder.

Despite these advantages, family and community pose three potentially serious hindrances to the effective treatment of psychiatric disorder in the primary-care setting.

Disadvantages to primary medical care caused by family and community factors

1. The relationship between physician and patient can be so close that the therapeutic frame necessary for effective psychotherapy may be virtually impossible to achieve. The patient may be a family member, friend, lawyer, golf partner, or even the doctor's doctor.
2. The doctor may be perceived as having divided loyalties, resulting in distrust that blocks open discussion of marital conflict: "If I tell him this, he might tell my husband when he goes fishing with him."
3. The setting is not conducive to regular visits at a fixed time since a fee cannot be charged that is commensurate with overhead costs.

The next case illustrates these points.

Case 20.1

■ Joan, a 32-year-old married legal secretary, tearfully tells her family doctor about her husband's dwindling affection. Her husband, Bill, a local policeman, has attended the clinic occasionally in the past for insurance examinations and minor ailments. Reluctantly, he agrees to an appointment with his wife.

At the joint interview, Bill expresses annoyance at Joan's irritability but insists he is committed to the marriage. When Joan stridently accuses Bill of lying, the doctor wonders whether Bill's complaints about her irritability have been correct. He reflects on this to Joan, who responds that since the doctor is a man he would not understand her point of view anyway.

Joan temporarily ceases her attendance. Bill, meanwhile, is conducting a secret love affair which he cannot discuss with anyone, despite his guilt and feeling of responsibility. Sensing Bill's withdrawal, Joan becomes despondent and threatens suicide.

Worried, Bill divulges his problems to another physician, who inquires why he had not previously sought help. Bill reveals that while he liked his former physician, he was concerned that the doctor might be too sympathetic toward his wife and therefore unable to help him. ■

Diffuse family boundaries and ethical quandaries

Such dilemmas abound in family practice. The high divorce rate, for example, has confounded the definition of *family* to the extent that the boundaries of many families are diffuse and ill-defined. Traditional doctor–patient loyalties can be strained by ambiguities and ethical quandaries.

Case 20.2

■ Sam, a young family physician, has recently established a new practice. He applies to the local bank for a home mortgage and for a business loan to build an office attached to his home.

Shortly thereafter, Sam sees in his office Vivian, a 40-year-old woman who complains of headaches. Vivian asks Sam to renew her prescription for fiorinal (a commonly used prescription drug containing a sedative, an analgesic, and caffeine) and diazepam.

Though uneasy with the diagnosis of migraine, Sam renews the prescriptions, but only for one week. He schedules Vivian to return for a complete history and physical examination; but just before the appointment, she calls to cancel and request further medication refills. This sequence repeats itself twice.

Even more uneasy, Sam learns from his staff that Vivian is the bank vice-president's wife and is rumored to be alcoholic. Against his better judgment Sam decides to refill the prescription, this time for 2 months.

The same weekend, still uneasy, he discusses the case with a visiting friend and colleague. Sam becomes acutely aware that his personal interests have influenced his management of the case, perhaps to the patient's detriment. He must now decide: should he reverse his decision and insist on good standards of care? If he does, he might lose the loan. Or, should he continue to fill prescriptions for the patient despite his compromised situation? ■

Clinical problems in the primary-care setting

Why is mental disorder so prevalent in primary care? There are several reasons:

Reasons for the prevalence of psychosocial problems in primary care

1. All the mental disorders described in DSM-III are seen in family practice, primary care medicine, and pediatrics.
2. Patients with psychiatric disorders that present with physical symptoms (e.g., somatoform disorder) usually seek care initially from primary-care physicians and not mental health professionals.
3. Many people seek help for life crises and life-style problems involving personal relationships, physical disorders associated with life-style, and the physical problems that are influenced by psychosocial factors (Houpt et al., 1980).

Opportunities for the primary-care physician to intervene

The primary-care physician should decide to what extent he or she is prepared to care for psychosocial problems. In the absence of clinical training, the extent of involvement is usually determined by the attitude and personality of patient and physician. However, the family physician has the opportunity to intervene in a broad spectrum of individual and family matters, each influenced by biopsychosocial factors and each carrying risk of later psychiatric disorder. Consider the following examples:

Case 20.3

Sexual dysfunction

■ A family practitioner notes that Nathaniel, a 65-year-old retired farmer, has checked "sexual dysfunction" on the history form. Further inquiry reveals Nathaniel has been impotent since his wife had surgery for prolapsed bladder, 3 years previously. After an appropriate history and physical examination, secondary erectile dysfunction is diagnosed: Nathaniel feared hurting his wife after surgery and his erection failed during their initial attempt at intercourse. Fear of failure then perpetuated erectile dysfunction. Practitioner and consulting psychiatrist jointly provide 10 sessions of sexual counseling. The couple's sexual functioning is restored and improved, and marital communication generally enhanced. ■

Case 20.4
Family planning

■ Before they have children, a couple in their mid-twenties ask about the transmission of diabetes, which runs very strongly in the wife's family. The physician outlines the genetics of this condition. He also helps them articulate their uncertainty about the marriage. ■

Case 20.5

Prenatal counseling

■ Jill, a young pregnant woman, is anxious about impending motherhood. The physician notes that she intends to bottle feed her baby. This surprises him, for he thought her to be up-to-date and well-informed. Inquiry reveals Jill would prefer to nurse the baby, but her husband opposes it, citing his mother's aversion to breast feeding. Subsequently, in joint interview, the couple use this issue to renew lapsed communication about another imminent change: Jill's mother has been more interfering lately, as she prepares for her first grandchild. ■

Other opportunities for effective intervention include:

1. Development assessment.
2. Marital tension.
3. Child rearing.
4. Learning disability.
5. Adolescent problems.
6. Contraception.
7. Drug abuse.
8. Life stress.
9. Adjustment to illness.
10. Illness behavior.
11. Death and dying.
12. Grief.

The primary-care physician knows the family and community in which these problems occur. This is the natural domain of the primary-care physician. Few of these patients attend a psychiatrist initially.

The aims of clinical practice in primary care

The need for psychological sophistication in managing severe physical disease

With respect to the care of psychosocial problems, the mission, aims, plans, and tactics of primary care may not be formally articulated. Unlike the settings discussed in other chapters, primary care has aims beyond the provision of psychiatric care, but even desperately ill patients who require the advanced biomedical technology of biomedicine may need psychosocial intervention. Consider, for example, the patient dying of cancer, the noncompliant patient with myocardial infarction, and the brittle adolescent diabetic. All these problems are associated with psychosocial disturbance that may affect compliance, response to treatment, and the health of other family members. The primary-care physician should be trained to provide comprehensive care to all patients and to involve allied specialists judiciously.

Mission

The mission of a family practice clinic providing all the medical care to a rural community might be: To provide comprehensive medical services to patients and to the community as a whole. The mission of an urban primary-care internist might be: To provide comprehensive primary-care and uncomplicated hospital care to all adults in the practice and to consult to associated medical facilities.

Aims

The rural practice might aim:

1. To provide comprehensive biopsychosocial care to all patients and their families.

2. To provide medical consultation to such community institutions as schools, nursing homes, social welfare department, courts and police, and the local community mental health center.

The aims of the general internist might be:

1. To provide comprehensive biopsychosocial care to all adults in the practice.
2. To provide consultation to the local nursing home.

Plans

General plans facilitate aims. For example, to facilitate the aim of providing biopsychosocial care, a family practice might plan:

1. To develop a charting system that includes a biopsychosocial data base.
2. To appoint a social worker to assist with psychosocial assessment and counseling.
3. To design a billing system that allows for psychotherapeutic intervention.
4. To develop an alliance with a general psychiatrist and a mental health center for providing inpatient and ambulatory services to patients with psychiatric disorder.
5. To develop alliances with social welfare and the Visiting Nurses Association to provide effective home services.

Clinical plans might include:

1. Designing clinical protocols for the assessment and management of common psychosocial disorders and problems in living.
2. Completing a genogram (Jolly, Froom, & Rosen, 1980) on all new patients (see the section on assessment in this chapter).
3. Completing a diagnostic net, flow chart, formulation, problem list, and goal-oriented management plan on all complex patients.
4. Preparing a biopsychosocial problem list on every patient.

Tactics

Tactics are the specific actions required to implement plans. Administrative tactics to implement the plan to record genograms might include:

1. Designing a form to record genograms.
2. Using standard notation.
3. Placing the form under the problem list on the inside of the front cover of each patient's chart.

Clinical tactics might include:

1. Recording a genogram at the end of each comprehensive history and physical.
2. Obtaining a genogram during the initial evaluation of all psychiatric disorders and psychosocial problems.

Protocols and algorithms

Equivalent aims, strategies, and tactics can be developed for all aspects of the biopsychosocial assessment and comprehensive management of primary-care patients. Protocols and algorithms are particularly useful in this setting. They enable the family doctor to be systematic while dealing with problems encountered relatively infrequently.

Special features of the diagnostic process and management planning

Diagnosis and management are continuous

Diagnosis and management interdigitate in all clinical settings. This is especially true in primary care, where time constraints and the patient's expectations may demand symptom management before diagnostic resolution. Other factors influence the clinical process in primary care:

1. Patients may not acknowledge personal problems.
2. Patients often present with hidden agendas.
3. Diagnosis relies on the patient's cooperation.
4. Diagnosis usually occurs over a series of brief visits.
5. Diagnosis requires an understanding of health, normal coping, illness, and illness behavior.
6. Diagnosis requires an understanding of the family and community.
7. Psychiatric disorder and psychosocial problems often present with physical symptoms.
8. A narrow biomedical doctrine impedes comprehensive care.
9. Primary care is pragmatic.
10. Primary care is multimodal.

Each of these factors in the clinical process will be discussed in turn.

Failure to acknowledge personal problems

Emotional disorder is detected in the context of general health care

In primary care, the diagnosis and management of emotional disorder occur within the context of general health care. The physician may note the symptoms and signs of psychosocial problems or psychiatric disorder in patients who seek care for physical complaints or reassurance about their health, for example, in an insurance examination or yearly health check.

Case 20.6

■ Orvil, a 52-year-old man, asks his doctor for a health insurance examination. There are no significant findings except for slight hand tremor and the odor of alcohol on his breath. The doctor does not mention his concern about alcohol abuse but decides to evaluate Orvil's drinking habits at a later date. Within a year, Orvil is admitted to the hospital for appendectomy. Four days later, he goes into delirium tremens resulting from alcohol withdrawal. ■

The strategy and technique of personal inquiry

The physician must consider how to inquire about personal matters that the patient has not acknowledged. Ill-timed or clumsy probing can rupture the therapeutic alliance; but by taking the easy course and avoiding the issue, the physician may be neglecting a medical time-bomb.

Hidden agenda

Nonphysical reasons for attending

Barsky (1981) outlines some of the more obscure, nonbiomedical reasons for which patients see their doctors. Amongst them are the following:

1. Life stress.
2. Psychiatric disorder.
3. Social isolation.
4. The need for information.
5. To seek help for someone else (e.g., spouse or child).

Clinical alerts that indicate the need for psychosocial inquiry

Barsky suggests that the physician should be alerted to inquire about psychosocial factors in the following circumstances:

1. When the patient suffers inordinate discomfort. The patient may distort or be confused about the nature of the illness.
2. When the biomedical diagnosis is already well-established or trivial and diagnosis is not the issue. The patient's fundamental need may be different from what is initially requested.
3. When the patient is dissatisfied with present or past medical care. Inquiry into the circumstances may reveal other agenda.
4. When the patient attends without apparent change in physical health. A recent life stress may be behind the visit.
5. When the patient attends more frequently than expected for a minor disorder or presents again and again with trivial complaints.

Diagnosis requires cooperation

The need for compliance with diagnostic procedures

The dangers of referral

The physician relies on cooperation during the diagnostic process. Patients are expected to report symptoms accurately and to comply with diagnostic procedures. Behavioral medicine techniques, such as the patient's recording of symptoms, require cooperation. If consultation is needed, the patient will be required to visit a psychiatrist in another office, hospital, or city. As mentioned in chapter 16, a request for consultation can provoke feelings of rejection or fear, and compliance may be poor. Thus, when appropriate, it is desirable to keep diagnosis and management within the primary-care practice.

The technique of diagnosis in successive brief visits

The goals of the initial visit

An initial visit to a family practitioner usually lasts 15 minutes or less. It is aimed at ruling out life-threatening pathology, relieving symptoms, and developing a relationship. Despite the brevity of the visit, a diagnosis must be entertained, and treatment, often of palliative or temporizing nature, provided. The doctor may then schedule further diagnostic visits as appropriate. Successive brief appointments can be closely spaced to provide support and to accumulate information. If the patient is already well-known to the physician, several brief notes may suffice.

The need for a longer psychodiagnostic interview

However, even a 30-minute interview, though usually long enough for categorical psychiatric diagnosis, is insufficient to assess the coping patterns and personality features important to successful intervention. It takes at least an hour to undertake a more detailed assessment and to provide the support needed in crisis.

Do not obscure diagnosis with premature treatment

Initial treatment should not be allowed to obscure diagnosis or put the patient at risk. Consider, for example, the patient who presents with depressed mood, insomnia, and agitation. Do not prescribe more than a few day's supply of benzodiazepine until you have confirmed or refuted the diagnosis of major depression and evaluated suicide risk. Antidepressant drug therapy can wait until then. Follow-up visits should be scheduled according to the patient's needs.

Health, illness, and sick-role behavior

Identify maladaptive or unhealthy coping styles and personal habits

The primary-care physician has an important role in illness prevention: to identify the personality types and coping styles that place patients at risk for illness, disease, and noncompliance. Physicians should be trained to include this assessment in their routine comprehensive evaluation of all patients. The following are examples of situational reactions or life-styles that could lead to psychiatric disorder:

1. Excessive drinking and inappropriate drug use.
2. Exposure to teratogens or poor nutrition during pregnancy.
3. Inappropriate child-rearing practices.
4. Type A personality, which is associated with driving, competitive ambition and an emphasis on deadlines.
5. Exaggerated denial of feelings following bereavement.
6. Confusion and impulsive behavior following divorce.

Illness behavior

Illness behavior and the sick role are reviewed in chapter 3. They affect the diagnostic process and management planning in all primary-care patients, including those with overt psychiatric disorder. The medical record should contain a place for recording this information (although there is no generally accepted nomenclature of health-related behavior). The diagnostic net is an initial step toward systematic record keeping.

The genogram

Assessment includes family and community

The primary-care physician, particularly the family practitioner, has more access than other physicians to the historical background and social context of the patient's illness. The medical record may contain a **genogram** (Jolly, Froom, & Rosen, 1980), which summarizes the patient's genetic background, significant illnesses and deaths of family members and the patient's reactions to them, and important past and current relationships. The genogram can guide the physician in planning an intervention that effectively mobilizes family resources (Sproul & Gallagher, 1982). The physician may also know patient and family through housecalls, community contact, and previous medical care and may know the community through having lived and practiced there.

The physical presentation of psychological distress

Chapter 10 describes how patients with physical disorder can present with symptoms of psychological dysfunction. Chapter 12 reviews the psychiatric disorders that commonly present with physical symptoms. In the primary-care setting, physical symptoms are often the presenting complaints of patients suffering from psychiatric disorder or struggling with psychosocial problems. For example:

Psychiatric disorders associated with physical symptoms

1. Patients with major depression often present without apparent depressive mood but with neurovegetative symptoms and signs. Chronic pain, weight loss, sleep disturbance, sexual dysfunction or excessive fatigue may dominate the clinical pattern.
2. Schizophrenic patients sometimes have vague or bizarre somatic complaints associated with delusions of persecution or bodily change.
3. Patients with anxiety disorders often present with such symptoms of autonomic arousal as palpitations or chest pain or with such physiological sequelae of hyperventilation as paresthesiae and light-headedness.
4. Drug and alcohol abuse underlie many medical problems.
5. Patients with somatoform disorders communicate emotional distress in physical terms. These patients take an inordinate amount of the physician's time because they provoke exhaustive but fruitless quests for physical disease. Early comprehensive diagnosis and management planning save time and money and avert iatrogenic complications.
6. Patients who are grieving or tense often have physical symptoms (*somatization*).

Case 20.7   ■ Four times during a 2-month period, Mrs. R. brings Ronnie, a 12-year-old seventh-grader, to the family practice clinic. Ronnie complains of abdominal pain. Other than an abdominal scar from a past appendectomy and mild epigastric tenderness to palpation, repeated examinations reveal no abnormality. At the third visit, Mrs. R. tells the resident that she is considering surgical consultation. Later, while reviewing the chart with her preceptor, the annoyed and perplexed resident notes that Ronnie's father, a heavy drinker for years, left the family 1 year ago. She schedules a 60-minute visit to take a psychosocial history.

Much useful information is revealed. The marriage was plagued from the start by Mr. R.'s erratic behavior and repeated desertions. Quite depressed since the most recent separation, Mrs. R. leans heavily on her son, not only for much of the "man's work" around the house, but also for emotional support.

The resident entertains the diagnosis of psychogenic abdominal pain and asks a consulting psychiatrist to review the case. The psychiatrist agrees with the preliminary diagnosis. To complete the formulation, he recommends that Mrs. R. record the timing and circumstances of each attack of pain and what she and Ronnie did to cope with it.

Reviewed 3 weeks later, the logs reveal that Ronnie often stays home from school in these circumstances. When interviewed alone, the boy mentions that he often lies awake worrying about his mother's health. Further inquiry reveals that Ronnie was hospitalized for appendicitis shortly after his father deserted the family on a previous occasion.

Psychiatrist and family practitioner formulate a dynamic diagnosis: the complaint of abdominal pain represents abnormal illness behavior derived from a past experience of surgery. Pain legitimizes Ronnie's desire to stay home when he is worried about his mother's well-being. He may blame himself for his parents' separation. His fear of his mother's fragility has prevented him from revealing his own anxiety.

The complete formulation is not communicated to Ronnie and his mother. Instead, a stress model is used to explain the symptoms. Ronnie and his mother are told that the pain is real, not imaginary, and that it is caused by worry, not disease. The analogy of muscle tension, fatigue, and pain is used. The rationale for treatment is presented as getting the worry out of Ronnie's stomach back into his head, where it belongs, then helping him deal with it properly. Mrs. R. is encouraged to send Ronnie to school despite pain if he has no fever. After one anxious telephone call on the following Monday morning, she is able to do so.

Further inquiry during the ensuing discussion supports the hypothesis that Mrs. R. suffers from a major depressive disorder. ■

In this case, the diagnostic process differs from that in a psychiatric clinic. By history, physical examination, and laboratory studies, the initial encounter aimed to exclude serious physical disorder. Despite repeated negative evaluations, a psychosocial diagnosis was not considered until the mother expressed her dissatisfaction by threatening to seek treatment elsewhere. The process is depicted in Figure 20.1.

The clinical process in Case 20.7 demonstrates several sins of omission:

Common flaws in the purely biomedical diagnostic process

1. Failing to search for further clues when no positive diagnosis was made.
2. Accepting a null hypothesis without hypothesizing alternative possibilities.
3. Failing to develop a diagnostic formulation.
4. Failing to evaluate the results of treatment, and instead relying on the patient to report either new symptoms or the failure to improve.

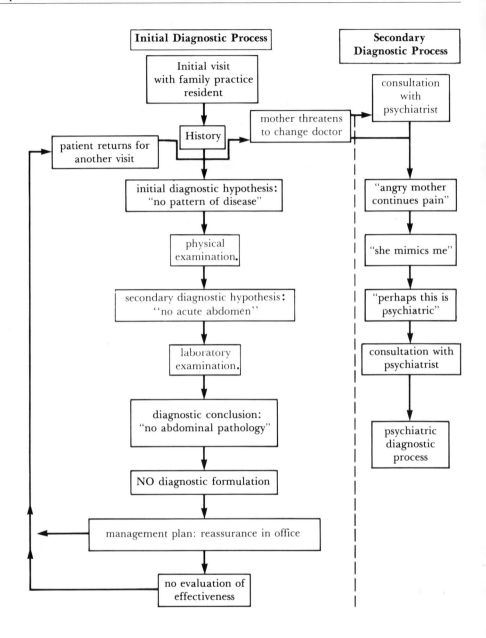

FIGURE 20.1
Psychiatric consultation in primary care: Ronnie (Case 20.7)

The inadequacy of the biomedical model

In Case 20.7, the resident failed to heed clear indications of the need for a psychosocial data base. Up to then, the resident's training had been in predominantly hospital settings, where a purely biomedical approach to diagnosis prevailed.

Training in the biopsychosocial model for primary care practitioners

After several years of practice, most physicians recognize the importance of psychosocial factors in illness behavior; but aside from Balint Groups (Balint, 1957) and similar, rather scattered efforts to convey the principles of modern psychiatry to primary-care physicians (Gallagher & Chapman, 1981), little systematic training in biopsychosocial medicine is available (Engel, 1982). This situation is in marked contrast to the scrupulous training of primary-care physicians in biomedical care.

The pragmatism of primary care

The need for diagnostic and management techniques that fit primary care

Primary-care physicians are not trained intensively in a restricted set of techniques, nor are they wedded to a unitary theory. They practice neither cardiac catheterization nor psychoanalysis. Given the brief patient contacts typifying office practice, they favor such techniques as pharmacotherapy that are expedient and fit the familiar biomedical model.

Modes of psychotherapy requiring regular appointments over a protracted time are not practical, for the physician must respond to a wide variety of clinical demands, often at a moment's notice. But techniques that can be applied during brief office visits, such as supportive or cognitive-behavioral psychotherapy, should be taught in primary-care training programs (Burns et al., 1983). Let us return to Ronnie, the 12-year-old boy with abdominal pain, to illustrate the point:

Case 20.7 (continued)

■ The resident does not share the complete diagnostic formulation with Ronnie and Mrs. R., but psychiatrist and resident design a management plan that fits the family practice setting.

Mrs. R.'s major depression responds well to antidepressant medication. She is encouraged to discuss her problems as a single parent. After her problems have been delineated, the resident helps her address each one in turn, beginning with the easiest. Consequently, Mrs. R. locates a day-care center for her preschool daughter, contacts a welfare social worker to help in financial planning, and begins job training at a vocational rehabilitation center.

At a meeting with his mother, sister, and the family practitioner, Ronnie is able to tell his mother how worried he is about her health. They agree to schedule a weekly evening meeting at home to communicate their individual concerns and administer the household. Ronnie bargains for time to participate in the social activities he has missed by staying home to protect his mother. Mrs. R. reassures Ronnie that she will attend the clinic for biweekly 15-minute appointments to get further counseling.

Ronnie's abdominal pain ceases, except for one episode coinciding with a favorite aunt's terminal illness. At that time, after examination reveals no biomedical disease, an adroit psychosocial history quickly reveals the family crisis. Ronnie is worried that his mother's grief signifies a return to her previous dysfunctional state. She, in turn, helps him distinguish her normal grief from the symptoms of the former depression. Effective communication is restored. ∎

The sequence of therapeutic results

In this case, psychiatrist and family practitioner collaborated. As a matter of urgency, Ronnie was sent back to school. Antidepressant medication and supportive psychotherapy relieved the mother's depression. She was then able to cope more effectively with Ronnie's separation anxiety and to take charge of her own life. Ronnie was given practical suggestions to normalize his adolescence. Mother and son begin to communicate more effectively.

A biopsychosocial grid

Table 20.1 is a Biopsychosocial Grid (Gallagher, 1982) representing the factors influencing symptom formation (see chapters 3, 4, 5, and 14). The grid helps the clinician comprehend how data important to several theories (biological, psychodynamic, and learning) relate, and it particularizes the cognition and emotion reflected by symptomatic behavior (Beck, 1976) (see chapter 12).

Using information from the diagnostic net, the physician categorizes physical, psychological, and social predisposing factors and precipitating stressors. Using the flow chart, the clinician can outline on the biopsychosocial grid how these factors influence the development of cognitive, affective, and behavioral responses. The psychotherapeutic interventions required become apparent.

Appropriate referrals

The patient can then be referred to the professional appropriate to that intervention. Thus, when psychodynamic psychotherapy is indicated it will not be attempted by a professional without adequate training.

Table 20.2 represents the grid used in planning psychotherapy for Ronnie and his mother. Note how the grid delineates stressors, thoughts, emotions, behavior, and consequences. Predisposing dynamic material is not indicated in this particular grid; but if unresolved predisposing conflicts interfere with cognitive-behavioral therapy, they can be considered and addressed, if required, in psychodynamic psychotherapy.

In Ronnie's case, the following sequence illustrates psychotherapeutic planning:

Stressor	*Thoughts*	*Emotions*	*Behavior*	*Consequences*
Mother's depression	Mother is fragile	Fear (of hurting her)	Avoids asserting himself or discussing feelings	Gets attention from mother
	I cannot leave her alone	Guilt	Misses school	Does not play with friends

TABLE 20.1
Biopsychosocial grid

	Predisposition	Stressors	Thinking	Emotions	Behavior	Consequences	Neuropsychiatric disorders
Physical	prophylactic psycho-pharmacology	biomedical treatment		psychopharmacology	psychopharmacology		psycho-pharmacology
Psychological		psychodynamic psychotherapy ←→		supportive psychotherapy	supportive psychotherapy		
		supportive psycho-therapy					
		cognitive-behavioral psychotherapy					
Social		behavior therapy	marital/family therapies		behavior therapy		

TABLE 20.2
Biopsychosocial grid, Peter (Case 20.1)

	Predisposition	Stressors	Thinking	Emotions	Behavior	Consequences	Neuropsychiatric disorders
Physical	previous appendectomy	puberty			provides support to mother	isolated from peers	
Psychological	pain experience; chronic anxiety and unresolved guilt about father's desertion	desire to be close to mother; fear of loss of mother	"I must be the man in the family"; "I am responsible for his leaving"	guilt; pain	complains of pain; stays home	medical attention; close to mother and reassured about mother's safety	
Social	father's alcoholism, unpredictability and desertion	mother's depression	"mother is fragile"	anxiety; fear of hurting mother	is unable to ventilate anxiety; desires to be with friends	isolated from peers	

The physician pursues the following successive therapeutic goals:

A sequence of thera-
peutic actions

1. Clarify Ronnie's distorted thoughts: "Your mother is not fragile; you will not hurt her by telling her what you think. You can safely leave her in the morning."
2. Modify the stressor by treating the mother's depression.
3. Eliminate the rewarding consequences of distorted thoughts, emotions, and maladaptive behavior: Ronnie is sent to school despite symptoms, thereby eliminating attention from mother and doctor.
4. Arrange for the reward of adaptive behavior: Ronnies's plan to play with friends is praised. His mother pays attention when he asserts his opinion or expresses his feelings.

The clinical process

A review of the clinical process in this case is instructive. The family practitioner became aware of the importance of psychosocial factors. The psychiatrist helped elucidate the psychosocial problem and recommended further evaluation. Subsequently, the family practitioner conducted the diagnostic family interview and intervened therapeutically to help mother and son communicate more directly.

The preventive poten-
tial of early psycho-
social intervention

It is difficult to predict how much the family's improvement will generalize to other areas of functioning. However, recalling the discussion of abnormal illness behavior in chapter 3, it is possible to conjecture the following complications if the mother's depression and the child's separation anxiety had remained untreated: continued depression; preoccupied, inadequate parental care; financial loss; alcohol abuse; medical illness; and even suicide. Meanwhile, Ronnie would have remained out of school, with devastating effects on academic progress and social development, and exposed to further unnecessary diagnostic procedures and laparotomy. As an adult, he would be likely to manifest continued abnormal illness behavior, for example, as somatoform disorder, or psychiatric disorder, such as agoraphobia, panic disorder, or dysthymic personality.

Multimodal care

The spectrum of dis-
orders in primary care
necessitates multidis-
ciplinary care

Primary care deals with life-style, the problems of living, psychiatric disorder, and combined physical and psychiatric disorder (Houpt et al., 1980). The treatment of such problems is provided by clinicians with different backgrounds – family physicians, psychiatrists, pediatricians, internists, social workers, psychologists and nurses, for example. Each setting has its own mix of clinicians. Each primary-care practitioner should strive to match the skills of different clinicians with the intervention required. Systematic biopsychosocial assessment and comprehensive management planning help the clinician specify the management required. Moreover, the practitioner's responsibility extends to the successful matching of a patient with a particular therapy and a clinician expert in that therapy.

The use of comprehen-
sive diagnosis in
multidisciplinary
management planning

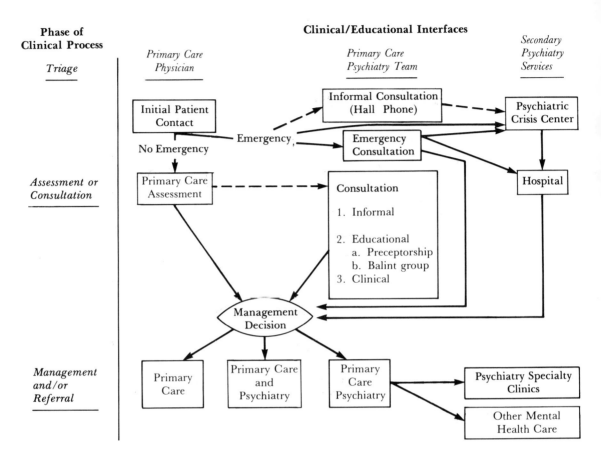

Phase of Clinical Process

Triage

Assessment or Consultation

Management and/or Referral

Clinical/Educational Interfaces

FIGURE 20.2
The psychiatric team in primary care

The coordination of psychiatry and primary care

In the College of Medicine of the University of Vermont, the Departments of Psychiatry and Family Practice have developed a model for clinical and educational collaboration (McMahon, Gallagher, and Little, 1983). The clinical process, depicted in Figure 20.2, shows how a psychiatrist can work with primary-care practitioners.

When patients are diagnosed, they are referred for appropriate treatment, preferably within the system. If necessary, external diagnostic consultation is sought, with the clear expectation that patient management will continue in primary care.

Intersystem linkage

Psychiatrists can facilitate external referral because they are familiar with mental health agencies. As a result of these intersystem links, patients are less likely to fall between the cracks. Susan (Case 17.1), the young woman with systemic lupus erythematosus discussed in chapters 17 and 18, illustrates coordinated care in a multidisciplinary primary-care setting.

**Case 17.1
(continued)**

■ A family physician is worried about his patient, Susan, a 32-year-old married woman with systemic lupus erythematosus. On her last visit, Susan seemed dissatisfied with her care; she looked more depressed than usual; and her blood pressure, 150/100, was unacceptably high. The physician decides to review her chart and revise the problem list.

The physician examines the problem flow sheets and notes that the hypertension, which formerly had been kept below 140/90 with hydrodiuril and methyldopa, has been fluctuating for 3 months between 165/110 and 140/85. He wonders why.

Susan's "depression/anxiety," a problem added to the list 6 months ago, has not improved despite a recent comment about "gains in assertiveness" by a nurse practitioner, who was providing supportive counseling. He considers this problem might need better definition.

Other progress notes reveal that in the past 2 months, Susan has made several unscheduled office visits and telephone calls to complain of headaches, fatigue, poor memory, and concern about a possible activation of her lupus (see Table 20.3).

TABLE 20.3
Susan's office visits 10/76–10/77 (Case 17.1)

10/ 2/76 – chest pain with palpitation treated with reassurance and antacid	3/11/77 – telephone call, "feeling funny"
	3/11/77 – counseling
	3/20/77 – hypertension
10/ 6/76 – no show	3/20/77 – counseling
10/15/76 – hypertension check	3/31/77 – counseling
10/24/76 – inquiries as to pregnancy	4/ 2/77 – conjunctivitis
10/29/76 – admitted to hospital with right retro-orbital headache and fever. Cardiogram, normal; CT scan, normal; blood culture, normal	4/15/77 – no show
	4/22/77 – counseling
	4/25/77 – headache; fiorinol, valium
	5/16/77 – hypertension
	5/27/77 – no show for counseling
11/ 5/76 – hypertension and back/buttock pain, thought to be secondary to multiple attempts at lumbar puncture treated with anti-inflammatory agents	6/13/77 – hypertension and wax removal, right ear
	6/17/77 – SLE and hypertension
	7/21/77 – counseling
	8/13/77 – counseling
11/10/76 – hypertension, amnesia, possible renal involvement: plans for memory testing and nephrology consult	8/19/77 – counseling
	8/26/77 – no show for counseling
	10/ 1/77 – migraine headache, hypertension, SLE
11/25/76 – phone call: headache, hypertension, sleep disturbance	10/ 6/77 – SLE, hypertension
12/12/76 – hypertension	10/22/77 – SLE, hypertension
12/20/76 – migraine headache	10/22/77 – foreign body removed (eye)
12/21/76 – refill compazine	10/23/77 – foreign body removed (eye)
1/22/77 – respiratory infection	11/ 1/77 – SLE, depression; consultation with SLE specialists
2/15/77 – upper respiratory infection	
2/18/77 – dislocated left shoulder, sent to Emergency Room for reduction	11/ 6/77 – SLE, hypertension, depression, headaches, fatigue, concern about medical judgment, continued marital difficulties; consultation-liaison psychiatrist
2/24/77 – hypertension, SLE, routine checks	
3/ 7/77 – hypertension, adjustment of chronic illness; plans for counseling by nurse practitioner	

The physician assures Susan that there is no evidence from physical examination and laboratory tests that the disease is active. Though Susan is somewhat relieved, the physician decides to schedule a 30-minute visit the following week. He plans to review Susan's progress in general and to discuss with her the possibility of consulting a rheumatologist and liaison psychiatrist at the health center.

The following Monday morning, Susan appears at the office, tearfully pleading for an appointment to get help for a headache she has had all weekend. Already overbooked, the doctor squeezes her in.

Susan's blood presure is 165/110. She cannot remember the details of the headache or whether she has been taking her antihypertensive medication regularly. She tearfully blurts out her fear that the doctor has "missed something." After all, hadn't his partner missed the diagnosis of lupus 3 years before?

Ruefully, the physician recalls his partner's extraordinary efforts to persuade Susan to consult a rheumatologist. Despite 18 months of negative laboratory inquiry, his partner had a hunch that there was a connection between Susan's repeated miscarriages and her other complaints, particularly polyarthralgia. When lupus erythematosus was finally diagnosed, her family, particularly her mother, had criticized the doctors for missing the diagnosis. "Here we go again," he thinks.

He glances at Susan's genogram (see Figure 20.3) and wonders whether problems with her husband and mother are stirring things up.

A screening physical and neurological examination uncover nothing new. Joints and skin show no abnormality. Cardiac examination reveals a systolic ejection click and a grade III/IV diastolic murmur at the upper left anterior chest, radiating to the apex. The murmur is of medium pitch, lasts through the diastolic phase, and is of plateau type. The same murmur was first noted during hospitalization 3 years ago. At that time, a thorough workup, including EKG, echocardiogram, and blood cultures, had been negative. Still uneasy, the physician diagnoses the headaches as tension-related, even though Susan has a history of migraine. He advises her to continue a regimen of regular rest and fiorinol. With Susan's permission, he requests consultation from two colleagues, a liaison psychiatrist who consults at the family practice and a rheumatologist at the medical center.

Susan's physician asks the psychiatrist to evaluate her behavior, mood, and adjustment to the illness and to recommend management. Subsequently, the psychiatrist reviews the progress notes, genogram, and hospital records.

The counseling notes contain valuable information about Susan's psychiatric history and illness behavior. She had complained persistently of memory lapses, which interfered with her daily activity but had no clear temporal pattern. Initially uncomfortable talking about herself, she eventually spoke of difficulty adjusting to the chronic illness. She also alluded to marital problems.

Susan and her husband had come from large families. Both wanted children, but Susan had not been able to carry a pregnancy to term without an exacerbation of lupus, leading to involvement of the central nervous system. After each miscarriage, Susan became depressed, a pattern which strained the marriage.

This combination of factors led to the hospitalization discussed in chapters 17 and 18 (Case 17.1). The notes indicated that Susan had unhappy memories of psychiatric hospitalization and an aversion to psychiatrists.

Susan realized she was too diffident toward her mother, husband, and others. Her father had died 4 years previously. Her mother had been unreasonably

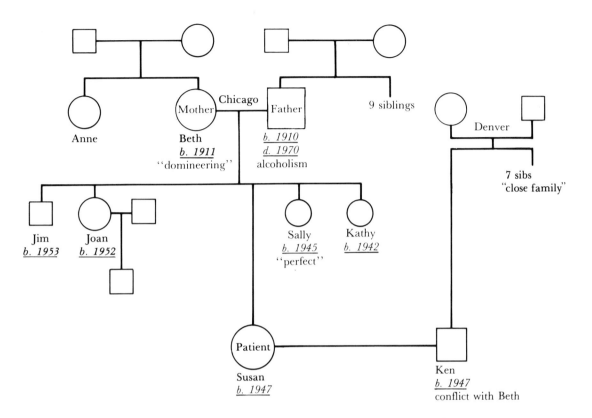

FIGURE 20.3
Susan's genogram (Case 17.1)

demanding since that time, expecting constant attention from her children. Because of conflict between her husband and her mother dating back to their marriage and exacerbated during her illness, Susan and her husband visited Chicago no more than once a year. Susan often felt "punished" by her mother's use of money to manipulate her family. Despite her mother's wealth, Susan had received nothing but occasional minor gifts, always with strings attached.

Two months before, Susan's husband opened a hardware store, an enterprise that has taken most of his time. Usually, he is working either at the store or in his office at home.

The psychiatrist concludes that the focus of Susan's counseling to date has been assertiveness training and emotional support. Having reviewed the notes, the psychiatrist next interviews the patient. Susan is a tall, fair-haired woman whose pale, rough skin and haggard face make her appear much older than 32. Susan looks ill, yet the interviewer is struck by her impeccable grooming and fashionable clothes. Her manner is polite, almost deferential. Although her conversation is cogent and fluent, she recalls events with difficulty, claiming poor memory.

TABLE 20.4
Diagnostic net: Susan (Case 17.1)

	Predisposition	Precipitation	Perpetuation	Pattern
Physical	• SLE • abortions ? CNS vasculitis	? worsening of SLE ? Fiorinol: sedation, regression ? Aldomet: depression • hypertension headaches	? Fiorinol: poor coping ? Aldomet: depression ? organic loss of memory function	• hypertension • fatigue • headache
Psychological	• memory disturbance since SLE • psychosis during SLE & after loss of child • always wanted children & can't have them ? low self-esteem *Coping style* Cognitive: denial (affect) vigilant focusing (physical symptoms) Behavioral: subassertive, avoids conflict, keeps busy	*Affect:* depression, anxiety ? grief (father's death, abortion) confusion about doctors' different opinions ? fear of abandonment by husband, mother, doctors *Cognition:* "I'm doomed." ? "I'm crazy." "I can't have babies."	? functional loss of memory ? attitude towards sex • conflict about pregnancy • minimization of emotion ? unresolved grief • fear of psychiatry *Behaviors* ? avoids grief dependency avoids referral maintaining behavior (memory aids, doctor visits, accepting gifts with "strings," from mother) capitulation subassertive behavior	• memory loss • depressed/anxious mood • minimization of conflict with husband over pregnancy • feeling of dependency *Behavior* no-shows at office ? noncompliance frequent contacts with medical system use of many doctors subassertive behavior

454

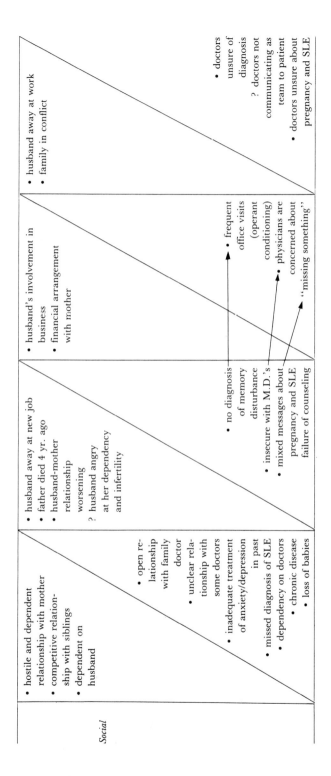

Childlike and tearful, Susan bemoans her mother's unfairness and her lost pregnancies. She is encouraged but frightened by the rheumatologist's suggestion that she try another pregnancy. Her gynecologist in Chicago thinks she might be able to have a baby if she moved there to be cared for by his high-risk team; but local gynecologists strongly disagree on the grounds that a further pregnancy might be fatal.

Susan refuses formal cognitive testing. Deciding that the highest priority is to establish a therapeutic alliance, the psychiatrist does not press the matter. He notes, however, that she is fully oriented, alert, fluent, coherent, and apparently neurologically intact. The impairment of short-term and long-term memory seems to be selective.

The psychiatrist's gentle, nonconfrontative strategy is effective. When the interview is finished, Susan schedules two further appointments, signs information release forms, and seems reluctant to terminate the conversation. ∎

Table 20.4 categorizes the data in a diagnostic net. Figure 20.4 is the flowchart that facilitates a dynamic diagnostic formulation. Table 20.5 presents the management plan in the form of goals addressed by diagnostic inquiry and therapeutic actions.

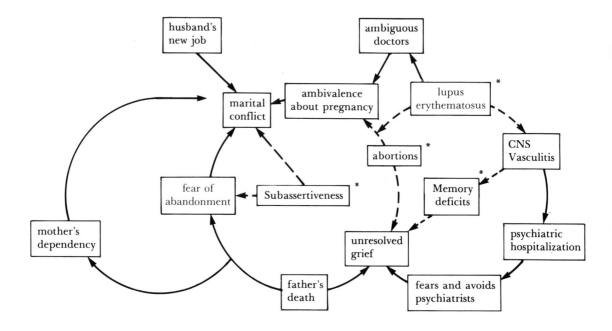

* Influence of predisposing factors represented by dotted lines.

FIGURE 20.4
Flowchart of problems: Susan (Case 17.1)

TABLE 20.5
Management plan: Susan (Case 17.1)

Pivotal problems	Goals	Treatment
1. Fear of psychiatric treatment.	1. Reduce fear and foster therapeutic alliance.	1. Schedule regular psychotherapy sessions for support and problem solving. 2. Empathic, directive stance.
2. Anxious, depressed mood.	1. Reduce medical uncertainty.	1. Schedule frequent office visits with physical and laboratory examinations when appropriate to reassure about the progress of disease.
	2. Clarify and modify stressors, particularly fear of abandonment.	1. Clarify roles of various physicians. 2. Enlist husband's participation in and support for the plan. 3. Encourage patient to set limits on mother's intrusive behavior.
	3. Increase control over anxiety.	1. Relaxation training.
3. Memory disturbance.	1. Clarify diagnosis.	1. Neuropsychological testing.
4. Marital conflict.	1. Modify perpetuating factors.	1. Explore the couple's individual feelings about abortions and pregnancy, SLE, family, etc. 2. Contract for marital therapy. 3. Recommend a more reliable work schedule for husband. 4. Set limits on mother's interference.

Long-Term Problems

1. Unresolved grief.	1. Mourn significant losses (father, babies, health).	1. Psychotherapy.
2. Subassertiveness and dependency.	1. Increase assertiveness and self-reliance.	1. Assertiveness training: learn new skills in relating to sisters, mother, husband, and doctor. 2. Encourage husband to reward her independence but not her sick role.
3. Ambivalence about pregnancy.	1. Resolve ambivalence.	1. Dynamic psychotherapy: focus on how religion, competition with siblings, her husband's anger, and oedipal issues with mother encourage a life-threatening pregnancy. 2. Encourage patient to seek prognostic clarity from doctors.

**Case 17.1
(continued)**

■ Susan is seen in individual psychotherapy by a male psychiatrist. The intermediate goal of establishing a supportive therapeutic alliance is difficult to achieve. Although Susan is eager to share her misery, she is also extremely angry at doctors who have been unable to give her babies, cure her terrible disease, and gratify her dependency needs. Because of her husband's recent "desertion" (to work), she is also very angry at men in general, an anger which spills out during interview. Susan experiences acute anxiety and abruptly leaves the office in tears, only to return when she has settled down, after 10 minutes.

The family practitioner and psychiatrist devise plans to reduce stressors and perpetuating factors immediately.

1. The system provides security, through the following goals:
   a. Clarify the tasks of all physicians involved. The family physician will attend to Susan's general health needs and provide support during regular office visits; the psychiatrist will work on Susan's depression and adaptation in psychotherapy; the rheumatologist will follow and advise on her systemic lupus when consulted by the family physician. Regular visits are scheduled. To return some control to her, Susan helps design this program.
   b. Enlist the husband's support for the plan and persuade him to reward Susan's independence and provide more support. The husband is interviewed and noted to be solid and responsible but angry at Susan's family. He is willing to participate.
   c. Set limits on Susan's mother's intrusiveness. Susan's ambivalent feelings about her mother (dependency and hostility) create anxiety when she attempts to resist her mother's interference. Ultimately, Susan benefits from role playing and rehearsing. This enables her to be more resolute and her husband rewards her with approval and attention.
2. The nature of Susan's memory disturbance must be determined. Once a strong therapeutic alliance is established, Susan agrees to neurological consultation and neuropsychiatric testing. The psychologist finds no organic memory disturbance and suggests that her memory losses are "manipulative." The psychiatrist diagnoses conversion disorder. However, he does not affront Susan's defenses but gently assures her that she has no permanent impairment and will gradually recover.
3. Susan's anxiety and depression must be relieved. Susan had learned some relaxation techniques in past. She practices these in the office and makes a tape to use at home.

Though treatment proceeds, Susan's relationship with the psychiatrist remains insecure and marked by hostile dependency. While completing a genogram with her, the psychiatrist notes that Susan concentrates on her family to the exclusion of her father. When her avoidance is noted, Susan becomes angry and tearful. The patient gradually relinquishes her defensive amnesia, and the psychiatrist explores, over several sessions, the events of her father's death. Susan expresses overwhelming feelings of loss, desertion, and anger, but she begins to recall some positive aspects of their relationship. Once she grieves for her father, her memory improves, and she becomes less anxious and depressed. She also begins to be more active in her marriage and her psychotherapy. She receives marital and sexual counseling for the sexual dysfunction secondary to chronic disease and emotional disturbance; her mixed feelings about pregnancy and birth control are clarified; she begins to accept the life-style changes necessitated by lupus; and she begins to come to terms with her inability to have children. Susan considers the possibility of developing other roles with children, begins to change her coping style from avoidance to tackling, separates emotionally from her mother, and stands up for herself with her husband.

Susan's lupus stabilizes and she accepts the disease. She chooses not to get pregnant but she avoids sterilization. Though her relationship with her mother is still problematic, she is much less dependent, and much more in control. Insurance runs out, so marital therapy is delayed until the following year. ■

A network of health care

The coordinated network of medical care described in this case assures continuity, comprehensiveness, specificity, and quality. Other administrative models have been developed to integrate mental health and primary care (Borus & Casserly, 1979; Adams et al., 1978; Pucees et al., 1983).

Summary

Primary care differs from other settings in which psychiatric disorders are recognized and treated. Primary care provides comprehensive care spanning the continua from health to disease and from conception to death. Primary care must be provided with an appreciation that the patient lives in a family and community and that the doctor–patient relationship is multidimensional.

The psychosocial problems encountered in primary care range from psychiatric disorder to the stresses of everyday life.

Though primary-care patients may need psychiatric care, they may not be seeking it when they visit the primary-care physician. Many patients attend with hidden agendas not directly related to their initial complaint. Diagnosis should include an assessment of illness and sick role behavior. The family and community factors contributing to the clinical problem should also be considered.

The primary-care physician should be aware that psychological disorder often presents with physical symptoms; a narrow biomedical model impedes comprehensive care. Primary-care physicians must be practical in their diagnostic procedures and management planning, and they should learn to coordinate consultants in a multidisciplinary team.

Selected Readings

Freeman, Sack, and Berger's (1980) *Psychiatry for the Primary Care Physician* is an excellent collection of papers about the presentation and management of the psychiatric and psychosocial problems in family practice.

Barsky (1979, 1981) has outlined some of the influences on illness behavior and (1979) succinctly reviewed psychiatric hypothesis-testing in primary-care settings.

Balint's (1957) classic description of his group meetings with general practitioners, *The Doctor, His Patient, and the Illness,* provides a psychoanalyst's perspective on the doctor-patient encounter in family practice.

21

The diagnostic encounter in child psychiatry: data gathering

Although the same fundamental strategy and tactics apply in all branches of psychiatry, three issues loom especially large in child psychiatry: the need to develop a relationship in order to understand a child, the need to understand current functioning from a developmental perspective, and the need to appreciate how the family interact. These considerations require the clinician to learn diagnostic techniques beyond those of adult psychiatry, and to add to the diagnostic net a third skein, the developmental, which interweaves with the biopsychosocial and temporal axes.

Differences from adult psychiatry

This chapter discusses the diagnostic encounter in child psychiatry and the methods by which a clinician gathers diagnostic information from parents, infants, children, adolescents, and others who are important in the case. Chapter 22 deals with the inquiry process, that is, the physical examination and special investigations used in child psychiatry. Chapters 23, 24, 25, and 26 are concerned with categorical diagnosis, the developmental axis, modes of treatment, case formulation, and management planning.

More specifically, chapter 21 discusses the following matters:

1. The clinical context of ambulatory child psychiatry.
2. Sources and methods of case referral.

460

3. The kinds of behavior problems that occasion referral.
4. Case intake and allocation.
5. Techniques of interviewing parents, observing infants, and interviewing children and adolescents.
6. The child mental status examination.
7. Clinical methods for the rapid screening of developmental level.
8. Family interviewing.

Need for a comprehensive evaluation

The term *child psychiatry* is a misnomer; the child is in continuous interaction with the social world, particularly the family. The need to view the patient from a comprehensive perspective is nowhere more apparent than when children and families are concerned. The following examples illustrate this point:

1. Many conditions manifest in childhood as psychological disturbance (attention-deficit disorder, for example) probably partly reflect physically determined developmental lags.
2. Overt neurological disorder such as epilepsy can present as a disruption of psychological processes.
3. Physical ill-health (acute infection, for example) generally has psychobehavioral consequences; social withdrawal, regressiveness, irritability, and lassitude are virtually universal.
4. Dysfunctions of information-processing and language will ultimately affect a child's self-concept and expectations of other people and the way the child relates to family, peers, and teachers.
5. Disturbances, distortions, or disruptions of early attachment due to deviant childrearing can affect physical health and development, the capacity to learn, self-esteem, personality development, and social competence.

In short, physical, psychological, and social factors are interwoven in every case.

The clinical context of child psychiatry

The different clinical contexts of child psychiatry

Child psychiatrists encounter patients in a number of settings: in pediatric wards; in consultation with community agencies; in association with lawyers and courts for investigating disputed child custody, child abuse, the termination of parental rights, and delinquency; and in the inpatient treatment of severely disturbed children and adolescents. For the most part, however, child psychiatrists diagnose and treat children and families in outpatient clinics or private offices. This chapter deals with the clinical process of child psychiatry in an ambulatory setting.

Team evaluation and solo practice

Psychiatrists who work in a clinic usually collaborate with child psychologists, social workers, and other clinicians; but even if a physician is in solo practice, the principles presented in this chapter apply. Some clinics have elaborate and extended diagnostic procedures; a social worker, for example, interviews the parents to obtain an extensive history of the presenting problem, previous health, early development, and family dynamics; a clinical psychologist administers tests for intelligence, school performance, and personality; and a child psychiatrist undertakes a series of diagnostic interviews with the adolescent or child.

The advantages of a team approach derive from the detailed information obtainable and the possibility of cross-validating clinical inferences. However, there are disadvantages. The traditional child guidance team is cumbersome and poorly adapted to urgent referrals. On the other hand, although solo practice is more flexible, there is a danger of intellectual isolation and stagnation. This chapter discusses the clinical process from the standpoint of a solo clinician who has access to allied clinicians when discretionary inquiry should be pursued or when collaborative treatment is indicated, but who is prepared to act alone when it is appropriate to do so.

Sources of referral

Families who attend a child mental health clinic usually come from a number of sources. The following list refers to 1 year of referrals to the Section of Child Psychiatry of the Medical Center Hospital of Vermont (in 1980–1981):

Self-referred	35.4%
From private physicians	23.8%
From schools	16.1%
From Department of Social Welfare & Juvenile Services	7.8%
From other sources in the Medical Center Hospital of Vermont	6.7%
From private psychiatrists	3.5%
From other sources	6.7%

Referral by parent

Why are children referred? Sometimes parents become aware of a child's emotional disturbance and seek help of their own accord. Sometimes they seek help preventively, during an emotional disruption such as divorce, for example.

Pediatric referral

Pediatricians and family practitioners are primary contacts for many patients. This is because emotional problems often present first with physical symptoms, because physical illness may cause psychological disturbance, and because some parents initially seek help from a primary contact physician for a clearly emotional disorder.

Case 21.1

■ On two occasions, Paula, an 11-year-old girl, was brought to a pediatrician's office for an attack of acute abdominal pain, headache, nausea, and vomiting. She had had several similar episodes during the previous 3 months and had been intermittently out of school for a total of 3 weeks over that period, due to abdominal symptoms.

On examination, vital signs were normal. Paula complained of colicky periumbilical pain. Her abdomen was generally soft, but she winced when her epigastrium was palpated. Rectal examination was normal, as were all other systems.

The pediatrician ascertained that the child had no siblings or close friends and that she was living with her mother, her parents having been divorced 2 years before. Paula and her mother were very close; both appeared to be anxious and somewhat depressed. Paula said she enjoyed schoolwork, but she complained of the way the schoolteacher shouted whenever other pupils in her class were unruly.

Having assured herself that the child had no physical disorder, the pediatrician diagnosed *separation anxiety disorder* in the form of school phobia. Her task was now to persuade mother and child that the abdominal pain, though real, was caused by tension, and that early referral to a child psychiatrist was required, lest the problem become intractable. ■

The need for an effective referral

An effective referral requires good collaboration between referring agent and child psychiatrist. The hesitation of a referring physician, for example, with doubts about the efficacy of child psychiatry or the credentials of mental health clinicians, will be apparent in tone of voice and attitude. If the clinician appears to be using referral to get rid of a problem case, the family are likely to feel dismissed or derogated.

Case 21.1 (continued)

■ As soon as the negative results of urinalysis, microurine, and complete blood count supported her primary diagnostic hypothesis, the pediatrician arranged to see Paula and her mother together. She explained that Paula's abdominal pains were not "imaginary" but, rather, the result of chronic tension caused by anxiety about leaving home to go to school. The mother said that she had suspected as much and asked the girl what it was that worried her about school. Paula could not say. The pediatrician explained that Paula's kind of problem was sometimes complex and that she recommended a psychiatric consultation.

The mother was startled by the suggestion, and Paula began to weep quietly. The pediatrician explained further that she did not mean to imply Paula was "crazy," but that both she and her mother might need specialized help to understand and solve the emotional problems at the root of Paula's difficulty in coping with the school environment. She briefly described what happens in a child psychiatry clinic. She added that if the pains recurred and Paula's temperature was normal, the mother should encourage her to go to school; there would be no serious physical or psychological result. Nevertheless, even if Paula were able to get to school, they should see the psychiatrist. Paula's and her mother's anxiety subsided. With their permission, the pediatrician telephoned the clinic to give information and alert the intake secretary that the mother would be requesting an appointment. ■

Behavior problems of referred children

Child psychiatry extends from infancy to late adolescence

What are the symptoms that occasion referral? To answer this question, it is necessary to divide children by sex and age (less than 4 years, 4 to 5 years, 6 to 11 years, and 12 to 16 years). There is no definite upper limit to adolescent psychiatry, but the end of high school is a suitable point to decide that the individual, though still in late adolescence, has entered the adult world.

The Child Behavior Checklist (Achenbach & Edelbrock, 1983) provides a standardized technique for gathering comprehensive information about symptoms and about both social and scholastic competence. The nature, number, and severity of symptoms exhibited by the patient are rated by the informant (usually one or both parents). The symptoms in this checklist have been factor-analyzed into a number of scales, and the individual can be compared with United States norms in regard to (a) total symptomatology; (b) internalizing or externalizing tendency; and (c) each of several symptom scales. A further refinement classifies children according to which of a number of configurations the individual's behavior problem profile most resembles.

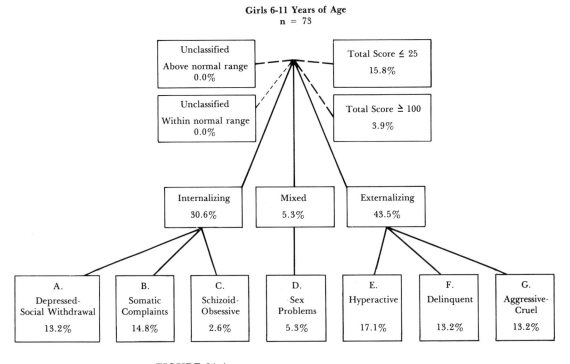

FIGURE 21.1

Patients referred to Section of Child Psychiatry, University of Vermont (1979–1980)

Figures 21.1, 21.2, 21.3, and 21.4 represent all girls and boys from 6 through 16 years of age who were referred to the Section of Child, Adolescent and Family Psychiatry of the University of Vermont, in the 2 years from 1979 to 1980. The children have been classified according to how closely they resemble the symptom profiles empirically identified by Achenbach and Edelbrock (1983). Note that classifiable profiles are divided first into internalizing and externalizing types (and mixed, in the case of girls). These global profile types are further divided into seven types for girls and six for boys. In general, profiles reflecting social withdrawal, depression, eccentric behavior, and somatic complaints are to the left of the array; overactive, aggressive, and delinquent profiles are to the right.

The behavior problem profiles in the Vermont survey are distributed in proportions roughly equivalent to those reported by Edelbrock and Achenbach (1980) in an analysis of 2,600 clinic cases. They appear to be a representative sample of patients referred to child mental health centers. In special settings, juvenile court clinics or pediatric referral centers, for example, different proportions of the profile types would be anticipated.

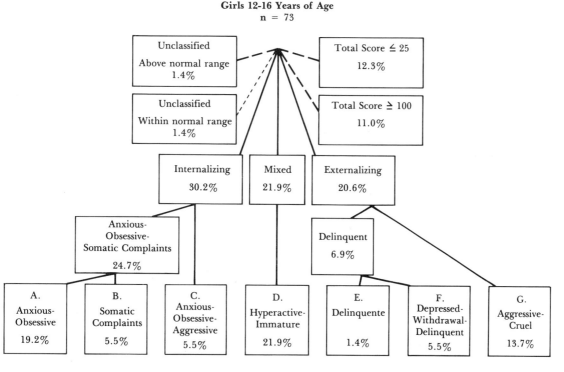

FIGURE 21.2
Patients referred to Section of Child Psychiatry, University of Vermont (1979–1980)

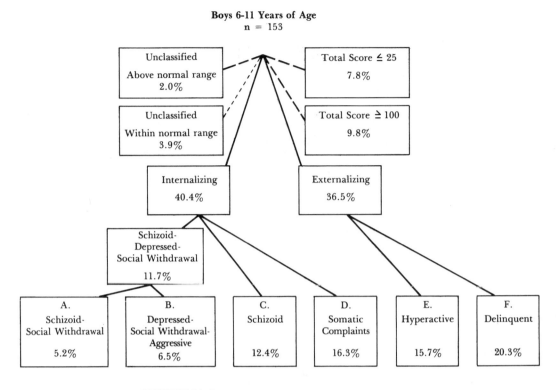

Boys 6-11 Years of Age
n = 153

Unclassified Above normal range 2.0%	Total Score ≤ 25 7.8%
Unclassified Within normal range 3.9%	Total Score ≥ 100 9.8%

Internalizing 40.4%

Externalizing 36.5%

Schizoid-Depressed-Social Withdrawal 11.7%

| A. Schizoid-Social Withdrawal 5.2% | B. Depressed-Social Withdrawal-Aggressive 6.5% | C. Schizoid 12.4% | D. Somatic Complaints 16.3% | E. Hyperactive 15.7% | F. Delinquent 20.3% |

FIGURE 21.3
Patients referred to Section of Child Psychiatry, University of Vermont
(1979–1980)

Collaboration with referring agent

The usefulness of personal contact with the referring agent

The psychiatrist should endeavor to speak personally with the referring agent. Exigencies of time often make this difficult, but there is no substitute for a telephone or corridor consultation before referral and after diagnosis is completed. Ask the referring agent the purpose of the referral: Is it for diagnostic advice? With or without options for further treatment? Can the referring agent describe, define, and explain the problem? What treatment has been attempted? With what effect?

The diagnostic encounter

The educative purpose of the initial encounter

Children and adolescents seldom initiate referral. Usually, adults become concerned and bring the patient for help. This practice has a number of consequences. Unless the patient is adequately prepared for what will happen, the

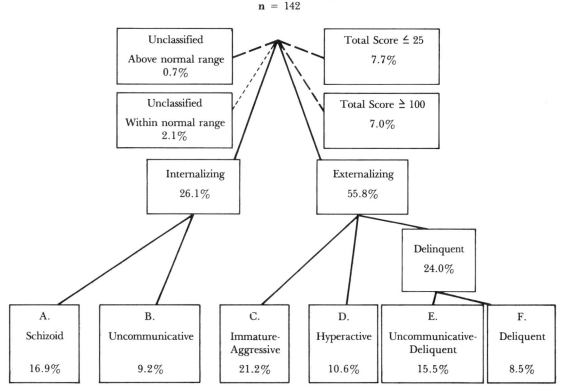

FIGURE 21.4
Patients referred to Section of Child Psychiatry, University of Vermont (1979–1980)

child may be mystified, fearful, or resistant. Unless the parents are aware that diagnosis and management are a family affair, they may wish to leave everything to an expert and stay on the sidelines. From one point of view, therefore, the initial encounter has educative purposes: to enlist the child's cooperation and to convey to the parents that they are about to embark on a collaborative venture.

The order of the interviews with child and family

Different clinicians approach the task of gathering information and enlisting collaboration in different ways. One method is to see the parents together, first, for a separate interview of from 1½ to 2 hours. A history can be taken and the parents helped to prepare the child for the next visit. The child is then interviewed for 1 to 1½ hours, and a decision made whether further interviews, examinations, or special investigations, are required. Sometimes the child does not need to be seen; the parental interview reveals a mild, transient, or developmental difficulty not requiring specialized attention. Most minor problems, however, are screened out and managed by pediatricians or school counselors; problems that get as far as a child mental health clinic are usually more intractable or complicated.

Once the inquiry process is complete and the clinician has a diagnosis and management plan, parents and child should be interviewed jointly. The diagnostic formulation is shared with the family, and the family's understanding and acceptance assured. A discussion of the management plan follows; the clinician explains the goals, tactics, anticipated duration, frequency, and cost of therapy. All family members are thereby given an opportunity during the negotiation to check, contribute to, and influence the clinician's opinion and recommendations.

Situations requiring the clinician to interview the entire family at once

In special circumstances, this order of interviews – parents first and child afterward – should be modified. If the family have come a long distance and require diagnostic evaluation within one day, it is appropriate to see them all together at first to ascertain the presenting problem from them and to explain how the appointments will be set up during the rest of the day. You may then interview the parents together and individually to obtain more detailed information on the child, siblings, and parents while the child in question is psychologically tested (if this is indicated). After a break, the child can be examined. Following this interview, discuss the evaluation, diagnosis, and management with the psychologist. This discussion will prepare you and the psychologist, working as a team, to consider with the family the strengths and problems revealed by your comprehensive assessment and to work out a management plan appropriate to a setting distant from your clinic (a plan which could be supervised by a local pediatrician, for example, or by telephone).

Emergencies

Another common circumstance demands flexibility and speed in response: the child psychiatry emergency. The most frequent emergencies are as follows:

1. Attempted suicide.
2. Homicide or attempted homicide.
3. Threats of suicide or violence.
4. Impending parental breakup or breakdown associated with inability to cope with a disturbed child's behavior.
5. Psychotic behavior or confusion (marked change of personality toward social withdrawal, secretiveness, excessive or eccentric fantasy life, impulsive behavior, gross overactivity, bizarre thinking, hallucinations, or ideas of reference, influence, or persecution).
6. Recent sexual trauma.
7. Grievous family loss with marked family disturbance.
8. Acute school refusal.
9. Running away from home.
10. Expulsion from school due to misbehavior.
11. Involvement with police due to recent misdemeanor, without previous history of antisocial behavior.
12. Substance abuse of recent origin.

Family crisis interviewing

In these circumstances, the child psychiatrist should see the entire family as soon as possible. In some cases, diagnosis becomes therapy. For example, if the communication between family members is poor, the clinician may be able to promote more candor than has been possible. In other circumstances, it becomes evident that the family system is so disorganized or so rigid that one or several members must be treated separately, at least to begin with. After emergency referral, the need to see an adolescent separately should be guided by your sense of how critical is the patient's need to be independent. The adolescent who fears being subordinated to disturbed, intrusive, restrictive or hostile parents and who has responded with a headlong rush into pseudomaturity will first need individual help. This does not preclude ultimate conjoint family therapy when improvement has occurred following individual treatment.

Reasons for seeing the child or adolescent first

Let us return to a consideration of the nonurgent diagnostic encounter. Different clinicians develop different styles. Some always see the child or adolescent first since they are concerned that the nominated patient will become resistant if convinced that the parents are having or have had a private conference with the clinician. This is a serious risk if the child is suspicious of or antagonistic to the parents. In that circumstance, the clinician may be perceived as yet another collusive adult authority (''We're taking you to a psychiatrist and we'll see what *he* has to say about your behavior''). If, from the background material, you strongly suspect such antagonism, arrange to interview the child or adolescent first at the initial appointment.

If there is no clear contraindication to doing so, there are definite advantages in seeing the parents initially. First, you get a full history, which is invaluable background when you assess the child. Second, the parents have the opportunity to check you out before they entrust their offspring to you. Last, you can help the parents prepare the child for seeing you.

The desirability of interviewing both parents

Note that it is desirable to interview both parents. Even if the parents are separated or divorced, endeavor to see them together for the initial encounter. If one parent is busy or absent, delay the first appointment until that parent is available (unless the referral is urgent), stressing the importance of both being present. The reasons for insisting on conjoint parental interviewing are as follows: more information is available; the parents can support, disconfirm, modify, or add to each other's impressions; both parents can form an opinion about your competence; and you will have indicated to them at the outset that treatment is a collaborative venture that starts with their preparing the child to attend.

At this point, it is appropriate to describe the components of the diagnostic encounter, in the following order:

1. Initial contact.
2. Intake questionnaires and checklists.
3. Interview with parents.
4. Interview with infant.
5. Interview with child.
6. Interview with adolescent.
7. Family interviews.

Initial contact

The need for a calm intake secretary

Initial contact is generally made by telephone. The importance of the secretary's calm, pleasant, welcoming telephone demeanor cannot be overstressed. In urgent or complicated cases, the referring agent, for example, will probably wish to speak to a clinician. The secretary must exercise discretion about whether to interrupt the clinician who is on call or leave a message for the clinician to call back.

Preliminary information

If the case is not urgent, the secretary gathers preliminary identifying information on an intake sheet, including name of pediatrician, previous medical and psychiatric treatment, and reason for referral. The secretary asks the referring agent to have the parent telephone. Further preliminary information can be gathered at that time, including a history of the duration and nature of the presenting complaint and associated phenomena.

Case 21.2

■ An adolescent's mother gives the following information to the clinic secretary. The referred patient is Pattie, a 14-year old girl, the oldest of three siblings of a divorced couple.

Pattie's father lives out of state and sees his daughter during summer vacations. The mother has not remarried. The child is in the ninth grade at the local high school.

Always somewhat moody, over the last 6 months Pattie has become negativistic and oppositional, seems to be "boy-mad," and has dropped in her school grades. Her mother, who referred her through the family pediatrician, is worried that she might have fallen in with bad companions and started to smoke pot.

Pattie's physical health has been excellent. The names, addresses, telephone numbers, occupations, ages, and dates of birth of all family members are obtained, along with relevant information concerning medical insurance. ■

Matching the clinician to the case

With this orienting information, the clinic intake team can decide who would be the most appropriate clinician for the family, a decision made on the basis of who is most suitable for a patient of that sex and age (in Case 19.2, probably a female therapist), what kind of special investigations are likely to be required, what kind of therapy is likely to be most appropriate, who is most skilled in that field, and who has the next available appointment time. If there is a potentially important physical aspect of diagnosis, a child psychiatrist is the most appropriate primary clinician; if an educational or cognitive component dominates the clinical pattern, a psychologist is the most suitable diagnostician. Often it is not possible to

Overlapping skills

determine a particular diagnostic emphasis; nevertheless, the overlapping skills of clinicians with different professional training backgrounds and the capacity for referral and consultation within the clinic allow wide discretion in case allocation. Note that in this model of clinic operation, staff are selected for common, overlapping competencies as well as for specialized diagnostic and therapeutic skills.

Waiting lists

Urgent referrals should be seen within 24 hours, and semiurgent cases within a week. It is unwise to have a waiting list of more than 4 weeks for nonurgent cases, since the family's motivation to get help may fade or the child's behavior worsen, causing insupportable personal or family distress.

Intake questionnaires and checklists

Preliminary data gathering

The clinician can be saved routine data-gathering during precious interview time by having the parents (and in some cases, the adolescent) complete checklists and questionnaires concerning a number of important matters. These data-gathering instruments can be mailed to the parents and returned in a self-addressed envelope. These instruments are comprehensive and less subject than direct interviewing to the limitations of parents' or clinicians' memory; moreover, the questions involved help orient parents to the child's development, behavior problems, and social and scholastic resources or handicaps.

A selection of useful instruments is as follows:

1. The Child Behavior Checklist for Parents.
2. The Teacher's Report Form.
3. The Child Information Intake Questionnaire.
4. The Minnesota Child Development Checklist.

The **Child Behavior Checklist for Parents** (Achenbach & Edelbrock, 1983) has two sections. The first deals with friendship patterns, academic performance, household responsibilities, and recreational involvement. The second section asks the parent to rate 118 different behavior problems on a three-point scale ("never," "sometimes," "often"). As already described, the social adjustment and behavior items can be compared with nonclinical norms. The behaviors have been grouped into scales from which patients can be classified according to how closely they resemble empirically derived profile types. At the present time, profile types are available for subjects of both sexes from 4 through 16 years of age. There is as yet no satisfactory parental questionnaire for children younger than four years, although one is in preparation.

The **Teacher's Report Form** (Achenbach & Edelbrock, 1983) requires parental permission. Like the Child Behavior Checklist, it has a section on social and scholastic competence and a section on behavior problems. It, too, has been factorized into behavior problem scales, and the child's profile of scales can be compared with empirically derived profile patterns.

An example of a general information form, the Child Information Intake Questionnaire (Ruoff, 1980) is provided in appendix IV. This is a convenient method for gathering routine information about the child's physical health; the mother's pregnancy; the child's birth, early development, temperament, early behavior and school history; family structure; parental health; and family history. If abnormalities or discrepancies are revealed in any of these areas, they can be further investigated when the parents are interviewed.

The **Minnesota Child Development Questionnaire** (Ireton & Thwing, 1972) is used with preschool children when a comprehensive parental review of the child's development is required. Development is divided into six subscales, and an age-normed profile is provided of the subject's attainment in each area.

The interview with the parents

What are the purposes of the initial interview with the parents? In general they are as follows:

Rapport

1. To form an alliance with the parents and help them prepare the child for the forthcoming interview.

History

2. To obtain a formal history of the presenting problem, past illnesses, general development, school performance and adjustment, peer relationships, recreation and interests, home and family environment, and family history.

Family background

3. To gather information about the relationship between parents and child, the methods of childrearing used, and the family's values and aspirations.

Marital relationship
Insight

4. To gather information about the current marital relationship and its history.
5. To determine how the parents comprehend the nature and cause of the problem in their family, and the kind of help they expect or would accept.

Allow 1½ hours for the first interview; however, it may not be possible to gather all this information in one session. If the initial history is incomplete, schedule a further joint appointment or appointments after the child or adolescent has been interviewed.

Before the parents arrive, familiarize yourself with the questionnaires they have completed. The Child Behavior Checklist will provide detailed information about the pattern of the child's symptoms together with systematic information about social and school adaptation. The Teacher's Report Form or the Child Behavior Checklist will alert you to the child's school progress and behavior. The symptoms manifested at school can then be compared with those described at home. Discrepancies are important. Sometimes, for example, the teacher perceives the child as more disturbed than the parents do. It may be that the parents are consciously or unconsciously minimizing the difficulty, or that the teacher is intolerant of the child's behavior, or that the child's behavior problems are limited to school.

Note discrepancies between the data-gathering forms

The Child Information Intake Questionnaire will alert you to problems in the past medical and psychiatric history, abnormalities of development and temperament, the structure of the family, and family history. Any features that are problematic, or potentially so, can be explored in direct interviews.

The Minnesota Child Developmental Inventory complements the developmental history by providing a younger child's developmental profile.

Inception

The general principles of interviewing are discussed in chapter 8. They should be modified to the extent that you will be eliciting information from a couple.

When the parents have arrived, greet them in the waiting room and usher them into your office, indicating the chairs or couch on which they should sit. Begin by telling them briefly what you already know and invite them to tell you their story:

> CLINICIAN: When Dr. Y. referred you to me, he told me you were worried about John's school progress and his behavior at home. Tell me how you first became concerned about him.

Reconnaisance

Let them proceed at their own pace, recounting events in their own order and stressing what they consider to be important. Listen and facilitate the flow of associations (see chapter 8).

The parents' behavior during the diagnostic encounter

While they provide the information, the interaction between the couple can be most informative. How do they sit in your office – side-by-side or separated by a space? Are they in tactile or nonverbal contact; or do they operate independently? Do they appear to come from similar or different social, cultural, or intellectual backgrounds? Which parent provides most of the information? Does one defer to the other or seek corroboration from him or her? Do they interrupt, contradict, complement, or support each other? Is there humor, warmth, coolness, remoteness, tension, irritation, or hostility between them? How do they relate to you? Are they bewildered, anxious, remote, tense, deferential, desperate, demanding? Are there points during the interview when one parent becomes discomposed? How does the other react at that time?

Detailed inquiry

When they have completed their account, you can ask about the following matters, if they are unclear. Did the problem have an onset? When? Did the onset coincide with a possible physical or psychosocial stressor? How has the problem evolved? Has there been any change over time? Is the problem persistent or intermittent? Do the exacerbations relate to vicissitudes in the child's personal life or physical health? How have the parents tried to help the patient? What was the effect of their efforts?

When the presenting problem has been fully explored, further topics can be considered according to appropriateness and the discretionary judgment of the clinician.

Other Problems:

Are the parents aware of any other problems in the child's behavior at home, at school, with adults, with children, or with siblings?

Parental attitudes are addressed by these questions:

1. How do the parents feel about having been referred?
2. How do they account for the child's problems?
3. What kind of help do they expect or want?
4. Why do they seek help at this particular time?

The medical history involves these questions:

1. Significant physical illness, surgery, accidents? Age and duration? Adverse reactions during or afterward?
2. Hospitalization? Age and duration? Adverse reactions during or afterward?
3. Physical disabilities? Epilepsy? Head injury?
4. Headaches, limb pains, abdominal pains, nausea or vomiting, fainting, eye symptoms, prolonged or frequent absences from school?
5. Previous psychological disturbance? Cause? Treatment? Outcome?
6. Current medication? Medication allergies?

The patient's developmental history includes these topics:

1. Pregnancy: Circumstances surrounding conception: motivation, acceptance, convenience, emotional turmoil, reaction of in-laws? Marital relationship during pregnancy? Maternal physical and emotional health during pregnancy? Toxemia, eclampsia, kidney disorder, hypertension, febrile illness, X-rays, medication, drug or alcohol intake? Excessive nausea, vomiting, vaginal bleeding? Maternal preparation for labor? Sex preference?
2. Delivery: Normal confinement, at term? Duration of labor, nature of delivery, complications? How soon was baby seen? Mother's initial thoughts on seeing infant?
3. Neonatal status: Birthweight, maturity, physical condition, intensive care, method of feeding, weight gain? Asphyxia, cyanosis, jaundice, convulsions, vomiting, rigidity, respiratory disorder?
4. Feeding: Breast fed? How long? Formula? Solids introduced? Weight gain? Vomiting, diarrhea, constipation? Colic, food allergies, eczema? Later conflict over eating, bulimia, hoarding? Present eating habits?
5. Motor development: Age in months of holding head erect, sitting alone, standing, walking alone? Coordination, gross and fine? Handedness? Repetitive motor habits?
6. Speech development: First words, two- and three-word phrases, sentences? Faulty articulation, stammering? Present language, vocabulary, and syntax?
7. Sphincter control: Timing, for bladder and bowel? Method of training? Child's response: resistance or acceptance? Regression? Enuresis or encopresis?
8. Sleep: Previous problems? Present habits? Deep, restless, or insomniac? Fear of the dark or of being alone, sleepwalking, nightmares, night-terrors, resistance to going to bed?
9. Sexual development: Early sexual curiosity or sex play? Sex education? Menarche, masturbation, nocturnal emissions? Gender-role identification, interest in opposite sex? Sex traumata?

Concerns about educational progress include:

1. Previous schools attended? Present school, grade, teacher? Current academic performance? Specific or general learning problems? Sports and recreations?

Relationship to peers, teachers, school rules? Capacity to concentrate? Truancy, fear of going to school, school refusal, attitude to homework? Antisocial behavior? History of drugs or alcohol?

2. Ambitions? Involvement in social and recreational activities?

A description of the home environment includes:

1. Location of home? Environment and neighbors? Layout of home? Sleeping arrangements?
2. Inside and outside space for play? Parental satisfaction with domestic arrangements?
3. Typical weekday and weekend schedule from rising to retiring?

Parent-child relationships involve consideration of:

1. Child's early temperament: easy or difficult? Any change in this with age? General mood; capacity for affection; tolerance for frustration; proneness to tantrum; aggressiveness; resentfulness; fearfulness; timidity; depression; sociability; acceptance of limits, rules, and discipline; response to punishment: stubbornness or compliance?
2. Parental methods of setting limits, discipline, consistency?
3. Time spent together: father–child; mother–child; family?
4. Child's attitudes to each parent: closeness, mutual understanding?
5. Conflicts about dependence and independence within child or between child and parents?

Concerns about the patient's social relations include:

1. Relationship with siblings, peers? Leader, follower, protector, dependent? Quarrels?
2. Able to win or lose at games? Favorite games?
3. Antisocial behavior? Relationship to authority figures?

The family history considers:

1. Parents: Age, occupation, physical and mental health? Drug and alcohol intake? Grandparents and relatives? Domestic, educational, and occupational background? Antisocial history?
2. Marital history: Previous marriages? Meeting, courting, acceptance by in-laws, early marriage, sexual adjustment, division of labor, management of money, settlement of disputes? History of competition, unfulfilled needs, hostility, abuse, separations? Parenting ability and capacity for affection? Motivation for child-care and child-rearing?
3. Siblings: Age, health, school or occupation, personality, relationship to patient?

4. Family values: Ethnic or sociocultural background? Emphasis on conformity or independence, authority or freedom, warmth or coolness, control or expression? Religion? Moral and esthetic values? Emphasis on education, money, success, prestige, gender differentiation?

5. Family and community: Relation to school, religious organization, cultural bodies, civic affairs.

Do not churn through these questions like a robot. The clinician using a hypothetico-deductive approach will pursue a discretionary route through this inquiry process. Much of it has already been touched upon in the Child Information Intake Questionnaire (see appendix IV).

After the interview with the parents, the child can be interviewed for 1 to 1½ hours, preferably at a different time. Since the technique of observing or interviewing must be modified in accordance with the patient's age, the observation of an infant and the interview with a child or adolescent are described under three separate headings, beginning with infant observation.

Observing the infant (birth through 3 years)

Need to evaluate infant in proximity to the primary attachment figure

An infant's existence revolves around issues of attachment to and individuation from the parent. The child can be examined as though he or she were a separate entity, but the child's need for a parent or parent surrogate is a central issue in the first 4 years of life. The infant can be regarded as functioning in an emotional envelope of more or less sensitive, responsive, stimulating, affectionate but nonrestrictive parental care, which gradually changes as the child grows, to foster autonomy and initiative. The developmental stages of psychosocial development in infancy have been described by Als, Tronick and Brazelton (1980) and Greenspan (1981b) and are discussed later in chapter 23.

Up to the age of 18 months (early infancy), the baby will be observed in the company of the parents. A number of points can be noted, in developmentally hierarchical order. These points represent overlapping developmental issues having an **epigenetic** quality. In other words, it is difficult for the child to pass from one step to the next unless the preceding steps have been adequately negotiated. For example, the earliest stages of human interaction (eye contact and smiling) are impossible if the baby cannot track and optically fixate on a visual stimulus.

1. Homeostasis: (0–3 months): Is the baby able to maintain control over sucking, respiration, cardiovascular function, skin circulation, and gastrointestinal function?

2. State regulation (0–2 months): Does the baby pass smoothly from deep sleep through dozing to quiet alertness, or are these states diffuse and the transitions between them excessively abrupt? Is the baby phlegmatic and hard to rouse, or irritable and too easily distressed?

3. Motor control (0–1 month): Are the baby's muscle tone and movements well regulated or are they disrupted by symmetrical or asymmetrical tremors, jerks, or clonus?

4. Distress and consolation (birth–onwards): What distresses the baby? How readily can it be distressed or consoled? How is the baby most effectively consoled?

5. Attention (1 week–onwards): Does the baby have the energy and interest to track an interesting spectacle visually or turn the head towards an interesting sound?

6. Habituation (1 week–onwards): When the child is presented repetitively with the same (originally novel) stimulus, does interest gradually or suddenly fade or does it persist?

7. Interaction (3 weeks–onwards): Does the baby make and sustain eye contact, smile, and seek tactile contact or accept it by molding body to caregiver? Does the baby vocalize in response to interaction?

8. Attachment (4 months–onwards): By 4 to 6 months, the baby begins to show preference for a primary attachment figure, usually the primary caretaker. How comfortable is the baby in your arms rather than the mother's?

9. Separation Anxiety (6 months–2 years): Does the baby show distress if the mother, the father, or both parents leave him or her in the room with you? Does the baby show recognition when the parents return? Separation anxiety is normal up to about 2 years.

10. Stranger anxiety (6–12 months): Does the baby show distress at an unfamiliar face? If distressed, can the baby be consoled by the primary attachment figure? This is normal up to 12 months.

During the first 12 months and afterward, temperamental features can be noted and checked for reliability against the parents' observations. One or two interviews in unfamiliar surroundings are clearly less than optimal for observations of this kind, but some temperamental features may be apparent during an office examination. The following features are taken from Thomas, Chess, and Birch (1968):

1. Activity level: Is the child very active, underactive, or normally active for his or her age? Is this characteristic?

2. Rhythmicity: Is the child predictable in sleep/wake/alert and hunger/feeding/satiety rhythms?

3. Approach: Is the child interested in the novel situation of your office, or timid or withdrawn?

4. Intensity of response: If the child shows excitement, pleasure, surprise, or distress in your office, how intense is this reaction?

5. Threshold: What intensity of visual, auditory, or other sensory stimulus is required to provoke a response in the child? Is the child phlegmatic, normal, or irritable?

6. Adaptability: Does the child fit in readily to the new situation or remain ill at ease and unhappy?

7. Mood: Is the child generally equable, happy, neutral, fretful, irritable, somber, or depressed during the interview? How characteristic of the child is this present mood?

8. Distractibility: Is the child distracted by random environmental stimuli (e.g., outside noises, waving curtains, buzzing flies) while engaged in a task such as block-building?

9. Persistence: When engaged in a task such as block play, does the child pursue it or, on the other hand, soon lose interest and move to something else?

Unrepresentative behavior samples

Remember that the sample of behavior you have observed might be unrepresentative. It is certainly invalid if the child is ill, in pain, fatigued, hungry, frightened or otherwise out of sorts at the time of the interview.

The CMSE for infants and toddlers

From 12 to 48 months, the infant demonstrates an increasing capacity to control behavior, assimilate and organize experience, and develop mental representations of the self, of other people, and of things in the external world. All of these rapidly increasing capacities are evident in behavior: in general motor activity; in interaction with familiar and unfamiliar adults, older children, and peers; in representational play; and in gestural and language communication. Thus, from 1 through 4 years, a rough child mental status examination is possible, covering most of the items described later in this chapter. The child of 3 years or more often can be separated from the parents and interviewed, using suitable play materials.

The interview with the child (4 through 11 years)

Goals

A clinical interview with a child in this age range has a number of possible goals, not all of which are attainable in every case. The following list is ideal; the priority of these goals varies with the particular patient:

Ascertain the child's attitude to the interview

1. To ascertain how the child feels about being interviewed and what the child believes to be the purpose of the interview. To correct misapprehensions and orient the child to purpose of the interview.

Ascertain the child's awareness of problem

2. To determine whether the child is aware of a personal or family problem and how the child accounts for the problem if it is acknowledged.

Complete CMSE

3. To complete a mental status examination of: the child's appearance, motor behavior and speech, relationship to the examiner, mood, cognitive functions, language development, thought process and content, quality of fantasy, salient fantasy themes and insight.

Explore self-concept and perception of key figures

4. To investigate the child's self-concept and to determine perceptions of, and the quality of relationship with, key figures in the interpersonal world: parents, siblings, extended family, peers, and other adults.

Judge developmental level 5. To estimate the level of the child's emotional, social, and moral development.
Coping 6. To gauge the nature and effectiveness of the child's current coping mechanisms.
Establish relationship 7. To establish a relationship with the child characterized by confidentiality, trust, and the potential to develop into a therapeutic alliance.
8. To determine the child's capacity for forming such a relationship.

Factors affecting the process of the interview

The importance of first impressions

The primary purpose of the initial interview with the child is diagnostic, but in child psychiatry, as in medicine generally, it is artificial to separate diagnosis from therapy. Adverse impressions formed by the child at first contact are often difficult to overcome, whereas a sensitive interviewer who helps the child relax enough to express thoughts and feelings leaves a powerful, even beneficial, impression.

The type of interview that evolves depends on a number of factors:

Factors influencing the interview

1. The child's developmental level.
2. The child's personality.
3. The child's expectations.
4. The environment.
5. The goals of the interview.
6. The interviewer's personality and interview style.

Age

To a large extent, the child's developmental level determines the content of the interaction. A preschool child is more likely to express ideas and feeling through action than words. A mature 11-year-old, on the other hand, may be prepared to spend an entire interview in conversation. Other children are comfortable with a mixture of play activity and verbal communication. The clinician thus must combine quiet observation, play, and conversation, in different degrees, with patients of different age and personality.

Openness

The well-adjusted child is normally cautious about sharing too much personal life with a stranger unless the child accepts the purpose for doing so. The psychologically disturbed child is even more inhibited from revealing frightening fantasies, secrets, or private fears at the interview, and initially, such material may find only oblique expression. In contrast, some disorganized children have such poor defenses against disruptive affects, memories, and fantasies that they release a torrent of psychopathological material before they have established a trusting relationship with the examiner.

Expectations

The child's expectation of the interview greatly influences its course. Children seldom come to a psychiatrist of their own accord, and those who bring them may not have prepared them well. Children's attitudes to the diagnostic encounter can be hostile, fearful, bewildered, blasé, or eager for help. Negative expectancies include the fear of bodily invasion in younger children (doctors in white coats with needles), the fear that secret inferiorities or shameful fantasies

Negative expectancies

Headshrinking

will be exposed, the fear of being induced to talk about matters so scary the child has never dared articulate them, and the universal adolescent fear of being rendered helpless on the couch of an exploitative sorcerer (head shrinker). Children with a history of antisocial behavior commonly expect a tricky cross-examination aimed to ferret out "the truth"; children with learning problems may be afraid of being tested and found wanting. The experienced clinician is sensitive to these possibilities and tries to ensure that the child's apprehensions are, at least in part, anticipated and mollified by parental preparation.

The office environment

The environment in which the interview takes place should be considered. An experienced clinician can be surprisingly effective in unpromising surroundings – perched on the edge of a sickbed in a noisy ward, for example. Nevertheless, adequate space and equipment are helpful. Large departments are likely to have separate playrooms with extensive equipment and fittings for sand and water play, cooking, and so on; but most clinicians must arrange their own offices to interview children as well as parents and families.

The arrangement of the office as a playroom

An ideal room will be spacious enough to have a carpeted section for seated interviewing, a section with linoleum-tiled surface for play, and a small table and chair. Play equipment should be stored in a lockable cupboard in which there is additional space to keep material or creations associated with particular patients in therapy. Most equipment is communal. A curious child can be told that it belongs to the hospital (or office) and may not be taken away.

Play equipment

Avoid clutter

Basic equipment

Different clinicians favor different play equipment, but it is preferable to err on the side of frugality. Remember that equipment is a means to the development of a relationship and the expression of thoughts and feelings. The less the clutter, the more the child must draw from inside. Here is a list of basics: easel, newsprint paper and felt pens; assorted blocks; assorted toy wild and domestic animals; matchbox cars; doll family of parents, brother, sister, baby, grandparents, plus nurse, and doctor; one or two stuffed animals; rubber ball; pack of playing cards; checkers. Add other items to the bare essentials, guided by your interests and what works for you: a small table and chair; puppets; toy pistols; other boardgames; doll's house furniture; plastic construction models. Avoid high-concentration games that preclude fantasy, such as chess or *Scrabble*. Finger paints, poster colors, and playdough are suitable only for fully equipped playrooms; but you may want to keep a soccer ball, football, and a baseball and glove for outdoor play.

Excursions

Do not be anchored to the office. An occasional visit to a soda fountain, outdoor construction site, nursery, or gymnasium can be very useful, especially with highly active youngsters who find a restricted environment tedious. In exceptional cases (for example, with extremely withdrawn patients), it can be productive to introduce a pet animal.

The style of the interview

The goals of the interview shape its style, to some degree. Sometimes it is essential to obtain from the child a veridical account of a past event, especially in medico-legal cases involving allegations of sexual abuse. These situations are much less common than those in which the clinician can allow the interview to evolve as the interaction dictates.

Structured and unstructured interviewing techniques

Two extreme interviewing styles are exemplified by the relatively unstructured approach advocated by Greenspan (1981a) and the highly structured DICA questionnaire (Herjanic & Campbell, 1977), which searches for symptoms pertinent to DSM-III. Structured interviewing is valuable for research purposes since it improves the interviewer's consistency, but it is not recommended for regular clinical interviewing.

Simmons (1981) recommends an approach a little to the right of Greenspan: an evolving interaction guided by a flexibly and sensitively applied system. This chapter advocates a similar middle-of-the-road style. Organize the interview according to your goals, using a hypothetico-deductive strategy (see the previous section on the interview with the child) but do not compromise a positive relationship for the sake of extracting information. In most cases, two to three 1-hour interviews are required to gather enough information to reach a reliable diagnosis.

The prerequisite for relating to children

The clinician who wishes to work with children should enjoy being with them. He or she should be sufficiently in touch with the past to be able to recapture and empathize with the sadness, tears, anger, frustration, puzzlement, excitements, and surprises of childhood. The clinician should be warm, accepting, and supportive but neither overidentified with the patient nor intolerant of children's natural messiness. Young clinicians with a high investment in verbal ability may be unnerved by the silent child or toddler. When interviewing children, the clinician has little more to offer than himself or herself. Nowhere in medicine is this clinical nakedness more apparent than in child psychiatry.

A variety of interviewing styles

Despite these cautionary comments and given a background of warmth and unintrusive interest, the interview allows room for a variety of styles. Some interviewers are active, engaging, and direct. Some are quiet, saying no more than is necessary to keep the child's associations flowing. Some use humor to spoof the fibber, relax the anxious child, and test the overactive, depressed, or psychotic child. In response to a joke, for example, the uninhibited child becomes even less controlled, the depressed child smiles wanly but soon fades, and the psychotic child is muddled.

The interview as a catalyst

The clinician should be unhurried, with no axe to grind; children are uncannily perceptive of intolerance or irritation cloaked by a watch-the-birdie brightness. The best interviewer is a kind of catalyst: able to attend when the child is freely associating or playing; able to interpolate a comment, question, or joke to get the interview started; able to get down on the floor and play beside or with the child when it is appropriate; able to appreciate physical closeness, messiness, and verbal aggression; but capable of setting reasonable limits to protect the child from breaking equipment, incurring physical injury, or hurting others. Skillful clinicians inject as much of themselves into the situation as necessary to allay anxiety and promote self-expression.

Personal reactions

The clinician should reflect upon his or her personal response to the individual patient. There may be some consensual validity in these reactions; but when they are predominant, inexorable, and overgeneralized, they disrupt the warmth and empathic acceptance required for effective interviewing. Some examples of these personal responses are described here as stereotypes, in somewhat caricatured form.

The intellectualizer is at a loss when confronted by the ambivalent, condensed, apparent chaos of childhood play. Overvaluing words, which sweep debris into little heaps (or under the carpet), this interviewer is defeated by the silent child and retires behind the *Archives of General Psychiatry*. The interviewer tells colleagues that play therapy is "boring" or "pointless."

The rescuer sees children as victimized by neglectful or abusive parents. Commonly, the mother is depicted as the villain, although the father has recently achieved more notoriety in this regard. The rescuer is determined to outmother the neglectful mother or wrest the child from the chauvinistic father's dominance. Self-righteous and unyielding, the interviewer sets up a tug-of-war with parents and allied workers and arouses in the child expectations that cannot be fulfilled without serious conflicts of loyalty.

The earth mother, a variant of the rescuer, seeks to heal all wounds with love, thus gratifying personal dependency needs. This interviewer can set no limits, and if the child wrecks the playroom or mounts a personal attack, the interviewer has nothing to offer but guilt ("How can you do this to me?")

The ear-boxer remembers his or her own father's stern (but "fair") admonitions. This interviewer guards against infractions of the rules and privately feels or openly contends that a good smack on the bottom would circumvent a lot of nonsense. Frequently perceiving children as "attention-seeking" and "manipulative," this interviewer is an especially pernicious influence in an inpatient unit.

The biologist is interested in children because through the child one can approach the central nervous system, close to the synapses, where the real action is. Children emit primitive behavior patterns similar to the animal experimental model. Biologists have great faith in the future of psychotropic medication. They despair of intervening with families.

The systems analyst believes the child is the wrong patient. A child is a member of a family system, which is the correct focus for diagnosis and treatment. Systems analysts are often refugees from adult psychoanalytic, social work, or behavior therapy training programs. They tend to overlook or deny the child's problems and, at worst, conduct an awkward version of marital couple therapy interrupted occasionally by children's protests or behavior ("What else is there to draw on?").

The mentalist conceives of all diagnosis and therapy in terms of intrapsychic issues. Physical, cognitive, and social factors are ignored in favor of an internal world peopled by hypothetical constructs. This kind of clinician usually needs to avoid parents, using such colleagues as social workers to keep them at bay.

The effect of reductionism on clinical interaction

These last three stereotypes (biologist, systems analyst, and mentalist) represent the reductionistic defenses of clinicians who restrict diagnosis and therapy to one paradigm at one systemic level and who seek explanations for all clinical problems in a unitary doctrine.

Conducting the interview

Precautions

First, a few precautions. Do not wear a white coat; it signals needles to some children. Wear sturdy trousers, pants, or leotards under a skirt so you can sit on the floor if you need. If you are worried about getting pigment or playdough on your clothes, consider donning a painter's coverall.

Never whisper to an adult about a child in the child's presence. Either speak openly or leave your comment to a later interview, when you can speak to the parent(s) alone.

Prevent destructiveness

Do not be misled; the mere expression of feeling in play activity, without reflection or understanding, is not helpful. The child who breaks things or attacks the interviewer is likely to be terrified afterward or overcome with remorse. The rules for the child are as follows:

> CLINICIAN: You may say or do what you want, except that you must stay with me for the allotted time, and I will not allow you to break things or hurt yourself or others.

Bear these precautions in mind; they need be stated only if the child seems likely to infringe them. You are now ready to start the interview.

Introduction

Go into the waiting room and greet the parent and child. Sit beside the child and introduce yourself. Tell the child what you plan to do – talk, draw, and play for about an hour – and invite the child to your room. If the child is resistant, wait a few minutes to see if the parent can reassure the child. If this is of no avail, ask the parent to bring the child to the room, indicating the parent will be leaving when the child is comfortable. Usually the parent can leave after a short time at a signal from you. If not, it is seldom necessary for the parent to be present for more than one or two interviews.

In the room, you will have set out suitable play materials for the younger child. The child of over 9 or 10 years can be ushered to an appropriate chair. Begin by asking the older child why the parents asked him to come and how he or she feels about it. If the child cannot or will not tell you, say what you already know and ask the child for a personal reaction to it.

Inception

> CLINICIAN: Hi. Have a seat.
> PATIENT: (*wide-eyed, uncertain, gives no answer*)
> CLINICIAN: You're Randy. I'm Dr. N. Your Mom told me you're 9 years old.
> PATIENT: Ten.
> CLINICIAN: Okay. Well, did Mom or Dad tell you why they wanted you to see me today?
> PATIENT: Yes.
> CLINICIAN: What did they tell you?
> PATIENT: I don't remember. Something about talking to you.
> CLINICIAN: About?
> PATIENT: About school or something.
> CLINICIAN: Things haven't been going well for you at school?

PATIENT: *(inaudible murmur)* . . . *(silence)*

CLINICIAN: Well, last week your parents came to see me. What they told me was that, over the last year, your schoolwork has been dropping off and you've had trouble getting along with other kids at school and on the school bus. Maybe you can tell me something about it?

PATIENT: They won't leave me alone.

CLINICIAN: Tell me about it.

If the child is younger, issue an invitation to use the play equipment. Don't push. Let the play theme emerge. Gently test if the child is prepared to tell you about it.

Topics that can be discussed

When the child is comfortable in conversation, the following topics can be touched on:

1. *Attendance at the clinic:* Reason for attendance. Feelings about attendance.
2. *School:* School, class, teacher. Best- and least-liked teachers. Reasons? Best- and least-liked subjects. Reasons? School grades. Homework. Liking for other school activities. Reasons? Changes of school? Reasons?
3. *Social background:* Neighborhood. Social groups. Clubs.
4. *Recreation:* Hobbies. Talents. Best-liked activity. Reason? Sports.
5. *Peer relations:* Best friend. Reason best friend is liked. Enemies. Reason enemies are disliked. Experiences of persecution or scapegoating. Opportunities and aspirations for leadership.
6. *Ambitions:* Occupation. Marriage and family. Travel.
7. *Health:* Recent illnesses; experiences of hospitalization.
8. *Family relations:* House: layout, yard space, bedroom. Chores. Parents; siblings; pets; family activities most enjoyed; relationship between parents; alliances within family; conflicts within family.
9. *Fantasy:* Dreams, good and bad. Three wishes. What to do with $1,000,000. Mutual story-telling technique. Drawings: of the family doing something together; of a person; of something nice and something horrible. The game "Squiggles" (see the section on eliciting fantasy in this chapter).
10. *Symptoms* (Take these from the Child Behavior Checklist): Fears, anxiety, obsessions, or compulsions, dissociation, depression, depersonalization. If indicated: hallucinations, ideas of reference, delusions, concern about death or suicide, difficulty controlling anger, antisocial behavior.
11. *Insight:* Recapitulation of reason for attendance, nature of problems, desire for help.

Use discretion

These 11 topics flow in a natural sequence from neutral to personal. Topics 1 through 7, though potentially informative, are ice-breakers. Topics 8 through 11 require more reflection and are likely to be more problematic. Do not follow the list in lock-step; rather, explore the topics in a discretionary manner. One child may be disposed to give a detailed account of peer and family relations; another will provide little information on anything beyond neutral topics; a third

Go at the child's pace

Develop trust

Don't use "Why?"

Explore what the child means

Avoid interrogation

prefers to play with toys and converse intermittently about them. Do not push; wait until the child is ready.

Remember that the primary aims of the first interview are to help the child relax with you and to lay the foundation of trust. Nothing should be allowed to compromise these aims, since without trust little can be achieved. If trust develops, it will be possible to clarify with the child the purpose of the interview, ascertain whether the child perceives problems in his or her life, evaluate the child's affect and capacity to relate to you, and catch a glimpse of the child's fantasy life. Further specific features of history and physical or mental status (e.g., family relations, capacity to concentrate, neuromotor integration) can often wait for a second or third interview, unless the child is especially cooperative at initial contact or unless the issue is urgent.

In general, many of the facilitatory interview techniques described in chapter 6 apply to children. There are some differences, however, that take account of the child's relatively more concrete, egocentric view of the world.

Do not ask "Why?" with children; this question puts them on the defensive; it has an accusatory tone and asks for an analysis of cause and effect that may be beyond the younger patient.

> PATIENT: The other kids pick on me all the time.
> CLINICIAN: Why?
> PATIENT: I don't know. They're mean.

Here are a number of alternatives:

> PATIENT: The other kids pick on me all the time.
> CLINICIAN: What do they say? What do they do? How do you feel about it? What do you do about it?

When a child uses an unusual word or phrase (particularly when it has an adult ring to it) do not assume it has the same meaning for both of you.

> ■ The patient, a pedantic 6-year-old only child in the midst of a postdivorce custody battle, has said that he thinks it would be preferable if he lived with his mother rather than his father, because his mother is more "sensible."
>
> CLINICIAN: How do you mean, "sensible"?
> PATIENT: Well, my father puts sugar on the cereal.
> CLINICIAN: Is that bad?
> PATIENT: Mom says it's bad for my health. ■

Avoid interviews in which you try to ferret out the truth from a child who has been involved in antisocial bahavior. Try to get in touch with the child's feelings about the situation and what led up to it. It can sometimes be useful to point out discrepancies or inconsistencies in the story to an older child who is evidently fabricating a story or holding back important details; but this technique is unlikely to be necessary except when the child has been involved in antisocial behavior.

> ■ The patient, an 11-year-old boy, has been accused of shoplifting.
>
> CLINICIAN: What do they say you took from the store?
> PATIENT: Chewing gum. Cigarettes.
> CLINICIAN: Tell me what actually happened.
> PATIENT: Everyone sticks his nose into my business.
> CLINICIAN: Everyone? ■

Buffer comments

When you introduce matters with an anxiety-laden connotation, especially if they seem to imply that the child is weird, crazy, or unique, it can be helpful to associate the issue with the difficulties of other children in similar circumstances. Simmons (1981) calls these "buffer comments."

> CLINICIAN: I see a lot of kids here who have problems after their parents get divorced. Many of them can't help blaming someone. I wonder if you ever felt like that?

Terminal recapitulation

At the end of the interview, recapitulate what you both have learned of the child's reasons for and feelings about seeing you. Never ask the child if he or she would like to return to see you; if a further interview is planned, indicate when it will be. Then, take the child back to the parent in the waiting room. As mentioned, avoid whispered hallway consultations with the parent. Either indicate clearly that the discussion will have to wait for a later appointment with the parents; if it is urgent, conduct it briefly in your office, preferably with the child present.

Notes

Should you take notes during the interview? Preferably not. If you cannot train your memory to stretch far enough, use a scratch pad on which to jot key phrases to remind you afterward of the order of events. Learn to use a dic-

Dictation

taphone. Record the interview, at once, after it has terminated.

The interpretation of play

The interpretation of childhood play is a specialized skill requiring extensive theoretical knowledge and supervised practical experience. This section only touches on the highlights.

Greenspan (1981a) provides a useful guide to the phase-appropriate

Normative fantasy themes

physical, affective, relational, conflictual, and cognitive phenomena and to the fantasy themes expressed during the first 10 years of childhood. Normative fantasy themes are summarized in Table 21.1.

Age-appropriate fantasies

Do not be surprised, for example, if an 8-year-old prefers to draw with a paper and pencil rather than poster colors or finger paints. No particular importance should be attached to the observation that a 4-year-old enjoys constructing

TABLE 21.1
Normative fantasy themes

Years	Themes
4	Anxiety over loss of approval of significant others; fear of bodily injury; omnipotent self-defense; curiosity about body differences and functions.
5 & 6	As with 4 years, but emerging capacity for guilt (''badness'') for transgressions, and increasing exploration of world. Polarities: love-hate, kind-mean, death-rebirth.
7 & 8	Fear of injury, especially in competitive interaction with peers. Emerging fear of inferiority in strength, speed, beauty, or intelligence, and concern with rules and conformity. Gender role differences.
9 & 10	Capacity for guilt and internal conflict. Black-and-white morality. Themes picked up from television serials and cartoons: invulnerability, pursuit and rescue, transgression and punishment. Gender role differences more imperative.

block towers and knocking them over, or that a 6-year-old recounts episodes of the television programs of ''Spiderman'' or ''Wonderwoman.''

Fantasy that reveals distortion or immaturity

The trick is to recognize deviations from, distortions of, or immaturity in the phase-related themes noted in Table 21.1. Children struggling to cope with an inner conflict between opposing forces (for example, between explosion and control, dependence and independence, activity and passivity, curiosity and avoidance, daring and injury, male and female, crime and punishment, invulnerability and helplessness, dominance and submission) are likely to express the theme in play over and over again like a phonograph stuck in a groove.

Repetitive family themes and unresolved conflict

■ A 4-year-old boy with psychogenic megacolon and encopresis constructs a railroad train of rectangular blocks on a flat platform of larger blocks. Making appropriate noises he slowly pushes the sections of the train over the edge, one by one. He plays this game over and over. ■

■ An obsessional 8-year-old with numerous tics and compulsive symptoms plays the same cops-and-robbers game at every interview. He is the thief; the clinician is the cop. The cop is cast as a clod whose gum-shoed pursuit is continually foiled by the robber's nimble strategems. The game ends when the criminal is ''electricuted'' by rotation in the office chair but escapes execution to rob again. At times, however, the policeman is cast as a ''murderer'' who stalks the child robber in order to liquidate him. ■

The idiosyncratic details, the repetitiousness, and the distorted, deviant, or grossly immature theme should alert the interviewer to fantasy material of diagnostic importance.

The child mental status evaluation

As the interview progresses, the clinician concurrently makes observations and may deliberately elicit information in order to complete a mental status assessment. The extended child mental status examination (CMSE) covers the following areas:

1. Appearance.
2. Motor behavior.
3. Sensory disturbances.
4. Voice, speech, and language.
5. Interaction with interviewer.
6. Relationship to interviewer.
7. Affect and mood.
8. Thought processes.
9. Thought content.
10. Quality of fantasy.
11. Insight.
12. Needs, pressures, and inner states.

Conducting the CMSE

See appendixes II and III for a complete list and glossary of CMSE items. For the most part, the CMSE is conducted in parallel with the interview. The interview goals and the topics addressed (see the beginning of this section and the list of topics) provide the data on which the CMSE is based. Only sections 9 (thought content) and 11 (insight) require specific investigation. Sections 9 and 11 are addressed only if cues from the parents or child have indicated that such discretionary inquiry would likely be fruitful. Developmental level should be screened specifically only if there is a suggestion of abnormality in language, cognitive development, or school performance. See Table 21.2.

Rating the CMSE

The form for recording a CMSE is included in appendix II. Although somewhat laborious to complete, the Child Mental Status Rating Scales provide a useful training experience and are a memory aid in an area sometimes treated rather skimpily. The items in the CMSE record are clinical inferences rated on a four-point scale (*not present – doubtful – moderate – marked*). The recorder should also note if the item is *not assessed* or *not applicable*. If the item is present, record the observation on which it is based.

Eliciting fantasy

Play, drawing, and action are the media through which the child communicates fantasy. The clinician can often help stimulate fantasy, encourage the child to articulate it, and catch a glimpse of the child's inner world.

As the child plays or draws with the equipment provided, invite verbalization of the action represented. You can ask who the characters are, what they are doing and thinking, and what will happen next. Sometimes, the child will allow you to join in and play, but do not push too soon and crowd the child.

TABLE 21.2
Items on the child mental status rating scales

A. Appearance and Behavior

1. Appearance

1.1	Height	1.7	Abnormality of physique
1.2	Weight	1.8	Lack of personal hygiene
1.3	Precocious physical maturation	1.9	Untidiness of dress
1.4	Delayed physical maturation	1.10	Inappropriateness of dress
1.5	Abnormality of skin	1.11	Other abnormality of
1.6	Abnormality of head, facies, or mouth		appearance

2. Motor Behavior

2.1	Hyperkinesis	e.	Choreiform movements
2.2	Hypokinesis	f.	Athetoid movements
2.3	Bradykinesis	g.	Ballismus
2.4	Abnormality of posture	h.	Mirror movements and motor overflow
2.5	Abnormality of gait		
2.6	Abnormality of balance	2.11	Motor impersistence
2.7	Abnormality of coordination	2.12	Torticollis
2.8	Impairment of power	2.13	Pronounced startle response
2.9	Abnormality of tone	2.14	Mannerisms
2.10	Abnormal movements	2.15	Rituals
	a. Tremor	2.16	Echopraxia
	b. Twitching	2.17	Stereotyped movements
	c. Tics	2.18	Repetitive habits
	d. Fidgetiness	2.19	Lack of sphincter control
		2.20	Other abnormality of motor behavior

3. Sensory disturbances

3.1	Abnormality of somatic sensation	3.4	Abnormality of special sense
3.2	Itching or paresthesia	3.5	Abnormality of body image
3.3	Synesthesia		

4. Voice, Speech, and Language

4.1	Absence of speech	4.11	Abnormality of syntax
4.2	Unusual accent	4.12	Babbling
4.3	Abnormality of amplitude	4.13	Idioglossia
4.4	Abnormality of pitch or tone	4.14	Echolalia
4.5	Abnormality of tempo	4.15	Difficulty in expressive language
4.6	Abnormality of phonation	4.16	Difficulty in comprehension
4.7	Abnormality of rhythm	4.17	Other abnormality of voice, speech, or language
4.8	Abnormality of articulation		
4.9	Abnormal use of words		
4.10	Obscenity or profanity		

5. Interaction with Interviewer

5.1	Aversion of gaze	5.5	Tense
5.2	Distant focus of gaze	5.6	Impulsive
5.3	Staring	5.7	Other abnormality of interaction
5.4	Unresponsive		

(continued)

TABLE 21.2 (*continued*)

B. Attitudes, Affect, Thought Processes and Thought Content	
6. Relationship to Interviewer	
6.1 Assertive	6.12 Invasive
6.2 Bewildered	6.13 Loquacious
6.3 Boastful	6.14 Overcompliant
6.4 Clinging	6.15 Preoccupied
6.5 Clowning	6.16 Seductive
6.6 Evasive	6.17 Shy
6.7 Fearful	6.18 Suggestible
6.8 Hostile	6.19 Suspicious
6.9 Impudent	6.20 Uncooperative
6.10 Indifferent	6.21 Withdrawn
6.11 Ingratiating	6.22 Other characteristic of interaction

7. Affect and Mood	
7.1 Angry	7.8 Histrionic
7.2 Anhedonic	7.9 Inappropriate affect
7.3 Anxious	7.10 Labile affect
7.4 Apathetic	7.11 Resigned
7.5 Depressed	7.12 Restricted affect
7.6 Euphoric	7.13 Silly
7.7 Flat affect	7.14 Other abnormality of affect or mood

8. Thought Processes	
8.1 Blocking	8.9 Looseness of associations
8.2 Circumlocution	8.10 Paralogia
8.3 Circumstantiality	8.11 Perseveration
8.4 Concretistic thinking	8.12 Poverty of thought
8.5 Defect in memory	8.13 Slowing of thought
8.6 Distractibility	8.14 Tangential thinking
8.7 Flight of ideas	8.15 Other disturbance in thought process
8.8 Incoherence	

9. Thought Content	
9.1 Compulsion	9.10 Illusion
9.2 Confabulation	9.11 Impulsion
9.3 Déjà vu	9.12 Malingering
9.4 Delusion	9.13 Obsession
9.5 Depersonalization	9.14 Phobia
9.6 Derealization	9.15 Preoccupation with own mental functioning
9.7 Dissociation	
9.8 Fabrication	9.16 Somatic preoccupation
9.9 Hallucination	9.17 Trance state

10. Quality of Fantasy	
10.1 Bizarreness	
10.2 Decreased productivity	
10.3 Increased productivity	

(*continued*)

TABLE 21.2 (*continued*)

11. Insight

11.1 Lack of understanding of reason
      for clinic attendance
11.2 Lack of understanding of nature
      of problems
11.3 Lack of desire for help

C. Salient Themes in Fantasy

12. Needs, Pressures, and Inner States

12.1 Achievement	12.27 Loneliness
12.2 Acquisition	12.28 Loss
12.3 Affiliation	12.29 Nurturance
12.4 Affliction	12.30 Optimism
12.5 Aggression	12.31 Pessimism
12.6 Alienation	12.32 Play
12.7 Antisocial	12.33 Preoccupation with body
12.8 Anxiety	function
12.9 Autonomy	12.34 Preoccupation with mental
12.10 Avoidance of blame	function
12.11 Change	12.35 Recognition
12.12 Compensation	12.36 Rejection
12.13 Conflict	12.37 Relaxation
12.14 Creativity	12.38 Resignation
12.15 Curiosity	12.39 Retention
12.16 Death	12.40 Revenge
12.17 Deference	12.41 Seclusion
12.18 Dominance	12.42 Self-pity
12.19 Exhibition	12.43 Sexuality
12.20 Exposition	12.44 Shame
12.21 Failure	12.45 Succor
12.22 Fantasy	12.46 Suicide
12.23 Guilt	12.47 Understanding
12.24 Inferiority	12.48 Vindication
12.25 Injury	12.49 Other salient theme
12.26 Lack	

Human figure drawing

Whenever possible, ask the child to draw. Have the child draw a whole person, using a number 2 soft pencil on 8½ " × 11" paper. Human figure drawings provide information about the child's developmental level (see Human Figure Drawing Test, in the next section) and body image. They may also provide information about self-concept, gender identity, ideal self, and bad self. These fragmentary images common to all children are likely to be distorted in the psychologically disturbed. After the drawing is completed, ask the child questions about it to test the capacity for fantasy.

Case 21.1 (continued)

■ Paula is an 11-year-old school-phobic girl. It is her first interview, and she is just beginning to relax. She has drawn a female figure with vertical lines attached to the arms.

CLINICIAN: Is that a boy or a girl, a man or a woman?

PAULA: It's a girl.

CLINICIAN: How old is that girl?

PAULA: I don't know.

CLINICIAN: Make it up like a story. How old would you guess she is?

PAULA: About ten.

CLINICIAN: What's she doing in that picture?

PAULA: Just standing there.

CLINICIAN: What are those lines going up from her arms?

PAULA: Strings.

CLINICIAN: How come?

PAULA: She's a puppet.

CLINICIAN: What is she thinking there, with strings on her?

PAULA: She's thinking that she hates it, being a puppet. It's dumb . . . .

Other questions helpful in eliciting fantasy about the figure are as follows:

*Question to elicit
fantasy from the
HFDT*

1. What makes her happy?
2. What makes her mad?
3. What makes her sad?
4. What makes her scared?
5. What does she need most?
6. What's the best thing about her?
7. What's the worst thing about her?
8. Tell me about her family.
9. What will she do next?

*Characteristics of the
KFDT*

A second drawing that is particularly helpful is the Kinetic Family Figure Drawing. Ask the child to draw the family doing something together. Note the child's conception of the members of the family; their relative importance (size) and power (configuration of arms and legs); their countenances (emotional expression, teeth, etc.); and suggestions of preferred attachments, rivalries, or coalitions within the family, as revealed by the relative distance between and grouping of family members. Ask the child to explain the drawing, using discretion in following the clues provided, according to the dynamic hypotheses you have already generated or those occurring to you when you see the drawing.

Another useful approach for eliciting desires and fears is to ask the child first to draw ''something nice'' and then to draw ''something horrible.''

''Squiggles''

The game of ''Squiggles'' introduced by Winnicott (1965), is an engaging technique that can generate a fruitful exchange of fantasy between child and adult. The clinician asks the child to draw a random scribble, then demonstrates how the scribble can be transformed into a figure, which is finally given a title. Next, the clinician makes a scribble and invites the child to transform it into a figure or scene with a title. Child and clinician then alternate in a series of titled scribble-transformations. In Winnicott's original technique, the clinician's drawings represent clarificatory comments or interpretations about the child's fantasy –

a sophisticated technique demanding considerable theoretical knowledge and technical skill. Even without such skill, however, you can stimulate a revealing interchange with a child who catches on. However, be careful your own drawings are not too good lest the exchange evolve into a contest in technical expertise. Instead, let your fantasy run free and allow your drawing to be a little blurred around the edges.

Several standard questions serve as ice-breaking overtures; for example:

Questions for eliciting
fantasy

1. "If you had three wishes, what would they be?"
2. "If you had $1,000,000 what would you do?"
3. "If you were wrecked on a desert island, who and what would you like to have with you?"

These questions test whether the child is capable of generating and discussing fantasy and reveal the salient themes in that fantasy (anxiety, independence, nurturance, succor, revenge, etc.).

Dreams
Earliest memory

It can be fruitful to ask for recent good and bad dreams. Finally, it is sometimes revealing to ask children for the earliest life-event remembered.

Clinical tests for the rough estimation of developmental level

Standardized psychological tests of cognitive, psychomotor, language and social development and tests of school performance are discussed in the section on special investigations (chapter 22). Their administration and interpretation is specialized and requires a clinical psychologist. However, a number of approximate clinical techniques can generate or screen diagnostic hypotheses about defects in these areas.

Routine screening for
developmental level
during the CMSE

Generally speaking, a child's vocabulary, syntax, grasp of the situation, comprehension of your questions, sensitivity to nuance, general knowledge, and capacity to abstract will point to normal or abnormal intellectual, language, and social development. If school progress is also satisfactory, there is no need for a formal psychological evaluation of cognitive capacity unless you have a hunch the child is exceptionally bright (and parents and school are unaware of it). Similarly, the child's motor development and the power and coordination of the child's fine and gross motor function will be referred to in the history and observable during the interview, particularly if the child is involved in play.

Precautions about
over- or under-
estimating ability

Several precautions should be kept in mind. Middle-class clinicians tend to view children of similar origin as normative and to underestimate the ability of those from different sociocultural backgrounds. Vivacious, loquacious, and charming children are typically overvalued; the reserved or somber child may leave a less favorable impression.

Administer clinical
screening tests in a
standard manner

The discretionary clinical tests to be described are no more than rough screens. Strive to administer them in a standard manner so the reliability of your evaluations will be enhanced. Try to ensure that the child is interested in the test and not distracted by extraneous stimulation, pain, fatigue, hunger, anxiety, or depression. Encourage the child when a response is given but do not give assistance with the answer. Remember: the tests to be described are screens; they determine whether formal psychometric evaluation is indicated.

The Minnesota Child Development Inventory (Ireton & Thwing, 1972) will already have been completed if the child is of preschool age.

A clinician can easily learn to administer the Peabody Vocabulary Test (PPVT) (Dunn & Dunn, 1981), which assesses the child's ability to point correctly, when given a word by the examiner, to one of four pictures on each page of a series of pages of increasing difficulty. It is essentially a test of denominative ability. The PPVT takes about ten minutes to administer, has norms for 2 to 18 years of age, and has the advantage of not requiring an oral response.

The Vocabulary List in Table 21.3 is a test of verbal ability requiring an oral response. The child should be asked, "What is an orange?" and so on until five consecutive words are missed. The child can be encouraged to explain or demonstrate the answer, but avoid asking leading questions. If the child is obviously incorrect, no questions should be asked; the examiner should pass on to the next word with a neutral "uh huh." The examiner can spell out or show the written word if necessary.

The Human Figure Drawing Test for children between 5 and 12 years of age is a test of drawing ability roughly correlating with intellectual development

TABLE 21.3
Vocabulary test

Words	Number Correct	Age (years – months)
1. Orange	5	6–0
2. Envelope	6	6–8
3. Straw	7	7–4
4. Puddle	8	8–0
5. Tap	9	8–8
6. Gown	10	9–4
7. Eyelash	11	10–0
8. Roar	12	10–8
9. Scorch	13	11–4
10. Muzzle	14	12–0
11. Haste	15	13–3
12. Lecture	16	14–0
13. Mars	17	14–3
14. Skill	18	14–6
15. Juggler	19	14–9
16. Brunette	20	Av. Adult
17. Peculiarity		
18. Priceless		
19. Regard		
20. Disproportionate		
21. Shrewd		
22. Tolerate		

TABLE 21.4
Human figure drawing test directions (after Koppitz, 1968)

1. Use number 2 pencil with eraser on 8½ ″ × 11″ paper.
2. Instruct child as follows: "On this sheet of paper, I would like you to draw a WHOLE person. It can be any kind of person you want to draw, just make sure that it is a WHOLE person and not just a stick figure or a cartoon figure." For a younger child who does not understand the meaning of "person," one can add. "You may draw a man or a woman, a boy or a girl, whichever you want to draw."
3. There is no fixed time limit on this test.
4. Note the order in which the child draws the parts of the figure, any last minute additions, or alterations, and spontaneous comments.
5. Ask the child to identify the sex and age of the figure. After the drawing is completed, ask the child: "Tell me about your person. How old is this person? What kind of person is this? What is the person doing?"
6. Score according to the Koppitz (1968) schedule.
7. Indicators of possible emotional disturbance are listed in Koppitz (1968).

(Koppitz, 1968). The child is asked to draw a whole person. Control the administration of this test by using a number 2 pencil with eraser and paper of standard size (8½ ″ × 11″). Test instructions are included in Table 21.4.

The Gesell Drawing Test is described in Table 21.5. It has norms for children as young as 16 months and a ceiling of 7 years.

It is useful to have in your drawer Word Recognition Cards classified in term of grade achievement. Glaser and Clemmens (1965), for example, provided word recognition lists of 20 words per grade level. The child should read each column to the end in order to be credited with that grade level. Partial grade achievements can be expressed as decimal points.

The reliability and validity of interviews with children

Test–retest reliability

Rutter and Graham (1968) investigated the reliability of semistructured playroom interviews with children of 7 to 12 years of age, conducted by trained assessors. Using the criteria "no abnormality," "some abnormality," and "definite abnormality," a 12-day test–retest reliability of .84 was obtained. The reliability of more detailed components of the evaluation was less impressive. An

Intertester reliability

intertester reliability of .74 was obtained when one interviewer watched as the other conducted the interview. Intertester reliability dropped to .64 when different evaluators examined the same child 4 weeks apart.

Validity

Compared with evaluations of abnormality from teacher or parent reports of the child's behavior, blind interviewers diagnosed as abnormal only 1.5% of the children assessed as normal by parallel means; but they detected abnormality in only 35% of the children regarded as abnormal by their parents or teachers.

From this study, it appears that brief test–retest and immediate intertester reliability is reasonable, but that interviews with children alone underestimate psychopathology. Much more work needs to be done in this area.

TABLE 21.5
The Gesell Drawing Test (16 months to 7 years)

16–18 Months

Procedure: Give paper and pencil to the child, saying, "Jimmy write." If there is no response, demonstrate what to do by scribbling with the same pencil; then repeat the instructions.

Credit 16 months: If the child scribbles after demonstration.

Credit 18 months: If the child scribbles before demonstration.

27–30 months

Procedure: Place the paper before child. Draw one vertical 3″ line and give the pencil to the child, saying "Jimmy make one like that." If the child makes a vertical motion, take the pencil back and make a horizontal line with the same instructions. If the child then makes a horizontal motion, take the pencil again and make two 3″ circles with same instructions. If the child fails any one of these attempts, start again from the beginning. If the child fails again, discontinue the test.

Credit 27 months: If the child makes a stroke rather than an aimless scribble.

Credit 30 months: If the child differentiates vertical, horizontal and circular *strokes*. (The quality of the drawing is unimportant.)

3 Years

Procedure: Place the paper before child. Draw a circle 2″ in diameter with the instruction, "Make one like this." Repeat this procedure twice more, allowing three tries.

Credit: If any of the three attempts is rounded and closed.

3½ Years

Procedure: Draw a cross (x) with lines about 2″ long instructing the child to, "Make one like this." Allow only one attempt.

Credit: If the two lines cross. (Be very lenient.)

5 Years

Procedure: Draw a 2″ square instructing the client, "Make one like this." Allow three attempts, repeating the demonstration and the instructions each time.

Credit: If any of the three attempts has (a) sharp corners, (b) one dimension less than twice the length of the other dimension, and (c) fairly straight lines.

7 Years

Procedure: Draw a diamond about 3″ high instructing the child to, "Make one like this." Allow three attempts, repeating the instructions each time. "Now make another one like this."

Credit: If any of the three attempts has (a) 4 definite angles, (b) is shaped more like a diamond than like a kite or a square and (c) has angles roughly opposite each other.

The interview with the adolescent (13 through 18 years)

Greater capacity for reflection about self and others

Interviews with adolescents have qualities intermediate between those with children and those with adults. The adolescent usually has the potential to sustain a face-to-face conversation for a full hour or more, although he or she may choose not to do so. Compared to children, adolescents are capable of greater self-reflection, a more objective perspective of themselves and others, and of recognizing a personal problem and deciding to do something about it.

Adult resistance to adolescence

The psychiatry of adolescence was a neglected field until the last 20 years. Even today, comprehension of this crucial epoch is sketchy and uneven. Beyond the theoretical issues, however, lie the problems of coming to terms with and involving oneself in a group of human beings who arouse powerful feelings in those who relate to them.

Popular speakers often draw attention to the historical record; the middle-aged have perennially complained that youth is going to the dogs and blamed adolescents for the shortcomings of a society. This century, however, has produced an uneasy counterbalance between a depreciation of age and a desire of the jaded to regain the vigor of youth. For the first time, perhaps, adolescents form a distinct subculture in which adults are out of place and from which they are excluded.

The extent of adult uneasiness, withdrawal, testiness, or envious spectatorship is greater than can be explained on the basis of social exclusion alone. The powerful and conflicting emotions of adolescence are denied, blurred, or repressed in the relative emotional flattening of adulthood. It is painful to resurrect one's earlier anxieties, confusions, and inner torments and to apprehend how less keen one's sensibilities have become. It is certainly upsetting to be reminded what a fool one once was, how shaky a painfully developed sense of self-esteem can be, and to what extent the exigencies of life have eroded an erstwhile idealism.

Emancipation

Meanwhile, crossing the developmental Rubicon, the adolescent must advance on several fronts. The adolescent must emancipate the self from dependence on parents and relinquish overclose attachments to them. This task may prove more difficult for the girl than for the boy if she has been more protected or restricted. Once freed, she can shift progressively towards heterosexual objects as she becomes capable of giving as well as receiving affection. Both the girl and the boy must reshape in more flexible form the more rigid superego of earlier years, and learn that the real world is colored in shades of grey. They must internalize controls, discriminate when to restrict and when to gratify needs, and tolerate tension.

Heterosexuality

Intimacy
Superego

Abstract reasoning

Their capacity to achieve these goals is supported by an increasing ability to reason and to think abstractly. Eventually, self-esteem is stabilized in the face of vicissitudes in personal relationships, and an identity is forged, the integration of many partial identifications from childhood and early adolescent years.

Identity

Adolescent coping strategies

Development is often attained by leaps and retreats and less commonly by smooth transition. The struggle to emancipate oneself and to achieve a more mature relationship with parents may be punctuated by displacement of affection to parent substitutes, an increase of narcissism and self-involvement, or a rebellion against parental restrictions and values. For a time, the adolescent may defend against drives by denial or asceticism but increasingly uses intellectualization, theoretical discussion, and idealism. These defenses against objects and drives are stabilizing and adaptive since they allow the breathing space necessary for a regrouping of strengths before further advances.

Psychopathology in adolescence

The disturbed adolescent, in contrast, typically has trouble breaking free of parents and assimilating drives within a stable self-concept. In these circumstances the normal defenses of adolescence become exaggerated and unbalanced: sweeping repression or denial, masochistic reaction formations, marked regression, and pathologically intense displacement of affection (for example, in "crushes") can be manifestations of psychological maladjustment in this age group.

Whatever the label applied to the adolescent patient who presents for treatment, the disturbance makes no sense unless it is viewed against the backdrop of normal development. The clinical case reveals the problems of adolescent development gone wrong, development arrested, diverted, or turned back from its normal course.

General characteristics of the emotionally disturbed adolescent

For this reason, it is possible to make generalizations that hold true for most of the clinical syndromes with which adolescents present. One can predict, for example, that an adolescent patient is having difficulty in accepting and constructively deploying sexual and aggressive drives. Adolescent patients will often wonder, in their anxiety, if they are going crazy. They may have retreated into neurotic inhibition of impulse; rather than reflect on their conflicts, they may act impulsively to express what cannot be assimilated; or they may hide behind a barricade of withdrawal and compensatory fantasy. Regardless of the apparent directness of her amatory experiences, the adolescent girl probably fears intimacy and is capable of little more than allowing herself to be used. In her attempts to emancipate herself, she may devalue her parents to an extreme degree or, more ominously, give up the struggle and allow herself to be manipulated like an automaton. Toward authorities in general, the boy is likely to be both contemptuous and demanding or, on the other hand, withdrawn and submissive. Both will be confused about the future. Their scholastic progress is probably affected. Futhermore, they wonder who they are, see themselves as shams, and attach themselves to others like buoys in a storm. In extreme cases of identity diffusion, there is such a loss of centrality and such a sense of dissolution that sexual identity, the sense of time, and the capacity to separate fantasy from reality are affected. Identity diffusion may represent a transient, reversible emotional disturbance or, on the other hand, foreshadow malignant psychotic transformation.

Factors affecting adolescent psychopathology

These are the basic factors influencing adolescent psychopathology: strong impulses; a fluid defensive structure; a fear of intimacy; a tendency to form intense but short-lived relationships; and a precarious sense of identity.

Achieving rapport

These developmental considerations are pertinent to the technique of interviewing adolescents. The clinician's attitude to the adolescent patient should be accepting and committed, avoiding seductiveness and not threatening the patient by overinvolvement. Pass beyond the acceptable limits of the relationship (by rejecting, withdrawing, or crowding the patient) and it is no longer tenable. The clinician must maintain surveillance over personal reactions in order to avoid exploiting or being exploited.

Choice of therapist

Generally, female therapists work better with adolescent girls, and male therapists with boys. Yet a man may be effective with girls who have lost or been rejected by a father. Among older adolescent girls with problems involving

Sex

homosexual feelings or bisexuality, a male therapist may become a useful bridge to heterosexual adjustment. A female clinician may represent a less threatening therapeutic figure for the borderline adolescent boy with sexual identity problems.

Age

Age can also be important. The therapist can be too young or too old for a particular patient. A therapist who is too old may be unable to jump the barrier of generations in order to be bothered with adolescent problems. A therapist who is too young may be threatened or seduced by the patient to gain vicarious pleasure from the patient's behavior. Adolescents can be extremely skillful in seeking out and exploiting adult vulnerabilities. The therapist who suddenly realizes how much he or she has contributed to and gained pleasure from the patient's maladaptive behavior may be frightened away from adolescents forever.

The need for genuine involvement

Before making an explicit or implicit contract, the patient may test what stuff the clinician is made of. This is no time for passive neutrality, long silences, or empathic grunts. Having already had experience of adults with personality defects, the patient is wise to have no respect for the phony, the autocrat, or the muddler. In contrast, the patient may relate quickly to a strong, decisive clinician who responds to deeper personal needs.

Therapeutic style

Various therapeutic styles are effective. Each clinician must develop an approach that suits, yet is adapted to the individual patient. The clinician's effectiveness is governed as much by attitude as by technical skill.

Candor

Holmes (1964) suggests that a conversational style characterized by unusual candor is often the most effective way of conducting the interview. This style shows the patient that the therapist can introduce matters of significance without anxiety and embarrassment. This approach applies to current conscious issues. It involves not beating about the bush and is equivalent to neutralizing an unspeakable secret by airing it.

Case 21.3

■ Tracey, a school-phobic, socially withdrawn 11-year-old girl, was admitted for investigation. During interviews with her female therapist Tracey was depressed and apparently struggling with a problem about which she was painfully conflicted; but she was able to give several clues that the issue concerned her father. The clinician remarked that there seemed to be a problem between her and the father. Tracey concurred but said that it was something she could not speak of. The therapist asked directly if her father had made sexual advances to her. Palpably relieved, Tracey wept and told the explosive story she had been forced to keep to herself. ■

If you have good reason for believing that something unspoken is true about the patient and the patient is aware of it, sometimes you had better say it. The directness of this approach can lead to a rapid cadence of communication, leaving the patient both interested in and challenged by the prospect of further contact.

Arguments

Holmes suggests that arguments are inevitable, even beneficial. Arguing can be a mode of conversation in which the hostile but frightened patient feels comfortable; but the clinician must learn to argue in a concerned manner.

Case 21.4   ■   Stu, an alienated and rejected boy of 14, has been admitted to an institution because of uncontrollability at home. In this interview, he is hiding his depression behind a facade of bitter resentfulness.

STU: (*contemptuously*) You're a fag.
CLINICIAN: What do you mean?
STU: You know what I mean. You're a faggot. (*He waits expectantly to see the effect of this bombshell.*)
CLINICIAN: Well, I could be a fag for all you know. But how could you know? You seem to be doing your best to avoid finding out anything about me. How come?
STU: People should mind their own business.
CLINICIAN: How do you mean?

Challenges

Holmes points out that the adolescent often uses an exclamation mark when a question mark is called for, expressing his questions as demands or assertions. "You can't stop me!" really means "Have you got the strength to stop me from doing this? Do you really care enough to try?"

Case 21.5   ■   Maureen, a 16 year old housebound phobic girl, passively acquiesced in her admission to the hospital. After 1 day, acutely distressed and sobbing, Maureen began to work on the clinician's guilt. She demanded to know why she could not go home at once. When this approach got nowhere, she tried to trap the clinician into setting a time limit to her stay in the hospital. "If I'm good can I go home in 1 week . . . 2 weeks . . . a month?" The clinician responded in this way: "Look, I know you're homesick; but we both know that your coming in here was necessary if you're going to get better. I can't tell you exactly how long you'll be here; you haven't even begun therapy yet. When the time comes for you to go home, we'll both know you're ready." Within a week, Maureen was able to admit the therapist was correct to insist she stay on and to tackle afresh her fear of public transport. This represented her most constructive step after 2 years of outpatient therapy.   ■

The crucial early task is establishing a dependable relationship. Be direct; indicate what you already know.

Inception

CLINICIAN: Your mother came to see me last week because she's been concerned about you. She told me something about your early life and how things are at home with your family. She's been worried because for the last year or so you've seemed very unhappy and you've not been able to concentrate at school. Maybe you could tell me something about it.

Reassurance and orientation

Confidentiality

The patient has heard about headshrinkers and has ideas about what is going to happen. If possible, these fantasies should be expressed and clarified at the outset. Reassure the patient about the confidentiality of the interview or, if it must be broken (as, rarely, it must), say so and why. For the same reason, if a parent must bring the patient for an initial interview, insist on seeing the patient first.

Expect cooperation

At some time during the first interview, you may need to explain that the interview must be cooperative. You may suggest that the patient must decide whether to obstruct you or to work on the problems. Long silences, ambiguity, and interpretive cleverness should be avoided, and neutrality and nondirectiveness laid aside; the adolescent is quick to spot when a clinician is using technique as a defense. Neutrality can be a cloak behind which a timid psychiatrist hides a fear of commitment, as can avuncularity or fraternization. Be yourself.

Avoid neutrality

It may be advisable to explain that the patient is free to say what he or she thinks, that you realize it is difficult to express everything that comes into the mind, and that often the most significant matters are held back. Convey the idea that diagnosis and therapy are collaborative.

Promote motivation

Although parental pressure may be necessary to get the patient to the first few interviews, therapy will not prosper unless the patient ultimately provides internal motivation. With patients capable of insight, one may allow the adolescent to decide whether to come back. In this situation, ask the parents to refrain from giving advice unless the patient seeks it. If the patient does so, they should express their opinion on the matter, without pressure.

Transference cures

Current involvements are often so immediate that there is little exploration of material from the past. Sometimes this is enough; one is impressed with the rapid transference improvements possible, given a potentially enriching external environment. As one would expect in view of the adolescent process itself, quick attachments to the clinician are common. Whether these relationships persist will be determined by the clinician's ability to help resolve the basic anxieties that impelled the patient into therapy in the first place. This is one reason why negative feelings at the beginning or in the course of the encounter should be taken up at once.

Let us return to the point made earlier. Different clinicians have different styles; the attitude, underlying philosophy, and approach are what matter, rather than the technical polish. Though there are few completely bad interviewers (anybody can help somebody), but some are more effective than others.

Characteristics of the effective interviewer

The effective clinician relates to a broad spectrum of people, creating an atmosphere that enables many patients to make significant choices. How is this achieved? Rogers (1951) suggests that the effective clinician is accepting, genuinely respecting patients and trusting them to go at their own pace without undue direction. The effective clinician empathizes with and has the ability to communicate empathic concern to the patient. Finally, the clinician is congruent, aware of personal responses, needing to play no role, and emotionally free to express personal feelings when it is appropriate to do so.

The family interview

It is important to interview the child or adolescent with the parents during the diagnostic phase. In the following circumstances, the entire family should be interviewed:

Rationale for inter-viewing an entire family

1. When there has been an emotional crisis affecting all family members, such as the attempted suicide or severe illness of one family member.
2. When it is apparent that there has been a significant breakdown in communication between two or more family members.
3. When it is important to mobilize all family resources in order to overcome an acute disturbance of one family member (for example, in acute school phobia).
4. When it is hypothesized that generally distorted communication within the family is perpetuating the emotional disturbance of one or more family members.

The timing of the family interview

It is important to decide whether one should involve all siblings and other immediate and distant family members; one should always interview the parents and the nominated patient together at some time in the diagnostic process to formulate a provisional family diagnosis. In the usual case, this interview can be arranged after the parental and child interviews are completed. The family interview can be merged with the negotiation of a plan for therapy or, if time and cost are less pressing, conducted as a separate diagnostic interview before diagnostic formulation. If the entire family are to be seen, the last arrangement is required.

What questions should be addressed in a family diagnostic inquiry? The following account is a simplified introduction to a complex area. For a more detailed discussion, see Hillman (1982), from whose diagnostic schedule this description has been adapted.

Family functioning can be viewed from a number of interlocking perspectives:

1. Family composition and external characteristics.
2. Developmental stage.
3. Functions, roles, and decisions.
4. Rules, beliefs, values, and aspirations.
5. Modes of communication.
6. Structural dynamics, coherence, and methods of coping with stress.

Family composition and external characteristics

Composition

Who are in the family, and what are their names and ages, educational backgrounds, occupations, and current physical and mental health? Are the children natural, adopted, fostered, or from a previous marriage? Who else lives at home? Do grandparents or other kin play a significant part in family life? Who are the pets, and whose responsibility are they?

Dwelling

Describe the setting, style, size, and apparent adequacy of the dwelling place for the family's collective and individual needs.

Demography

What are the combined income, social class, ethnic tradition, cultural background, and religion of the family?

Community

Does the family fit in to the immediate environment in terms of housing, social background, ethnic tradition, cultural interests, and religion; or is it markedly different?

Developmental stage

Families can generally be classified according to how far they have progressed along the following sequence of stages:

Developmental stages

1. Establishment (newly married, no children).
2. New parents (oldest child 0 to 2 years).
3. Preschool family (oldest child 3 to 5 years).
4. School-age family (oldest child 6 to 12 years).
5. Adolescent family (oldest child 13 to 19 years).
6. Young adult family (oldest child 20 or older and all other children still at home).
7. Family as launching center (as children depart one by one).
8. Postparental family (all children gone, but parents still working).
9. Aging family (after retirement).

Each stage makes different demands on the family in terms of communication, roles, functions, and methods of collective coping.

Functions, roles, and decisions

Distribution of work, power, responsibility

How are labor, responsibility, privilege, and power distributed in the family? Who are the breadwinners? Who are the nurturers? Who does the inside and outside work at home? Who mends things when they go wrong? Who cooks, who cleans up, who disciplines, and who comforts?

Decisions

How are decisions made about the house, money, vacations, rules, and discipline? Is the prevailing mode of decision-making authoritarian (maternal, paternal, or both), permissive, democratic, educational, lax, or chaotic? The more chaotic the family, the less coherent the leadership, the lines of communication, and the manner in which decisions are made.

Emotional Roles

What are the emotional roles of different family members? Can you characterize them? In many instances, these roles serve to maintain a kind of homeostasis; for example, the illness of a child with anorexia nervosa may help involve parents who would otherwise drift apart.

Rules, beliefs, values, and aspirations

Rules

Family rules may be explicit (for example, bedtime, table manners, tolerance for back talk, and the allocation of tasks), or implicit (for example, ''Never upset mother''; ''Make allowances for baby''; ''Father knows best''; and ''Keep your fingers crossed that father won't be drunk tonight, but don't talk about it'').

Examples of explicit beliefs are as follows:

1. Attitudes to formal education.
2. Community responsibility.
3. Friendship.
4. Loyalty.
5. Desirability of hard work.
6. Patriotism.
7. Religion.

Shared beliefs

Less easy to determine, yet no less binding, are the implicit beliefs conveyed more by parental modeling and attitude than by direct education. Some examples of the latter are: ''Big boys don't cry''; ''Girls should be sweet''; ''If you can get away with it, it's worth a try''; and ''Arguments are won by whoever shouts loudest.''

Shared values

The values of the family, like its shared beliefs, are conveyed by direct education within the family, by example, and by reinforcement or the threat of exclusion. Values represent superordinate principles in regard to the relationship between people, of people to nature, and of people to supernature. Family values are expressed in its moral and ethical code; its commitment to esthetic, artistic, and cultural expression; and a set of shared concepts that convey the meaning and purpose of life.

Values overlap with aspirations, the commitment of the family to the collective and individual future.

Modes of communication

Decisions

Conflict-resolution

How does the family make decisions about communal matters (such as recreation and vacations) and resolve conflicts between siblings, parents, and child, or parents? Is there a clear leader? Do the family talk matters out or act them out? To what degree do they discuss matters in a group, hold family meetings, give direct advice or lectures to each other, or, on the contrary, avoid direct confrontation on communal issues? How rigid, flexible, spontaneous, impulsive, reserved, or constricted are they? How do they express affection, praise, criticism, anger, sorrow, and joy?

Structural dynamics, coherence, and methods of coping with stress

Coherence

Does the family have coherence? Is it reasonably flexible in regard to individual differences? Can it cope with change? Does it share socially effective principles, define the roles of family members, and distribute responsibility clearly?

Inflexibility and
vulnerability

Pathological families are likely to be inflexible yet vulnerable. They can be seriously imbalanced by blurring of role boundaries between family members or by inappropriate role reversals (for example, when a son adopts a protective, possessive, husbandly attitude to his mother). Other disturbed families are rift by open conflict or emotional divorce between family members. Coalitions can form; for example, between mother and son against father and daughter.

Boundaries

Minuchin (1974) describes families according to their boundaries (clear, diffuse, or rigid), subsystems (spouse subsystem, parental subsystem, and sibling subsystem), style of transaction (enmeshed, normal, or disengaged), and mode of coping with stress (resolution or continuing conflict, coalition formation, triangulation, detouring, or emotional disengagement).

Transactions
Mode of coping
with stress

Enmeshment refers to a blurring of boundaries between two or more family members, resulting in a sharing of psychopathology between the people involved. In school phobia, for example, it is common to find that mother and child have an intensely involved, mutually reinforcing, anxious attachment and that the mother has many fears about the world external to the home.

Disengagement refers to a defensive lack of communication between two or more of all family members amounting to an emotional divorce between parents or an estrangement and remoteness between other family members. In one case, for example, a father and son did not converse for several years following an argument about religion.

Detouring refers to the manner in which conflict between two family members, particularly between parents, is avoided and diverted onto another family member. In this manner, scapegoating can arise.

Case 21.6

■   On three separate occasions, Rhoda, a 9-year-old girl, confided in her mother that her father had repeatedly sexually interfered with her. The mother did nothing about it, saying, on one occasion, that it happened to every girl. Eventually, the secret leaked out through one of the child's friends, and the father was convicted of incest. The family then rejected Rhoda because she had broken up the family.   ■

Detouring is a form of triangulation through which a particular child becomes involved in a conflict-laden relationship between the parents.

The composition of the family, its external characteristics and developmental stage, and its explicit rules, beliefs, and decision-making methods are probed in the parental interview. Conjoint interviews of the entire family, sometimes supplemented by special techniques for investigating transactional patterns, will be required to illuminate the precise modes of communication and the structural dynamics of the family as a whole. The parental interview alone can only provide hints about these more intimate matters; but exigencies of time and cost may preclude a more exhaustive family investigation.

Summary

This chapter describes the reasons for and modes of referral to a child psychiatrist or child psychiatric clinic. Intake procedures include the routine collection of a minimum data base from questionnaires and forms. After the basic information is analyzed, the clinician is free to pursue a discretionary inquiry.

The techniques and content of interviewing and observing parents, infants, children, adolescents, and families are described. Exhaustive protocols are provided, not to direct the clinician on a mindless routine search, but to serve as a set of tools that can be drawn on in a discretionary inquiry directed by an array of categorical and dynamic hypotheses.

The Child Mental Status Examination is derived from the interview in most cases, except when abnormal thought content must be assessed and clinical screening tests for the rapid estimation of developmental level are indicated. Both of these areas are discretionary.

By this stage in the diagnostic encounter, the clinician can decide whether and how physical examination and special investigations are required to complete the inquiry process, reach a diagnostic conclusion, and formulate a comprehensive diagnosis. The physical examination and special investigations are discussed in the next chapter.

Selected Readings

The use of behavioral ratings and multivariate approaches to classification is discussed in Achenbach's (1982) *Developmental Psychopathology*.

The semistructured approach to interviewing children is described in Simmons's (1981) *Psychiatric Examination of Children*. The unstructured approach is presented by Greenspan's (1981a) *The Clinical Interview of the Child*. Lippman (1962) is also very helpful. Greenspan's (1981b) *Psychopathology and Adaptation in Infancy and Early Childhood* is a useful guide to the evaluation of infants and toddlers.

The technique of interviewing adolescents is described by Holmes (1964) in a classic work, *The Adolescent in Psychotherapy*. Meeks (1980) and Lamb (1978) are also helpful in this regard.

Among the techniques for eliciting fantasy, the reader should refer to Gardner (1971) for the mutual storytelling method and to Winnicott (1965) for the technique of "Squiggles."

For assessing family functioning and interaction, see Glick and Kessler (1980) and Minuchin (1974).

22

Diagnostic inquiry in child psychiatry: the physical examination and special investigations

The inquiry mode
After preliminary information has been gathered from referring agent, parents, and teachers and interviews have been completed with parents, child, and family, the clinician will have constructed a tentative pattern of clues and inferences and generated an array of categorical and dynamic hypotheses. The diagnostic process then moves into an inquiry mode, the clinician seeking evidence to confirm or disconfirm hunches made on the basis of the cumulative pattern or patterns of clinical phenomena. This chapter first considers the physical examination as a screening and as a discretionary procedure, although it may have been completed before the family interview.

After the child has been interviewed, a physical examination should be conducted. Most patients referred to a child psychiatry clinic have already been physically assessed by a pediatrician or are under regular pediatric care. If not, a pediatric check should be arranged.

Routine physical parameters
Vital signs (pulse rate, blood pressure, respiration rate, and temperature) should be taken, and growth parameters (height, weight, and head circumference) plotted on standard curves.

507

Discretionary physical examination

If the diagnostic encounter yields clues indicating the need for a discretionary physical examination, this should be conducted at once. Some children, for example, look dysplastic, with developmental asymmetries (e.g., of facial features), distortions (e.g., webbed neck), or disproportions (e.g., unusually long arms). Unusual features of this sort might prompt one to investigate the child's chromosomal makeup. There is evidence (Rappaport et al., 1979) that the following minor physical anomalies are associated with developmental problems, especially hyperactivity in boys:

Minor physical anomalies

1. Head of abnormally small or large circumference.
2. Hair fine and electric.
3. Epicanthic folds.
4. Hypertelorism.
5. Ears low-set, malformed, asymmetrical, or with adherent earlobes.
6. Palate high.
7. Tongue furrowed.
8. Fifth finger incurved.
9. Third toe long.
10. Syndactyly.
11. Abnormal gap between first and second toes.

The significance of these anomalies is not clear; they may be the result of congenital toxic insult or genetic predisposition.

Central nervous symptoms

The following symptoms are referable to disease of the central nervous system:

1. Headache.
2. Ocular or visual symptoms.
3. Deafness.
4. Tinnitus.
5. Imbalance.
6. Episodic disruption of consciousness.
7. Recent memory defects.
8. Intermittent confusion.
9. Anesthesia.
10. Paresthesia.
11. Weakness.
12. Abnormal tone or incoordination.
13. Tremor.
14. Abnormal movements.
15. Regression in sphincter control.

These symptoms prompt immediate neurological consultation.

Brief neurological screening observation

The psychiatrist can perform a brief routine neurological screen during the interview by observing the child's speech, gait, posture, balance, gross and fine motor tone, power and coordination, facial symmetry, and ocular

Routine neuro-logical screen

movements and by checking for tics, tremor, clonus, or choreatiform move-ments of the fingers and hands. The routine screen can be extended by baring the child's feet and forearms and examining the following:

1. Cranial nerves.
   a. Movement of eyes, face, and tongue.
   b. Pupillary reflexes.
   c. Visual fields.
   d. Hearing.
   e. Fundi.
2. Motor power and tone.
3. Reflexes.
   a. Biceps.
   b. Triceps.
   c. Supinator.
   d. Patellar.
   e. Ankle.
   f. Plantar.

Leave examination of the reflexes and fundi to the end.

The benefits of a physical examin-ation outweigh its disadvantages

Some child psychiatrists avoid physical examination. The clinician may worry that an upsetting examination will impede a positive relationship or tilt the spontaneous development of the child's transference. There may be some point to these considerations, but the potential benefits of a nonintrusive physical ex-amination outweigh its disadvantages.

Soft signs

Much ink has been expended on the topic of soft signs in neuropsychiatric disorder. Soft or nonfocal signs are neurological phenomena thought to have no clear locus of origin, to be developmentally normal up to a certain age, and to reflect uneven neurological maturation in older children. Soft neurological signs include the following:

1. Choreatiform or athetoid movements, especially of the outstretched fingers and hands.
2. Synkinesis.
3. Dysdiadochokinesis.
4. General clumsiness.
5. Dysgraphesthesia.

Can these signs be consensually identified and elicited in a standard manner? Do they have significant test–retest and intertester reliability? Do they occur fre-quently enough in an at-risk population to make them worth eliciting? Are they singly or in clusters associated with such disorders as learning disability, attention deficit, or schizophrenia? Do they predict which hyperkinetic children will re-spond to stimulant medication? None of these questions has been clearly answered.

Criteria for a reliable and valid set of soft signs

The items of an ideal neurological schedule for nonfocal signs would have the following characteristics: (1) frequency, (2) reliability, and (3) the capacity to discriminate between children with neuropsychological abnormalities and normals. No such definitive schedule exists. Age norms have not been established for the various nonfocal signs that have been proposed (although many are thought to be age-related); the significance of the signs in relation to neurological functioning is unclear; the predictive validity of the signs is disputed; the signs may be related to IQ and sex (being more common with low IQ and in boys); and it is unclear whether the signs are activated or accentuated by emotional arousal.

Close (1973) proposed a 43-item examination schedule for soft signs; but Werry and Aman (1976) found that many of Close's items occurred too infrequently to be useful, that intertester reliability was unsatisfactory unless the items involved the counting or timing of a performance rather than its subjective rating, and that the discriminative power of the signs was dubious. The evidence for the predictive validity of these signs is inconclusive (Shaffer, 1978). We cannot confidently recommend that an examination for nonfocal signs should be included routinely in the physical examination.

Special investigations

Many inquiry procedures described in chapter 10 are appropriate for children; but a number of special investigations are specifically designed for them. These investigations are the main subject of this section.

Could a special investigation contribute significantly to diagnosis, preferably in such a way as to influence treatment? This criterion should determine whether a particular test will be chosen. Special investigations are either (1) screening tests that are part of a minimum data base, or (2) part of a discretionary inquiry plan derived from an array of diagnostic hypotheses the clinician has generated. Special investigations are conducted in four areas:

Types of special investigation

1. Physical.
2. Neurological.
3. Psychological.
4. External consultation.
   a. Speech pathology.
   b. Audiology.
   c. Physical therapy.
   d. Occupational therapy.

The first three of these are discussed in this chapter.

Physical and neurological investigations

Physical investigations are usually undertaken in consultation with a pediatrician. The physical disorders most likely to require differentiation in child psychiatry, and the investigations most likely to contribute to excluding physical disorders are considered under the following headings:

Clinical patterns requiring investigation

1. Pervasive developmental problems.
2. Acute or subacute disintegration of behavior and development.
3. Delay in speech and language development.
4. Attention deficit and hyperactivity.
5. Depression.
6. Conversion symptoms.
7. Anorexia.
8. Sleep disturbance.
9. Delay in speech and language development.
10. Learning problems.
11. Abnormal movements.
12. Episodic lapses of awareness.
13. Episodic violence.

Pervasive developmental problems

During infancy or afterward, the child manifests a severe arrest or retardation of language, intellect, and social development. Additional features may include unexplained episodes of panic or rage, marked resistance to environmental change, hyperactivity, repetitive motor phenomena, and deviant speech. The onset may be in early infancy (before 30 months) or afterward (up to about 7 years). Sometimes the child regresses from a state of relatively normal development to such a condition; but more often, the child's development has always been abnormal. Organic causes must be excluded. The following conditions should be considered and special investigation ordered:

1. Hearing impairment: Acoustic testing.
2. Aphasia: Speech pathology consultation; language testing.
3. Seizure disorder: Electroencephalography.
4. Chromosomal anomaly: Chromosome analysis (especially if the child looks dysplastic).
5. Hypothyroidism: Thyroid function tests.
6. Metabolic disorder: Tests for amino acids in the urine (especially phenylketonuria).
7. Intracranial lesion: Skull X-ray; CT scan (but only if there is additional evidence for an intracranial space-occupying lesion).

8. Herpes encephalitis: Virologic studies of the cerebrospinal fluid; immunologic testing (if there has been an acute or subacute regression), electroencephalography, CT scan.

Acute or subacute disintegration of behavior and development

After a period of normal or relatively normal development, the child fails to make developmental progress and loses such recently acquired skills as sphincter control, coordination, dexterity, attention and concentration, memory, language, capacity for problem solving, school performance, emotional control, and social competence. In some cases, the child demonstrates abnormal motor patterns, hallucinations, delusions, and disorganization of thinking. Consider the following:

1. General systemic disease.
    a. Thyroid disorder: Thyroid function tests.
    b. Adrenal insufficiency: Adrenal function tests.
    c. Porphyria: Urinary porphyrins.
    d. Disseminated lupus erythematosus: Examination for LE cells.
    e. Wilson's disease: serum ceruloplasmin.
2. Toxic factors.
    a. Delirium due to systemic infection, electrolyte abnormality, or physiologic toxins: Electroencephalography; specific biochemical, bacteriologic or virologic tests.
    b. Drugs (e.g., intoxication with sympathomimetics, hallucinogens, or anticonvulsants; withdrawal from sedatives): Urine drug screen; blood toxicology.
3. Disease of the central nervous system.
    a. Seizure disorder: Electroencephalography with nasopharyngeal electrodes.
    b. Space-occupying lesion: Skull X-ray; CT scan.
    c. Herpes encephalitis: (see pervasive developmental disorder).
    d. Metabolic or subacute viral encephalitis: Electroencephalography; examination of cerebrospinal fluid; immunology.
    e. Degenerative diseases: Urine amino acids, electroencephalography; biopsy.
    f. Demyelinating disease.
    g. Leukemic infiltration of central nervous system: Examination of blood and cerebrospinal fluid.

Attention deficit and hyperactivity

Before or after starting school, the child demonstrates poor concentration, distractibility, and a tendency to impulsiveness, with or without hyperactivity and learning problems. The following disorders should be considered and special investigations ordered if the clinical features suggest that one or other is a real possibility:

1. Hyperthyroidism: Thyroid function tests (if there is other evidence of hyper-dynamic cardiovascular function and sympathetic overactivity).
2. Plumbism: Urine lead levels; examination of blood for stippled cells; X-rays of long bones.
3. Seizure disorder: Electroencephalography with nasopharyngeal leads.
4. Sleep apnea: Otorhinolaryngological examination; sleep electroencephalography and observation.
5. Sydenham's chorea: Blood antistreptolysin-O antibody titre.

Depression

The child becomes underactive or overactive; insomniac or hypersomniac; impaired in thought tempo, concentration, and energy; readily provoked to tantrum or weeping; socially withdrawn; and preoccupied with thoughts of low self-esteem, guilt, and loss. The differential diagnosis includes virtually any physical disorder that could sap energy, impair thinking, and disrupt the child's capacity to cope. Consider the following disorders:

1. General systemic disease.
    a. Malignancy.
    b. Chronic infectious disease.
    c. Viral infection (e.g., influenza, infectious hepatitis, infectious mononucleosis).
    d. Hypothyroidism.
    e. Hypoadrenalism.
    f. Chronic anemia.
    g. Subnutrition (e.g., anorexia nervosa).
2. Toxins: Chronic intoxication with anticonvulsants or sedatives: urine drug screen and blood levels.
3. Central nervous disease: Degenerative central nervous diseases: neurological examination; specific tests.

It is often difficult to determine to what degree a child's depression is part of a pathophysiologic process or how much it represents a secondary psychological reaction to loss of function, hospitalization, restriction of freedom. lack of stimulation, and loneliness.

Conversion symptoms

The child develops a set of symptoms that mimic physical disorder. Common conversion symptoms are loss of consciousness, loss of phonation, motor impairment, abnormal movements, seizures, special sensory defect, anesthesia, pain, loss of balance, or such gastrointestinal complaints as vomiting and abdominal pain. Conversion disorder can mimic many physical conditions. The inquiry plan should both exclude the hypothetical physical disorder and establish positive criteria for conversion (e.g., emotional trauma coinciding with onset; absence of organic signs; pattern of symptoms representing the patient's naive idea of pathology; contact with a model for the disease; pattern of symptoms fulfilling a communicative purpose; and gain for the patient in the sense of nurturance, security, and avoidance of difficulty). The following physical disorders are especially likely to be mistaken for conversion disorder:

1. General systemic disease
   a. Disseminated lupus erythematosus: Examination for LE cells.
   b. Hypocalcemia: Blood calcium.
   c. Hypoglycemia: Blood sugar (e.g., with insulinoma).
   d. Porphyria: Urinary porphyrins.
2. Central nervous disorder
   a. Multiple sclerosis.
   b. Movement disorders (chorea, dystonia musculorum deformans, Tourette's syndrome, Wilson's disease).
   c. Spinal cord tumor.
   d. Intracranial space-occupying lesion (especially in brain stem, cerebellum, frontal lobe, or parietotemporal cortex): Neurological examination; CT scan.
   e. Seizure disorder.
   f. Migraine.
   g. Dystonic reactions produced by neuroleptic drugs.

Anorexia

The child or adolescent loses weight markedly as a result of voluntary restriction of food intake. The following conditions should be ruled out:

1. Chronic systemic infection (especially tuberculosis).
2. Systemic malignancy (especially pancreatic, mediastinal, retroperitoneal, pulmonary, lymphatic, or leukemic malignancy).
3. Hypothalamic or pituitary tumor: Skull X-rays; CT scan; tomogram of sella turcica; pneumoencephalography.
4. Diabetes mellitus: Urinalysis; glucose tolerance testing.

5. Hyperthyroidism: Thyroid function tests.
6. Drug addiction.

Sleep Disturbance

The child can present with hypersomnia, insomnia, nightmares, night terrors, restless sleep, or sleepwalking. Consider the following:

1. Seizure disorder: Electroencephalography (including polysomnography).
2. Delirium (e.g., in acute febrile illness or toxic states).
3. Narcolepsy.
4. Intoxication with sedative, opioid, anticonvulsant, neuroleptic, or antidepressant drugs.
5. Hypoglycemia.
6. Any debilitating disease, especially disease associated with chronic hypoxia (e.g., congenital heart disease, pulmonary insufficiency, anemia).
7. Sleep apnea: Polysomnography; otorhinolaryngological examination.

Delay in speech and language development

The child manifests a relative delay in comprehending speech or in expressing and correctly enunciating words, phrases, and sentences. Exclude the following:

1. Deafness: Acoustic testing.
2. Palatal abnormality: Otorhinolaryngological examination.
3. Cerebral palsy: Neurological examination.
4. Mental retardation: Physical examination; psychological testing.
5. Seizure disorder: Electroencephalography.
6. Aphasia: Consult with speech pathology.
7. Developmental articulatory dyspraxia: Consult with speech pathology and pediatric neurology.
8. Pervasive developmental disorder (see inquiry plan for pervasive developmental problems).

Learning problems

The child manifests a general or specific difficulty in learning, particularly in reading, writing, written expression, calculation, or spatial skills. Exclude the following:

1. Visual defect: testing visual acuity and visual fields; ophthalmoscopy.
2. Deafness: acoustic testing.

3. Inability to attend in class due to debilitating illness, fatigue, hunger, pain, or drug use.
4. Cerebral palsy: Neurological examination.
5. Mental retardation.
6. Seizure disorder.
7. Dementia due to intracranial space-occupying lesion or cerebral degeneration.

Abnormal movements

The child manifests repetitive movements that can be brought partly under control. Exclude the following:

1. Attention-deficit disorder.
2. Tourette's syndrome.
3. Sydenham's chorea: Antistreptolysin-O titre.
4. Huntington's chorea.
5. Wilson's disease.
6. Paroxysmal choreoathetosis.
7. Dystonia musculorum deformans.
8. Cerebellar tumor or degeneration.
9. Drug effects, for example: Caffeinism or the extrapyramidal effects of neuroleptic medication.

Episodic lapses of awareness

Recurrent episodes during which the patient, usually an adolescent, has the sense of being abruptly altered, different, or unreal and of observing the self like a spectator. The patient may perceive that the world is unreal and different or that conversations and scenes have been experienced previously in precisely the same manner. Consider the following:

1. Seizure disorder: Electroencephalography.
2. Cardiac arrhythmia: Electrocardiography.
3. Narcolepsy: Electroencephalography.
4. Migraine.
5. Hallucinogenic drugs: Urine drug screen.

Episodic violence

The patient periodically loses control, assaults others, or destroys property. The explosions may be unheralded but usually arise from an emotional context of tension with or without alcohol intake, and are disproportionate to the apparent provocation. The patient may or may not have an antisocial personality. Exclude:

1. Temporal lobe seizures: Electroencephalography with nasopharyngeal leads.
2. Herpes encephalitis: Electroencephalography, immunologic study, examination of cerebrospinal fluid for viral culture, and immunology.
3. Drug effects (alcohol, phenylcyclidine, hallucinogens, amphetamine): Urine drug screen.

Psychological investigations

This section does not attempt to introduce the reader to all the tests clinical psychologists use with children. It deals, instead, with the kinds of questions a child psychiatrist might usefully ask a psychologist to address and with the kinds of tests relevant to diagnostic inquiry in child psychiatry.

In general, four areas of psychological assessment are relevant to child psychiatry:

Areas of psychological assessment

1. Neuropsychological function.
2. Cognition, language, and educational achievement.
3. Personality.
4. Behavioral analysis.

The first area is the least highly developed and will probably expand rapidly in the near future. The second is highly developed, complex, expanding, and associated with a sophisticated application of statistical mathematics. The third, having been a field of intense activity until about 1960, has receded somewhat, as many clinical psychologists have become preoccupied with behavioral approaches to assessment and treatment.

Neuropsychological testing

Neuropsychological testing

1. Is there any evidence of brain dysfunction from the pattern of test performance?
2. Is there any evidence of a deterioration in test performance that could be caused by a progressive brain disorder?
3. Is there any evidence of previous, non-progressive, damage to the brain?

The psychiatrist is most likely to ask these questions in the following circumstances:

Indications for neuropsychological testing

1. The child appears to have deteriorated in cognitive performance and emotional control, and a progressive brain disorder is hypothesized.
2. The child manifests pervasive developmental disorder, and diagnosable brain disorder must be excluded.
3. There is a delay or abnormality in speech and language development, and a progressive brain disorder must be excluded.
4. The child has sustained an insult to the brain (e.g., head trauma or neurosurgery), and it is important to determine how serious and irreversible the damage is and what areas of mental functioning are most affected.

Neuropsychological testing is most helpful in the fourth circumstance. In the first three situations, neuropsychological testing should never be relied on to clinch or reject a diagnostic hypothesis; it should be considered only as corroborative evidence. It is of most use when a baseline of functioning is required for future comparison.

The **Halstead-Reitan Neuropsychological Test Battery** (Reitan & Davison, 1974), a composite test originally designed for adults, has been modified for children from 5 through 8 and from 9 through 14 years. The test yields an impairment index, according to the number of subtests in which the subject performs within the range characteristic of brain-damaged people.

The **Bender Gestalt Test** has a developmental scoring system (Koppitz, 1975) and is suitable for children over 5 years of age. The child is asked to copy a number of geometric designs. Children with brain dysfunction make characteristic errors, with rotations, omissions, perseveration, poor angulation, and lack of integration.

The **Graham-Kendall Memory-for-Designs Test** (Graham & Kendall, 1960) is similar to the Bender-Gestalt Test, except that the subject must reproduce geometric designs from memory. Both tests are highly correlated with mental age up to 10 years, which is taken into account in the scoring system.

The **Frostig Developmental Test of Visual Perception** (Maslow et al., 1964) consists of five subtests: eye-hand coordination, figure-ground perception, form constancy, position in space, and spatial relations. A perceptual age level and perceptual quotient can be obtained (equivalent to mental age and intelligence quotient).

Tests of intelligence such as the **Wechsler Intelligence Scale for Children** (Wechsler, 1974) sample a range of verbal and nonverbal cognitive functions and provide a test score profile that may suggest brain dysfunction.

The **Luria-Nebraska Neuropsychological Battery** (Golden, Hammeke, and Purisch, 1978), a composite test of neuropsychological functioning, has recently been introduced.

Further advances await a better understanding of how the developing brain can be disrupted by acute and chronic, reversible and irreversible, and progressive and static pathoanatomic lesions and biochemically determined disorders. The brain may be affected on a particular side, in one or several areas, or diffusely. Only when these matters are better understood will it be possible to design psychological tests yielding more than global impressions of organic dysfunction.

Intelligence, psychoeducational and language testing

Testing cognitive performance

1. What is the level of general intelligence?
2. Is this estimate a good reflection of potential?
3. Is there any evidence of an interference with cognitive function by physical or psychosocial factors?
4. Is there an unevenness in functioning, suggesting the need for more detailed cognitive or psychomotor testing?

The psychiatrist is likely to pose these questions in the following hypothetical circumstances:

Indications for cognitive testing

1. The child's specific or general developmental delay, poor school progress, poor social adaptation, or lack of intellectual grasp suggest below average intellectual functioning.
2. The child, despite unimpressive school progress, gives evidence from the history (e.g., unusually mature interests) or interview (e.g., preternatural curiosity, grasp of abstraction, or facility in technical matters) of being especially bright.
3. The child appears to have deteriorated in cognitive performance (e.g., to have become more forgetful, absent-minded, or dreamy and to have deteriorated in school grades).
4. The child is doing poorly at school, and the question has been raised of a specific developmental cognitive disability rather than a general lack of intelligence.

The **Stanford-Binet Test** has been widely used since Terman's 1916 revision. It was recently brought up to date (Terman and Merrill, 1973). The Stanford-Binet provides an IQ based on age-normed means and the distribution of scores around the mean; a score of one standard deviation below the mean for that age is equivalent to an IQ of 84. The components of the Stanford-Binet test are of less use than those of the Wechsler tests in suggesting areas of specific dysfunction.

The Wechsler Tests; the **Wechsler Adult Intelligence Scale-Revised,** WAIS-R (Wechsler, 1981); the **Wechsler Intelligence Scale for Children,** WISC-R (Wechsler, 1974); and the **Wechsler Preschool and Primary Scale of Intelligence,** WPPSI (Wechsler, 1967), provide IQ scores based on age-normed distributions, 15 points being equivalent to one standard deviation from the norm. Six subtests of the Wechsler have a significant verbal content (general information, general comprehension, arthmetic, similarities, vocabulary and digit span), and six subtests tap perceptual, spatial, and motor skills (picture completion, picture arrangement, block design, object assembly, coding, and mazes). Verbal, performance, and full-scale intelligence quotients are calculated from the subtest scores. The unevenness of the subtests may suggest areas of dysfunction that can be pursued with more specific tests of verbal or psychomotor ability.

Other tests of intelligence performance include the **McCarthy Scales** (McCarthy, 1972) and a number of tests that can be conveniently administered to classroom groups, such as the **Slosson** (Slosson, 1975).

When it is important to minimize the importance of language, as with deaf or foreign-language subjects, such tests as **Raven's Matrices** (Raven, 1960) or the **Leiter International Scale** (Leiter, 1948) can be used.

A number of areas of specific dysfunction can be assessed; for example:

1. Attention and concentration (e.g., subtests on the **Wechsler Tests**).
2. Figure-ground discrimination (e.g., the **Frostig Test,** Maslow et al., 1964).
3. Immediate memory and intersensory integration (e.g., **Visual-Aural Digit Span Test,** Koppitz, 1977).
4. Eye-hand coordination (e.g., the **Frostig Test,** Maslow et al., 1964.
5. Spatial reasoning (e.g., object assembly and block design subtests on the **Wechsler Tests**).
6. Sequencing ability (e.g., digit span and picture arrangement on the **Wechsler Tests**).

Tests of language function

When should the child psychiatrist request an evaluation of language functioning?

Indications for language testing

1. When the child has a developmental delay in verbal comprehension, articulation, the acquisition of a vocabulary or in expressive syntactical competence. Several or all of these competencies may appear to be defective, according to the developmental history and the interview with the child.
2. When there is a marked discrepancy between verbal and psychomotor abilities (verbal being significantly lower), as may occur in partial deafness, cultural disadvantage, or a developmental disorder of language development.

Receptive verbal comprehension can be tested with the **Peabody Picture Vocabulary Test** (Dunn & Dunn, 1981), and expressive vocabulary through a subtest of the **Wechsler Tests.** The **Illinois Test of Psycholinguistic Abilities** (Kirk, McCarthy, & Kirk, 1968) is based on a comprehensive theory of language functioning. This test analyzes language functioning in terms of receptive, associational, and expressive phases, and auditory, vocal, gestural, and graphic modalities.

Testing Educational Achievement

When should the psychiatrist question the child's academic competence?

Indications for psychoeducational testing

1. When the child's academic progress has always been slow, in all areas.
2. When the child's performance has deteriorated; for example, following an emotional trauma such as divorce.

3. If a child appears to be underachieving; that is, if school performance is inconsistent with the child's apparent ability.
4. If the child has particular problems in special areas of learning, such as reading or calculation.

Different functions related to learning

If the psychiatrist poses questions in this form to the psychologist, different combinations of tests can be applied. When the child's performance has always been slow, for example, intelligence testing and a test of general academic performance, such as the **Wide Range Achievement Test** (Jastak & Jastak, 1978), can be used. If there has been a recent decline in performance, then intelligence, general achievement, and personality testing can be combined to determine whether the child's capacity to attend, register, retain, or retrieve information and solve problems has been affected by emotional disturbance. A combination of intelligence and achievement testing will determine whether the child is an underachiever. To pinpoint special disabilities, global intelligence testing is required, after which the psychologist may explore cognitive functioning in detail. In reading retardation, for example, the following areas may be investigated with special tests: attention, impulsivity, auditory and visual perceptual discrimination, the capacity to attack an unfamiliar word by using phonic skills, language function, short-term memory for simple and complex sequences of symbolic information (e.g., digits, words, phrases, or narratives) presented aurally or visually and expressed orally or graphically. The **Woodcock-Johnson Psychoeducational Battery** (Woodcock & Johnson, 1977), is comprised of a number of cognitive, achievement, and educational interest subtests. It is often used for detailed assessment of academic functioning.

The field of educational achievement and of the attentional, perceptual, memory, abstracting, linguistic, and sequencing skills that underlie it are of great importance in developmental psychopathology. The intertwining of intellectual problems, learning disability, language dysfunction, and emotional disturbance make this a field of vigorous research.

Personality testing

Test of personality

Tests of personality are based on two sets of propositions – trait theory and psychodynamic theory.

Trait theory stems from the contention that people have more or less stable dispositions to behave in certain ways, dispositions that can be measured as continuous dimensions. An example of a trait is neuroticism. Neuroticism is measured in the **Eysenck Personality Inventory** (Eysenck & Eysenck, 1963), for example, by a questionnaire concerning the subject's tendency to react

Trait Questionnaires

habitually with anxiety, tension, or fear. Most trait-oriented tests are structured questionnaires with relatively objective, standardized methods of scoring. Other traits that can be assessed are, for example, anxiety, extroversion, locus of control, aggressiveness, and depression.

Projective tests

Psychodynamic theory depicts personality as an everchanging flux and balance between (1) unconscious and preconscious drives, images, and affects; (2) ego defenses that block, divert, or rechannel the unconscious drives; and (3) the ego processes through which the drives are expressed, given the constraints of the external world and the moral imperatives of conscience and ego ideal. Tests derived from this theory are likely to be relatively unstructured, and to rely on the assumption that the more ambiguous the stimulus, the more liable the individual is to respond in a way reflecting the personal inner world. This tendency is known as **projection,** and the tests that depend on it are called projective tests. The relatively ambiguous stimuli used with children include inkblots (**Rorschach Test,** Exner, 1978); pictures of human figures, usually in some sort of interaction (**Thematic Apperception Test,** Murray, 1943; **Michigan Picture Completion Test,** Hutt, 1980); pictures of animals interacting (**Children's Apperception Test,** Bellak & Bellak, 1974); and drawings of the human figure or family (**Human Figure Drawing Test,** Koppitz, 1968); **House–Tree–Person Test,** Buck, 1966). With these tests, the psychologist, like the clinician in a play interview, attempts to catch a glimpse of the subject's fantasy world and to make inferences about the subject's capacity to cope with current pressures from the environment, from the unconscious, and from the superego.

Social cognition

A third area of personality testing is in its infancy insofar as clinical application is concerned. These tests derive from a general theoretical field known as self-theory, social cognition, and moral development. For example, tests have been designed to tap self-concept, the difference between perceived and ideal self (self-image disparity) and the capacity to identify, predict, and reason about the feelings of other people. This is likely to be an area of increasing research activity in the near future.

When should a psychiatrist ask for personality testing, and what kind of questions and answers are likely to be constructive? The following situations exemplify those to which personality testing could contribute.

Indications for personality testing

1. The clinician has formed certain dynamic or trait-oriented hypotheses from the history and clinical interviewing and seeks independent confirmation, disconfirmation, or elaboration of them.
2. The clinician is considering implementing exploratory psychotherapy but has doubts about whether the patient has the fundamental resources (ego strength) to benefit from it or whether interpretive work will be too disturbing for the patient to tolerate.
3. The clinician has decided that expressive psychotherapy is indicated and seeks a prediction of the kind of material likely to emerge in therapy.
4. The patient has been referred for forensic evaluation, and the motivation for dangerous or bizarre antisocial behavior (such as rape) is in question. In this case, the clinician is usually seeking information that will expand, confirm, or refute the dynamic hypotheses formed as a result of clinical interviewing.

Questions posed the projective tester

Some questions that may be posed the psychologist are as follows:

1. What are the dominant current fantasies, needs, wishes, fears (e.g., needs for sustenance, nurturance, protection, attachment, sex, affiliation, independence, achievement, power, dominance, or submission; fears of annihilation, loss, abandonment, rejection, neglect, injury, disintegration, inferiority, failure, nonconformity, loss of identity, sexual disorientation, or sexual dysfunction)?
2. What are the conscious and unconscious mental representations of significant people: parents, siblings, peers, spouse, children, authority figures?
3. What are the dominant ego-defenses? How effective are they? What is the likelihood of decompensation in the near future, for example, during psychotherapy?
4. What is the level of moral development? How differentiated and favorable are the patient's self-concept and self-esteem? Is there a significant disparity between perceived self and ideal self? What is the patient's gender identity? Can the patient identify personal feelings, identify the feelings of others, and reason causally and predictively about others' feelings?

Behavioral assessment

Behavioral analysis

If a child manifests disturbed behavior (e.g., tantrums) in a particular setting (e.g., the classroom), it can be helpful to observe the child directly. What events precede the behavior in question? What precipitates it? How do others (e.g., parents, teachers, peers) respond? Is there any evidence that the behavior is precipitated or perpetuated by the environment? Such observations could lead to practical management plans enabling those in the natural setting to respond more effectively to the distressed, uncontrolled, or coercive child.

At this point, however, the use of trained observers is an expensive proposition and has been restricted to specific behaviors in research settings. An alternative approach is recommended by Achenbach & Edelbrock (1983), who discuss the use of parents and teachers as observers. High test–retest reliability (.80–.90) has been found for parent and teacher checklists of children's behavior, and interparent and interteacher reliabilities have varied between .70 and .90. Teachers and parents, however, agree only at a .30–.40 level, undoubtedly because they view the child in different settings.

Using parents as observers

It is recommended that the **Child Behavior Checklist for Parents** be used routinely, and that, if permission is given by parents, the **Child Behavior Checklist for Teachers** be completed routinely before the initial interview with the parents. The use of the Child Behavior Checklist to determine a child's problems and competencies is discussed in chapter 19.

When it is important to determine the antecedent circumstances, concomitant events, and consequences of a particular behavior (e.g., tantrums), the

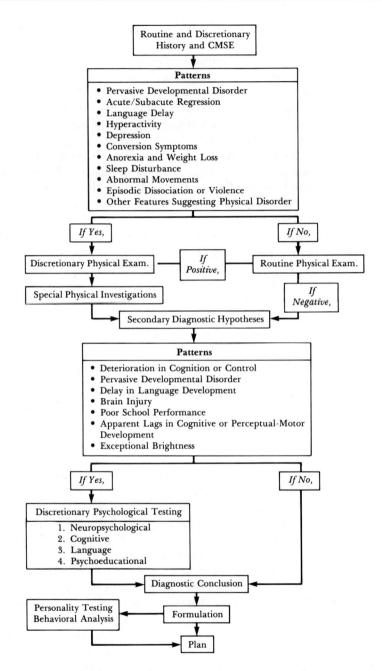

FIGURE 22.1

Routine and discretionary inquiry in the clinical process in child psychiatry

Parental logs   child's caretakers can be asked to keep a log of problem incidents. Such logs can be a useful source of information for planning a behavioral intervention and monitoring its effectiveness.

Summary

In a flow chart, Figure 22.1 summarizes how routine and discretionary inquiry are sequentially incorporated in the clinical process. After the routine data base has been gathered, and history and mental status examination completed, a clinical pattern will have emerged. A number of patterns (such as one suggesting central nervous dysfunction) listed in the diagram, indicate the need for discretionary physical examination and, possibly, discretionary physical investigations (e.g., biochemical, hematological, or radiological). If the clinical pattern does not suggest the need for further discretionary inquiry, a routine physical examination should suffice.

At this point, the clinician should have refined the array of hypotheses, and will have discarded some hypotheses. Another group of patterns, listed in the diagram, indicate the need for psychological testing of neuropsychological, cognitive, language, or psychoeducational functioning. If not, the clinician can proceed to a diagnostic conclusion.

A comprehensive diagnosis can then be formulated. If exploratory psychotherapy is being considered, personality testing would be useful. If the clinician decides to modify a specified behavior, behavioral analysis might be required.

Selected Readings

The physical examination and special physical investigations in pediatric psychiatry are described by Herskowitz and Rosman (1982) in *Pediatrics, Neurology and Psychiatry – Common Ground.* Achenbach (1982) provides a good summary of psychological testing in *Developmental Psychopathology.*

23

Categorical diagnosis in child psychiatry

Categorical diagnosis: DSM-III

Chapter 23 deals with categorical diagnosis in child psychiatry. Chapters 24, 25, and 26 deal with the biopsychosocial, temporal, and developmental axes of diagnosis, and with diagnostic formulation, modes of treatment, and goal-directed management planning.

The utility of categorical diagnosis

Chapter 7 reviews the philosophical, ethical, scientific, and practical issues surrounding psychiatric classification. We noted that categorical diagnosis is more pertinent and perhaps more reliable the closer the diagnostic entity to the organic end of the diagnostic spectrum. The categorical approach is of most use for scientific classification and statistical purposes; its utility for individualized management planning is more limited. For individualized management planning, a comprehensive diagnostic formulation is required. Nevertheless, the clinician inevitably seeks to identify biopsychosocial patterns in order to relate a particular case to others of comparable nature.

In DSM-III, an attempt has been made to classify the psychiatric disorders of childhood and adolescence and to define each entity as precisely as possible. The five main groupings of disorders are as follows:

I. Intellectual.
II. Behavioral.
III. Emotional.
IV. Physical.
V. Developmental.

The reader is referred to the source for precise and detailed definitions of each disorder. This chapter summarizes and reviews the child and adolescent section of DSM-III and compares it with alternative approaches.

Intellectual disorders

Mental retardation can be of mild (educable), moderate (trainable), severe, or profound degree. In these disorders, intellectual, social, and adaptive functioning have been persistently delayed since early childhood. It is conventionally associated with an IQ of less than 70.

Behavioral disorders

Attention-deficit disorder

This disorder involves persistent lack of concentration, distractibility, poor emotional control, impulsivity, or overactivity. It may be diagnosed in the preschool years or, in less severe cases, remain latent until the child begins school. These children seem to have particular difficulty concentrating when they are expected to attend to tasks imposed by others, as in the classroom. Some of these children have all the symptoms listed except hyperactivity. Learning problems and social immaturity are common in this disorder. Attention deficit disorder may lead to social inadequacy, poor organization, and impulsiveness in adulthood. The boundary between attention-deficit disorder and conduct disorder is indefinite.

Conduct disorder

This disorder is associated with persistent behavior counter to the rules of family and society, involving such antisocial actions as lying, stealing, truancy, running away from home, sexual misconduct, and aggressiveness.

Conduct disorders are classified on two dimensions: *aggressive* versus *nonaggressive* and *undersocialized* versus *socialized*. The first dimension is self-explanatory; the second requires inferences about the child's capacity to feel, offer, and accept affection, friendship, and loyalty. The child with socialized conduct disorder is likely to belong to a gang, to be capable of affection, friendship, and guilt and to have come from a home in which there was consistent early affection. In contrast, the undersocialized delinquent shows little affection, loyalty, or guilt, is fundamentally egocentric in orientation, and may manifest antisocial personality disorder in adulthood.

Emotional disorders

Separation anxiety disorder

This disorder leads to distress at leaving home, sometimes manifest as a phobia of attending school. The fear of school is usually a reflection of underlying anxiety about parting from an attachment figure and of fears that the figure (usually the mother) will abscond or be harmed. The anxiety is commonly somatized, for example, as abdominal, limb, or head pain; nausea; vomiting; and diarrhea. Anxiety may also be expressed in dysphoria, clinging, nightmares about separation, and low frustration tolerance.

Avoidant disorder of childhood or adolescence

This disorder causes persistent shyness, avoidance of strangers, and a tendency to hang back in peer relations.

Overanxious disorder

This disorder involves persistent self-consciousness, anxiety about competition and behaving appropriately in company, and worry about the future. Somatic concomitants are likely.

Reactive attachment disorder

This disorder occurs in infants in response to emotional and physical neglect, usually due to institutionalism, or to maternal rejection, depression, or substance abuse. The infant, who is deficient in ocular tracking, smiling, and interest in the environment, fails to respond to human contact, fails to thrive, and becomes physically weak, hypotonic, and vulnerable to intercurrent physical disease.

Schizoid disorder of childhood or adolescence

This disorder involves avoidance of peer contact and a preference for being alone. The schizoid child is socially gauche and uncomfortable, absent-minded, and prone to excessive daydreaming.

Elective mutism

This disorder typically occurs at the beginning of elementary school. The child, who is quite communicative at home and evidently has normal comprehension of speech, refuses to talk to anyone outside the family and may show other negativistic or oppositional behavior.

Oppositional disorder

This disorder occurs after 3 years of age and is characterized by persistent disobedience, tantrums, provocativeness, and negativism directed towards parents and teachers.

Identity disorder

This disorder occurs in late adolescence and is characterized by confusion and uncertainty about career goals, friendship, loyalties, sexual orientation, religion, and morality. This disorder stops short of psychosis but commonly leads to a deterioration in academic, occupational, and social functioning.

Disorders associated with physical symptoms

Anorexia nervosa

Anorexia nervosa usually begins in adolescence. It is more common in females than in males, and is associated with an intense fear of gaining weight, voluntary restriction of food intake, loss of at least 25% of original body weight, an apparent distortion of body image, and numerous physical sequelae to subnutrition (for example, amenorrhea, growth of fine hair on body, hypoproteinemic edema, and anemia).

Bulimia

This disorder is characterized by recurrent, episodic, secretive eating binges terminated by self-induced vomiting, repeated dieting, or laxation. It is associated with marked fluctuations of weight.

Pica

Pica usually occurs in children from 1 to 5 years of age, rarely later, and is associated with the persistent eating of such nonnutritive material as dirt or clay.

Rumination

Occurring in infancy, this disorder is associated with repeated, persistent regurgitation of food, often preceded by a thrusting forward of the mandible or the insertion of a fist into the mouth. Rumination can lead to cachexia. It is usually associated with emotional neglect.

Transient and chronic motor tic disorder

This disorder involves sudden, jerky, repeated, and purposeless movements of one or more circumscribed muscle groups. The two conditions are distinguished by their duration.

Tourette's disorder

The onset of this disorder is sometime between 2 and 13 years of age, with recurrent, involuntary, purposeless movements of many muscle groups, vocal tics (including swearing), and echokinesis. The patient usually has the capacity to control the movements for brief periods.

Stereotyped movement disorders

Headrocking, headrolling, headbanging, body rocking, hand wringing, finger clicking, and other purposive, repetitive, voluntary, rhythmic movements of different parts of the body characterize this disorder.

Stuttering

Stuttering is an interruption of speech by persistent, repetitive, hesitations, pauses, or repetitions of sounds, syllables, or words.

Functional enuresis and encopresis

These disorders involve delay of normal sphincter control, in the absence of organic disease of bladder or bowel.

Sleepwalking and sleep terror disorders

These sleep disorders occur in sleep stages three or four (as does nocturnal enuresis).

Pervasive developmental disorders

Early infantile autism

The onset of this disorder is usually before 30 months. It is characterized by a marked incapacity to relate to other people, an absence, delay, or deviation in speech and language development, insistence on the maintenance of sameness, delayed or markedly uneven intellectual development, eccentric repetitive movements, and attachment to inanimate objects. In later life, a residual state may be diagnosed.

Childhood onset pervasive development disorder

In this disorder, the onset is after 30 months and before 12 years. It causes impairment in social relations, episodes of inexplicable panic or rage, resistance to environmental change, eccentric movements, abnormal speech patterns, and self-mutilation or injury.

Atypical pervasive developmental disorders

These disorders are associated with social impairment, intellectual unevenness, and other features that resemble, but are insufficiently distinctive to indicate, an unqualified diagnosis of early infantile autism or childhood onset pervasive developmental disorder.

Specific developmental disorders

This group of disorders is characterized by arrests or delays in one or more of such areas of development as expressive or receptive language, speech articulation, reading, calculation, and manual dexterity.

The reliability and validity of categorical diagnosis

Unsatisfactory reliability

Field trials of the reliability of the DSM-III for childhood and adolescent disorders have not revealed acceptable agreement in diagnosis between clinicians, even when disorders were grouped into broad categories. The lack of agreement may have arisen because the clinical phenomena included in DSM-III are too inferential in nature, or because its diagnostic criteria are too imprecise and the boundaries between the different disorders too unclear, or because the clinicians tested were inadequately trained to use the system.

As Achenbach (1980) points out, the diagnostic categories in DSM-III were derived from the accumulated wisdom of a committee. The categories thus have clinical face validity but have not been refined by trial-and-error research or substantiated by empirical studies of clinical phenomenology.

Empirical taxonomies

Other diagnostic systems, such as that proposed by the Group for the Advancement of Psychiatry (1966), have not proven any more reliable. This is one reason multivariate approaches to taxonomy, as exemplified by that of Achenbach and Edelbrock (1983), are receiving increased attention. Intertester and test–retest reliability of an empirical system is much more impressive than that of the clinically derived taxonomies. Much more work must be done, however, to determine the validity of multivariate taxonomy.

Need for validation studies

To illustrate the scientific problem of establishing the validity of a clinically intuited or statistically derived taxonomic category, let us consider the scientific disputes that currently abound in the area of depression in childhood.

Until recently, the question seldom arose. Children were regarded as having a mental organization too immature to generate and sustain the complex psychic phenomena of adult melancholia. About 30 years ago, Spitz, Bowlby, and others described the pathetic state of institutionalized infants and the reactive unhappiness of children who were abruptly separated from their parents. The word *depression* began to be applied to children more freely, particularly in situations involving neglect or disruption of attachment. Subsequent studies of juvenile suicide and antisocial behavior suggested that depression could be "masked" by other behavior (a concept borrowed from adult psychiatry). By the 1970s the term was used in so many ways that confusion reigned:

The reactivation of the diagnosis of depression in childhood

Reaction to separation

1. The term *depression* was applied to a clinically observable state of emotional distress, social unresponsiveness, and habit-regression found in toddlers and preschoolers, and to a state of developmental arrest, social unresponsiveness, and psychosomatic vulnerability found in infants, both subsequent to separation from the primary caretaker after about 6 months of age.

Dysphoria

2. The term *depression* was applied to a dysphoric mood observable in, or complained of, by unhappy children and adolescents.

A clinical syndrome

3. *Depression* was loosely applied to a syndrome clinically observable in older children or adolescents, characterized by sadness, sense of loss, low self-esteem, anger, emotional lability, suicidal ideation, and failure to concentrate and learn, following acute or chronic loss of, or rejection by, parents, or the exposure to severe family disruption.

Masked depression

4. In association with the previous category, the hypothetical psychopathology of depression might be "masked" by school failure, antisocial behavior, substance abuse, or in other symptoms.

An internal dynamic

5. *Depression* was applied to a hypothetical psychic state characterized by identification with a lost or unattainable object and the turning inward against the self of anger originally directed toward the ambivalently regarded object. In Kleinian Theory, this hypothetical condition was described as a position that was, up to a point, a normal stage of development in early infancy;

however, if circumstances prevented the child from negotiating this stage, fixation would be likely, and the child would subsequently be vulnerable to depression.

During the 1970s, the term *depression* was used in three further distinct ways:

Learned helplessness

6. The experimental work of Seligman (1975) suggested that the "learned helplessness" of laboratory animals who had no control over when they were punished might be analogous to human depression.

Pathological attitudes

7. Kovacs and Beck (1977) suggested that children are predisposed to depression when, as a result of adverse early experience, they have developed the following cognitive triad:
   a. The self is viewed as bad, inadequate, and unworthy.
   b. The environment appears to make exorbitant demands.
   c. The future seems bleak and unchanging.

Major depressive disorder

8. Recent genetic, biochemical, and pharmacological research into adult major depressive disorders of bipolar and unipolar type has led to a trickling down of interest to child and adolescent psychiatry. Researchers are now attempting to identify major depression, mania, and bipolar depression in children and adolescents. The term depression in this context refers to a categorical diagnostic entity equivalent to the adult DSM-III diagnosis of the same type.

The ubiquity of sadness

In their multivariate approach, Achenbach and Edelbrock (1983) found that parents reported between 43% and 86% of clinic-referred children and adolescents to be "unhappy, sad, or depressed," particularly in older children. The statistical analysis revealed a factor in 6- to 11-year-old children strongly suggestive of a depressive dynamic. It included the following symptoms:

A depressive cluster in childhood

1. Afraid of doing something bad.
2. Needs to be perfect.
3. Feels unloved.
4. Feels persecuted.
5. Feels worthless.
6. Tense.
7. Self-conscious.
8. Sulky.
9. Tearful.
10. Unhappy.
11. Worrying.
12. Guilty.
13. Lonely.

A cluster analysis of behavior profiles revealed a group of 6- to 11-year-old boys with peaks on *depression, social withdrawal,* and *aggression* and a group of girls with peaks on *depression* and *withdrawal.*

Lack of a clear syndrome in adolescence

Achenbach and Edelbrock (1983) found that adolescents were different. The childhood symptoms that suggested a symptom cluster of depression seemed to spread out across three factors in adolescent boys (*schizoid, uncommunicative,* and *hostile withdrawal*) and across two factors in girls (*anxious-obsessive* and *depressed withdrawal*).

This empirical study suggests that though sadness is common in childhood and adolescence, and though there is some support for a depressive syndrome in childhood, sadness is so widespread among adolescent patients that there is little support for a syndrome and even less for an entity of depressive disorder. This comparatively unbiased research is preferable to the narrow approach, in which the child or parent is asked questions framed according to preconceptions about adult melancholia or manic depressive disorder. In a narrow approach, the child may be regarded as guilty of depression, so to speak, until proven otherwise.

The search for biochemical markers

It will be difficult to pursue the matter any further unless a biochemical or physical correlate can be found in association with a depressive symptom cluster. Unfortunately, there are many unhappy, lonely, and despairing children; probably no more than a minority have a genetic-biochemical anomaly beneath their sorrows. Most of the children and adolescents who complain of sadness are unhappy for obvious reasons. Whether chronic despair in childhood can lead to physiological exhaustion and depression remains to be seen.

Summary

This chapter summarizes the most important diagnostic entities in the childhood section of the DSM-III. Unfortunately, field trials of DSM-III have not revealed satisfactory reliability among clinicians who use the system to categorize children. For this reason, empirically derived multivariate taxonomies have been promoted. Up to this time, neither clinical, categorical nor empirical, taxonomic systems have been validated.

Selected Readings

For a complete description of the DSM-III categories of psychiatric disorder in childhood, the reader is referred to the original *Diagnostic and Statistical Manual of Mental Disorders* (1980). Achenbach (1980) presents a critique of this approach.

24

The developmental axis

The three axes of diagnostic formulation

Three axes of diagnosis As already discussed in chapters 10, 13, and 14, a comprehensive diagnostic formulation – the prerequisite for management planning – requires the interweaving of two axes: the vertical, **biopsychosocial** and the longitudinal, **temporal.** This chapter deals with the biopsychosocial and temporal axes in childhood and adolescence and describes how a third axis, the **developmental,** is essential to understanding psychopathology in children and adolescents.

As in adults, the biopsychosocial axis in children can be subdivided as follows:

1. Physical systems.
    a. Peripheral biosystems.
    b. Control biosystems.
       Autonomic.
       Neuroendocrine.
       Subcortical.
2. Psychological functions.
    a. Information processing and motor control.
    b. Communication.
    c. Images, attitudes, and emotions.
    d. Internal controls, rules, and aspirations.

        e. Social competence.
        f. Coping techniques.
    3. Social systems.
        a. Intimate support systems (e.g., family).
        b. Institutional systems (e.g., medical).

Behavior has different implications at different ages

All physical and psychological systems are subject to developmental change. A particular behavior, such as tantrums or truancy, is likely to have different implications at different ages, depending on the subject's level of biopsychosocial development. The physical and psychosocial drives and needs that energize the apparatus are expressed in different forms as development proceeds. The reactions of family and such social systems as school or hospital are also likely to vary according to the child's developmental level.

Development, therefore, affects all levels of biopsychosocial functioning and can be inferred from advances in the following areas:

1. Physical dimensions and functioning.
2. Information processing and motor control.
3. Communication.
4. Images, attitudes, and emotions.
5. Internal controls, rules, and aspirations.
6. Social competence.
7. Coping techniques.

Aside from physical and motor development, which are dealt with in pediatric texts, each of these areas will be described in this section and included in synoptic tables (Tables 24.1 to 24.5). First, however, a set of general principles will be presented. These principles apply to all levels and areas of development.

TABLE 24.1
Antenatal and perinatal hazards to development

Antenatal development

Hazards which may disrupt intrauterine development or cause perinatal morbidity:

1. Chromosomal abnormality (e.g., Down's syndrome)
2. Abnormal hormonal environment (e.g., diethylstilbestrol)
3. Malnutrition (e.g., protein-calorie subnutrition)
4. Smoking
5. Alcohol
6. Drugs (e.g., thalidomide, heroin)
7. Infection (e.g., syphilis)
8. High temperature (e.g., fever)
9. Premature delivery
10. Lack of oxygen (e.g., obstructed labor)
11. Maternal emotional stress

TABLE 24.2
Synopsis of development during infancy

Infancy 0 to 18 months

1. *Developmental Tasks.* Mutual attachment, trust, and separation.
2. *Context.* Mother-infant dyad. Extrauterine gestation.
3. *Sensorimotor Milestones.* Focuses on object (4 weeks). Smiles at face (6 weeks). Holds head up (3 months). Sits (6 months). Reaches for and grasps object (6 months). Crawls (8 months). Stands (9 months). Walks (12 months). Points (13 months). Throws (15 months). Feeds self (18 months).
4. *Information Processing.* Thinking inseparable from sensation and action. Early perceptual discrimination. Attention to patterns (2 months). Recognition of familiar face (5 months). Repetitive actions (6 months). Means and ends (12 months). Object permanence (12 months). Self-identity (12 months).
5. *Communication.* Acoustic discrimination. Prelinguistic babbling (3 months). Single-word phrases (12 months). Comprehension ahead of expression.
6. *Attitudes and Emotions.* Symbiosis. Discrimination between self and not-self (6 months). Unstable images of self and mother. Separation and individuation. Ambivalence. Confusion of personal feelings with feelings of others. Transitional object (18 months).
7. *Regulation.* Internal threshold for stimulation. Withdrawal and habituation. Primitive mental mechanisms: denial, splitting, introjection, projection.
8. *Social Competence.* Early attachment: sucking, clinging, following, crying, smiling. Recognition of mother, separation anxiety (6 months). Stranger anxiety (7 months). Fear of strange objects (10 months). Preference for primary attachment figure (12 months). Response to siblings (12 months).
9. *Psychosocial Hazards.* Neglect, abandonment, abuse. Lack, loss, insensitivity, unresponsiveness of care-giver. Multiple care-givers without continuity. Overstimulation.
10. *Signs of Maladjustment.* Excessive crying, insomnia, digestive disturbance, colic, failure to thrive, depression, excessive separation anxiety, failure to attach to others.

The principles of growth and development

Normal development

1. Growth and development are dynamic, propulsive, evolving processes associated with the maturation of the individual. Growth refers to structure, development to function.
2. Growth and development involve the increase, multiplication, differentiation, articulation, and hierarchical integration of structure and function.
3. Developmental trends are in the following directions: small to large; global to specific; diffuse to organized; rigid to flexible; and unstable to stable.
4. Growth and development result from an interaction between genes selected by the evolution of the species and the physical and social environment.
5. Growth and development affect all levels of systemic functioning, from biochemical to psychosocial.
6. Structural change is coordinated with adaptational requirements during growth and precedes new functional capacity.

TABLE 24.3
Synopsis of development during early childhood.

Early childhood 1½ to 5 years

1. *Developmental Tasks.* Separation, individuation, autonomy, initiative.
2. *Context.* Family.
3. *Sensorimotor Milestones.* Kicks, runs (2 years). Sphincter control (2½ years). Puts on shoes (3 years). Stacks 9–10 blocks (4 years). Dry at night (4½ years). Dresses and undresses (5 years).
4. *Information Processing.* Stable internal representations (1½ years). Imagination, fantasy, egocentrism and animism (2½ years). Difficulty estimating time, dating past events, and gauging distance and volume (3–5 years). Classification and serial order (5 years).
5. *Communication.* Vocabulary of 300 words in 2–3 word phrases (2 years). 1,000 words in simple sentences (3 years). Knows most regular and irregular grammatical rules (5 years).
6. *Attitudes and Emotions.* Need for independence from primary caretaker. Need to explore. Struggle for autonomy. Sense of personal worth and loveability. Core gender identity (2 years). Resolves feelings of possessiveness and rivalry in family circle (5 years). Gender role (5 years).
7. *Regulation.* Unconscious defenses of repression, reaction formation, displacement and symbolization. Primitive concept of right and wrong, truth and lie, transgression and punishment (4 years). Conscience and ideal self (after 5 years).
8. *Social Competence.* Parallel play (3 years). Cooperative play (4 years). Sympathy and affiliation (4–5 years). Imitation of adult role behavior (5 years).
9. *Psychosocial Hazards.* Neglect. Abandonment. Separation from or loss of attachment figures and familiar surroundings. Divorce. Excessive restrictions or punishment. Inconsistency of care-giver. Inability of care-giver to allow separation and independence. Physical illness and other threats to bodily integrity. Physical abuse.
10. *Signs of Maladjustment.* Excessive or frequent negativism, tantrums, resistance to training, disturbances of sleep, separation anxiety, fears, depression, aggressiveness to or withdrawal from peers.

7. Growth and development proceed in a predictable, genetically determined order and sequence, at a predictable pace, in a predictable direction.
8. Each biopsychosocial system has its own nonlinear pattern of growth. The growth patterns of different systems toward peak functioning may be asynchronous.
9. Sensitive periods occur during the growth and development of all systems. At these times, specific internal or external factors are required to stimulate or promote a normal functional outcome.
10. It is possible to identify leaps or spurts in growth or development, preceded and followed by plateaus or periods of slower growth and consolidation.
11. Each period of development is more than an accumulation of functions from those of the preceding period. Each period is an hierarchical reintegration of previous developmental achievements, which enables the individual to adapt more effectively to the demands of the environment.

TABLE 24.4
Synopsis of development during late childhood

Late childhood 6 to 11 years

1. *Developmental Tasks.* Toleration of separation, learning from others, industry.
2. *Context.* Family, peer group, neighborhood.
3. *Physical and Sensorimotor Milestones.* Rides bicycle (8 years). Nipple buds (9½ years). Team sports (10 years). Female preadolescent growth spurt (9–14 years).
4. *Information Processing.* Concrete reasoning: keeps two aspects of an object in mind at once, mentally reverses operations, can be more objective in reasoning and classifies by more than one characteristic (7–9 years). Uses rehearsal (7 years) and meaning (10 years) to enhance memory. Dates events by relating them to personal experiences (9 years).
5. *Communication.* More complex syntax, analysis of language, association between symbols and sounds, word recognition, blending of sounds, reading, and writing.
6. *Attitudes and Emotions.* Develops liking for adults outside the family and capacity for friendship with peers. Represses immature dependence on family and may reject it in other children. Strives for independence but fears abandonment.
7. *Regulation.* Change from a morality based on proscriptions (6 years) to one based on reciprocity and cooperation (8–11 years). Definition of right and wrong changes from one based on rules (6 years) to one based on the common good (11 years). Sense of fairness and injustice (10 years). Further development of conscience, ego ideal and values.
8. *Social Competence.* Capacity to infer the thoughts, feelings and intentions of others (7–10 years) and to consider alternative solutions to interpersonal problems (10–11 years). Friendship, reciprocity, sharing, teamwork (8–11 years).
9. *Psychosocial Hazards.* Physical differences, impairment or disfigurement. Learning problems. Poverty. Parental discord, separation, divorce, and physical or mental illness. Physical or sexual abuse.
10. *Signs of Maladjustment.* Learning disability, hyperactivity, lack of sphincter control, aggressiveness, stealing, lying, truancy, school refusal, gender role confusion, excessive anxiety and fears, hypochondriasis, depression, social withdrawal.

12. In successive periods, immature functions from earlier periods must be inhibited in order to allow the expression of new functions appropriate to the subsequent period.
13. It is necessary for earlier periods of development to have been negotiated satisfactorily if later periods are to proceed normally.

Abnormal growth and development

1. Abnormal growth or development can occur locally or generally.
2. Abnormality is manifested by precocity, delay, regression, exaggeration, diminution, absence, duplication, or distortion.
3. Abnormal growth or development in one system tends to affect the growth or development of adjacent or related systems.

TABLE 24.5
Synopsis of development during adolescence

Adolescence 12 to 21 years

1. *Developmental Tasks.* Emancipation from parents, career choice, sexual orientation, control of sexuality, sense of identity and capacity for fidelity and intimacy.
2. *Context.* Family, peer group, neighborhood and city or district.
3. *Physical Milestones.* Female growth spurt (9–14 years). Male growth spurt (11–16 years). Menarche (9–14 years). Scrotal and testicular enlargement (9–13 years). Pubic hair (12 years). Axillary hair (14 years). Mature sperm (15 years). Male facial hair, acne (16 years). Arrest of female skeletal growth (17 years), and male skeletal growth (21 years).
4. *Information Processing.* Abstract thinking: propositional, inductive and deductive logic, symbolic reasoning, algebra and metacognition. Estimates time and distance accurately, and uses calendar to date events.
5. *Communication.* Mature language expression and comprehension. Artistic expression. Capacity for debate, rhetoric, irony, satire, dissimulation and complicated lying.
6. *Attitudes and Emotions.* Resurgence of unresolved conflicts. Increased self-involvement (12–16 years). Shift toward heterosexual relations (15–16 years). Crushes, infatuations, rivalry, jealousy, rejection. Early adolescence likely to be smooth, erratic or turbulent. Initial challenge to parental values (12–16 years).
7. *Regulation.* Resurgence of old, unresolved conflicts dealt with by displacement to parent substitutes, or the reversal of affect from exaggerated regard to disrespect. Introversion. Periodic regression to immature behavior. Denial of sexual drives and asceticism. Intellectualization and idealism. Interest in abstract values.
8. *Social Competence.* Has a best friend and seeks to join social groups. Loyalty, teamwork, altruism and idealism.
9. *Psychosocial Hazards.* Enforced passivity. Threats to identity and self control. Loss of, or rejection by, close friends. Lack of career choice. Antisocial companions. Drugs and alcohol. Pregnancy.
10. *Signs of Maladjustment.* School failure or dropout. Exaggerated rebelliousness. Antisocial behavior. Alcohol or drug abuse. Premature sexual activity. Pregnancy. Social withdrawal. Abnormal eating patterns. Depression. Hypochondriasis. Excessive anxiety. Suicidal behavior. Psychosis.

4. Excessive stimulation of a developing system can lead to hypertrophy or increase of function up to a point, after which atrophy or reduction of function ensues.
5. At a sensitive time in the development of a system, lack of appropriate stimulation or exposure to inappropriate or excessive stimulation may lead to irreversible functional impairment in that system or related systems.
6. Decline from peak function proceeds by destabilization, diminution, dedifferentiation, disintegration, dissolution, or diffusion.
7. Functional regression involves the reappearance of immature phenomena that formerly were inhibited, incorporated within, or superceded by more complex modes of behavior.
8. Developmental failure, arrest, delay, distortion, deviation, or precocity are due to genetic abnormality, or adverse environment, or both. In effect, genetic program and environment either fail to interact or interact in an appropriate manner.

The periods of psychosocial development

This section discusses the following periods of psychosocial development:

Periods

   I. Early infancy (0 to 18 months).

  II. Early childhood (18 months to 5 years).

 III. Late childhood (6 to 11 years).

 IV. Adolescence (12 to 21 years).

Within each period, the following issues are described:

Issues

  1. Developmental themes.

  2. Information processing.

  3. Communication.

  4. Images and emotions.

  5. Internal controls, rules, and aspirations.

  6. Social competence.

  7. Coping techniques.

Finally, Tables 24.2 to 24.5 synopsize the biopsychosocial changes associated with each period of development, together with the clinical phenomena associated with psychopathology during each period.

Early infancy (0 to 18 months)

The hazards that may affect intrauterine development or perinatal health are summarized in Table 24.1.

Developmental themes

Innate self-regulatory capacities

The normal infant is born with the capacity for thermal, respiratory, and cardiovascular control and for regulating internal electrolytes and acid-base balance. The neonate is able to suck and ingest milk. Diurnal rhythms soon stabilize, with predictable changes from the states of deep and light sleep, through quiet alertness, to fussing and distress.

Early motor responses

Motor control and repertoire develop rapidly. As primitive grasping, clasping, and withdrawal reflexes disappear, the baby begins to exhibit the reflexes and movements that foreshadow standing and walking. The timing of these familiar sensorimotor milestones is fully described in pediatric texts and summarized in Table 24.2.

Attachment

Soon after birth, the baby begins to exhibit behavior that is the basis of human **attachment:** sucking, grasping, clinging, orienting to human vocal and

Attachment responses

visual stimuli, ocular fixation and eye contact, smiling, crying, and vocal responses. The baby's attachment has a powerful effect on the parent, promoting mutual emotional bonds within which each reciprocate. In this context, the baby becomes aware of the difference between self and nonself, and between parents and other people.

Reciprocity

Mother and infant develop an intimate relationship characterized by an intricate reciprocity. In face-to-face interaction, the baby's level of affective involvement waxes and wanes about four times a minute. The sensitive mother adapts the intensity of her stimulation to the infant's alternations.

Stranger anxiety

By age 6 months, the baby recognizes the chief caretaker or primary attachment figure, and between 6 and 10 months often begins to show distress at the approach of a stranger. Quite early, the baby recognizes and is entertained by siblings and responds to both parents. By 12 months, the baby is likely to move preferentially to one or the other parent, particularly if distressed.

Primary attachment

Extrauterine gestation

The first 12 months have been likened to an *extrauterine gestation,* the mother enveloping the baby in a protective envelope and responding promptly and appropriately to needs for food, interaction, and consolation. Repeated satisfying interactions create a sense of confidence and fulfillment in the parent and are the origin of a sense of trust in the infant, a **basic trust** in the goodness and predictability of human relationships.

Basic trust

The origins of parental behavior

The capacity for loving, protective parental bonding is ultimately instinctual, a biologically determined potential derived from the evolution of the species. But mothering and fathering involve attitudes and skills picked up from models during formative years and refined by previous experiences of caring for children. In short, parents make babies into children, and babies make parents of adults. Biological inheritance provides the framework, but parental skill is learned. Learning accrues as a consequence of innumerable developmental transactions in the course of which each partner – parent and infant – is changed.

Symbiosis

The early mother–infant relationship has been likened to a symbiosis, the psychosocial welfare of each partner being dependent on that of the other (Mahler, Pine, & Bergman, 1975). Symbiosis reaches its peak at about 5 months. Thereafter, satisfactory mutual experiences in earlier infancy and the development of the child's mobility and communication allow the mother to relax her protectiveness and encourage the older infant to explore the environment. For the first 6 months, however, mother and infant are so intensely involved that the mother virtually is the nurseling's environment. The child's sense of self emerges from this intimate reciprocating relationship.

Information processing

Though infant perception is difficult to study, there has been considerable progress in the last 20 years, using as indexes the following phenomena: visual fixation, cortical evoked potentials, ocular electrical patterns, reaching, directional crawling, searching, testing, attention, and habituation.

Neonatal perceptual capacities

It is apparent that the neonate explores the environment and that the capacity for attention to and discrimination among sensory stimuli develops rapidly. Newborns attend preferentially to edges with high contrast, scan visual patterns, prefer sweet tastes and smells, and turn toward pulsating noise. They show a special preference for sounds with the tone and rhythm of the human voice; neonates have been observed to move in rhythm to vocal intonations. By 2 months, the infant begins to attend to patterns and color, and to make phonological distinctions. By 3 months, the infant has shape constancy and shows a preference for complex visual patterns. By 5 months, the infant is capable of responding to complex multisensory stimuli as *Gestalten,* foreshadowing recognition of the parent and 7-month stranger anxiety. The latter probably reflects distress at the discrepancy between a new face and the memory of a familiar face. Cross-modal transfer, eye to hand for example, is also apparent by 6 months, the infant visually fixing on an object, then reaching accurately to grasp it. By about 8 months, a crawling infant will hesitate and show fear when confronted by the visual illusion of a cliff.

Sensorimotor period

Piaget entitled the first 18 months of life the **sensorimotor period** of development because thought is not yet separable from perception and action. Not until 12 to 18 months do true mental operations begin as the infant begins to form stable inner representations of the external world.

The reflexive subphase

The first 6 weeks are described by Piaget as *reflexive* (subphase I), the infant's life being dominated by diurnal cycles of sleep, waking, feeding, and eliminating. Nevertheless, the very young infant is already beginning to attend to interesting stimuli, to habituate to stimuli that are repetitive, and to interact with caretakers.

Piaget describes the following subsequent subphases of the sensorimotor period:

Subphases of the sensorimotor period

II. Primary circular reactions (2 to 4 months): The infant tries to make interesting experiences recur by repeating actions that coincided by chance with the original experience.

III. Secondary circular reactions (5 to 8 months): After eye-hand coordination has been achieved, the infant can produce a perceptible effect on an object by repetitive activity (e.g., shaking a rattle). Thus, different action schemes are coordinated and become the basis of the concept of object permanence, which develops in the next subphase.

IV. Coordination of secondary schemes (9 to 12 months): The coordinated schemata of the third substage are themselves coordinated. The infant uses one object or action (means) to get another object (end). This subphase is the basis of later concepts of causality.

V. Tertiary circular reactions (13 to 18 months): The infant uses trial-and-error to get what is wanted, thereby discovering new effects on objects and new means for achieving desired ends.

Habituation

By 3 months, the infant habituates to a familiar visual object or sound several hours after it was initially presented. By 3 to 4 months, the infant will

Object permanence

smile selectively at a familiar person. However, by 5 months, if an object in which the infant is interested is covered, the baby will at once lose interest. The first signs of **object permanence** do not appear until about 12 months, as the infant becomes capable of following a hidden object through a transformation. For example, at 9 months, if an interesting object is hidden first behind screen A, then moved behind screen B, the baby will search behind A; whereas, at 12 months, the baby will go to screen B. The development of object permanence depends on the gradual acquisition of stable memories that are independent of action.

Self-identity

The beginnings of self-identity are noted at about 9 months, when infants will pluck an object from the forehead while viewing themselves in a mirror. At 18 months, some children can name their own images.

Imitation

Within the first 2 months, some babies will spontaneously imitate facial movements. At about 13 months, deferred imitation is exhibited. Between 18 and 24 months, the infant will strive hard to imitate an adult model and may be distressed if the performance falls short of the adult's.

Prerequisites for language development

By 18 months, therefore, several prerequisites for language development have appeared:

1. The ability to form a mental representation of an object (schema) or action (scheme).
2. The stability of the schema or scheme in the absence of the object or action.
3. The ability to apply the schema or scheme to new instances (generalization).
4. The ability to imitate others.

Communication

At 2 months, the prelinguistic infant can utter about 7 distinct sounds; by 18 months, about 21; and by 30 months, about 27. In general, vowels are acquired in advance of consonants. Phonological progress is from back-of-the-throat to front-of-the-mouth, with the emergence, at 18 months, of voiced, plosive, and fricative consonants. At 13 months, the infant shows a preference for two-syllable words (e.g., *da-da*) whereas one-syllable words (e.g., *go*) predominate at eighteen months.

Phonological development

Acoustic discrimination

The neonate possesses discriminative acoustic perceptual skills, some of which may be innate. Jakobsen (1941) suggested that voice production develops because the infant becomes progressively more able to discriminate between the contrasting features of speech sounds; for example, between vowel and consonant; stop (e.g., /p/) and continuant (e.g., /m/); stop (e.g., /p/), and fricative (e.g., /f/); labial (e.g., /p/) and dental (e.g., /t/); diffuse (e.g., /p/) and concentrated (e.g., /k/); voiced (e.g., /b/) and unvoiced (e.g., /p/); and affricative (e.g., /ch/), and liquid (e.g., /l/).

The acquisition of language

Language is acquired through human interaction. The child brings innate potentials to the process, but others significantly influence it. Early language acquisition is guided by, and probably dependent on, the infant's cognitive development. Adults address infants in a simplified form of language (motherese), which may help the child decipher and establish grammatical rules; moreover, the semantic context in which the adult addresses the child is a simple and interactive one, involving concrete objects and their qualities in the present, in direct association with the infant. Parents also tend to impute curiosity and intention to their prelinguistic infants, thus shaping linguistic interaction in that direction.

The interactive context of language acquisition

Single-word phrases, the first primitive speech acts, appear before 12 months. The typical 13-month-old infant has a vocabulary of about 10 words, referring usually to objects or actions. Different infants may be more oriented to objects (referential) or to personal needs (expressive) in their language. Comprehension is thought to be generally in advance of expression.

Images and emotions

Freud described the ego, the executive aspect of mental life, as differentiated from the id, the source of unconscious drives. Hartmann modified Freud's original theory, contending that nuclei for the ego functions of perception, memory, learning, language, motor control, and defense are present at birth. Given an "average, expectable environment," these **ego apparatuses of primary** autonomy develop rapidly in infancy and early childhood. In addition, however, the ego develops controls against excessive external or internal stimulation. Primitive controls differentiate into the numerous **ego defenses,** which are expressed in combination as **coping techniques.** Some of these coping techniques become secondarily autonomous and eventually function in a manner independent of their original defensive purpose (**ego apparatuses of secondary autonomy**).

The development of the ego

It is probable that by 18 months, the infant has stable mental schemata of self, parents, siblings, other people, and inanimate objects. Some images, that of the mother for example, are invested with intense contradictory emotions. Love for and anger toward the one person is known as ambivalence, a dilemma inevitable in all close relationships.

Ambivalence

Internal controls

The normal infant is born with some capacity to regulate internal and external stimulation, but parents must provide the baby's chief protection against stimulus overload. Infants differ in **stimulus threshold** and in the intensity and predictability of their reactions (Thomas, Chess, and Birch, 1968). Some infants, for example, respond to repetitive stimulation by losing interest (habituating) or even by falling asleep. Others do not habituate readily to continual stimuli. The

Stimulus threshold

Ego defenses

temperamentally more difficult infant is readily distressed by minor acoustic, tactile, or kinesthetic input.

The primitive ego defenses of habituation, denial, splitting, introjection, and projection develop during infancy, antedating language development.

Social competence

Empathy

The normal baby is born with the capacity for attachment, but babies differ in the degree to which they tolerate and seek human interaction and the degree to which they respond to cuddling. By 4 to 6 weeks, social smiling develops. Visual, vocal, and tactile interaction are the chief modes of social exchange in the first 6 months. After about 6 months, the infant can recognize changes in the mother's emotional state, responding to maternal distress by crying, or to depression by withdrawing.

Individuation

Mahler depicts the infant up to 4 months of age as in a **symbiotic phase** of development: closely attached to, but not differentiated from, the mother. From 4 to 7 months, the infant enters the phase of **differentiation.** From 7 to 15 months, in the phase of **practicing,** the infant becomes increasingly exploratory. A temporary pause occurs from 15 to 24 months, with a reversion to episodes of separation anxiety and clinging, the phase of **rapprochement.** Parents who are uninvolved, rejecting, unempathic, or unable to tolerate the infant's separating from them are likely to impede individuation and the child's emerging sense of selfhood (Mahler, Pine, & Bergman, 1975).

Coping techniques

In stressful situations (for example, in physical pain or deprived of contact with a primary attachment figure), the infant has only a limited repertoire of responses. The neonate's potential is exhausted by expressing distress, seeking consolation, and falling asleep.

Maladaptive coping during infancy is manifest in such psychophysiological disturbances as:

Failure of coping or maladaptive coping in infancy

1. Infantile colic.
2. Excessive crying.
3. Restless and unpredictable sleep.
4. Excessive vomiting.
5. Diarrhea.
6. Rumination.
7. Excessive separation or stranger anxiety.
8. Reactive attachment disorder (the infant's reaction to traumatic separation from a primary attachment figure).

9. Lack of social responsiveness due to emotional neglect.
10. Failure to thrive due to neglect.

Early childhood (18 months to 5 years)

Developmental themes

Basic developmental tasks of early childhood: autonomy

From 18 months to 3 years, the infant's central task is to develop a **sense of autonomy,** mastery, and individuality, in contrast to helplessness, doubt, and shame. The effective parent therefore welcomes and encourages the toddler's exploration, while protecting the child from harm and setting reasonable, consistent, nonintrusive limits.

Initiative

From 3 to 5 years curiosity expands, and the healthy child develops a **sense of initiative,** in contrast to inhibition, guilt, and anxiety. During this period, the child learns to emulate the parent of the same sex while retaining affection for the parent of the opposite sex. By the end of this period of development, the child has the physical, intellectual, emotional, and social capacity to cope with formal schooling.

Information processing

Presymbolic, nonverbal and symbolic thought

After 18 months, the child develops stable internal representations of external actions, objects, or events. Presymbolic knowledge antedates representational thinking and persists as nonverbal action thought. (Picture yourself executing a tennis backhand stroke, for example.) But the symbolic representation of objects greatly facilitates mental operations.

Concretism and egocentrism

Though 3-year-olds are often very imaginative and may sometimes have difficulty distinguishing vivid fantasy from reality, they are comparatively concrete, have difficulty thinking relatively or changing perspective, are easily distracted, and have difficulty planning ahead to cope with unfamiliar problems.

A 3-year-old's **egocentrism, animism,** and **anthropocentrism** can be seen in the tendency to attribute the origin of night to the need to sleep and the movement of clouds to men driving engines. The child may regard a dream as external, real, and substantial, and a bicycle as alive because it moves. At this age, children have difficulty estimating time, distance, and volume.

Failure to conserve

The preschool child is likely to be distracted by a single salient feature of a perceptual array. For example, the child will think there is an increase in the volume of water if it is poured from a short, wide glass into a taller, narrower one. Thus, unable to conserve mass, volume, or number, the preschooler is regarded by Piaget as being in the **preoperational stage** of development. Nevertheless, the beginning of concrete operational mental structures is manifest in the

Early classification and seriation

5-year-old's ability to classify objects according to their perceptual qualities (size, color, etc.) and to place objects in serial order (according to one characteristic, such as size).

Communication

Syntactic development

Language development is very rapid during this period. At 12 months, the infant has about five words and speaks in single word phrases. If a child's first word has not appeared by 18 months, diagnostic evaluation is indicated. At 2 years, the normal child has about 300 words and speaks predominantly in two- and three-word phrases. At 3 years, vocabulary has expanded to about 1,000 single words used in complete sentences, despite characteristic syntactic mistakes due to the overgeneralization of inferred grammatic rules (e.g., *mans* instead of *men*, or *goed* for *went*). Irregular, complex, and idiomatic syntax is acquired during the elementary school years.

Innate language competencies

Impoverished language environments

It appears that the normal child is inherently primed to develop the intent to communicate, to acquire the rules of the ambient language and to apply the inferred rules generatively in appropriate contexts of communication. Operant conditioning probably plays a part in language acquisition, but the process is too rapid, extensive, and general to be explained on the basis of stimulus-response learning. Initially, the child appears to imitate the parent in an interactive context, learning to name objects and to distinguish between concrete polarities such as *you/me*, *there/here*, *give/take*, and *to/from*. Syntax appears to be acquired by exposure to repeated examples of a particular form and by generalization from word position and semantic context. An impoverished language environment is likely to be associated with deficient intellectual stimulation and diminished cognitive development.

Images and emotions

From 18 months to 3 years, the child learns to be more independent of the mother, a task greatly aided by motor development, sphincter control, and the acquisition of language; but the child's venturing must sometimes be limited by the parents. The stage is thus set for power struggles.

Negativism

When there is a conflict around toilet training, the child may respond by holding on, refusing to use the receptacle provided, and depositing feces in less convenient places. Similar struggles can occur over eating, talking, and going to bed and staying there.

Confidence; impulsiveness; overcontrol

The child who successfully negotiates this phase will develop confidence and a sense of personal worth. The child who does not do so may remain ambivalent, self-doubting, and overcontrolled, or impulsive, negativistic, and prone to feelings of badness. More fundamentally still, a normal sense of self depends ultimately on whether the child is able, or has been allowed, to complete the period of separation-individuation. Uncaring, unempathic, or absent parents,

Core gender identity

or parents who themselves have an unstable sense of identity may impede individuation.

Between 18 months and 2 years, the child develops a sense of **core gender identity,** of being a *he* or a *she* (Money and Ehrhardt, 1972). Gender identity, the child's imagination and curiosity about sexual differences, the maturing endogenous erotic excitability of the clitoris and penis, together with the loves, jealousies, and fears of family life, all set the stage for the **oedipal** or **phallic period** of development, between 3 and 6 years of age.

The male oedipus complex

The boy is thought to enter the oedipal period both primarily attached to the mother and primarily identified with her. His affection for her, together with vague erotic fantasies of possessing her exclusively, lead to rivalry with, and fear of retaliation by, the father. Awareness of anatomical sexual differences, together with a fear of damage to the erotically charged penis, lead to **castration anxiety.** This causes a boy to repress his sensual longing for the mother and identify with the father. Thus, the boy resolves oedipal conflict by internalizing from the father a **superego** or conscience comprised of taboos and moral principles, an **ego ideal** or set of guiding aspirations, and a **masculine gender role.**

The female oedipus complex

The girl also begins this period primarily attached to the mother and identified with her. Repeated, unavoidable frustrations at the mother's hands, culminating in the fantasy that she once had a penis but was deprived of it by the mother, cause the girl to displace her sensuous attachment from mother to father and to wish the father would give her a baby. Thus, in contrast to the boy in whom castration anxiety ends the phallic period, the girl's oedipus complex is initiated by **penis envy.** Like the boy, however, the girl identifies with the same-sexed parent (though, perhaps, more ambivalently) and develops a superego, ego ideal, and **feminine gender role.**

Feminine gender role

Internal controls, rules, and aspirations

Ego defenses

During this phase of development, the ego defenses of repression, denial, reversal, reaction formation, displacement and substitution develop.

Fear, anxiety, guilt, moral development

Transgressions against parental authority first cause fear of being apprehended and punished; later, anxiety emerges about losing affection; and, by the end of the oedipal period, a sense of guilt, the result of an infringement on internalized standards. The oedipal superego is harsh. Not until adolescence is there much room for shades of gray in moral judgment. Four-year-olds regard an act as good or bad according to its result: What gets punished is bad, and what is rewarded must be good. The 5-year-old is likely to interpret untoward events (such as accidents or illness) as punishment for personal transgression, a phenomenon Piaget called "immanent justice." Between 5 and 7 years of age, the child evaluates an act according to the moral label others have attached to it: Some things are good and others are bad. Lying, for example, is always bad. It is not until early adolescence that the child learns to judge acts against an abstract standard and to comprehend the reason and justification for rules.

Social competence

Preschool children with secure parental attachment are more responsive to other children and more sociable and sympathetic than those with insecure attachment. Irritable and impulsive children are more likely to come from homes that are either coercive or lax and inattentive.

Social cognition

By 4 years of age, the child can recognize personal feelings of pleasure or displeasure but is likely to interpret others' feelings according to what he or she would feel in that situation, rather than from the facial and word cues presented. After observing a dramatic event, preschool children seldom discuss causation or emotion and are more likely to concentrate on situation and action. Nevertheless, preschoolers recoil from the anger of others and try to console parents or friends who are distressed.

Psychosexual development involves the adoption of appropriate gender identity and gender role. It is likely that gender role is the result of an interaction between physical characteristics, hormonal effects, social reinforcement, and the child's construction of the meaning of these influences.

Psychosocial differences between the sexes

What sex differences have been firmly established? Not as many as one might think. Males are biologically more vulnerable than females and tend to be more variable in all cognitive skills. Before adolescence, girls are more advanced in verbal ability whereas boys have begun to perform better in spatial and mathematical tasks. Girls are perceptually more sensitive (for example, to pain) and have better finger dexterity. Preschool boys are physically more active than girls in same-sexed groups; girls express more fear. There are no sex differences in sensitivity, nurturance, or sociability, but boys are directly and indirectly more aggressive, somewhat more competitive and dominant with peers, and relatively less compliant to adult direction.

The differences described are not spectacular; the overlap between the sexes during childhood is very apparent. However, it is likely that stereotypic sex roles originate from a coordinated interaction of biological and social influences in accordance with a sexual specialization of evolutionary origin.

Coping techniques

Preschool children have many more coping techniques than infants. They can plead, charm, demand, cajole, or even attack to get what they want. They can cooperate with or resist others. They can show sympathy and concern or withdraw into self-absorption. Play and fantasy are used to assimilate new experiences, particularly emotionally distressing ones.

Common signs of maladaptive coping are as follows:

Maladaptive coping techniques

1. Frequent tantrums.
2. Breath-holding episodes.
3. Refusal to eat.

4. Food fads.
5. Resistance to toilet training.
6. Unwillingness to go to bed.
7. Nightmares.
8. Night terrors.
9. Unwillingness to sleep alone.
10. Excessive fears.
11. Bed-time rituals.
12. Excessive separation anxiety.
13. Hyperactivity.
14. Depression.
15. Excessive aggressiveness to peers.
16. Avoidance of peer interaction.

Late childhood (6 to 11 years)

Developmental themes

The concept of the latency period

This developmental period was originally entitled **latency** by Freud since he believed that, following the family drama of the oedipal period, sexuality subsided for physical and psychological reasons. It is now apparent that sexual interests continue during this period, but that children, aware of adult disapproval, are more discreet in their behavior.

Industry, inferiority, and self-esteem

Nevertheless, the elementary school years are often more peaceful than those preceding them. The child moves gradually beyond the home and becomes increasingly involved with the peer group. The central developmental task of latency is to develop **a sense of industry,** in contrast to a sense of inferiority and failure. The child acquires physical skills, learns the rules of social intercourse, and learns how to learn. Anything impeding these processes is likely to cause feelings of unhappiness and incompetence. The mentally or physically handicapped child, the chronically sick child, the disfigured child, the socially isolated child, and the child with learning disability are at a severe disadvantage and likely to need help if they are not to suffer irreparable loss of self-esteem.

Information processing

Concrete operations

Between the ages of 5 and 7 years, the average child is in transition from the egocentric preoperational period of thinking to the **stage of concrete operations.** Able now to keep two or more aspects of a perceptual array in mind, the child discovers, for example, that volume is constant despite the fact that the fluid level rises when water is poured from a wide container into one taller but narrower (*conservation*). During this period, the child learns to **reverse transformations**

Reversal

mentally; for example, the child can determine equivalence of volume by pouring the water back to the original container in the mind's eye.

Decentering

The child **decenters** during latency, becoming more objective about concrete problems, less dominated by immediate perceptual configurations, and less restricted by a personal viewpoint. Seriation and classification by more than one perceptual characteristic (e.g., color and shape) become possible, as does grouping according to such categorical qualities as function (e.g., correctly classifying all the tools from a heap of mixed objects). However, the concrete operational child tends to be limited to immediate perceptual data and unable to conjecture about the merely possible. Not until about 12 years of age does abstract reasoning (formal operations) develop.

Seriation and classification

Concrete operations depend on attention and memory. It is likely that attention is not a unitary faculty but rather a composite of:

Attention

1. The capacity to scan the environment systematically.
2. The capacity to divide attention among stimuli.
3. The capacity to attend selectively to stimuli.
4. The capacity to ignore distraction.
5. The capacity to be perceptually flexible, if required.
6. The capacity to inhibit random or impulsive responses.

Research evidence suggests that compared to the preschooler, the school-aged child scans the environment and more efficiently ignores distraction, inhibits impulsive responses, and remains on task. This may be partly due to the older child's capacity to discern the critical features of a problem and develop a mental plan to deal with it. Attentional capacity is reduced in attention-deficit disorder and some forms of learning disability.

Memory

Immediate, recent, and remote memory (with registration, short- and long-term storage, and retrieval) are probably not unitary phenomena. When presented with a stimulus requiring more than immediate registration, a 7-year-old uses control techniques to transfer information to long-term storage. The first of these **mnemonic techniques** to appear is rehearsal. The second strategy, semantic encoding, becomes more prominent in preadolescence. Semantic encoding involves the assimilation of new information into preexisting cognitive structures – memory by association of meaning. Thus, the child actively constructs a personal memory (and may even distort it somewhat according to the meaning superimposed on the original perceptual data). Formal schooling fosters semantic encoding.

Rehearsal
Semantic encoding

Communication

Language production and comprehension advances during the school years in two leaps: from 5 to 8, and from 10 to 13, years.

Children must learn to distinguish phonemes (e.g., /k/ or /t/) from syllables (e.g., *cat*). As they advance, they use more complex syntactic forms (e.g., auxiliary verbs and conjunctions) to express complex relationships. By preadolescence, they are aware that words convey multiple meanings and can have an abstract connotation.

Language stems from knowledge, and knowledge begins with action in the real world. Not until preadolescence does the child think abstractly (using symbols to manipulate symbols) and reason in a hypothetico-deductive manner about the possible, in contrast to the actual. Language is the medium of abstract thought and metacognition, by which the subject thinks about thinking.

Metacognition
Knowing and reading

The importance of the interaction between language and knowledge can be illustrated by the development of the capacity to read. The mature reader does more than decode a series of alphabetical symbols. The reader makes predictions about the ends of words, phrases, and sentences, given their initial elements, automatically imposing on the written medium an understanding of the structure of language and the semantic context of what is being read. Unable to read other than word by word or syllable by syllable, like many dyslexics, the reader is liable to forget what has gone before and lose the sense of the passage.

Reading skills

Reading requires the coordination of a number of subskills. The child must learn (a) to segment sentences into phrases, words, syllables, and phonemes; (b) to associate particular alphabetical symbols or graphemes (e.g., *c*, *a*, and *t*), with particular phonemes (/k/, /a/, /t/); and (c) to blend the phonemes phonically (/k/a/t/). Eventually, familiar words are recognized in toto. Poor readers often reverse letters and spelling, probably not because of impaired perceptual discrimination, but because they are struggling with the differential encoding and decoding of visual symbols.

Having decoded graphemes, blended phonemes, and recognized familiar words, the advanced reader uses clues from the syntax of the sentence and from punctuation and capitalization to decipher the meaning of phrases, sentences, and passages. The child thus requires a reasonable memory span and grammatical awareness in order to decipher written symbols according to the structure of language and finally to automatize the whole process.

Reading retardation

The process can break down at a number of points. Intellectual retardation, sensory handicap, social disadvantage, poor language development, emotional disturbance, lack of motivation, and poor teaching can impede reading. More specific causes of developmental reading disorder are as follows:

Developmental
reading disorder

1. Inability to segment words and syllables into phonemes.
2. Inability to encode phonemes as graphemes and to decode graphemes to phonemes.
3. Failure to automatize the matching of graphemes to phonemes and phonemes to graphemes.
4. Impairment of the ability to analyze sequential language by applying an intuitive knowledge of its semantic and grammatic structure.
5. Delay in automatizing these subskills.

Images and emotions

Learning the culture

The shift towards concrete operations and symbolic memory provides the latency child with the capacity to bind tension and plan ahead imaginatively. Thus, the child is freer to learn from peers and adults other than the parents and to acquire from schoolyard, classroom, and media a knowledge of the culture in which he or she must live. From peers, the child learns to get along with others; from parents, the child learns morality and gender role expectations; and from school, the child learns the formal structures of the society and the intellectual tools necessary to function within it.

Fantasies of late childhood

Oedipal fantasies about parental sexuality are repressed and controlled by identification with the same-sexed parent. Fears of premature independence are commonly expressed in fantasies of abandonment, abduction, or attack by alien beings. The preadolescent defiance of parental rules can lead to Cinderella and return-of-the-conquering-hero fantasies; while residual anxieties about castration or penis envy heighten the child's natural curiosity about sex differences, impregnation, and giving birth.

Regression

From time to time, a regression occurs, and the child becomes messy or babyish. A whole classroom can behave in this way – disintegrating by contagion. An interest in swearing and off-color jokes is part of the same process.

Internal controls, rules, and aspirations

Moral development

The latency child knows the difference between right and wrong actions and is capable of feeling guilt if internal standards have been transgressed. There is a gradual movement from a morality based on rigid moral restrictions in early latency to one based on reciprocity, friendship, and the common good. Thus, internalized parental restrictions are tempered by the need to cooperate with others.

Ego defenses

Repression, denial, and reaction formation become more effective. The more mature defenses of rationalization and substitution develop, helping the child to bind tension, delay gratification, inhibit impulsive action, and impersonalize aggression.

Social competence

Social inference

During this stage, children develop the capacity to infer the thoughts, intentions, and feelings of other people and to consider the causes and consequences of their own or others' actions. By 12 years of age, the child is able to conjecture about another's inferences concerning a third person. At the same time, the child becomes increasingly able to discriminate among and express finer shades of personal feeling and to consider alternative ways of resolving interpersonal dilemmas.

Coping techniques

Common causes or indications of failing or maladaptive coping in the grade-school years are as follows:

Maladaptive coping

1. Learning disability.
2. Attention deficit disorder with hyperactivity.
3. Enuresis and encopresis.
4. Excessive aggressiveness toward peers.
5. Withdrawal from peers or inability to relate to them.
6. Stealing, lying, and running away from home.
7. Separation anxiety disorder, with school phobia.
8. Gender role confusion, with effeminancy in boys.

Adolescence (12 to 21 years)

Developmental themes

Adolescent hormonal changes

Puberty is heralded by a decreased sensitivity of the hypothalamopituitary axis to inhibitory feedback by gonadal steroids, by an increased production of gonadotrophin releasing factors, and a subsequent release of gonadotrophic hormones.

Preadolescent growth spurt

Primary and secondary sexual development

The adolescent growth spurt begins between 9.5 and 14.5 years of age in girls and between 10.5 and 16 years in boys. Female breast buds and pubic hair appear at 11.5 ± 2.2 years and menarche at 12.7 ± 2 years. Male scrotal and testicular enlargement begin at 11.2 ± 2 years. Not only are onset of puberty and rates of growth different in boys and girls, but fat and muscle development also differ in proportion. Approximately 17% of the female body mass must be fat before menses begin, and 22% of body fat is required for regular ovulatory cycles.

For reasons that are unclear, the median age of puberty has been dropping in recent decades. Meanwhile, the requirements of education have led to such an extension of the upper age of adolescence that it is now indefinite. Other social factors that have influenced adolescence are the rising divorce rate, unemployment, and the availability of contraception.

During early adolescence, from 12 to 14 years, the relative calm of latency is disrupted by the emergence of new feelings and needs. Tension, irritability, tears, moodiness, and defiance are common, though usually transitory. In middle adolescence, 15 to 17 years, the adolescent regains composure. Peer relationships and career goals become more important. In late adolescence, the individual should complete the development of a **sense of identity,** move toward **social intimacy,** and choose a career.

The main **developmental tasks of adolescence** are as follows:

Developmental tasks of adolescence

1. To control and channel sexuality and aggression in accordance with sociocultural expectations.
2. To relate sexually to someone of the opposite sex.
3. To emancipate oneself from excessive social, emotional, and economic dependence on parents.
4. To choose a career.
5. To develop a mature sense of identity and the capacity for commitment and fidelity.

Information processing

Formal operations

By 12 years of age, many adolescents are capable of **formal operational thinking.** Formal operations involve hypothetical, propositional logic and the ability to use symbols (such as verbal concepts or algebra) to think about other symbols. The capacity to reason in this way is greatly influenced by education. Only about 30% of the adult population can do so.

Piaget postulated that formal operations depend on cognitive structures that are equivalent to algebraic or logical concepts. There is evidence that powerful generic structures of this nature underlie the combinatorial thinking involved in systematic experimental reasoning. Formal operations also allow the adolescent to entertain and evaluate philosophical and political ideas, thus adding an abstract dimension to moral development.

Images and emotions

Early male adolescence

Boys enter adolescence intensely involved with the same-sex peer group. An increasing interest in the opposite sex leads to a new concern about dress, hair, and skin. Adolescent heterosexual contacts have an egocentric quality at first, each partner being as interested in his or her own performance and control as in the other person. Infatuations can be intense but brief. A revival of castration anxiety leads to fears of masculine inadequacy expressed as concerns about impotence or homosexuality. The boy is often embarrassed by displays of maternal affection and tends to challenge the father's authority, seeking partly to exert his own power and partly to test the father's resolve. In a group, early adolescent boys can be boastful, exhibitionistic, and competitive, telling obscene jokes that serve the purpose of relieving communal tension about sexual competence.

Early female adolescence

The adolescent girl enters adolescence closely involved with her intimate friends who form a smaller affiliation group than the boy's. She defends herself against becoming too dependent on her mother by intermittent defiance of authority and by developing a confiding relationship with a best friend. Often, she becomes more distant toward her father as well. Welcoming the physical changes of puberty, she begins to direct her sexual interest toward boys but may use pop stars and other rather distant heroes as bridges to closer personal relations. When she begins to attract boys, a new and disturbing source of rivalry with her own sex becomes apparent. Feminine roles are changing. Today, there is increasing pressure for women to train and compete with men in the job market. Some girls see themselves as trailblazers in this regard.

Erotic arousal

In comparison with boys, girls do not so readily relate their yearning for affection to genital sensation; before adulthood, female genital masturbation is not universal. This may be because of a stronger social prohibition, in girls, against touching the genitals. In contrast, the adolescent boy who never masturbates is uncommon and likely to be suffering either from pathological lack of desire or pathological overcontrol.

Internal controls, rules, and aspirations

During the latency years, the child represses oedipal feelings and infantile dependency on the parents. The effectiveness of this repression and the adequacy of the child's self-esteem depend on early emotional security.

Regressive tendencies

The relative calm of latency is disrupted by the surge of pubertal sexuality and aggression. The adolescent reexperiences the ties of early childhood and must control these regressive tendencies if development is to continue in the direction of independence, identity, and intimacy. For these reasons, early adolescence can be a period of inner turmoil with moodiness and resistance to parental authority. The advantage of this mild disequilibrium is that the normal

The resolution of old conflicts

adolescent has a chance to resolve old problems derived from the preschool years. The psychologically disordered adolescent, on the other hand, restates these conflicts as psychological symptoms or disruptive behavior without resolving them.

How does the adolescent cope with regressive images and feelings? All the patterns to be described can be discerned, in normal adolescents, in various combinations. They are displayed in exaggerated, unbalanced form by emotionally disturbed patients of this age. The patterns can be summarized under two headings, as follows:

Defenses against old ties and impulses

1. Defenses against old object ties.
   a. Displacement.
   b. Reversal of affect.
   c. Introversion.
   d. Regression.
2. Defenses against impulses.
   a. Repression.
   b. Reaction formation.
   c. Intellectualization.
   d. Idealization.

Displacement

Defenses against old object ties.   In displacement, dependency needs are often transferred to parent substitutes, heroes, or idealized contemporaries. These new attachments are often overstated as romantic crushes or allegiances to philosophical or religious leaders. Detached from parental control, so to speak, the adolescent may be involved in intermittent acting out, in the form of vandalism or speeding, for example. More extreme detachment is manifest in running away from home, the premature assumption of a pseudo-adult personality, delinquency, and the espousal of cult religions.

Reversal

In reversal of affect, the adolescent who cannot detach may reverse dependency, turning love to resentment, attachment to revolt, and respect to derision. This defense is normally manifest in a cocksure disregard for parental opinion on the ground that the adults are hopelessly out of date. It is exaggerated and prolonged in some disturbed adolescents who remain tied to their parents in a mutual hostile dependency.

Introversion

In introversion, feeling that has been detached from parents may be invested in the self as an increase of narcissism. This gives rise to the typical adolescent absorption in dress, grooming, skin, figure, beauty, and strength. It is also manifest as an increase of self-assurance and in fantasies of power, beauty, suffering, or heroism. In exaggerated, pathological form, it is manifest in the body preoccupation of anorexia nervosa, the hypochondria of anxiety disorder, and the obsessive mirror-gazing of incipient schizophrenia.

Regression

In regression, the maturing adolescent intermittently reverts to childish interests, play, or dependency on parents. However, the emotionally arrested adolescent may become locked into a rigid conformism to authority or shift from one unstable identity to another, as in borderline personality.

Repression

Defenses against impulses.   In repression and denial, the inhibited adolescent is likely to postpone development by repressing and denying sexual and aggressive feelings and attempting to maintain an image of being good that originated in latency. This phenomenon, when exaggerated (as in the personality that predisposes to anorexia nervosa), is likely to have been fostered by the family.

Reaction formation

In reaction formation, some adolescents attempt to control their impulses by dedicating themselves to asceticism. This trend sometimes dovetails with athleticism (especially endurance sports, body building, and ballet). Extreme examples of the defense are manifest in anorexia nervosa, obsessive-compulsive neurosis, and early schizophrenia.

Intellectualization

Intellectualization combines the capacity for formal operations with the need to control impulses in a search for a set of abstract principles that can regulate behavior. The adolescent, however, is likely to be somewhat inflexible in applying the principles arrived at. Sometimes the adolescent is unable to act, being paralyzed, so to speak, by incompatible moral ideas.

Idealization

Idealization is the last defense against impulse to be discussed here. Unlike the adult who sees the shades of grey in moral arguments, the adolescent can be a purist; once established, a principle is absolute and must be applied regardless of the situation. Thus, the adolescent may view the more realistic adult as hopelessly compromised.

Gradually, ideals and principles are tested, discarded, or internalized as the final layers of the **ego ideal** and **superego.** To begin with, the superego is somewhat harsh and conventional; later, it is tempered by concepts of reciprocity and relativity. Peer group sanctions for sexual and other experimentation are of importance in this regard.

The sense of identity

The adolescent forges a new **sense of identity** out of the numerous partial identifications of the previous developmental periods. Adolescence is not complete until all these partial identifications are subordinated to an inclusive sense of uniqueness, bridging what the adolescent was with what will become and reconciling an individual's conception of the self with the community's conception. Thus, the adolescent attains a sense of inner continuity and social belonging. Only when identity formation is consolidated will the individual be capable of the fidelity of late adolescence and the intimacy of early adulthood.

Some examples of abnormal variants of identity formation are as follows:

Variants of identity formation

1. Identity diffusion.
2. Identity foreclosure.
3. Negative identity.
4. Psychosocial moratorium.

Identity diffusion

In identity diffusion, the adolescent can find no sense of wholeness but feels fragmented or empty, alienated from others, and bereft of a future. In more extreme cases, the adolescent loses a sense of the continuity of time.

Identity foreclosure

In identity foreclosure, such circumstances as poverty, divorce, or chronic illness or the death of a parent, force the adolescent to grow up before a mature sense of identity has been forged. Such individuals may feel cheated of their youth, and have difficulty allowing their own children the freedom to experiment that is necessary for optimal development.

Negative identity

A negative identity develops when the adolescent assumes a persona that directly contravenes the expectations of parents and society. Thus, the renegade develops, repudiating parental values by ostentatiously going to the dogs.

Psychosocial moratorium

In a kind of psychosocial moratorium, the normal adolescent takes, or is allowed, an extended opportunity to experiment before social and vocational commitments are expected. Extreme examples are the perennial graduate student and the aging hippie.

Normative adolescence

Adolescent turmoil

Earlier accounts of adolescence were derived from the observation of patients and undoubtedly exaggerated the turbulence of normal adolescence. Recent observations have stressed the comparative smoothness of this developmental period for many adolescents. Adolescent turmoil (beyond transient anxiety and mild depression) is usually a sign of psychopathology.

Offer and Offer (1975) describe three normative routes through adolescence:

1. Continuous growth.
2. Surgent growth.
3. Tumultuous growth.

Continuous growth

    Adolescents characterized by continuous growth have a relatively smooth transition from childhood to adulthood. They get on well with their parents, share parental values, have stable friendships with either sex, and work effectively for a future they keenly anticipate. They tend to come from stable homes in which there is trust and affection, and they have few psychological symptoms.

Surgent growth

    Adolescents with surgent growth have more problems in their families. They develop in spurts preceded by plateaus of apparent immobilization. Less action-oriented than the continuous group, they are more prone to anxiety, depression, anger, and turmoil, slower to make heterosexual contact, and less stable in self-esteem.

Tumultuous growth

    The tumultuous growth group have many problems. Conflict with parents, unstable peer relationships, early heterosexual contact, academic failure, self-doubt, and psychological symptoms or inhibitions are characteristic. Their families are the least stable of the three groups and more prone to divorce, illness, and other disruption.

Coping techniques

During adolescence, the failure of coping techniques or the expression of maladaptive coping techniques are manifest in the following developmental problems:

Maladaptive coping

1. Hypochondriasis.
2. Mild depression or anxiety, often related to vicissitudes in personal relationships or to the demands of schooling.
3. Loneliness or rejection by peers.
4. Insecurity about attractiveness or sexual performance.
5. Premature sexual involvement and adolescent pregnancy.
6. Failure to emancipate socially and emotionally from parents.
7. Eating disorders (e.g., anorexia nervosa).
8. Anxiety disorders (especially school phobia).
9. Antisocial behavior.
10. Poor school progress.

11. Dropping out of school.
12. Rebellious behavior at home or school.
13. Failure to plan for a future career.
14. Involvement in drugs or alcohol.

Summary

This chapter brings together the work of Heinz Werner, Sigmund Freud, Heinz Hartman, Anna Freud, Jean Piaget, Margaret Mahler, John Bowlby, Roger Brown, Jerome Bruner, and other developmentalists. The reader should refer to their original works for details of their distinguished contributions to the science of child development. Do not be misled by the condensed nature of the chapter; a unified account of human development is not yet possible. Inevitably, the field (and this chapter) is a pastiche.

The chapter is summarized in Tables 24.1 to 24.5, a series of synopses of the four developmental periods.

1. Prenatal development and infancy.
2. Early childhood.
3. Late childhood.
4. Adolescence.

Tables 24.2 to 24.5 are divided into the following themes, milestones and functions:

1. Developmental tasks.
2. Context.
3. Sensorimotor milestones.
4. Information processing.
5. Communication.
6. Attitudes and emotions.
7. Regulation.
8. Social competence.
9. Psychosocial hazards.
10. Signs of maladjustment.

By keeping in mind the issues summarized in these developmental charts, it will be possible for you to diagnose the relative development of a child or adolescent in the first seven developmental lines and to determine if there is any evidence of general or specific arrest, delay, precocity, or deviance. If so, you may decide to specify such an abnormality as a goal in a comprehensive management plan (see chapter 25).

Selected Readings

The principles of growth and development discussed in this chapter have been strongly influenced by Heinz Werner's (1948) *Comparative Psychology of Mental Development*, which presents the organismic theory of human development.

There is a wide choice of introductory texts in child development. Mussen, Conger, and Kagan's (1979) volume is one of the best. Achenbach (1982) has a useful comparative analysis of the biological, cognitive, social-emotional, and educational perspectives on development.

Authoritative reviews by different authors on life-cycle development can be found in the *Handbook of Developmental Psychology* edited by Wolman (1982). Refer to this text for detailed and critical accounts of the techniques and problems of longitudinal research and the development of perception, language, cognition, social competence, moral judgment, and sex-role differentiation.

Like Freud's, Piaget's theory evolved over a lifetime. For that reason, it is helpful to get an overall perspective of his work before reading the original. Ginsburg and Opper's (1969) review is one of a number of useful introductions to this classic theorist.

The concept of psychosocial themes associated with successive periods of development originated with Freud and was elaborated by Erikson (1950) in *Childhood and Society*.

The following authors present useful syntheses of child and adolescent psychosocial development, from a clinical point of view: Lewis (1982), Shafii and Shafii (1982), and Bemporad (1980). Greenspan and Pollock (1980) have edited a multiauthored text, *The Course of Life*, which presents contemporary psychoanalytic thinking about child development.

25

Modes of treatment in child psychiatry

In general, there are three modes of treatment in child psychiatry:

1. Physical.
2. Psychological.
3. Social.

Nonspecific treatments   Within each mode are specific techniques. Unfortunately, research into the outcome of treatment in child and adolescent psychiatry has far to go, partly because children and families differ widely in regard to developmental level, temperament, psychological characteristics, and sociocultural background. It is not possible to recommend specific treatments for particular disorders. In most cases, the clinician must rely on clinical experience in order to recommend a combination of treatments keyed to goals derived from the comprehensive diagnostic formulation (see chapter 26).

This chapter summarizes each of the more common forms of treatment under the following headings:

1. Nature.
2. Aims.
3. Indications.

    4. Contraindications.

    5. Dangers.

The indications, contraindications, and dangers described are meant not as rules but guidelines. For more details, the reader should consult standard reference books on somatic, psychological, and social treatments.

Physical treatments

The only physical treatments used today in child and adolescent psychiatry are pharmacological. Pharmaceutical agents in common use can be divided into four types:

    1. Major tranquilizers.

    2. Minor tranquilizers.

    3. Tricyclic antidepressants.

    4. Neuroanaleptics.

      As the individual moves into late adolescence, the pharmacokinetics, dose levels, and medication effects approximate those of adults (see chapter 12).

      Generally speaking, the clinician should prescribe the lowest effective dose of medication. Compared to adults, children have less capacity to store and metabolize drugs. Thus, the onset of drug action may be more rapid and the duration of drug effect less predictable.

Major Tranquilizers

Nature

    1. Phenothiazine and butyrophenones.

    2. The most frequently used of these drugs are: chlorpromazine, thioridiazine, trifluoperazine, fluphenazine, and haloperidol.

Aims

    1. Reduce psychotic hyperactivity, affective explosiveness, or self-injurious behavior.

    2. Control psychotic thought disorder.

    3. Counteract social withdrawal in psychosis.

4. Reduce abnormal movements in Tourette's syndrome (haloperidol).
5. Sedation and anxiolysis (e.g., chlorpromazine).

Indications

1. Adolescent-onset schizophreniform disorder or schizophrenia.
2. Latency-onset schizophreniform disorder or schizophrenia.
3. Early onset pervasive developmental disorder (in order to reduce hyperactivity and self-destructive behavior).
4. Organic brain disorder with severe aggressive behavior toward self or others.
5. Very severe anxiety (rarely; only if other treatments have proven ineffective).
6. Very severe hyperkinesis (rarely; only if other treatments have proven ineffective).

Contraindications

1. Bone-marrow depression, liver disease, cardiovascular disorder.
2. Central nervous depression, epilepsy.
3. History of personal or family hypersensitivity.

Dangers

1. Impairment of learning.
2. Anticholinergic effects.
3. Orthostatic hypotension (especially chlorpromazine).
4. Urinary disturbance (especially thioridiazine).
5. Parkinsonism, akathisia, dystonic reactions, tardive dyskinesia, akinesia.
6. Seizures (especially chlorpromazine), delirium.
7. Hyperpyrexia, malignant syndrome.
8. Leukopenia (especially thioridiazine).
9. Photosensitivity (especially chlorpromazine).
10. Pigmentation of lens and cornea.
11. Cholestatic jaundice (rare nowadays).
12. Increased weight (especially thioridiazine).
13. Breast enlargement, galactorrhea, amenorrhea.

Minor tranquilizers

Nature

1. Diazepam, chlordiazepoxide, diphenhydramine, hydroxyzine.

Aims

Reduce anxiety, panic.

Indications (for temporary symptom relief)

1. Separation anxiety disorder.
2. Overanxious disorder of childhood.
3. Hyperventilation syndrome.
4. Insomnia caused by tension (diphenhydramine).
5. Night terrors, somnambulism (diazepam).

Contraindications

1. Depression.
2. Psychosis.
3. Hyperkinesis.
4. Asthma (diphenhydramine).
5. Pyloric or urinary neck obstruction (diphenhydramine).
6. Glaucoma (diphenhydramine).

Dangers

1. Paradoxical excitement (chlordiazepoxide).
2. Drowsiness (hydroxyzine).

Tricyclic antidepressants

Nature

Imipramine, amitryptyline.

Aims

1. Counteract depression.
2. Reduce phobic anxiety, separation anxiety.
3. Prevent nocturnal enuresis, somnambulism, night terrors.
4. Increase attention span.

Indications

1. Depressive syndromes (dubious effectiveness under 12 years of age).
2. School phobia.
3. Nocturnal enuresis, somnambulism, night terrors.
4. Attention-deficit disorder.

Contraindications

1. Glaucoma, urinary tract obstruction.
2. Cardiac disorders, renal disease.

Dangers

1. Anticholinergic effects, electrocardiographic abnormalities.
2. Insomnia, tremor.
3. Hypo- or hypertension.
4. Nausea, constipation, flatulence, abdominal pain.
5. Thrombocytopenia, agranulocytosis.
6. Acute psychotic episodes (hypomania or toxic delirium).

Neuroanaleptics

Nature

D-amphetamine, methylphenidate, magnesium, pemoline.

Aims

1. Increase attention span.
2. Decrease impulsivity and hyperactivity.

Indications

1. Attention-deficit disorder.
2. Narcolepsy.

Contraindications

1. Prepsychotic conditions.
2. Hyperthyroidism.

3. Epilepsy.
4. Renal insufficiency (pemoline).

Dangers

1. Anorexia.
2. Insomnia (transient).
3. Headache, abdominal pain, nausea.
4. Tachycardia (methylphenidate).
5. Tremors, increased hyperactivity (D-amphetamine), restlessness.
6. Acute hallucinosis.
7. Depression, irritability.
8. Rash (pemoline).
9. Growth retardation (probably due to depression of appetite; recovers when medication is ceased).

Psychological treatments

These therapies include a variety of techniques in four main groups:

1. Individual psychotherapy.
2. Behavior modification.
3. Social and cognitive behavior therapy.
4. Remedial therapies and remedial education.

Individual psychotherapy

The different forms of individual psychotherapy vary in accordance with the following dimensions:

1. Brief versus protracted.
2. Supportive, directive, and reality-oriented versus expressive, exploratory, and oriented to unconscious material.
3. Structured, interpretative versus unstructured, client-centered.
4. Play-oriented versus verbally oriented.

Supportive psychotherapy

Nature.   A loose collection of techniques without clear theoretical basis derived from humanistic understanding and personal experience.

Aims.

1. Establish an identificatory relationship.
2. Define current problems.
3. Consider and implement problem solutions.
4. Suppress ego-alien, unconscious material and restore status quo ante.

Indications.

1. Adjustment disorders.
2. Temporary emotional crises due to situational stress.
3. Remitted psychotic disorders when the patient is in need of rehabilitative help.

Contraindications.   Severe disorders requiring more specific or more extensive therapy.

Dangers.   Excessive dependency on therapist. Otherwise relatively safe. The development of an undesirably intense relationship with the therapist is a potential problem with any therapeutic technique, but it is more likely in intensive psychotherapy of long duration.

Client-centered therapy

Nature.   A form of play therapy or verbal psychotherapy in which the patient is gently encouraged to explore personal feelings and attitudes. In client-centered therapy, the therapist empathically reflects the feelings explicit or implicit in the patient's play and verbal or nonverbal communications. The pace of therapy is generally determined by the patient and is usually brief to intermediate in duration. Based on the work of Rogers (1951).

Aims.

1. Establish an empathic, accepting relationship.
2. Encourage self-exploration by judicious reflection of feeling.

Indications.

1. Children and adolescents with adjustment reactions and mild anxiety disorders.
2. Adolescents with problems involving career choice, academic commitment, or mild identity confusion.

Contraindications. Severe disorders, especially psychosis or prepsychosis, conduct disorder, borderline personality.

Dangers. Excessive or unresolved dependence. Otherwise, relatively safe.

Exploratory psychotherapy

Nature. A form of play therapy or verbal psychotherapy in which the patient's unconscious conflicts, usually in a specified area, are resolved by interpretations based on the patient's play and verbal and nonverbal behavior. Usually extended in duration (6 to 12 months) and moderately intensive (1 to 2 times per week). Derived from the work of Freud (see child and adolescent psychoanalysis).

Aims.

1. Establish relationship.
2. Help patient to become aware of unconscious wishes or defenses by judicious interpretation of wishes or defenses.
3. Terminate relationship when treatment objectives are reached.

Indications.

1. Anxiety, somatoform, and dissociative disorders.
2. Personality disorders and interpersonal difficulties related to neurotic conflict.

Contraindications.

1. Conduct disorders.
2. Schizoid, schizophreniform, or schizophrenic disorders.
3. Borderline personality.
4. In patients who fear intimacy.

Dangers. Intense transference reaction with severe emotional turmoil.

Child and adolescent psychoanalysis

Nature. An extensive (e.g., 1 to 5 years) and intensive (e.g., 3 to 5 times per week) form of exploratory therapy in which a radical resolution of unconscious conflicts is sought by using interpretation and, in some older adolescents, by analyzing the transference relationship between patient and analyst. Based on the work of Freud.

Aims.

1. Establish relationship.
2. Encourage spontaneous expression of thoughts and emotions (through play and conversation).
3. Aid resolution of unconscious conflict by interpreting unconscious wishes, transference, and ego defenses.
4. Support patient in working through personal solutions to problems that have been rendered conscious in analysis.
5. Terminate relationship.

Indications.

1. Anxiety disorders.
2. Somatoform disorders.
3. Borderline personality (if not severe).

Contraindications.

1. Psychotic disorders.
2. Pervasive developmental disorder.
3. Conduct disorders.
4. Severe personality disorders.
5. Patients who cannot tolerate intimacy.

If this form of therapy is to succeed, the patient must have a reasonable capacity to tolerate tension, the ability to express emotions in words, the motivation to seek help, and considerable economic resources.

Behavior modification

Nature

A group of loosely associated therapeutic techniques derived from the principles of learning.

Aims

1. Systematic desensitization. Exposing the patient to progressively more anxiety-provoking stimuli, while at the same time teaching the patient to relax, or pairing the phobic stimuli with a pleasant activity (such as eating), or associating the stimuli with pleasant fantasy.
2. Reinforcement of coping responses. Rewarding responses that counteract or are incompatible with the problem behavior.

3. Implosion. Forced entry into the phobic situation.

4. Shaping. Rewarding progressive approximations to desired responses, especially in habit training.

5. Token reinforcement. Poker chips, stars on a calendar, and so on, that can be exchanged at stipulated times for reward, such as money or privileges. The tokens are used for immediate reinforcement of desirable behavior.

6. Aversion. Interrupting undesirable behavior (e.g., self-destructive head banging) by applying a noxious stimulus (e.g., an electric shock) whenever the behavior is expressed.

7. Time out. Deprivation of anticipated reinforcement (e.g., attention) by consistently isolating the child when the undesirable behavior (e.g., tantrums) is expressed.

8. Massed practice. Multiple repetitions of an undesired behavior (e.g., a habit spasm) in order to weaken its association with an underlying emotional state (e.g., anxiety).

9. Substitution. Replacing an undesirable behavior (e.g., smoking) with a neutral one (e.g., chewing).

Indications

1. Phobic disorders.
2. Eating disorders.
3. Habit training (e.g., functional enuresis or encopresis).
4. Preschool management problems (e.g., tantrums).

Contraindications

1. Psychosis.
2. Situations in which the patient has a fear of or resistance to being controlled.

Dangers

1. Deterioration (reported after implosion).
2. Appearance of new undesirable behavior (e.g., if desensitization is too limited in scope).

Social and cognitive behavior therapy

Nature

A group of techniques focusing on intermediate cognitive responses as the primary target for intervention.

Aims

1. Participant modeling. Combining the observation of a model who behaves in a desired way with the opportunity to practice the desirable behavior.
2. Interpersonal problem-solving. Teaching the subject to infer the causes and consequences of interpersonal events and actions and to consider alternative solutions to interpersonal dilemmas.
3. Cognitive-behavior therapy. Helping the patient to define and alter the self-defeating expectations and attitudes underlying maladaptive behavior.
4. Self-instruction training. Teaching the child to reflect on a problem rather than act impulsively.

Indications

1. To encourage behavior that will counteract a phobia.
2. To overcome social impulsiveness or inhibition.
3. To counteract the pessimism that predisposes an adolescent to depression.
4. To replace motor impulsiveness with reflectiveness.

Contraindications

Psychosis.

Dangers

As with behavior modification.

Remedial therapies and education

Nature

A large group of remedial or rehabilitative programs designed to help the child or adolescent overcome chronic physical, educational, or social handicap.

Aims

Remedial therapies and technologies have been designed for a variety of handicaps, including:

1. Cerebral palsy.
2. Orthopedic impairment.

3. Blindness.
4. Deafness.
5. Aphasia.
6. Learning disability.

These therapies may be provided in a separate institution (such as a school for the hearing impaired) or incorporated in a regular school program (mainstreaming). The current trend is toward mainstreaming whenever possible.

Dangers

1. The child may be labeled and discriminated against in a separate (categorical) program.
2. The child's needs may exceed the teacher's competence or capability in a mainstream program.
3. The child may not be accepted by unimpaired classmates.

Social therapies

Group therapy

Nature

Groups of six to eight children or adolescents, with a group leader, meeting between once per week and daily. Groups for preschool children emphasize social stimulation. Activity groups for latency-age children emphasize socialization. Groups for adolescents focus on mutual support and common problems. Group therapy often is used as an adjunct to other forms of therapy (particularly during hospitalization).

Aims

1. Provide social experience.
2. Allow expression of feeling in an accepting environment.
3. Foster awareness of common experience and allow group to consider solutions to common problems.
4. Promote group cohesiveness during hospitalization.

Indications

1. During hospitalization of latency-age children or adolescents.
2. Social isolation.
3. Adolescents with a common problem (e.g., after divorce, physical handicap, alcoholism).

Contraindications

Patients who are disturbed by forced intimacy.

Dangers

The group should be well balanced, with a judicious combination of aggressive instigators, compulsive neutralizers, and dependent followers. If there are too many aggressive children, the group will explode. If there are too many neutralizers or followers, group process will stagnate.

Role play

Nature

A subtechnique of group therapy, commonly used in hospital treatment, in which a recent social incident is reenacted, usually with role players different from those involved in the incident but with the help of those actually involved.

Aims

1. Insight.
2. Consideration of common problems and alternative solutions.

Casework with parents

Nature

Casework extends from intermittent contact with the patient's parents (to keep them informed about progress) to intensive counseling (e.g., in regard to marital problems, child management, or health care).

Aims

1. Provide information.
2. Promote more consistent child management or health care.
3. Institute a behavior modification program at home.
4. Resolve marital problems.
5. Prepare one or both parents for referral to another therapist.

Indications

1. Whenever the child is in intensive individual therapy.
2. Behavior modification in a natural environment.

Contraindications

If the parents are very antagonistic, they may need to be interviewed separately.

Conjoint family therapy

Nature

A form of group therapy in which the patient's family is treated. The family meet with a therapist (or male and female cotherapists) for intensive, brief therapy in order to promote crisis resolution, or for a more extended period if radical changes in family interaction are proposed.

Aims

1. Resolve family conflict.
2. Promote a common understanding of family problems.
3. Encourage consideration of alternative solutions to common problems, especially when the family have reached an impasse.
4. Foster a common awareness of previously unexpressed family rules, roles, and expectations.
5. Alter long-standing maladaptive interaction patterns (e.g., coalitions, rifts, scapegoating, enmeshment, or skewing) and abnormal patterns of communication.

Indications

1. When the patient is recovering following hospitalization for severe mental illness.
2. When the patient's problems are perpetuated by family interaction patterns.

Contraindications

1. When family members are excessively hostile or intrusive toward the patient.
2. When the parents are on the verge of separating.
3. When the patient is seeking to become independent of a severely pathological family system.

Dangers

1. Tension in other family members as the homeostasis of the family changes.
2. The accentuation of a preexistent rift between the parents.

Psychiatric hospitalization

Nature

Psychiatric hospitalization involves a severely disturbed child or adolescent in a psychiatric inpatient unit with special programs and a therapeutic milieu designed for children or adolescents. The special program coordinates pediatric, psychiatric, psychological, social work, nursing, educational, and occupational therapies. Placement may be brief (e.g., less than one month) or extended (e.g., six months to one year), depending on the patient's needs.

Aims

1. Separate disturbed patient from family.
2. Undertake comprehensive diagnostic workup.
3. Control suicidal, aggressive, or disorganized psychotic behavior.
4. Institute treatment programs requiring coordination and intensive monitoring.

Indications

1. Suicidal, aggressive, destructive, disruptive, or dangerous behavior beyond the control of the family and caused by mental illness (especially schizophreniform, schizophrenic, and affective disorders).
2. Severe anorexia nervosa.
3. Severe anxiety, somatoform, and dissociative disorders.
4. When the patient's severe emotional disorder is perpetuated by complex family interaction pathology.
5. Severe adjustment disorders with depressed mood secondary to emotional stress.
6. Organic mental disorder (e.g., substance-induced delirium or hallucinosis).
7. Comprehensive diagnostic evaluation of complex cases, especially those requiring the coordination of a number of specialties (e.g., an adolescent who has a chronic physical illness associated with a serious psychiatric disorder and family interaction problems).
8. Pervasive developmental disorder (for diagnosis and management planning).

Contraindications

1. Conduct disorder of undersocialized, aggressive type.
2. Chronic substance abuse or dependence, without other complications.
3. Some cases of personality disorder (especially of borderline type) in which there is a danger of training the patient to be chronically ill.
4. When hospitalization will aggravate alienation between family and patient.

Dangers

1. Accentuating dependency and training the child or adolescent to be a patient.
2. Scapegoating and permanent extrusion by an alienated family.
3. When added pressure on staff could lead to communication breakdown and deleterious effects on all patients.

Safeguards

1. Clear but nonautocratic psychiatric leadership.
2. Staff selected for defined but overlapping roles.
3. Clarity of general aims and individual treatment goals.
4. Good coordination of and clear communication among staff.

5. Early planning for postdischarge disposition.
6. Family involvement in admission, diagnosis, management planning, and continuing treatment.
7. As far as possible, an environment approximating that of the average child of that age (in schooling, social opportunity, and recreation) and deemphasizing chronic invalidism.
8. Day hospitalization for less severely disturbed patients.
9. Planned discharge to outpatient or day hospital care as soon as possible.
10. Good coordination between regional inpatient unit and community mental health agencies.

Specialized day-care or residential units

Nature

Residential units usually based on an educational (rather than a medical) model, with programs designed for children or adolescents with special problems.

Examples

1. Preschool day-care programs for children with special physical, educational, or psychological needs (e.g., underprivileged children or children with pervasive developmental disorders).
2. Residential units for children and adolescents with severe physical handicaps or disorders.
3. Pediatric hospital units for infants and children who have experienced physical neglect or abuse.
4. Residential units for adolescents with substance dependence (usually emphasizing behavior control).
5. Residential units for adolescents with conduct disorder (usually emphasizing behavior control).
6. Residential units for the mentally retarded.
7. Boarding schools for adolescents with learning problems.

Other placements away from home

Nature

Temporary or permanent placement of a child or adolescent in a foster or group home.

Aims

1. Temporary fostering while parents and child are in treatment preparatory to the return of the child.
2. Permanent fostering, with or without view to adoption, after disintegration of home of origin or when parents are unable to provide adequate care.
3. Group home placement for children and adolescents too disturbed to cope with the emotional vicissitudes of foster home placement.
4. Community group home placement designed to promote independent living skills for mentally retarded adolescents or adolescents with pervasive developmental disorders.

Summary

This chapter summarizes the physical, psychological, and social therapies commonly used in child psychiatry. In almost every case, combinations of techniques will be used; the patient's biopsychosocial needs demand multifaceted management. An adolescent hospitalized for anorexia nervosa, for example, is likely to require a combination of the following forms of therapy:

1. Pediatric treatment to correct subnutrition and fluid and electrolyte imbalance.
2. Behavior modification to counteract voluntary restriction of food intake.
3. Individual expressive psychotherapy to provide insight and promote conflict resolution.
4. Family therapy to help the family undo the parent–child enmeshment and hidden interparental conflict commonly associated with this disorder.

These therapeutic interventions should be provided in a therapeutic milieu offering opportunity for peer group interaction, group therapy, schooling, and recreation.

A sophisticated, multifaceted, individually designed management plan requires a comprehensive biopsychosocial, temporal, and developmental diagnostic formulation. The diagnosis should be shared with the patient and parents at a negotiation interview, and the parents' and patient's collaboration sought in the management plan. The derivation of a goal-directed management plan from a comprehensive diagnosis is described in the next chapter.

Selected Readings

The association between diagnosis and treatment is discussed in *From Diagnosis to Treatment in Child Psychiatry* (Group for the Advancement of Psychiatry, 1974).

Useful introductions to pharmacotherapy in childhood and adolescence are found in Klein et al. (1980) and White (1980). In this field, the enthusiasm of clinicians often exceeds the empirical evidence. Werry (1978) presents a critical review of the effectiveness of different pharmacological agents in different disorders.

The following books are useful to the clinician seeking an introduction to individual psychotherapy with children and adolescents: Axline (1969), Adams (1982), Lippman (1962), Reisman (1973), Holmes (1964), Meeks (1980), and Lamb (1978). Introductions to the use of behavioral techniques with children and adolescents are found in Leitenberg (1976), Rutter and Hersov (1977), and Achenbach (1982). Family therapy is described in Glick and Kessler (1980) and Minuchin (1974), and group therapy in Slavson and Schiffer (1975) and Rose (1972).

The residential treatment of children and adolescents is discussed in Stone (1979), Zinn (1979), Holmes (1964), and Meeks (1980).

26

Comprehensive planning in child psychiatry: a case example

Case 26.1 ■ Matthew M. was referred to the intake secretary of the Child Psychiatry Clinic by his mother, after the family pediatrician advised it. She reported to the secretary that Matthew, who is aged 9 years, lives with his parents in a small rural town. She also told the secretary that the pediatrician had ruled out physical disorder and advised her that Matthew had an emotional problem:

Matthew cried "at the drop of a hat," seemed to have difficulty relating to other children at school, was fearful of sleeping at night, and had "a poor self-image." These symptoms had become noticeable during the previous summer vacation. Since school began, they had become worse. Mrs. M. could give no reason for Matthew's disturbance. She thought her son might prefer to see a female clinician but readily accepted an appointment with a male psychiatrist.

A telephone call to the child's pediatrician revealed that Matthew was in excellent physical health aside from hay fever, and that there had been no serious childhood illnesses, surgery, head injury, or history suggestive of epilepsy. The pediatrician thought there might be a problem between the parents and noted that the father was a rather "testy" man.

Mrs. M. completed a Child Behavior Checklist and Child Information Form. Matthew's teacher completed a Conner's Teacher's Questionnaire.

In the social competence items of the Child Behavior Checklist, Matthew's mother reported the following:

I. Sports: skateboarding, bike-riding, swimming. In the first two, he is involved with "average" frequency and skill; in the third, he is "less than average."
II. Recreations: reading and drawing ("above average" frequency).
III. Organizations: "Quit Cub Scouts after 1 year."
IV. Chores: firewood, trash ("average") "Must keep after him constantly to do chores; sometimes I give up."
V. Close friends: Four or more. Sees them three times a week.
VI. Gets on with: Siblings and other children, "worse" than others of the same age; parents, "about the same;" plays by himself "better than others."
VII. Current school performance: Reading, writing, and spelling – "average;" arithmetic, "below average;" geography, "above average."

He has never been in a special class or repeated a grade.

In the Behavior Problems section of the CBCL, the mother checked the following behaviors as evident during the last 12 months.

Very or Often True	*Somewhat or Sometimes True*
Allergy	Acts too young for his age
Clings to adults	Argues a lot
Cries a lot	Can't concentrate
Demands attention	Can't get his mind off certain thoughts ("outer space")
Fears certain animals, situations, or places ("Nightmares about creatures from outer space")	Complains of loneliness
	Day-dreams
	Destroys own things
	Disobedient
Feels he has to be perfect	Doesn't eat well
Feels no one loves him	Doesn't get along with other children
Feels worthless or inferior	Doesn't seem to feel guilty after misbehaving
Gets teased a lot	Fears going to school
Likes to be alone	Fears he might do something bad
Nightmares	Feels others are out to get him
Poorly coordinated	Gets in many fights
Self-conscious	Lying or cheating
Stubborn, sullen, irritable	Not liked by other children
	Too fearful or anxious
	Plays with own sex parts too much
	Poor schoolwork
	Prefers playing with younger children
	Refuses to talk
	Screams a lot
	Secretive
	Showing off
	Sulks a lot

Somewhat or Sometimes True
Talks too much
Unhappy, sad, or depressed
Whining
Withdrawn
Worrying

The scoring of the social competence profile reveals that Matthew has the following T scores: Activities (55), Social (48), and School (52). He is therefore in or above the normal range in social competence.

The scoring of his behavior problems indicates a raw score sum of 62 ($T = 71$), which is in the clinical range. The T score for internalizing behavior is 73; and for externalizing, 65. The difference between these scores is insufficient for him to be regarded as predominantly either an internalizing or an externalizing child.

T scores on the following behavior factors are in the pathological range: anxious ($T = 79$); depressed ($T = 80$); uncommunicative ($T = 75$); and withdrawal ($T = 79$).

Based on intraclass correlation, he most closely resembles the following profile types: anxious-schizoid (0.779); anxious-schizoid-withdrawal (0.727); and depressed-withdrawal-aggressive (0.288).

On the Conner's Teacher's Questionnaire, the following items were checked:

1. "Very much": Overly sensitive to criticism; appears to lack leadership.
2. "Pretty much": Makes inappropriate noises; unpredictable behavior; submissive toward authority; appears to be easily led by other children; no sense of fair play; childish and immature; denies mistakes; does not get along with other children; uncooperative with classmates; easily frustrated.
3. "Just a little": Demanding; disturbs other children; pouts and sulks; mood changes; quarrelsome; excessive demands; appears to be unaccepted by the group; fails to finish things he starts; uncooperative with the teacher; difficulty in learning.

The teacher added the following remarks:

> "Often cries in class for little or no reason. Manipulates situations to put himself down. Recently, Matthew seems to be enjoying the added attention and is going out of his way to show that he needs it."

In the Child Information Form, the mother noted no medical problems during pregnancy. Delivery was normal and at term. Matthew's birthweight was 8 lbs., 15 ozs.

During infancy, he was easy and predictable. The milestones of his motor development, language development, and sphincter control were within normal limits, although toilet training was regarded as difficult and he had trouble separating from his mother to go to kindergarten.

Other than diarrhea (at 18 months) and hay fever, he has had no serious childhood illness. His only surgery was for circumcision. He takes rynaton for allergy. His eyesight was normal at a recent check. His hearing has not been checked but is not regarded as defective.

Interview with parents

The parents attended the child psychiatrist together on the day before Matthew himself was to be interviewed.

Mr. M. is a tall, gaunt, graying 50-year-old man dressed in a gray suit and vest. His face is deeply lined and he walks with limitation of movement in both hips. At the inception, he said little; but after 5 minutes, he interrupted his wife and thereafter tended to be the dominant influence during the interview.

Mrs. M. is a plump, conservatively dressed woman, with fading red hair. Where the husband was direct and matter-of-fact, Mrs. M. made a softer and more sensitive impression. The parents seldom looked at each other during the interview, but they told complementary stories about Matthew's present behavior and development.

They began by giving the ages and names of those in the family. The father is 50 years of age, and the mother is 48. There are four siblings: Donald, age 21; Linda, age 20; Erin, age 16; and Matthew, age 9 years.

To the psychiatrist's question about what it was that concerned them most in Matthew at the present time, Mrs. M. said:

"He is upset with himself. People hurt his feelings all the time. He cries a lot and thinks his friends don't like him, whereas they really do. He has red hair, is teased about it, and hates it. The children call him 'carrot-top.' He can't take teasing.

"At school, he cries a lot. At home, he often cries if he has been pushed during play. Sometimes he provokes the teacher by saying to him, 'I suppose you think I can't do this problem.' He puts himself down all the time.

"Recently at school he told the teacher that his dog had died and that he had got a new dog. This is untrue. Afterward he admitted that he just wanted attention. Actually, his sister owns the dog. He wishes her dog were dead so that he could have his own dog."

At this point, the father broke in, forcefully, to say:

"He is supersensitive. He tries hard to be perfect. He wants his parents' approval. Really, he's been babied and spoiled. He's just got to outgrow it. Everybody has to – and soon."

Mrs. M. went on to say she thinks she has done more little things for Matthew than she did for the older children. For example, she tied his shoes until he was 7 years of age, much longer than she did for the older children. His two oldest siblings have also tended to baby him. Sometimes Matthew will call to his mother to come in and see him when he is lying in bed on Sunday morning and she is making the breakfast. At such times, she usually accedes to his request. "It's a habit. I have to get out of it. I seem to have had more time to do things for him. Yet, if he can't do things he gets furious and throws up his hands. If he makes one little mistake with his homework, he'll get mad and tear it up."

The psychiatrist asked how the parents felt about this.

MOTHER: I feel very badly for him that he can't correct it. It's agony for him.

FATHER: I'm not as involved, from moment to moment, as my wife is. I feel zero. He's got to learn to live with himself as I have had to with myself.

MOTHER: Matthew's father works 5 days a week until 9:00 at night. He also works on Saturdays and Sundays. Yet when he is home with Matthew, it is good quality time. He has been in business for 7 years in a hardware store.

Mr. M. mentioned that he and his wife sleep in separate bedrooms and that Matthew often comes in to sleep with him at 2:00 in the morning.

The psychiatrist asked how long they had been sleeping apart.

FATHER: Seven years.

MOTHER: It is significant. One day Matthew said to me, "How come you two don't smooch?" He must know there is something wrong between us. Donald, his older brother, is in Oregon and Linda is at school in Texas. Matthew misses them very much. He is upset that they are so far away. It's hard on him. He makes me promise I will take him to the airport with me when I pick them up from the plane and when they depart. Matthew said to me one day, "How come I always fight with Donald before he is going to leave?" Matthew and Erin don't get on. She is 16 and ridicules him. He put a sign on his door saying, "Keep out from your so-called baby brother." Really, if I need a baby-sitter I would rather hire one than ask Erin to look after him. Sometimes she goes overboard when she criticizes him. There is more than a touch of cruelty in her. We've been through this before. She resents her younger brother.

Mr. M. then mentioned that he used to be a commercial traveler, working out of Boston, and that Matthew was conceived just before they left Boston to come to Rhode Island 9 years before. There was a big change after leaving Boston. From being away for weeks at a time, the father was now home every night. For 2 years in Rhode Island it was a good life, but then he went into business for himself and has had to work, over the last 7 years, 7 days a week in order to keep his business afloat. In addition to that, he has had severe osteoarthritis in both hips with chronic pain, culminating in two hip-replacement operations. The final operation was carried out 6 months before. He has been much better physically since that time.

FATHER: Some things you just have to accept. Like me being a cripple. It takes time to get going in the morning, but I'm not fighting city hall any more.

MOTHER: It was harder for him than anyone realized. He lived with one hip for 35 years. It was broken when he was 14 years of age.

FATHER: I put it off for a long, long time. I begged the doctor for a glue job, and then he agreed to do it. Then I had to defer the operation twice because of severe business difficulties. Finally, 5 years ago, I couldn't work and had the right leg done. It was a big relief, but then the new hip began to feel better than the old left hip and I had to have the second hip done 6 months ago. Life hasn't been a picnic, but I don't expect as much from it as my wife does.

(*Mrs. M. agreed, nodding her head.*)

FATHER: You're not entitled to happiness like my children think, only the pursuit of happiness. The last 10 years have been hard for us. Until then, I'd been successful in Boston. I shouldn't have left, but my wife was unhappy. I had a work problem, so I decided to leave Boston. My wife wanted New England, so we came here. It turned out that I made a false business move, then I had to open my own business, which required much more time and capital than I expected and has paid less than I expected. Yet what project is different from that? We are just here and have to make the most of it.

MOTHER: He worked a miracle. He has always had a driving ambition to own his own hot dog stand. But we lost a lot of happiness and a normal home.

FATHER: There is no wife-beating but my wife shouldn't be married to a business man. Dollars and cents worry her. She should have been married to a social worker or a child psychiatrist.

MOTHER: It's hard to bring up children when you're alone with them. At night he's exhausted and in such pain and agony. Kids need both parents, but it's not his fault.

FATHER: It's a luxury to have both parents. Many families don't have both parents always available. Maybe that's why we have more psychiatrists now than we used to.

At this juncture, the psychiatrist asked the parents if there was anything else they were concerned about in Matthew's development. They could add nothing else except that he has many allergies. The father interjected that he was more concerned about Matthew's allergies than his frame of mind. ''Matthew is on pills. He can't go through life taking pills all the time.''

FATHER: I didn't feel it was necessary for Matthew to be here but, after all, his mother has more time to think of these things than I do. I'm here because my wife wanted me to be here. But I'm resigned to it now, particularly since I have been able to run the conversation. (*They both smiled at this.*)

MOTHER: I feel I should have taken Erin to see you 3 years ago. I've made mistakes with my children. One day Matthew told me that he was ''mental.'' He is very unhappy.

FATHER: He is not terribly unhappy. He just has to accept it. What about Donald? Donald is fourth year at college. He blew his first year at college, but now he has done quite well. He has survived pretty well on his own and asks for nothing from us except when he is broke. He has always had a job, saved his money, and got grants. Both kids, Donald and Linda, have done this. Linda is at a university in Texas. She works hard, is on the Dean's List, and is determined to be an engineer. Erin is something else. This month, she is 17 years of age. She is hard, determined, and incorrigible.

MOTHER: That's not the right word. Erin and her father are alike. They are bright and have a will of iron. If we directed her, Erin could move mountains. She is a junior in high school and doing well at her work. Really, she is brighter than Donald and Linda. Three years ago Erin was fat, had greasy hair, and was sloppy and causing problems at school. I made my husband go down to discuss this with the school, and after that she picked up, lost weight, and began to work. Now she does her home assignments before she goes out at night, although she still resents authority.

FATHER: I was really upset about her, but she buckled down until last semester, when she bombed out.

MOTHER: I still think she has come a long way.

FATHER: I'll have to wait and see. I'm afraid she's turning into a queen at home, and we don't have room for queens. Yet, she'll clean the house out on Saturday mornings pretty well, provided you don't look behind the bookshelves.

MOTHER: One night she reported me to the police for child abuse. I was arguing with her, shook her by the shoulders, and she threatened to telephone the police and tell them that I was abusing her. I told her to go ahead and she did. The policeman came over and had a long talk with her.

The psychiatrist asked about past physical illnesses. The parents indicated that, apart from allergies involving nasal congestion caused by sensitivity to pollen, Matthew has been physically healthy. He has no history of surgical operations, accidents, fractures, head injuries, fainting attacks, or seizures. He is not well-coordinated physically and not particularly good at sports.

The psychiatrist then asked the parents about Matthew's early development. He was the fourth pregnancy and unplanned. No contraceptive precautions had been taken, for religious reasons. In the father's words, he was "The Cincinnati Kid," conceived on Friday night, after the father returned from a business trip to Ohio. Mrs. M. initially resented being pregnant, but the pregnancy was uneventful. After the birth of their son, the parents were pleased, particularly the father.

Confinement was at term, and birthweight 8 pounds, 15 ounces. The delivery was normal after a 2-hour labor. Both baby and mother were in good health after delivery.

Matthew was bottle fed. He made good physical progress during the first 2 years. He was a "good" baby: predictable, neither excitable nor sluggish, regular in his cycles, and generally happy in mood. He adapted well to new situations and showed no marked stranger anxiety. In fact, he was much friendlier as an infant and toddler than he is now. He was handled a great deal by the older siblings and treated rather like a doll.

The milestones were normal: He walked before 12 months, and spoke early quite intelligibly. Nowadays, however, he sometimes reverts to babytalk and has to be told, "Knock it off and shape up."

MOTHER: He's really anxious to talk to you so that you can help him with his crying.

FATHER: I think my wife has waited too much on all the kids and that is wrong. I'm happier with my lot than my wife is with hers. After all, I'm on the downhill now, over 40 years of age, and on the short end of life.

MOTHER: Maybe I haven't had my crack at life yet.

Returning to Matthew's development, Mrs. M. said that there were no problems with toilet training aside from a brief period at 18 months, following an attack of gastroenteritis. There has been no enuresis or soiling.

The parents could remember no emotional problems before Matthew went to school. In fact, they had not been concerned about him until about 12 months before. The only fear he had before that time was of heights. The mother remarked that she herself has a fear of heights and probably transmitted it to her son.

The family have lived in the same house since Matthew's birth, and he has attended the same school. He is now in grade 4. His school achievement is adequate, although he has a slight problem with mathematics. He reads a great deal, enjoys encyclopedias, and loves to pore over maps. He has little interest in sports and quit the Cub Scout group "because it was like a bedlam."

He has many friends. Children often come to the house, but Matthew is considered to be rather shy.

To the psychiatrist's questions, the father said he was 50 years of age. He was born in the same suburb of Boston in which his wife lived. Though they both attended the same high school they did not keep company until later.

The paternal grandfather, alive at 85 years, is a retired plumber. Mr. M. is the elder of two siblings. He can remember how, during the depression, the paternal grandfather would go to town in the morning with his lunch and trolley-car money, looking for a day's work. He said that, like himself, his father was a good but hard man who believed in discipline, "very different from parents today." He repeated that he considers his wife is too soft with the children.

In the father's early adolescence, the paternal grandfather contracted empyema. His medical care expended all his family's resources and forced the paternal grandparents to start again from scratch to save money to buy a house.

Mr. M. graduated from business school. He has always been a salesman, starting door-to-door, and moving up through retail selling to managing a territory, first for a steel company, and then for a company that marketed wood products throughout the United States. At the time he left Boston, he was a successful senior salesman.

The mother, aged 48 years, has lost both her parents. She described them as "very happy." She was the middle of three siblings. Her father had also been a salesman.

The parents began to court in their mid-twenties, having been introduced by the father's sister.

FATHER: It's not all bad, but we tear ourselves apart trying to raise a family.

MOTHER: The last 5 years have been too much for me. I feel I've had it with his illness, the pain, and the business problems. (*At this point she began to weep.*) After he had the first operation, I used to refer to it as his "nice-time operation." He was so much more relaxed afterwards. But the pressures have been unreal.

FATHER: We play games. I earn the living and she runs the house. I'm sure if I knew how much it cost to run, I would blow up. But I'm not involved in the day-to-day operation of the house. My job is to put food on the table. Yet winters are a business disaster. My business is good only for 9 months.

MOTHER: I don't love him. It's been gradual, maybe over 5 years.

FATHER: I love Sheila as a person, but we've had no sex life for 5 years. It wasn't a hell of a sex life before because we were Roman Catholic and had too many children.

MOTHER: When Erin was small, by the time she was out of grammar school, I used to think that I would leave him. I can't put my finger on when I stopped loving him. It wasn't because he was unfaithful to me. We've been faithful to each other.

FATHER: I worked too many hours for that.

The parents then began to describe an argument they had recently had about whether the father should buy a new truck, as the mother thought, or whether his old, beat-up vehicle was good enough.

Mr. M. said that he has always been a hard worker. He used work "for escape." He did not understand what had happened to their marriage but thought it began to "fall apart" when he was offered a promotion and took his family to a new suburb without consulting his wife. She has never forgiven him. Mrs. M. agreed that she was still angry about the move because it took her away from her parents and sister; but she thought that the rift between them had been more gradual.

Neither parent had ever seen a doctor or psychiatrist for emotional disorder or tension-related problems. However, Mrs. M. thought that she should have attended somebody 5 or 6 years before, and that Erin should have been seen by somebody.

The interview terminated at this point, the parents indicating that they had explained to Matthew why they wanted him to see the psychiatrist and that Matthew was eager to talk to somebody.

Interviews with the child

Next day, the psychiatrist entered the waiting room and greeted Matthew and his parents. Matthew was a slight, red-headed, freckled boy of average stature. He willingly entered the psychiatrist's office and sat in a comfortable chair. Though quiet at the beginning of the interview, he soon became more animated as he entertained the psychiatrist with imaginative stories. He was verbally fluent and had a good vocabulary, using such phrases as "I feel threatened." He was aware that he had emotional problems but not how they originated.

Matthew began by expressing an interest in the psychiatrist's foreign accent. He described all the foreign people that he knew. He had Irish and Korean friends at school. He attended the fourth grade of the local elementary school.

THERAPIST: Why have you come to see me?

MATTHEW: 'Cause I cry a lot, that's all. When people make fun of me, call me "Hot-hair" and "Carrot top," I get upset. One boy stole two cars from me and I got upset. Sometimes I cry when I do something stupid, like spilling my lunch.

THERAPIST: How do you feel when people call you names?

MATTHEW: Terrible sad and angry. Once during a kickball game, a bully got one of my friends on the ground and hurt him. I gave the bully a bloody nose, but I cried myself. People make more fun of me when I cry. They call me "Cry-baby." I tell the teacher, but that doesn't stop them from teasing me. Usually they are older kids and sometimes kids in groups. Sometimes when I'm sitting at the lunch table, 5 kids will start teasing me.

(*At this point, there was a pause. The therapist waited until the patient began to speak again.*)

MATTHEW: I would like to be a doctor and work on kids like the allergist who sees me. I'm allergic to everything except dogs. I have a machine in my room every night to take the dust out of the air, and sometimes I can't get to sleep.

THERAPIST: What do you think keeps you awake at night?

MATTHEW: I'm scared of the dark. I think of "Close Encounters of the Third Kind." I think of a naked lady with no bosoms, with long arms and 6 fingers. In the movie, they talked of kidnapping, and that could happen to me. If that happened, I would just go "Bye-Bye" in a spaceship.

THERAPIST: What would happen then?

MATTHEW: I would be tortured on a planet, put in a thing like a box with electricity going through it. I bought a UFO comic and saw a scary being in the comic with a long, pointy head and triangular eyes. I think about the beings sometimes, that they could kill me. When I get scared by these things, I put my head under the pillow and under the blankets. I also have bean-bag teddy bears.

THERAPIST: What do you do with the teddy bears?

MATTHEW: I put them on the bed so that the beings will think that the teddy bears are human and take them to the planet instead of me. Sometimes I get out of bed and turn the light on. Sometimes I go in and sleep with Dad.

THERAPIST: You go to sleep with your father?

MATTHEW: I stay with him for about an hour, and he is asleep and doesn't know I'm there.

THERAPIST: Why do you not go in to sleep with your mother?

MATTHEW: Why? Because Mom sleeps downstairs. I'd rather go to Dad's bed because it is warmer, has an electric blanket, and I'm not scared any longer.

THERAPIST: Do you have any dreams?

MATTHEW: Yes. I dream of two girls I'm in love with. Amy and Kathy in my class. Kathy is prettier and Amy is skinnier. Sometimes Kathy kicks me 50 times hard before I step on her foot. Amy was in my class last year. Her Uncle Joe is a race car driver and I can get his autograph. His cousin John is one of the ones who picks on me.

(*There is a pause*)

THERAPIST: Do you have any unhappy dreams?

MATTHEW: No, I just have happy dreams, just their faces and they disappear when I'm afraid.

THERAPIST: What would you like to be when you grow up?

MATTHEW: I'd like to be a children's or an animal doctor. I wouldn't want to be a surgeon because I might make a mistake.

THERAPIST: You worry about accidents?

MATTHEW: Yes. I saw three car accidents, and in one a guy almost died. I trip a lot and sprained my heel and ankle, and once I fell off a horse. I sometimes worry that something bad will happen. This year I wanted straight A's at school, but I got an A and some B's, a C and a D and felt terrible.

THERAPIST: Do you find any of your subjects difficult?

MATTHEW: Reading is difficult, and this year I had only 10 100's and only 5 smiling faces in my book. I am the second worst reader in my reading group.

THERAPIST: Your mother tells me how much you like to read maps and encyclopedias.

MATTHEW: Yes, I like to look up foreign countries and states. And I like to know all the states in the United States.

THERAPIST: If you took an airplane from here to Texas, what states would you fly over?

MATTHEW: New York, West Virginia, Pennsylvania, Kentucky, Missouri,

Kansas, Texas. I think I missed Illinois. I like looking at atlases and pictures, and finding out where things are.

THERAPIST: If you could make three wishes and the wishes would come true, what wishes would you make?

MATTHEW: I would like to be a doctor. I would like to have all the atlases in the world. And I would like to not be made fun of any more. It really hurts because I have too much feelings.

THERAPIST: Do you know where the feelings come from?

MATTHEW: No.

THERAPIST: Do you have other worries?

MATTHEW: Yes, when I fall off a skateboard.

THERAPIST: How are things at home for you?

MATTHEW: Fine.

THERAPIST: Are you happy there?

MATTHEW: Yes.

THERAPIST: Do you get along with your family?

MATTHEW: I don't get along with Erin. I hide the cigarettes from her because I want to trick her and stop her from smoking. She has a cigarette habit. I have a lot of arguments with Erin.

THERAPIST: What do you argue about?

MATTHEW: Crying. She says "You're the biggest baby in the whole world;" and I go ahead and try to kill her. I throw the teddy bears around the room when I'm angry.

THERAPIST: When do you get the most angry?

MATTHEW: When Erin makes fun of me. Sometimes when Mom tries to kiss me. I don't like that mushy stuff. Mom tries to kiss me too much and I feel threatened. I feel it's a gun in her mouth and that it's dangerous to get kissed.

THERAPIST: Are they loving kisses?

MATTHEW: They're loving kisses but dangerous.

THERAPIST: How do you get along with your Dad?

MATTHEW: Pretty good. We're good friends sometimes. Sometimes he and I go for drives together.

THERAPIST: How do your Mom and Dad get on together?

MATTHEW: They're good friends, but they have disagreements about the kids. Dad is the punisher and the bad guy and Mom is the good guy.

THERAPIST: Do Mom and Dad ever have fights together?

MATTHEW: Yes; sometimes I think they might get divorced.

THERAPIST: What would happen then?

MATTHEW: I would have to go to a foster home. I wouldn't like that. But I don't think they will really break up. If they did break up, Dad would take the two sons and Mom would get the girls.

THERAPIST: What do you do when they fight?

MATTHEW: I would like to say, "Stop fighting." I haven't really said it, but I'd like to. I would like to make a come-back at them and yell at them. I get angry at them, but I get scared that if I'm angry I'll just get "pow-pow-pow" from them.

THERAPIST: What's the biggest worry you have apart from crying and being scared?

MATTHEW: Just tripping, nothing else. Mostly my problems and sometimes the family problems.

THERAPIST: I've enjoyed talking to you, Matthew. I think I understand some of your problems a lot better now. You are very good at describing the things that worry you. Maybe there's a connection between the things you've told me about.

MATTHEW: I like talking to you. I think it helped.

THERAPIST: I want to have a talk with your Mom and Dad and then we will work out a time when you can come back to see me again.

MATTHEW: Would you like to hear three jokes?

THERAPIST: Yes.

MATTHEW: Once upon a time there was a papa bull who ate three bales of hay, a baby bull who ate one bale of hay, and a mama bull. How much did the mama bull eat?

THERAPIST: I don't know.

MATTHEW: Nothing, because there's no such thing as a mama bull. If the wind is blowing from west to east, which way would the peanuts fall off the peanut tree?

THERAPIST: Towards the east.

MATTHEW: Wrong. There is no such thing as a peanut tree. A man had three wishes, and genie said that she would give him his wishes. He wished for a car, and suddenly a car appeared. He wished for a million dollars, and a million dollars appeared. He was driving around in the car with a million dollars in his pocket, and he began to sing, "I wish I were an Oscar Meyer Wiener," and he got turned into a wiener.

The interview terminated at this point.

One week later, Matthew and his parents returned to the clinic. Matthew was greeted in the waiting room and entered the psychiatrist's office cheerfully. He brought with him, as a gift, a folder of drawings. The psychiatrist thanked the child for the gift, perused the drawings briefly, and said he looked forward to seeing them later, in more detail.

At the clinician's request, Matthew drew a person. He produced a figure with large round head, short black hair, rudimentary eyes, a nose, and smiling mouth. The body was oval in shape. Legs and arms protruded stiffly but symmetrically from the body. There were three stubby fingers on each hand. Collar-, sleeve-, and trouser-lines were marked on the neck and limbs. On the front of the chest, Matthew wrote ZAP! (reversing the Z), with parallel jagged inclined lines above the exclamation.

Asked to tell a story about the figure, Matthew recounted the following tale:

"He is pretend . . . . He almost got blind. He thought his wall was a door. He went through his magic wall to the Land of the Animals. It cleared his seeing. He stayed with the bear family. Behind the woods there was a big monster that came out when it was dark and went, "ZAP!" His voice stuck on the kid's stomach . . . on his shirt . . . the roar came out first. It didn't go on at first. His favorite show at home was "Zapman." He went "Zap" on his shirt . . . the kid went through the wall again. Then he was blind . . . real handicapped. He was deaf before."

Matthew then drew a picture of a dinosaur, its large body and flipper under the ocean, and its neck, head, yellow eyes, and teeth protruding above the waves. From its mouth, large purple drops are falling. Ahead of the monster is a diminutive man in a boat. The man holds a pistol, which is discharging in the direction of the monster.

"Zapman was in the boat. The Zapmonster came ashore to trick Zapman. Zapman took the Zapmonster out to the ocean. But Zapmonster surprises Zapman; he goes down and comes up. But Zapman had his Zapbelt and shot Zapmonster with bullets. The monster bled purple blood."

Matthew was asked to draw "something nice" and "something nasty." For the first, he drew a flower. For the second he drew a set of buttocks from which feces were falling, saying:

"It's nasty. Poop in the water. It pees on the target and uses poops for a large bomb."

Matthew and the psychiatrist then played "Squiggles" together. To demonstrate the game, the psychiatrist first drew a frightened face, in profile, entitled "Boy Scared of Alien Creature." Matthew, in turn, drew a four-legged creature behind bars, entitled "A Zoo." The psychiatrist drew "A Bandy Eagle." Matthew laughed and replied with "A Boney Camel" (reversing the "B"). The psychiatrist drew "Two Ghosts," and Matthew drew "A Duck Man Rabbit."

At the end of the interview, the psychiatrist met the parents briefly. The father said: "Matthew is making the most out of this. He began to stutter at school, but it was an act. He told his mother he should go to the eye doctor because sometimes the letters are blurry. I asked him 'When?' and he said 'Just before I cry.' He still gets out of bed during the night, but not because he is frightened."

Mrs. M. added: "I'm as tense as a drum. He's been crying at home more than ever. He's hard to wake. When I try to get him up he says: 'Don't yell at me. There are different yells. That's an angry yell.'"

After the interview terminated, the clinician examined the contents of the folder that Matthew had prepared for him. In it, stapled together, were six cartoon-like adventure stories signed by the author, each about five numbered pages long. The stories were entitled as follows:

"A Tweetle Bettle Adventure," "The Tweetle Bettle Battle," "Tweetle Bettles have Battles over Water," "Tweetle Bettles have Battles Underwater," "Tweetle Bettles have Battles in the Air," and "Tweetle Bettles in Space."

These cartoon-stories depicted black bugs escaping in boats from dinosaurs, engaging in aerial dogfights, firing cannons and rockets at each other, manning submarines, launching a spacecraft, and arriving at a celestial body with a cratered surface.

Child Mental Status Examination

Matthew presented as a physically attractive child of average stature, with red hair and freckles. He manifested no hyperactivity, no abnormality of gross or fine movement, and no motor habits. His speech was normal in articulation, rhythm, pitch, and tone.

He made excellent eye contact with the interviewer, was highly communicative, even loquacious, and demonstrated friendliness, warmth, and a sense of fun. He was emotionally very responsive and showed no dysphoria, anger, anxiety, or fear.

His attention span was normal. He manifested no distractibility and no disturbance of sensorium, abnormal thought process, or abnormal language. His vocabulary was somewhat advanced for his age. His comprehension and verbal expression appeared to be at least average.

He did reveal abnormality of thought content. Magical thinking abounded, involving alien "beings," obsessive-compulsive rituals with teddy bears, "Zapman," "Zapmonster," and the "Tweetle Bettles." However, he had no illusions, hallucinations, delusions, or ideas of reference. Salient themes in the content of his thought included anxiety, fear, loss, abandonment, helplessness, the threat of physical attack, and physical injury. His fantasy was productive and original, even bizarre; but its elements were well integrated. He was able to differentiate fantasy from reality (except perhaps at night). Aware that he had emotional problems, he wanted and appreciated psychological help. ■

The diagnostic net

Sufficient information has been obtained to complete a diagnostic net (see Table 26.1).

The diagnostic formulation

Biopsychosocial axis

Physical

Normal physical health and development

Matthew is a 9-year-old child who is in good physical health (aside from allergic tendencies). His physical development is within normal limits for his age. He has no neuroendocrine or central nervous abnormalities aside from an alleged clumsiness not apparent on gross examination.

Psychological

Normal information processing

His capacity for information processing (attention, concentration, perception, reasoning, and judgment) and communication are clinically normal. His creativity and expressive language are above average for his age.

Disturbance in images, emotions and attitudes

Matthew has multiform fears of loss of, abandonment by, and abduction from his parents, particularly his father. He fears helplessness and physical injury if abandoned. Even though he dreads a catastrophic separation from both

TABLE 26.1
Diagnostic net: Case 26.1: Matthew

	Predisposition	Precipitation	Perpetuation	Pattern
Physical	Allergies	? Cumulative stress		Allergies "Clumsy"
Psychological	Last-born child Rivalry with sister Fear of separation		Senses mother's anger at father Aware of possibility of parental separation Worries about father's health	Separation anxiety Fears abandonment Fears injury Depressed Anger at mother Fears loss of father Rivalry with sister Poor self-esteem Clinging Weeping Attention-seeking Fearful Perfectionistic Often teased Irritable Argumentative Sulking Obsessive rituals
Social	Oldest two siblings have left home Sister jealous of him Parents estranged Father in chronic pain Mother babies him		Parental arguments Parental estrangement Father's pain Mother's preoccupation Hostility from father to sister	Mother very concerned Father wants to ignore his symptoms Sister teases him

Family problems →

Treatment for allergies

parents, he harbors conscious anger and resentment toward his mother. He has deficient control over his anger, depression, and fear. His moral development seems relatively immature, and he does not seem to experience guilt as much as shame and a lowering of self-esteem.

Behavioral

Maladaptive coping

He displays a mixture of coping styles involving dependency (clinging, fear of school, immature behavior), manipulativeness (demanding, argumentative, stubborn, disobedient, screaming, sulking, whining), dysphoria (weeping, loneliness, feeling rejected and inferior, self-consciousness, fearfulness, depression), and withdrawal (likes to be alone, poor concentration, daydreaming, poor schoolwork, secretive, withdrawn, worrying).

Social

Parental dissension and family tension

His parents are emotionally estranged. The tension between them explodes from time to time in arguments and threats of divorce. The father is almost totally involved in keeping his marginal business solvent. This and his chronic arthritic pain have left him grimly overcontrolled. The mother resents the lack of satisfaction in her life and is often preoccupied with thoughts of leaving the father. An older sister has a strained relationship with the father and a mutually rivalrous relationship with Matthew.

Temporal axis

Predisposing and perpetuating factors in family environment

There were no clear predisposing factors aside from Matthew's having been an unplanned child, the last born to middle-aged parents whose marriage was already strained. There were no acute precipitating factors, aside from the cumulative effect of family tension and the departure of protective older siblings, who may have ameliorated the tension between the parents. The current pattern of his emotional disorder is perpetuated by interparental tension, paternal absence and illness, maternal overprotection and preoccupation, and his sister's rivalry with him.

Developmental axis

Physically and intellectually, Matthew is developing normally; in fact, his language development is advanced for his age.

Unresolved conflicts

Psychosocially, he is still struggling with the psychological tasks of early childhood: trust, autonomy, self-control, mastery, and initiative. Consequently, he is unable to cope with the emotional demands of school for persistence and industry and of the peer group for the control of aggression. His ability to do so is impeded by unresolved conflicts of oral, anal, and oedipal nature.

The dynamic interaction of the biopsychosocial pattern and perpetuating factors is depicted in the flowchart in Figure 26.1.

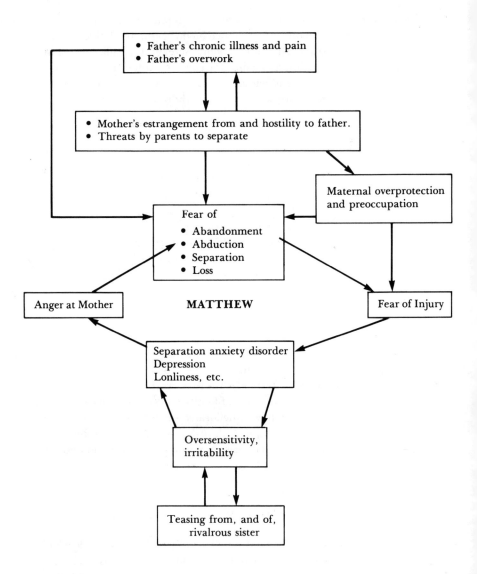

FIGURE 26.1
Flowchart: Case 26.1: Matthew

The management plan

Categorical diagnosis

It can be readily seen that no diagnostic label could capture this network of interactions. Nevertheless, to provide a diagnostic title for the records, Separation Anxiety Disorder of Childhood would suffice.

The flowchart in Figure 26.1 can now be used to generate a set of problem issues that can be restated as goals for a treatment program. Referring to the flowchart, the following pivotal problems emerge:

Pivotal problems

1. Paternal absence and preoccupation due to pain and overwork.
2. Maternal estrangement from and hostility to father.
3. Maternal overprotection.
4. Matthew's separation anxiety from both parents and his anger at mother.
5. Sister's hostile, rivalrous relationship.

Problems 1, 2, and 3 are clearly interrelated and in turn interact with problem 4. Problem 5 is subsidiary. How can these problems be rewritten as goals?

Goals

Goal 1. Encourage father to spend more relaxed time with Matthew.
Goal 2. Help parents to reduce their emotional distance and tension.
Goal 3. Reduce maternal hostility to father and her preoccupation (?depression) leading to overprotection of and manipulation by the patient.
Goal 4. Reduce Matthew's separation anxiety, associated fears, and depression related to his conflicts around the parental figures.
Goal 5. Reduce Erin's hostile interaction with Matthew.

None of these goals is urgent. Goals 1–4 are equivalent in priority and of intermediate status.

Management

A convenient approach to all goals would be to treat parents, Erin, and Matthew in conjoint family therapy. In favor of such an approach would be its relative economy of effort, time, and expense. Against it, might be the severity of the interparental tension and the possibility that this would dominate therapy and distract attention from Matthew's disturbance.

Another approach would be as follows:

Goal 1. Paternal psychological absence.
Goal 2. Maternal hostility to father.
Goal 3. Maternal overprotection.
Therapy: 1. Marital counseling
2. With some individual counseling sessions with each parent.
Frequency: Once per week.
Duration: 3 to 6 months.

There is a possibility that counseling could catalyze actual parental separation. Even if this occurred, provided the parents separated after due consideration of all the issues involved, and provided Matthew were adequately prepared for it, the outcome might be preferable to an irreconcilable domestic climate of frigidity, emotional divorce, and impending disaster. The marital counseling should be conducted in parallel with individual help to Matthew.

> Goal 4. Reduce Matthew's separation anxiety.
> Therapy: Individual expressive psychotherapy.
> Frequency: Once per week.
> Duration: 6 months.
> Goal 5. Reduce hostile interaction between Erin and Matthew.
> Therapy: Unclear. This matter could be dealt with during marital therapy. It might be necessary to invite Erin to join a parental counseling session. On the other hand, Erin's problems, particularly her hostility to her father, might be so serious as to indicate the need for individual therapy.

If both marital therapy and individual therapy were to be recommended, it would be preferable for separate therapists to conduct each mode of intervention. This would help diffuse questions of trust and confidentiality that would be likely in Matthew's therapy. Ultimately, conjoint family therapy might be indicated. Alternatively, intermittent family conferences involving the parents, children, and both therapists could be arranged.

Evaluation   How will the therapeutic team know when the goals of therapy have been attained?

Goal 1. Counteract parental absence.
Goal 2. Alleviate maternal hostility.
Goal 3. Reduce maternal overprotection.

These three goals could best be evaluated by the parents themselves, who should determine their own marital goals during counseling.

Goal 4 (alleviate separation anxiety) could be evaluated by readministering the parental Child Behavior Checklist at three-month intervals and by obtaining parallel information from the child's teachers.

Negotiation

Negotiation   Before therapy begins, the clinician responsible for diagnosis should meet with Matthew and his parents and outline for them the diagnostic formulation. The family will then have the opportunity to question and modify the diagnosis. The management plan can then be introduced and the family can consider it. Questions of time, cost, and convenience can be discussed. If the first plan is not possible (e.g., for reasons of expense), a modified form of treatment may be feasible. The main purposes of this phase of the clinical process, negotiation, are to give the family an opportunity to influence diagnosis and planning and to establish an informal contract involving an agreement on the nature of the problems and the goals, methods, expense, and estimated duration of treatment.

Summary

This chapter applies the concepts discussed in chapters 13, 14, and 15 to diagnosis and planning in child psychiatry. Note that the developmental axis has assumed great importance. It is also apparent that the social level of biopsychosocial axis is crucial in childhood and adolescence, due to the intense, continuous interaction among child, family, peers, and school. Temporal diagnosis is no less relevant; predisposing, precipitating, and perpetuating factors are all involved in the current pattern of biopsychosocial responses.

The diagnostic net and flowchart aid management planning. In child psychiatry, management goals virtually always need to address problems in the family system as well as in the child's functioning. The clear statement of physical, cognitive-educational, psychological, or sociofamilial goals enables the clinician to choose among alternative therapies, to nominate and determine a means of evaluating outcome, and to estimate the time required to reach each goal.

PART VI

A review of research into clinical reasoning

prepared by
Barry Nurcombe and Ina Fitzhenry-Coor

27

Clinical reasoning in
psychiatry: research
and education

Introduction

How do clinicians think? How do they discern the distinctive features of a case,
consolidate the features in a pattern, and reach accurate conclusions? Can students be taught to do so? This chapter reviews research into medical reasoning
and describes a series of studies in psychiatric reasoning carried out at the
University of Vermont. The chapter also describes a teaching program, The
Diagnostic Process, that was involved in several of these studies.

The study of expert reasoning, particularly medical reasoning, is complicated by a number of explicit controversies and implicit tensions:

1. Intuition versus systematization.
2. Clinical reason versus actuarial formula.
3. Description versus prescription.
4. Man versus computer.

Controversies between the clinical and statistical approaches to diagnosis

The diagnostician has been regarded on the one hand as dynamic, and sophisticated, and on the other as hazy, subjective and unscientific. Proponents of the statistical approach to clinical decision-making regard human reason as limited and fallible and point to many studies demonstrating the superiority of machine algorithms to human rationality (Meehl, 1954, 1974). The inflammatory polemics that have arisen provoke denial, counterattack, or disregard. The following comment from a textbook on bedside diagnosis (DeGowin & DeGowin, 1976), illustrates the dismissive approach: "Statistical methods can only be applied to a population of thousands. The individual either has a rare disease or doesn't have it; the relative incidence of two diseases is completely irrelevant to the problem of making the diagnosis" (p. 7). Others (e.g., Holt, 1958; Elstein, 1976; Blois, 1980) recommend a more balanced conclusion, which is elaborated later in this chapter.

The mystique of diagnostic reasoning

Clinicians have great respect for the power of reason. They are proud of their theoretical knowledge and clinical acumen and remember with pleasure past diagnostic masterstrokes. So mercurial and rapid is clinical intuition, they think, that it can never be directly understood or taught. Indeed, excessive scrutiny might render it self-conscious and faltering. Leave it alone, they say; let physicians acquire it in their own way, as they always have.

Fear of the machine

Meanwhile, looming behind the intuitive thinker is the spectre of the machine advancing with inexorable logic to annex medicine and relegate the physician to a subsidiary role in the clinical enterprise. How realistic is this fantasy? Will computers replace the physician? Could machine logic supplant human judgment? Can clinical reasoning be analyzed and taught? These are the central issues of this chapter.

Research into medical decision-making

In extensive reviews of the field, Elstein and Bordage (1979) and Shulman and Elstein (1975) define three research enterprises in clinical decision-making:

1. Clinical judgment.
2. Decision theory.
3. Information processing.

Three theories of clinical reasoning

Clinical judgment research attempts to identify the criteria a clinician uses in reaching a specific conclusion and to determine the proportionate weight accorded each criterion. In **decision-making** theory, the clinician is viewed as one called on to make probabilistic decisions when relevant information is incomplete. The unreliability of human reason in these circumstances is analyzed. **Information processing** traces the natural route of clinical reasoning by analyzing its progressive elements.

Prescription vs. description

The first two approaches are prescriptive; they propose to supplant (or at least supplement) human reasoning with machine algorithms. The third is descriptive; it attempts to analyze clinical reasoning, improve the natural process, and accelerate its acquisition.

Clinical judgment

The lens model

Figure 27.1 illustrates the theoretical model (Hammond, 1955) derived from Brunswik's (1955) concept of a determinative lens. A patient, let us say, presents a number of symptoms and signs the clinician selects as criteria. These criteria are weighed and combined to reach a judgment (for example, a diagnostic conclusion, outcome, prediction, or management decision). One example would be the way in which a clinician combines clinical features in a case of attempted suicide (e.g., past history of suicide, presence or absence of major depression, the nature of the recent attempt, and the quality of emotional support available) to judge the risk of further self-induced injury. Researchers attempt to capture the policy of an expert by determining the relative importance of each criterion the expert uses. The mathematical model can then be used in a computer program that combines data like an expert but with cast-iron reliability.

Capturing an expert's policy

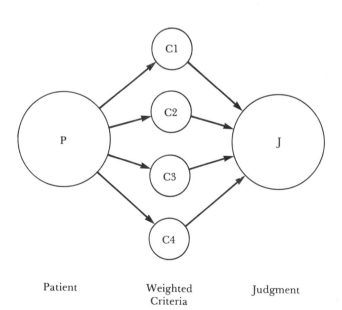

Patient   Weighted   Judgment
                 Criteria

FIGURE 27.1
The lens model of clinical judgment

Decision theory

Risky and probabilistic decision-making

Medicine is risky. Decisions about diagnosis or management must often be made before all relevant information is available. Medicine is also probabilistic. The clinician must infer diagnosis from data (symptoms, signs, laboratory findings, X-rays, psychological tests, etc.) that are subject to varying degrees of error since they are conceptually distant from the pathological structures or functions at the heart of medical problems. In this sense, no branch of medicine is more risky or probabilistic than psychiatry.

Bayes' theorem

To be an efficient decision-maker, it is suggested, the physician should be thoroughly steeped in Bayes' theorem. Bayes' theorem relates:

1. The probability that a disease is present, given a finding or set of findings, $P\left(\dfrac{D}{F}\right)$, to

2. the probability of the finding in that disease, $P\left(\dfrac{F}{D}\right)$,

3. the base-rates of the disease, PD, and

4. the base-rate of the finding, PF, in a specified population.

$$P\left(\frac{D}{F}\right) = \frac{P\left(\dfrac{F}{D}\right) \times PD}{PF}$$

$$\begin{array}{c} \text{The probability of a} \\ \text{disease given a finding} \end{array} = \frac{\begin{array}{c}\text{The probability of that} \\ \text{finding given the disease}\end{array} \times \begin{array}{c}\text{The probability} \\ \text{of the disease*}\end{array}}{\text{The probability of the finding*}}$$

(*in a specified population)

A variation of Bayes' theorem allows the medical gambler to calculate the odds involved in distinguishing between two diseases. (D_1, D_2) when a test could be positive $(T+)$ in either disease but is more likely to be positive in one (D_1) than the other (D_2):

$$P\left(\frac{D_1}{T+}\right) = \frac{P\left(\dfrac{T+}{D_1}\right) \times PD_1}{\left\{P\left(\dfrac{T+}{D_1}\right) \times PD_1\right\} + \left\{P\left(\dfrac{T+}{D_2}\right) \times PD_2\right\}}$$

Assume that the dexamethasone suppression test (DST) is positive in 70% of cases of melancholia and positive in 5% of all psychiatric cases admitted to the hospital that are not diagnosed as melancholia. Assume it is known that 5% of admissions to an inpatient unit suffer from melancholia, and that 95% do not. What is the likelihood that a diagnosis of melancholia is correct if the DST is positive? According to Bayes' theorem,

$$P\left(\frac{D_1}{T+}\right) = \frac{.70 \times .05}{(.70 \times .05) + (.05 \times .95)}$$

$$= \frac{.035}{.035 + .045}$$

$$= .44$$

In other words, the odds are less than 50–50 that the diagnosis of melancholia is correct.

Erroneous reasoning caused by lack of knowledge of base rates

Medicine is seldom taught in these terms. The intuitive diagnostician gauges $P\left(\frac{F}{D}\right)$ from theoretical knowledge and clinical experience with patients who have that disorder. Strictly speaking, $P\left(\frac{F}{D}\right)$ should then be combined with local base-rates for (1) the disease and (2) that set of findings. Systematic errors are likely to creep into the subjective estimation of and allowance for base rates (Tversky & Kahneman, 1974, 1981; Kahneman, Slovic & Tversky, 1982; Arkes, 1981). Examples of erroneous thinking are as follows:

Representativeness

1. If a set of clinical features resembles a textbook disease syndrome, clinicians tend to overestimate the probability that the disease is present, without adequately taking base rates $\left(P\left(\frac{D}{F}\right) \text{ and } P\left(\frac{F}{D}\right)\right)$ into account.

Subjective base rates

2. In medicine generally and in psychiatry in particular, there is a dearth of knowledge about base rates. Clinicians must fall back on subjective estimates that are often erroneous. Furthermore, they are likely to be overconfident in the reliability of their subjective estimates.

Salience

3. Clinicians tend to overestimate base rate (*PD*) as a result of previous salient experiences; for example, an encounter with a recent, an exotic, or a serious case. Serious diseases also are likely to be overdiagnosed, for obvious reasons.

Conservatism

4. Clinicians are conservative thinkers. They are slow to correct subjective base-rates in the light of new information. They have particular difficulty incorporating negative evidence and evidence available late in the diagnostic process (Edwards, 1968).

Therapeutic fads

5. Clinical experience cannot control for the placebo effect. Clinicians are liable to be overconfident in the efficacy of favorite treatment techniques that have not been scientifically evaluated.

The utility and value of treatment

6. In evaluating the desirability of an outcome, clinicians have difficulty separating utility and value. There is a trade off, for example, between longevity and quality of life. One patient may be prepared to accept a greater surgical risk in the hope of more mobility; another may not.

The framing of options

7. The way in which problems are framed influences the attractiveness of options. Losses loom larger than gains.

Stereotypical bias

8. Preconceptions, particularly stereotypical ones (see chapter 5), bias the recall of information and the collection of new evidence.

Premature closure

9. Early preference for a diagnosis impedes the collection or consideration of evidence that might invalidate it.

Hindsight bias

10. Hindsight is easier than foresight. It is easier after the event than before to find predictive evidence for an outcome.

Machines lack common sense

This catalog of errors refers us to an earlier question. Will the computer supplant clinical judgment? Blois (1980) has reviewed the dispute between clinicians and actuaries. He concludes that when identified data must be weighted and combined to reach a reliable decision, the machine is superior. However, Blois goes on to say that machines are dumb and restricted to specified microworlds. Even if we could program one to deal with the two million or so interlocking facts in medicine, we still could not instruct it to use common sense to elicit and sift salient clues from a patient. The idea that the semantic world can be reduced to elementary facts leads to an infinite regress. The technical problems of merging programmed microworlds, even those of elementary nature, have proven insuperable.

The potentially complementary roles of clinician and machine

Automated history formats, even those using branching logic, provide information that must be sifted, validated, and combined with other clinical information in order to form the clusters of clues and inferences that are the grist of hypothesis generation. The clinician is indispensable at the outset of the clinical process, when the world must be confronted; clues elicited, sifted, and validated; inferences drawn; and clusters assembled. At the end of diagnosis and planning, if a problem can be stated in formal terms, a machine may be more efficient. The clinician discerns; the machine computes.

The next section examines the process of clinical discernment.

Information processing

Using experts from different fields that require complex problem-solving, cognitive psychologists have attempted to analyze the steps involved in human reasoning. Among those who have been studied are chess players (DeGroot, 1965), physicists (Larkin et al., 1980), neurologists (Kleinmuntz, 1969), family practitioners (Feightner et al., 1975), and internists and medical students (Elstein, Shulman, & Sprafka, 1978).

The steps of sequential reasoning

Much of this research has been inspired by the pioneering work of Bruner, Goodnow, and Austin (1956) and Newell and Simon (1961). Typically, subjects are requested to describe the progressive stages of their thinking about a problem. From these accounts of sequential cognitive tactics, the psychologist generalizes about the elements and steps involved. An attempt is sometimes made to validate the model by designing a computer program that simulates the problem solver.

Pattern storage
and retrieval

A chess grand master, for example, has an experiential memory of perhaps 50,000 board patterns. Using experience and the capacity to conserve short-term memory by chunking perceptual clues, the grand master can reproduce nonrandom 25-piece board configurations with near-perfect accuracy. If the disposition of pieces on the board is random, the master's recall drops to that of a novice. The retrieval of patterns from long-term memory gives the chess master access to strategic options based on predictions about the future course of the game.

List structures

Memory is indexed by the patterns stored therein, and each pattern is associated with an action or set of possible actions. Memory patterns have been likened to list structures, that is, to organizations of nodes (items and their components) connected by links (the relations between items and their components) (Larkin et al., 1980). A clinical syndrome, for example, might be stored as a memory structure; that is, as a set of clinical features linked by temporal, spatial, and causal relations. The memory of the syndrome is also connected to tactics for eliciting, discerning, evaluating, and assembling missing elements of the structure and, subsequently, to therapeutic options.

Tracing the process of medical reasoning

Bounded rationality

Elstein and Bordage (1979) characterize clinical reasoning as a species of rationality (Newell & Simon, 1972) ''bounded'' by the absolute limits of working memory. To cope with these constraints, a clinician transforms an **open problem** (one with no clear end-point) into a number of **closed problems** (each with an end point), by generating diagnostic hypotheses (Bartlett, 1958). Data are then elicited and processed according to the hypotheses generated.

The lack of a
formal system for
diagnostic reasoning

Feinstein (1967, 1973a, 1973b, 1974) maintains that clinical medicine lacks a formal system for diagnosis. Diagnosis, he contends, proceeds from eliciting and designating the manifestations of disease to identifying disease entities; that is, from effect to cause. He describes three levels of reasoning in the diagnostic process:

Three levels of
diagnostic reasoning

1. Symptoms and signs.
2. Simple or multiple clusters of symptoms and signs.
3. Underlying structural abnormality.

Feinstein can find few criteria for reasoning at any of the three levels.

Feinstein considers that diagnosis is not an end in itself but rather the means to an end, and that interrelated causal explanations are more pertinent to management planning than are categorical tags. Consequently, the logic of diagnostic thinking should involve graduated decisions on a pathway to management. Feinstein recommends the following decision path:

The sequential logic of diagnostic decision-making

1. Perceive salient data.
2. Verify salient data.
3. Designate data as symptoms and signs.
4. Decide whether designated data are significantly deviant from the normal range.
5. Select data pertinent to diagnosis.
6. Assemble a list of pertinent manifestations for formal reasoning.
7. Refer manifestations to a clinical domain and to a disorder in the domain by generating the array of domain/disorder candidates that best explain the clinical manifestations.

The schema seems plausible, but does it correspond to the actual thinking of experienced clinicians?

Support for Feinstein's concept of graduated decision-making has come from work at Michigan State University (Elstein, Shulman, & Sprafka, 1978). The Michigan group studied experienced physicians and medical students who were presented with a number of cases in the form of simulated patients and patient management problems. From the responses of their subjects, Elstein and coworkers identified three units of analysis that made clinical sense and were compatible with generic research in information process-tracing: cues, hypotheses, and information search units.

It was found that clinicians elicit salient cues from the patient. These cues are combined so as to delineate a clinical problem; for example:

> This is an ill-looking, sallow, unmarried woman with a low fever who complains of back pain, rigors, and night sweating.

Clinical problems are then resolved through a process of hypothesis generation and verification.

Hypothetico-deductive reasoning in the diagnostic process

Hypotheses are generated early in the interview, when only a limited data base has been acquired. Each diagnostic candidate is tested during the inquiry process by collecting evidence from discretionary and routine history, physical examination, and special investigations. Thus, the clinician can revise, delete, or add to the hypothetical array if indicated, and reach a conclusion about the most likely diagnosis. The eventual decision is reached according to which hypothesis yields the maximum number of positive evidential cues or which shows the maximum difference between positive and negative evidence.

Limited capacity for hypotheses

Due to the limitations of short-term memory, the number of hypotheses considered at any time rarely exceeds five. Depending on the content of the problems, initial hypotheses may be general and move gradually toward specificity; at other times, they consist, from the outset, of an array of specific alternatives.

Pattern recognition

From a cognitive standpoint, medical problem-solving is a series of operations involving pattern recognition, probability estimation, and decision making. The generation of hypotheses is analogous to the retrieval of files via an index. An incomplete pattern is associated with a number of possible complete syndromes. The hypothetical complete patterns are retrieved from long-term memory, presumably by association with key features in a configuration. The subsequent inquiry process aims to collect evidence that will complete (or not complete) the hypothetical patterns. Thus, the array of hypotheses acts as a problem space that organizes the gathering of further information in order to cull and refine the array of hypotheses. The capacity to interpret evidence and evaluate hypotheses is stored in memory until needed. It depends on general cognitive ability and specific experience with the class of problems to which the problem at hand belongs.

The array of hypotheses forms a problem space

The specificity of medical reasoning

Elstein, Shulman, and Sprafka found little individual consistency across problems. In other words, a clinician's experience with the problem appeared to have the greatest influence on the style of reasoning used. If familiar with a particular kind of problem, the clinician functioned in a sophisticated manner; if unfamiliar, less efficient methods of reasoning might appear. Subsidiary experiments demonstrated that sophomore medical students could be trained to generate hypotheses early in their contact with patients (Allal, 1973). However, instructors found it difficult to provide subjects with well-timed, constructive feedback.

Early hypothesis generation

Support for the Michigan State research is available from parallel studies at McMaster University by Feightner et al. (1975) and Barrows (1979), who originally used simulated patients for research and evaluation. These workers showed that family practitioners and internists were comparable. Both types of clinician generated an initial hypothesis less than 1 minute after first contact with a patient. The average number of hypotheses was six. All hypotheses emerged by 5 minutes. Routine questioning and physical examination were used in order to rule out remote possibilities, buy time, and scan for further information, particularly when hypothesis-related inquiry had reached a dead end. More than half the relevant information was collected before the first quarter of the interview had passed.

Inefficient styles of reasoning

Barrows (1979) has described a number of problem-solving "pathologies" associated with novice clinicians. "Eureka" is characterized by spot diagnosis with premature closure and failure to consider later evidence one way or the other. "Buckshot" scatters a wild profusion of unsystematic inquiries. "Basket" pursues the search in an unfocused, interminable, no-stone-unturned manner, waiting for something to appear. "One-at-a-time" juggles only a single hypothesis, pursues it to the end, and starts again if it must be discarded. "Cookbook" has a mania for algorithms and works mechanically down a predetermined sequence of binary choices. "Disengaged" generates hypotheses but the inquiry process is uncoordinated. "Disease-of-the week," a variant of "Eureka," finds evidence for a vogue diagnosis in every patient until a new exotic diagnosis captures the imagination.

Tracing the process of psychiatric reasoning

Research into psychi-
atric reasoning

Relatively little research has been ventured in the process of psychiatric diagnosis and none in psychiatric management planning. The best known investigation in this field, by Gauron and Dickinson (1965), studied clinicians of different levels of experience, using standard case files as diagnostic problems. Subjects could request further information from a variety of sources (e.g., reason for referral, mental status, laboratory findings). After each request, the subject's rationale was investigated. Gauron and Dickinson uncovered a number of cognitive styles, such as hypothetico-deductive logic, premature closure, indecisiveness, lack of selectivity, and disorganization. Some of these styles are comparable to the pathologies referred to by Barrows (1979). However, this study was based on nonnaturalistic problems (case files rather than actual patients) and depended on impressionistic (rather than empirically derived) conclusions. Other studies of psychiatric diagnosis (Kendell, 1973; Sandifer, Hordern, and Green, 1970) are consistent with the hypothetico-deductive nature of clinical reasoning in psychiatry.

Diagnostic process research at the University of Vermont

The logical system suggested by Feinstein (1974), Elstein, Shulman, and Sprafka (1978), and Barrows (1979) has guided initial research into diagnostic reasoning at the University of Vermont (Nurcombe & Fitzhenry-Coor, 1982; Fitzhenry-Coor & Nurcombe, 1983). To provide material for inductive analysis, we investigated the reasoning of different health professionals with varying levels of experience: medical students, social work students, psychiatry and family practice residents, and experienced psychiatrists, psychologists, and social workers. Thus, we hoped to determine:

1. Whether experienced clinicians, regardless of discipline, used similar diagnostic tactics.
2. Whether experienced clinicians used more sophisticated and efficient diagnostic tactics than did students and residents.

To do so, we used two investigative techniques:

1. Printed narrative case problems.
2. Videotaped case problems.

Printed narrative case problems

Segmentation

Narrative cases provide a written account of the initial diagnostic encounter between the psychiatrist and a patient. Preliminary information is fully reported and followed by a transcript of the dialogue between patient and clinician. The narrative is divided into six segments. After each segment, subjects are asked to write down the state of their reasoning at that point. This technique has the advantage of being standardized, portable, and applicable to large groups; however, it lacks fidelity to the natural diagnostic encounter.

Videotaped case problems

Segmentation

The videotaped case problem is a videotape of a similar diagnostic encounter. The case is filmed to heighten the viewer's identification with the clinician. The camera is directed over the interviewer's shoulder to focus on the seated patient, zooming in on the face at times of heightened emotion. Like the narrative case problem, the tape is divided into segments, after each of which subjects are asked to record their state of thinking. The tape has more fidelity than the narrative problem and similar advantages of standardization and portability. After some preliminary studies, all our analyses have been conducted on responses to videotaped problems.

Appendix I illustrates a modification of the videotaped case technique. Here, an experienced clinician has been asked to view a tape, stop it at any point, and record on dictaphone the progressive development of his reasoning about the case. Thus, he was not constrained by arbitrary case segmentation, and his dictated comments are likely to be closer to the actual process of thought.

Diagnostic process recall

A third approach, diagnostic process recall, has not yet been used in our studies. It involves the retrospective analysis of an interview between the subject and an actual patient or an actor simulating a patient (Barrows, 1979; Elstein, Shulman, & Sprafka, 1978). This technique (stimulated recall) has high fidelity, but it is unwieldy, cannot be standardized, and cannot be used with large groups.

The content analysis manual

From the raw material provided by clinicians in response to narrative and videotaped problems, we have developed a manual for the content analysis of written (or dictated) responses (Fitzhenry-Coor & Nurcombe, 1983). In the manual, we have defined:

1. The unit of analysis.
2. Descriptive content-analysis categories.

The unit of analysis is a phrase or sentence that embodies a unitary idea. Each unit can be assigned to a particular content-analysis category. In accordance with the manual, subjects' responses are parsed into units and then assigned to the appropriate category. Interrater reliability, in regard to units and categories, can be established, and the concurrent validity of the analysis investigated further by comparing the results with other estimates of diagnostic performance. In all the studies to be described, written responses were first typed and coded by number. The protocols were then analyzed by raters trained to high levels of reliability and unaware to which group the subjects belonged.

The following components seem to appear sequentially in the process of diagnostic reasoning:

The sequence of reasoning

1. Salient cues.*
2. Clinical inferences.
3. Preliminary hypotheses.
4. Inquiry plans.
5. Diagnostic conclusions.
6. Management plans.

Salient cues

The experienced clinician first notes information considered important to diagnosis. This commences at the beginning of the initial interview and includes information transmitted in the referral, if available. These bits of information are called salient cues and derived by the clinician from the following sources:

The sources of salient cues

1. The history given by the patient.
2. The history obtained from other sources.
3. The mental status examination.
4. The physical examination of the patient.
5. Physical and psychological tests.

Clinical inferences

The clinical problem as a pattern of cues and inferences

The clinician abstracts from single cues or combinations of cues, first-cycle clinical inferences. These inferences may also include the subjective impact made by the patient on the clinician. For example, ''Thinks he is Jesus Christ'' and ''Speaks in Messianic tones'' and ''Illogical connections between thoughts'' may be transformed into an inference, ''Grandiose delusional thinking.'' A clinical problem is identified from a pattern of cues and inferences, a pattern which, though often incomplete, suggests one or more possible explanations.

Preliminary hypotheses

This step involves generating one or more early hunches called preliminary hypotheses, based on cues, inferences, or a combination of both. Hypotheses can also be derived from relationships among the cues and inferences, including inferred discrepancies, inconsistencies, gaps, contrasts, and parallels in the history

---

*The term *cue* is used interchangeably with *clue* in this section.

(see chapter 5). Hypotheses serve the purpose of organizing subsequent inquiry. The flexibility and complexity of the clinician's thought are reflected in the efficiency and organization of the array of preliminary hypotheses.

Categorical and
dynamic hypotheses

       Hypotheses apply to two domains: categorical and dynamic. The categorical domain refers to summary categorizations of current psychiatric disorder patterns. The dynamic domain has to do with inferences concerning predisposition to the current disorder and its precipitation, pattern, and perpetuation, together with analyses of interaction of vulnerability, resources, stress, and social environment.

Inquiry plans

Probes and alerts

Based on each preliminary hypothesis, the clinician generates systematic probes (or alerts) designed to elicit (or be ready for) evidence verifying or refuting the initial hypotheses. The contributory evidence acquired by the clinician at this

Second-cycle cues and
inferences

point is in the form of second-cycle cues or inferences of negative or positive nature. On this evidence, the clinician makes a decision to:

1. Discard a hypothesis
2. Test it further with additional inquiry, thus repeating the cycle; or
3. Come to a conclusion concerning diagnosis.

Diagnostic conclusions

Assuming the clinician has tested the hypotheses fully, he or she will formulate a diagnostic conclusion and determine whether the evidence satisfies criteria for inclusion in a unitary diagnosis or whether more than one diagnosis is required.

Management plans

The clinician will generate management plans based on the diagnostic conclusion.

The effects of experience

Our first studies (Nurcombe & Fitzhenry-Coor, 1982; Fitzhenry-Coor & Nurcombe, 1983), investigated the association between clinical experience and logical, complex diagnostic reasoning. At the same time, we validated a profile of diagnostic competency composed of the following indices.

Content analysis
performance scores

1. The onset of hypotheses score. This score reflects the percentage of the subject's hypotheses generated during the first segment of the videotape test.

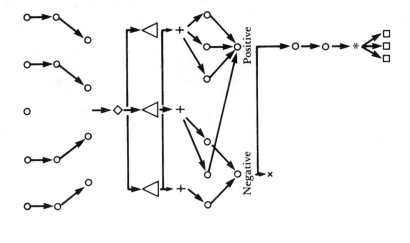

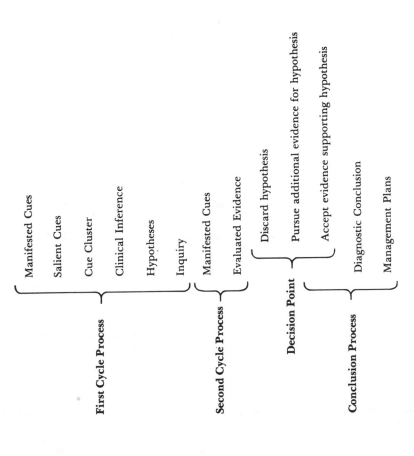

First Cycle Process
- Manifested Cues
- Salient Cues
- Cue Cluster
- Clinical Inference
- Hypotheses
- Inquiry

Second Cycle Process
- Manifested Cues
- Evaluated Evidence

Decision Point
- Discard hypothesis
- Pursue additional evidence for hypothesis
- Accept evidence supporting hypothesis

Conclusion Process
- Diagnostic Conclusion
- Management Plans

FIGURE 27.2
Diagnostic decision-making process model

Based on research findings in nonpsychiatric medical diagnosis (Elstein, Shulman, & Sprafka, 1978), we expected experienced clinicians to generate an array of working hypotheses relatively early in the test.

2. The hypothesis tracing score. This score reflects the subject's consistency in repeatedly testing working hypotheses during each segment of the videotaped case. The score is derived by counting the number of times each discrete hypothesis is reevaluated in the protocol. A weighted score reflecting the quantity of evaluations is then assigned to each hypothesis, and these scores are summed to produce a total score. The hypothesis tracing score is designed to reward a subject who systematically reviews hypotheses, in contrast to one who generates many hypotheses but tests few of them.

3. The tactical justification score. This score is designed to measure yet another aspect of clinical reasoning: the subject's expression of rationales and explanations for specific steps in diagnosis. For example, the subject may provide a justification for a certain hypothesis or a plan for inquiry. The frequency of such rationales in the protocol is calculated and the total becomes the tactical justification score. Because rationales and explanations are associated with complex reasoning, we expected this score to be greater among experienced clinicians or students who had received the training program.

4. The diagnostic accuracy score. A measure of the subject's accuracy in nosological diagnosis forms another part of the profile of competency. Several methods of deriving this score have been piloted, the most satisfactory of which seems to be assigning numerical weights to the subject's diagnosis. The most likely diagnosis for a specific case is decided by the consensus of a panel of experienced clinicians. This diagnosis is given the greatest numerical value. Alternate but plausible diagnoses (as in a differential diagnosis) are assigned lesser weights. The score is then determined by summing these weighted values in any single protocol.

The experience gradient in performance scores

In initial studies, we found that experienced clinicians generated hypotheses earlier than did residents or medical students (Nurcombe & Fitzhenry-Coor, 1982). Residents and clinicians were more likely to reevaluate earlier hypotheses than were students. Residents and experienced clinicians were more likely to offer rationales than were students. Residents tended to state rationales for their inferences and hypotheses, whereas experienced clinicians tended to justify inquiry strategies and management plans. Finally, experienced clinicians were diagnostically more accurate than were residents and students. Thus, the validity of our profile of diagnostic competence was supported by these preliminary studies.

The effects of training

Having shown that the four performance scores were sensitive to the difference between subjects of varying experience, our next task was to determine whether the scores of medical students and psychiatric residents were sensitive to training (Fitzhenry-Coor & Nurcombe, 1983).

The medical students who participated in this study completed an 8-week clinical rotation in the Department of Psychiatry, while the residents participated in a course specifically designed to improve diagnostic reasoning. This course is described later in this chapter in the section on teaching diagnostic reasoning.

The impact of training

A comparison of pretests and posttests revealed a tendency for both groups to improve in all indices except diagnostic accuracy. Medical students' pre- to posttest scores for hypothesis tracing and tactical justification reached statistical significance. Aside from diagnostic accuracy, the performance scores seemed to be sensitive to both specific training and general experience.

Production of rationales

A more detailed analysis of the complexity of tactical justification scores revealed that the improvement following training was associated with an increase in the justification of clinical inferences and working hypotheses, not with the explanation of diagnostic conclusions or management. It is possible that this preliminary version of the training program in diagnostic reasoning had effectively stressed the earlier stages of the diagnostic process but inadvertently neglected the later stages of diagnostic conclusions and management planning. Conversely, it is possible that in the short training period, subjects had acquired justification skills in making inferences and hypotheses but had not refined those skills in the more complicated areas of diagnosis and management planning.

Experimental vs. control groups

The initial investigations summarized here were pilot studies primarily designed to establish the validity of a profile of diagnostic competence. They were not, in a sense, true tests of the effectiveness of the training program. Such tests would have required the systematic comparison of students who received the diagnostic process training with students who did not receive it. To evaluate the teaching program properly, we subsequently undertook a carefully designed experimental versus control study in which several groups of students in psychiatric rotation who received this training were compared with other groups who did not. The results of this study vindicated both the organization and content of the training program and the effectiveness of our assessment measure, the University of Vermont Diagnostic Process Test.

Design of the study

Sixty-seven medical students participated in the study; 33 of them were members of rotations receiving our training course, and 34 of them were in the traditional psychiatric program. Each group was tested before the 8-week rotation and again after its completion. Both groups were tested using the standard open-ended test format and videotape cases.

As in our earlier studies, the subjects' protocols were typed, coded by number, and content-analyzed by raters unaware of the subject's group or the pretest–posttest status of the protocol. Again, as in earlier studies, a high degree of interrater reliability (more than 90% agreement) was attained. Numerical subscores were calculated by raters without knowledge of the subject's status. The four profile scores described earlier in this chapter were calculated for each subject, along with several subscores designed to explore high or low performance.

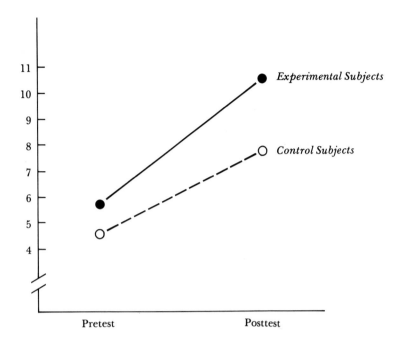

FIGURE 27.3
Mean number of hypothesis generated: pretest–posttest comparisons of experimental and control subjects

Results of the experimental vs. control study

Initial analyses of variance indicated no significant differences between the pretest scores of the experimental and control subjects. Thus, we could assume that both groups entered the study with comparable diagnostic skills. Analyses of posttest performances yielded highly significant differences in posttest scores for most of the components of the profile. Trends toward improvement were greater among experimentals than controls on all measures but one.

Experimental subjects generated a greater number of hypotheses than did controls on the posttest (see Figure 27.3). Furthermore, experimental subjects tested hypotheses more systematically (hypothesis tracing score: $p < .001$) (see Figure 27.4). The latter finding was extremely encouraging in that consistent reevaluation of hypotheses was a central goal of the training program. Experimentals also exerted significantly greater care in offering rationales for their hypotheses (tactical justification score: $p < .006$) (see Figure 27.5). Finally, experimental subjects' diagnostic accuracy on the DSM-III was significantly higher ($p < .004$) (see Figure 27.6). The only component of the diagnostic competency profile that did not produce significant posttest differences between experimentals and controls was the onset of hypotheses score, in which the control group performed slightly better.

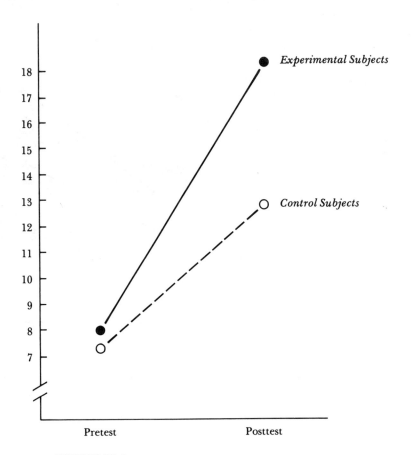

FIGURE 27.4

Mean hypothesis-tracing scores: pretest–posttest comparisons of experimental and control subjects

More stringent multivariate tests that covaried pretest performance with posttest performance replicated the results just discussed, corroborating the impact of the training program.

Results of subscores   Subtest scores tended to substantiate better performance of the trained subjects, with one exception. There were few complex rationales for diagnoses/management planning among both experimentals and controls, and no significant differences were found between groups on this subscore. These results do replicate a finding in one of the earlier studies: Even though new students of psychiatry may generate complex rationales for inferences and hypotheses, they fail to do so for the later (and perhaps more difficult) steps of diagnosis and management (Fitzhenry-Coor & Nurcombe, 1983). The replication of these results in the experimental versus control study suggest that even though the training program was designed to promote this skill, it was too demanding for the still inexperienced clinician.

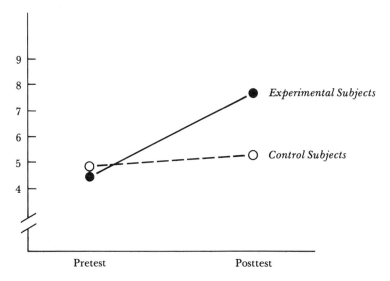

FIGURE 27.5
Mean tactical justification scores: pretest–posttest comparisons of experimental and control subjects

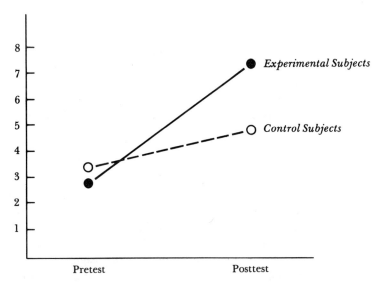

FIGURE 27.6
Mean diagnostic accuracy scores: pretest–posttest comparisons of experimental and control subjects

In summary, the experimental versus control study suggests that systematic clinical judgment can be taught to medical students. Like Elstein's (Elstein, Shulman, & Sprafka, 1978) and Feinstein's (1974) models, even novices gather information, formulate inferences, generate hypotheses, and test their hypotheses by asking for specific additional information about the patient. As they move toward a diagnostic conclusion, even novices consider management plans for the individual case.

The validity of the hypothetico-deductive model in psychiatric diagnosis

Thus, the basic hypothetico-deductive model has been supported. Furthermore, it can be taught in the classroom. The only exception to the findings conveyed in earlier studies in medical diagnosis and studies of highly experienced psychiatrists is that students-in-training do not necessarily learn to generate a major portion of hypotheses early. This skill seems to be a function of years of experience and familiarity with a wide array of possible diagnoses. Alternatively, it may reflect the student's hesitancy to move from cues and inferences in the open problem space to a more closed problem space, for fear of prematurely shutting out other diagnostic possibilities.

Teaching diagnostic reasoning

The use of videotape to promote diagnostic reasoning

Early in our experience using videotaped case problems to investigate diagnostic reasoning, we realized that a segmented tape might be the basis of a new technique for teaching the tactics and strategy of clinical reasoning. Instead of merely testing reasoning with the tape, we thought, it might be possible to teach small groups of trainees to assemble the patterns and generate the hypotheses that are the basis of effective clinical problem-solving.

Experience with successive rotations of medical students helped sharpen course objectives and improve teaching technique, particularly the method of using the group to enhance the strategy of reasoning. Students also significantly influenced the style and content of this book, which provides the theoretical base of the course.

Objectives

The objectives of the course are set out in chapter 2. As with any professional expertise, clinical problem-solving involves the application of theoretical knowledge and procedural skill to stepwise reasoning, guided by a set of appropriate attitudes. The different components of the diagnostic process are elaborated in the course objectives under the following headings:

A. Knowledge (see chapters 3, 4, 5, 6, 11, 12, 23, 24, 25).
B. Procedures (see chapters 8, 9, 10, 14, 15, 16 to 26).

C. Tactics (see chapter 7).

D. Strategy (see chapter 7).

Learning experiences

Every 8 weeks at the University of Vermont, a new group of from 12 to 15 third-year medical students enters the Department of Psychiatry for a full-time clinical core experience. During the first and eighth weeks of their rotation, they complete pre- and posttests. From the second through the seventh week, they meet as a group to undertake the course for 1½ hours each week.

A number of teaching videotapes have been prepared. The case problems scheduled on the six weeks of the course are as follows:

The videotape case problems

Week 2: A young man who asserts that he is the reincarnation of Jesus Christ.

Week 3: A young woman recovering from an acute psychotic breakdown.

Week 4: A socially withdrawn young man who thinks his family are making noises to annoy him.

Week 5: An agitated middle-aged woman who is convinced her husband has divined she has a guilty secret.

Week 6: A 35-year-old man who is agitated, depressed, and insomniac.

Week 7: A late-middle-aged man with acute amnesia of recent onset.

As described, the videotapes are of actual interviews between a psychiatrist who has never seen the patient before and a patient recently admitted to the psychiatric unit of the Medical Center Hospital of Vermont. The tapes are filmed to heighten the illusion that the viewer is not a mere spectator but actually encountering the patient. Each tape is from 30 to 40 minutes in duration.

Room arrangements

The lecture room is provided with chairs arranged around the periphery of the room and oriented toward a video screen on one side and toward a long chalkboard on an adjoining wall. A number of DSM-III manuals are available for reference on a central table.

Reading guide

Students are asked to read particular chapters of this book before each session. It is stressed that rereading will be required. The following reading guide indicates the progressive change in emphasis of the teaching sessions:

Week 2: The process as a whole. Recognizing cues and drawing inferences. Chapters 1, 2, 6, 7.

Week 3: Clarifying the problem: cues, inferences, and patterns. Chapters 6, 7, 8, 9, 11.

Week 4: Clarifying the problem and generating hypotheses. Chapters 6, 7, 8, 9, 11.

Week 5: Generating hypotheses and planning inquiry. Chapters 6, 7, 8, 9, 10, 11.

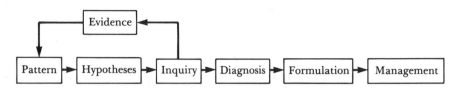

FIGURE 27.7
The tactics of clinical reasoning: chalkboard categories

Week 6: Generating hypotheses, planning inquiry, and reaching diagnostic conclusions. Chapters 6, 7, 8, 9, 10, 11, 14, 15.
Week 7: Diagnostic conclusions, formulations, and management plans. Chapters 6, 7, 11, 12, 14, 15.
General Reading: Chapters 3–5, 13, 16–27.

The use of a chalk-board flowchart

Before each session, the flowchart in Figure 27.7 is drawn at the top of the long chalkboard. The purposes of the flowchart are to remind students of the process as a whole and to organize the recording of the class's weekly deliberations. Thus, although the teacher progressively changes the focus of teaching, the flowchart flags the entire process and its ultimate purpose. Again, using the flowchart, the teacher can indicate the tactics to be dealt with in each session, review tactics at the end of the session, and foreshadow the focus of next week's class.

The session commences with a brief discussion of the step or steps of clinical reasoning to be emphasized that day. Students then view the initial segment of the tape (that is, about 6 minutes). They may wish to jot notes as they watch. After the segment is viewed, they divide into subgroups of three or four to work collaboratively on the following tasks:

The focus of the weekly sessions

Week 2: Recognize cues and draw inferences.
Week 3: Assemble cues and inferences into patterns.
Week 4: Assemble patterns and generate hypotheses.
Week 5: Generate hypotheses and plan inquiry.
Week 6: Reach diagnostic conclusions based on evidence derived from hypotheses.
Week 7: Reach a diagnostic conclusion and prepare a diagnostic formulation.

Weeks 6 and 7 involve viewing of the first segment and then the whole tape. By the final two weeks, students are expected to work alone rather than in subgroups.

Small-group deliberation

As the subgroups discuss the problem, the teacher moves from one to another, encouraging those who are on the right track and asking Socratic questions of those who have completed their deliberations or seem to be at an impasse.

Large-group discussion

Next, designated students from the three or four subgroups summarize the collective decisions of their subgroups. The teacher records their decisions on the chalkboard under the headings of the flowchart. Figure 27.8 represents a chalkboard record of the collective deliberations of a class (concerning the patient involved in Appendix I).

When information from each subgroup is reported, students are asked to discuss it. Do they agree? Would they want to alter, amend, or change any of it? Why? During this discussion, the teacher conveys by example the strategic objectives of the course:

Strategic objectives

1. Keep cues and inferences separate.
2. Tolerate uncertainty and avoid premature closure.
3. Consider alternatives.
4. Look for negative as well as positive evidence.
5. Be prepared to revise hypotheses.
6. Be prepared to commit yourself when you have enough evidence.
7. Be aware of your personal reactions to the patient.

The following suggestions are aimed to help the instructor promote the strategic objectives:

Techniques of reinforcing the strategic objectives

1. Move from the individual to the group and back to the individual again. Try to draw out the quieter members. Use verbal and nonverbal encouragement.
2. When a student provides an inference (e.g., "This man is hallucinated"), ask the student to cite the cues on which it is based (e.g., "He says he hears voices"). Then ask if alternative inferences could be drawn from those cues.
3. When a hypothesis is generated from a pattern of cues and inferences, encourage the generation of alternative hypotheses as well.
4. Give special emphasis to arrays of hypotheses that are efficiently organized in hierarchical fashion (see Figure 27.8).
5. Never reject an inference or hypothesis as incorrect, even if you personally disagree. Accept it, ask for the evidence on which it is based, and ask the student for an alternative inference or hypothesis. Be explicit about this ground rule if students begin to discount each other's ideas.
6. Relate each hypothesis to an inquiry plan involving discretionary history, MSE, physical examination, or special investigations.
7. Stress the use and significance of negative evidence (e.g., "If the dexamethasone suppression test were negative, what is the likelihood that your diagnostic hypothesis of major depression is correct?").
8. Give your own ideas only when the students have exhausted theirs. Rather than tell students the answers, refer them to texts (e.g., DSM-III or a reference text on psychiatry).
9. Encourage commitment in the last two weeks of the course by asking for provisional diagnostic conclusions and formulations. Instruct the students to select a final inquiry plan to prove the diagnosis they think most likely.

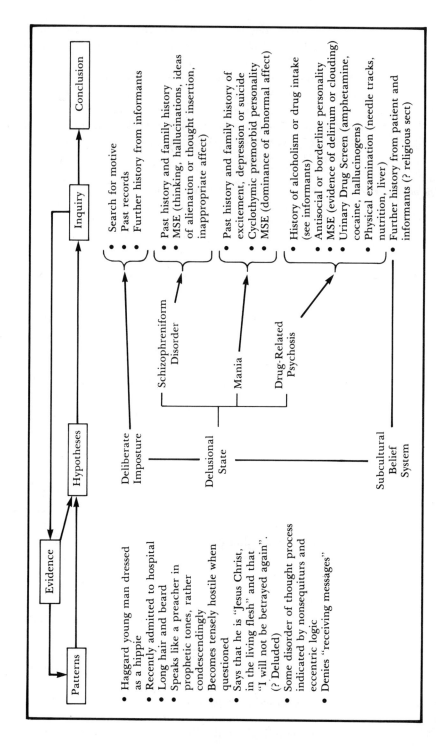

FIGURE 27.8
The chalkboard record of the deliberations of a class

10. The class can be encouraged to become aware of (and, if they wish, to disclose) their personal reactions to the patient. Tell the students to watch the patient and try to become aware of how they react. Heighten their awareness by turning off the sound. What feelings arise? Can they remember being in such a situation before? Of whom does the patient remind them? What would they like to do next? Invite the participants to reveal any of these matters in the group, but make it clear that self-disclosure is voluntary.
11. Solicit criticism from students during and after the course.
12. Try to ensure that residents and other clinical teachers also address the objectives of this course by referring to its key concepts when they teach students on the wards and in the clinics.

Summary

The scientific study of clinical reasoning has been impeded by a polarization of attitudes. Physicians often regard diagnosis as an inscrutable art naturally acquired and risky to probe. Statisticians, on the other hand, point to the fallibility of human decision-making and seek to supplement (if not supplant) the clinician with machine algorithms. Two of the three research models in this field, clinical judgment and decision theory, are prescriptive and actuarial in nature. Only the third model, information processing, attempts to trace the natural steps of clinical reasoning.

The clinical judgment model identifies the ultimate criteria used in reaching a specific decision and determines the proportionate weight accorded to each criterion in that decision. Thus, an expert's judgment can be represented in a mathematical formula that affords complete reliability.

Decision theory explores the frailties of the human computer confronted by problems requiring probabilistic decisions when the data to be dealt with – the clinical features of the case – are at a distance from their source (the abnormality and derangement of structure and function). Decision theory derives its impetus from Bayes' theorem, a mathematical device which takes base rates into account when considering the probability that a particular disorder is present, given a clinical finding or syndrome.

Repeated studies have clarified that when data must be formally combined to reach specific decisions, machine logic is superior to human judgment. But clinical problems are seldom clear-cut. The clinician is indispensable for the eliciting, sifting, and evaluating of information and the individualizing of management plans.

The information processing model investigates the natural steps of clinical problem-solving. From a number of studies of expert reasoning, a hypothetico-deductive process has emerged: The clinician transforms an open problem into an array of closed problems, first by stating alternative solutions in hypothetical form and next by seeking evidence for or against each hypothesis.

Research at the University of Vermont has demonstrated that experienced psychiatrists naturally use a hypothetico-deductive approach to clinical problem-solving. They discern salient cues, draw inferences, assemble patterns, generate hypotheses, select an inquiry plan, gather evidence, and weigh it to reach diagnostic conclusions. We found that, compared with novices, experienced clinicians generate hypotheses earlier, are more consistent in evaluating them, and more likely to provide rationales for their inquiry plans. They also reach more accurate conclusions. We found that indices of early hypothesis generation, consistency in evaluating hypotheses, and the rationalization of tactics were all sensitive to change in association with training. Carefully controlled subsequent research demonstrated the efficacy of a new training program in diagnostic reasoning aimed to enhance the tactics and strategy of diagnostic reasoning identified in previous studies. Highly significant statistical differences between experimental and control subjects' performances on our indexes of diagnostic competence substantiated our belief that systematic hypothetico-deductive reasoning can be taught and applied in the clinical setting.

Research is never conclusive. These findings should be replicated with other subjects in different settings. The rather intricate measures of clinical reasoning used in our research must be simplified if they are to be useful to teachers who wish to evaluate the progress of their students, and the general efficacy of the teaching technique described should be tested in other settings. Many other areas are worthy of study. The natural process of management planning, for example, has never been clarified; the method of planning propounded in chapters 14 and 15 was not derived from empirical research. A potential problem exists with formal systems of this sort; if they are not perceived as enhancing natural processes, they may be discarded as unnatural or unwieldy.

What is the future of the clinical process? Closer interaction between clinician and computer should be fruitful, particularly in the planning of management; but contemporary machines cannot incorporate sufficient knowledge of the social and clinical worlds to tailor comprehensive, multifaceted, individualized plans of management. In this regard, the clinician is indispensable; clinical judgment will be enhanced by the computer, not superceded. In the collaboration predicted, the clinician will elicit, discern, and sift information; the computer will combine the data to calculate the probability and utility of different outcomes; and the clinician will design an individualized plan according to a comprehensive diagnostic formulation that includes an awareness of the patient's needs, wishes, and values. Reconsidered from this perspective, the ideological disputes described early in this chapter seem very simplistic.

Envoi

Like research, books are never finished. There is always more to say, another chapter to revise, new paths to pursue. Yet, just as the diagnostic process should be concluded when enough information has been gathered and the therapy terminated when patient and clinician agree that the goals of treatment have been attained, this book must be brought to a close. Its ultimate virtue will depend on whether it helps teachers and students become more aware of their inherent rationality and whether it helps them think systematically and constructively about the diagnosis and management of patients in their care.

Selected Readings

The contemporary debate between clinicians and actuaries is reviewed by Meehl (1954), Elstein (1976), and Blois (1980).

An excellent comparative review of the clinical judgment, decision theory, and information processing models of clinical reasoning is found in Elstein and Bordage (1979). The statistical fallacies that undermine the intuitive thinker are exhaustively reviewed in Kahneman, Slovic, and Tversky (1982). Weinstein et al. (1980) describe a technique of rational clinical decision-making in *Clinical Decision Analysis*.

The most distinguished research into clinical reasoning follows the information processing model. It is described in Elstein, Shulman, and Sprafka's (1978) *Medical Problem Solving*.

The use of simulated patients to teach hypothetico-deductive reasoning is described by Barrows and Abrahamson (1964). The use of videotape for educational feedback to novice clinical interviewers was pioneered by Kagan (1975).

Appendixes

I

Process-tracing of the diagnostic reasoning of an experienced clinician

Introduction

This appendix contains a typescript of a videotaped initial interview between a clinician, Dr. B. Nurcombe, and a patient, Mr. R., who had recently been admitted to the psychiatric ward of a hospital associated with the University of Vermont School of Medicine.

The videotape was observed by a second clinician, Dr. F. P. McKegney, who was instructed to interrupt it at will in order to express the content of his diagnostic thinking as the interview progressed. Dr. McKegney stopped the videotape 19 times to comment on the progress of his thinking about the patient. He presented his final conclusions at the end of the interview. His comments during these interruptions have been inserted at appropriate points in this typescript, allowing the reader to follow the development of his diagnosis.

The purpose of this appendix is to permit the reader to trace and analyze the tactics and strategies of an experienced clinician in response to one of our videotaped cases. To facilitate the reader's understanding of the process of diagnostic reasoning as a hypothetico-deductive sequence, the author has inserted notes next to each of the experienced clinician's commentaries.

These notes contain the following information:

1. The tactics (see chapter 7) the observing clinician used in consolidating evidence, generating hypotheses, and drawing conclusions. These tactics are shown in italics adjacent to each of the 20 responses.
2. An abbreviated analysis of the case-specific steps demonstrated by Dr. McKegney as he used each tactic (chapter 27). These analyses are shown in lower-case italics adjacent to each of Dr. McKegney's responses.

The reader may wish to maximize the learning experience with this transcript by keeping separate notes of the diagnostic process demonstrated by Dr. McKegney. To do this most effectively, the reader should organize a system like the chalkboard flowchart illustrated in Figure 27.7 of chapter 27, on which cues and inferences, hypotheses, inquiry strategies, diagnosis, and management are written down as the case progresses. In this manner, readers can compare their clinical responses to the case with that of the experienced clinician. Readers can also compare their analyses of the clinician's reasoning with the author's analysis.

Following the typescript, two additional components of appendix I summarize the experienced clinician's process of diagnostic reasoning.

The first component (Figure I.1) summarizes in graphic form the interaction among evidence, inquiry, hypotheses, and diagnostic conclusions apparent in Dr. McKegney's reasoning. The second component (Figure I.2) summarizes an aspect of the hypothetico-deductive method by tracing the evaluation of each hypothesis generated by the experienced clinician.

All three parts of this appendix are designed to illustrate and reinforce the particular method of clinical diagnosis presented in this textbook.

Typescript of videotaped interview, with commentary by an experienced clinician

The case of Mr. Matthew R.

Case I.1   Mr. R., a 24-year-old, single, white male, was brought to the hospital by a friend, one day before this interview, because he was claiming to be Jesus Christ. He was admitted to a psychiatric ward. He has never before been interviewed by the interviewer, Dr. B. Nurcombe.

At interview, Mr. R. is an emaciated man in his early twenties, with a ravaged face and long, wavy auburn hair and beard. He is dressed in a denim vest without undershirt, denim trousers, thongs, and hat. When he sits, he puts his hat on the floor and looks for an ashtray in which to rest his cigarette.

He speaks in measured, rhythmical, cadenced tones, as though preaching, and adopts a helpful, somewhat condescending approach to the examiner. However, he becomes increasingly irritated as the interviewer persists with questions. After 9 minutes he bursts into tears saying, "Will you please understand me? I don't know, I'm just a man;" but he regains composure quickly. Toward the end of the interview, he smiles impishly as he describes his experiences with drugs.

(*The timed progress of the interview is indicated to the left of the dialogue in minutes and seconds.*)

The interview

0:00   Dr. N: Mr. R., could you tell me why it is you've come to the hospital? I understand you came yesterday.

    Mr. R: Yes.

    Dr. N: Why is it that you've come to the hospital?

    Mr. R: To assure my friend, *Paul,* that he could *sleep* well, while I was at the same time not *crazy,* which he believes somewhere I am. Now he *knows* I'm not and I know I'm not.

0:30   Dr. N: I see.

    Mr. R: Okay?

    Dr. N: So your friend, Paul, brought you to the hospital?

    Mr. R: Yes.

    Dr. N: And you came to demonstrate to him that you weren't crazy?

    Mr. R: *Right.*

    Dr. N: I see. Can you tell me some more about that?

    Mr. R: Uh, what do you *need* to know about that and I will tell you, but I have to know what you *need* to know.

    Dr. N: In some way, Paul felt that you were not well?

1:00   Mr. R: Right. Although he knew that I was well and he was well, I proved to him without a shadow of a doubt I am Jesus in the living flesh.

#1. Patient's voice was very calm, steady, well controlled, with contradictions already in well *and* sick. *Already the possibility of denial of problems and potentially unreliable subjective data base.*	1. *Discern and evaluate salient cues.*
	2. *Interpret cues.*
	3. *Assemble clusters to define a pattern.*
	  • *Moves to clinical pattern using limited cues*
	  • *Interprets content of patient's responses*
	  • *Questions reliability of patient's history*

But my name will *always* remain Matthew, just as I told him. *No one* but *no one* can betray me this time. The only man that could was stone deaf. *He* is your witness as a doctor. You can examine Gary *anytime* you want, and when you do, you will find he is stone deaf.

    Dr. N: But you're, you're . . . .

1:30   Mr. R: He is Gary M. is his name and he is a Saint, the only one.

    Dr. N: He is a friend of yours?

    Mr. R: He sure *is* my friend. Remember, they're all my friends *this* time. Okay?

    Dr. N: Stone deaf, he didn't hear what you were saying?

2:00 Mr. R: Right. Until he *knew* he could, and then he, now he does hear me. Only when I'm within his visual range. Believe me, I do not send *messages* or receive *messages*.

#2. Some dissociation, some contradictions, some mixing of visual and auditory parameters, increasing pressure – perhaps lessening control. Diagnostic possibilities include organic mental syndrome, schizophrenia, paranoid reaction, possibility of malingering. Unreliability is becoming more likely in terms of what actually happened prior to hospital.

1. *Interpret cues.*
   - *Interprets characteristics of patient's thought processes*
   - *Notes midinterview changes in patient's affect*
2. *Generate an array of alternative hypotheses to explain patterns.*
   - *Generates four hypotheses early, contrasting functional vs. organic psychoses*

I do not hear *voices*. I do not see things that aren't real. Everything I believe I believe because I *had* to believe because I would not be deceived even by my own self. *Christ in the flesh.* I would not *let* me deceive myself. That is why I am sitting here now and that is why *you* are interviewing *me* and all the people that are seeing my face are hearing exactly what they *need* to hear; and what they *don't*, they just *won't* hear. Okay? Now, what do I need to say next?

2:30 Dr. N: I would like to hear as much as I can about what you mean. Would you tell me more about being Jesus in the living flesh?

#3. Increasing concern about control, controlling himself, being controlled by others, not being deceived, not deceiving himself; begins to suggest ideas of reference or projection, and raises the possibilities of hallucinations, auditory or visual – not clear.

1. *Assemble clusters of cues and inferences to define a pattern.*
2. *Generate hypothesis to explain pattern.*
   - *Associates control and deception to form tentative clinical inference of projection, generating hypothesis of hallucinosis*

Mr. R: Okay. Now, you *know* I came and I was crucified, right? When I was crucified, was it not that I came for the sins of the world, right? To deliver man . . .

Dr. N: Two thousand years ago?

Mr. R: . . . from his own evil. Well, I *guess* it was. I don't *know* the exact day and I won't tell you anything I *don't* know. But I *know* I do not bear any marks on my body from **3:00** where those nails went into me. Okay? Anywhere. If you would like to see it, I will remove my shoes. Okay?

Dr. N: I believe you. I believe you. There are no marks.

Mr. R: Which everybody thought should be there when I come again, right? Well, they're not, and they won't be, there. And the long hair that he had, well look. Okay? **3:30** The beard – look, it's growing back finally. Okay? It's *always* been a part of me. I've never changed *me*. Okay? I'm still Matthew, I'm still just a man.

#4. Increasing pressure of speech, sharper movements and more challenging to the interviewer. I begin to feel some anxiety in terms of patient's controls or lack thereof. Content is beginning to fill out; a possible, probably delusional scheme about being Christ.

Discern, evaluate, and interpret cues.
   - *Notes midinterview changes in patient's affect*
   - *Interprets these changes*
   - *Alert to patient's level of self-control*
   - *Reexamines evidence to support inference of delusional scheme*

And when my *heart* stops, I will die just as assuredly as *you* will, but I will *not* be betrayed.

DR. N: But you're saying that you're a man even though you're Christ?

MR. R: And I was a *man* that time, too. And this is the *third* time I am coming to you. I will not spare *anyone* if I *must* come *again*. Not that I *have* to, but if I do, I will not *spare* all those who will not accept what they must.

4:00

DR. N: Matthew, there is something I don't quite understand.

#5. Patient is using numbers in a confusing fashion. His train of thought is more dissoci-ated – raising paranoid schizophrenia as the most likely diagnosis; but all other possibilities mentioned earlier still remain quite possible.	*Search for evidence to support or disconfirm hypothesis.* • *Evaluates cognitive functioning as evidence for paranoid schizophrenia* • *Does not discard other hypotheses*

MR. R: What's that?

DR. N: This is the second time you've returned?

MR. R: *Right.* And the *third* time I am coming to *you.*

DR. N: I don't follow you.

MR. R: Of *course* not. I'm speaking plain, *right?* You're not supposed to understand what you can't, *right?*

DR. N: Yes.

MR. R: I *told* you that.

DR. N: Yes.

MR. R: *Now* you *do* know. Okay? Now what *else* must I explain?

4:30

DR. N: This is now the second time you've returned right now, but there will be a third time?

MR. R: No, this is the *third* time I am coming to *you.* Upon my *second* time here, I was crucified as surely as you can believe as a Christian. Are you a Christian?

DR. N: No, I'm not.

MR. R: Okay, well you don't *have* to be, but you are okay, *too,* because *God didn't damn a soul* and *He will not damn anybody* unless I have to appear again.

DR. N: I see. But if you have to return again . . .

5:00

MR. R: And the twin prophets in the Revelation, I *will* be one. My twin, Paul, who doesn't look like me but is my twin because I was the *only begotten* son, *begotten* - not the *only* son - but *begotten.*

#6. Patient's fixed stare and hypervigilant at-tention on the interviewer speak against a delirium; other organic mental syndromes remain a possibility since some of the confusion in dates and time could well be reflective of an organic mental syndrome; probably couldn't be ruled out until tests of biological function are done. However, the anger and challenging of the interviewer more strongly reinforces the paranoid qualities and with the dissociation make it more likely that this is a paranoid schizophrenic reaction.	*1. Search for evidence regarding hypothesis.* *2. Develop an inquiry plan to test hypothesis.* • *Notes negative evidence for delirium* • *Notes need for biological tests* *3. Revise hypothesis if evidence warrants it.* • *Combines two patterns, anger and dis-sociation, to form hypothesis of paranoid schizophrenia*

5:30 I was, *yes.* Okay. Now, Paul, no matter what, if you guys do not leave me, let me leave here because you somehow think I am *insane,* well, *any* of you have that right reserved because *that is your self-doubt, not mine.* I do not doubt myself any longer. And if you hold me back, believe it or not, the Scriptures will be fulfilled no matter *what* anyone is ever held true to a *God,* not a *man,* a *God.*

6:00 DR. N: How will Scriptures be fulfilled? In terms of what? The apocalypse or what. . .

MR. R: *Read* the *Revelations,* my friend. You can understand it now and only you can now when you read it. Those who need to read it, they too will come to me with a Bible. In their own time, now, believe me, I don't want *everybody* that sees this come running to me with a Bible.

DR. N: Yes.

MR. R: When they believe, when they believe that I will not deceive them, I'm not the

6:30 *Antichrist* which everyone knows is alive. Well, Richard Nixon is the *Antichrist.*

#7. Dissociation very clear with an overinclusiveness and shifting of topics. Diagnostic possibility of paranoid schizophrenia sufficiently strong that I would begin to not inquire any further about content per se but try to key in on patient's affective state and attempt to develop a relationship and reduce the anger and probably anxiety the patient is likely to be experiencing.

1. Reach a conclusion about which hypothesis is best supported by the evidence.
- *Uses dissociation in thought process to begin to close on diagnosis of paranoid schizophrenia*

2. Design a management plan.
- *Chooses to move to management based on patient's immediate needs, rather than pursuing firm diagnosis*

Six, six, six was in Revelations.

DR. N: Uh-uh.

MR. R: That number identifies that need and believe me, tell me in your own heart that he is not *every bit* the Antichrist that you have been led to believe. The *tea of Babylon* in the Book of Revelations is *oil* – right? We have enough coal in this country to sustain us for a

7:00 *thousand years* – right?

DR. N: Um-hmm.

MR. R: Why do we need OPEC's oil? It is the *tea of Babylon* which the world will *feed* upon, okay?

DR. N: What effect will that have upon us to do that?

MR. R: To do what?

DR. N: To feed upon the tea of Babylon? What effect will. . .

MR. R: Nothing. Nothing. It will have no effect on you.

DR. N: But you feel Nixon and the oil crisis was predicted in the Revelations?

MR. R: Of *course* it was. Read the book, N.D.C.C., ''None Dare Call It Conspiracy.'' It

7:30 was published, put out in 1971. Read it. One year before he became president. Okay?

DR. N: Um-hmm.

MR. R: Now I do not lie and you know that. Okay? I am *Jesus* in the living *flesh. When* and *only when* somebody wants to come with that Bible to me, then *they're* okay, too.

DR. N: Yes.

MR. R: Okay? But I will not leave here. I will *always* be here. This is where I belong. But believe me.

8:00 DR. N: The world you're in?

MR. R: Here in the world, that's right. *Believe me you,* it *will* happen and it *will* come to pass whether or *not* you are a Christian or not. Believe me, *you* are not damned and you never *have* been. Okay, you want to use my name in vain? Go right ahead. Do not ever say goddamn because you know full well now that he never damned anybody.

8:30 DR. N: Um-hmm. Okay. Could I ask you a few questions about the experiences that you've had? When did you become aware that you were Christ incarnate?

MR. R: You know, I really didn't know until I was up on that ward delivered by a friend who knew he could take me away as a friend and my own self-doubt (*snap of fingers*) just like that.

DR. N: That was yesterday?

MR. R: Yes.

DR. N: So you first became aware of this yesterday?

MR. R: Yes. I removed my own self-doubt; *I* didn't remove it, my *Creator* did, my *Father* removed it. At the time, he knew I didn't have to doubt even me any longer.

9:00 DR. N: Did you have any thoughts that you might be Christ before yesterday?

MR. R: No.

DR. N: Tell me how the revelation came to you that you were. Can you tell me the moment it came?

MR. R: No. Will you *please* understand me. (*His face contorts.*)

#8. Patient's more demonstrated anguish is a sign of strength which I would then respond to directly rather than the delusional content surrounding the anguish.

Design a management plan.
* *Comments on management of affect*

I don't know, *I'm just a man.* (*Weeps*)

DR. N: I know. I know. I know. Come on, now.

MR. R: I don't know. (*Weeping, face contorted with grief, he holds his head, looks up at the ceiling, and regains composure.*)

9:30 DR. N: That's okay. All right. The thought first came to you yesterday?

MR. R: No. The *thought* didn't.

DR. N: I see.

MR. R: The *doubt* left me.

DR. N: I understand.

MR. R: And now you are *all* left endowed by the same Creator with that doubt. *Test yourselves,* don't test *me.* I'm up there for anybody on Baird 6. Right?

#9. Sort of klang associated in doubt-endowed *only reinforces the presence of a thought disorder. Time and historical content unreliable. Deal with the current anguish. Establish a relationship; should be both therapeutic and a further diagnostic thrust to see how well he is able to relate to the interviewer as a real physician rather than one of "them."*

Search for evidence to support or disconfirm the hypothesis.
* *Continues to gather data on thought disorder*
* *Expresses concern about need for management and its therapeutic as well as diagnostic goals*

DR. N: Can you tell me when the thought first came to you? How long ago was that mainly? How did it first come?

10:00 MR. R: I don't know. I know all my life though, all my life here, not that I have lived again as a man. . .

DR. N: Yes.

MR. R: to die again as a man, but *Christ* I am *Christ,* but my name is *Matthew* will never change.

DR. N: Okay.

MR. R: Okay?

DR. N: I have to ask some detailed questions. Do you understand?

10:30   MR. R: And *I'm* not angry with *anybody.*

DR. N: I understand, and if you don't want to answer, you say no.

MR. R: Well, you *know* I'm going to answer.

DR. N: So, what I would like to ask you is when the first, the very first time the thought came to you that you were Christ.

MR. R: Just as soon as I looked at Gary and I said, "Gary, do you hear me? Am I Jesus?" Gary said, he *didn't* say because he's *mute.*

DR. N: Yes.

MR. R: Okay?

DR. N: Yes.

11:00   MR. R: He could only have *betrayed* me by writing down "Matthew is Jesus."

DR. N: Yes.

MR. R: He *didn't* betray me.

DR. N: No.

MR. R: Okay? And *he* is living proof for anybody else too.

DR. N: When was that? How long ago?

MR. R: Two nights ago, maybe three, I can't be sure, okay?

DR. N: So, it's very recent . . .

MR. R: Yes.

DR. N: that this thought came to you?

MR. R: Yes.

DR. N: Do you remember the very first time it came into your mind, I am Jesus?

#10. The lack of clarity around the awareness of time frame is unusual in terms of the possibility of paranoid schizophrenia and it raises again – makes more strong – the possibility that we are dealing with a posttoxic or even toxic state despite the alertness and even hypervigilance of the patient.

Search for evidence to support or disconfirm hypothesis.
- *Notes negative evidence for paranoid schizophrenia*
- *Considers the same evidence as supporting possible organic psychoses*

MR. R: Yes.

DR. N: When was that?

MR. R: Convinced?

DR. N: Convinced.

11:30   MR. R: *Yesterday* when my *doubt* was removed.

DR. N: I see. And before, say a week ago, this thought had never come to you?

MR. R: No, I just felt that I was Matthew with a dream, but I told everybody who could believe that that dream would come true because they knew I was their friend. I never lied to them.

DR. N: What was the dream that you had?

MR. R: I don't know.

DR. N: That you were Matthew . . .

MR. R: I just knew that somehow this would all come to pass.

DR. N: That something very fine, something very important would happen?

12:00   MR. R: Right. And I have always told all of my friends that *home* for me is ———. Okay? And home it is.

DR. N: Okay. So, you've always lived in ———?

MR. R: No. I haven't.

DR. N: Tell me about where you've lived.

12:30   MR. R: Well, I've lived in Pennsylvania because that's where I was born.

DR. N: Um-hmm.

MR. R: I've lived in Vermont twice in my life. Once I moved away from ———, once I returned to ———. I've lived in Massachusetts, about 16 years of my life in a town called ———, Massachusetts . . .

DR. N: Um-hmm.

MR. R: in which my brother of the flesh from the same two parents that I was born of here, John, still resides; okay?

DR. N: Um-hmm.

13:00   MR. R: Now I am here, I am home, I guess that never was my home, but I believed it then, too; now I don't believe it.

DR. N: How long have you been in ———?

MR. R: Whew! This time?

DR. N: Yes.

MR. R: For sure, I can't tell you, but I know I've been here . . .

DR. N: Approximately.

MR. R: for at least a month this time, month and a half, but I have been commuting back

13:30   and forth from ——— on a bus. You can check *that* out, too. I don't fly.

DR. N: And where have you been living?

MR. R: Where?

DR. N: Um-hmm.

MR. R: I can't lie. ——— Street is my legal address. Okay? That is where *Paul* resides, my brother and my twin.

DR. N: I see.

MR. R: Okay? That is my legal address.

DR. N: He's your twin brother who resides there?

MR. R: Yes, but he doesn't *look* like my twin.

DR. N: Was he born of the same parents?

MR. R: No, he wasn't.

14:00   DR. N: I see. But he lives in a house there?

MR. R: Oh, yeah, it's a definite house just like you live in, don't ya?

#11. Identity of siblings and time are making the data rather meaningless for objective assessment; full of contradictions and vagueness. That means that information has to be gathered from others regarding actual living situation, interpersonal relationships, ability to function, care for self, etc. Patient's anguish again has come up, particularly around the fact that he "cannot lie." I might pursue the feelings behind that statement, again primarily for relationship building and not for reliable data.

1. Develop an inquiry plan.
   • Perceives family history as unreliable
   • Generates a plan for obtaining data from other sources
2. Design a management plan.
   • Notes affect and its exploration as a tactic of management

DR. N: And he's been, you've been living with him as a guest in his house?

MR. R: Right.

DR. N: I see. Have you been working recently?

MR. R: I haven't worked; only what I *had* to do. Not recently, no. My job is what I'm doing now and *believe* me; if anybody in their heart wants to stop me, they can stop me from leaving here; but when I do leave here when Paul comes as my friend, unless that is the day I must too die, as assuredly I know I will, because I am a *man*.

14:30

DR. N: I see.

MR. R: I will go to school to become a *psychiatrist*.

DR. N: Um-hmm.

MR. R: Okay? And now you know why none of the doctors here that know in their own hearts as a psychiatrist they couldn't let me leave here if I was insane.

15:00

DR. N: But you wish to become a psychiatrist?

MR. R: I sure do. That is what I want to be.

DR. N: Why is that?

MR. R: I don't know, I didn't know that for sure yet until just it came to me just like everything else comes.

DR. N: When did it come to you that you would like to be a psychiatrist?

MR. R: For sure?

DR. N: Yes.

MR. R: I don't know, I guess, ah, I can't answer that one honestly.

DR. N: How did it come to you? In what form?

MR. R: Just, um, my own thought, my own thought, believe me. I've never had a message sent to me.

15:30

DR. N: You've never had messages sent to you?

MR. R: No, and I do not *send* messages. I do not *receive* messages.

DR. N: You've had no communication with anybody else?

MR. R: No.

DR. N: From God?

MR. R: No. I do not hear voices.

#12. The flatness of the affect is prominent in this segment, and the content about being a psychiatrist is spontaneous and inappropriate and probably rules out malingering since it's too far out. The shift to the psychiatrist from previous religious content probably reinforces the diagnosis of paranoid schizophrenia rather than a posttoxic state since the patient is now focusing in on the interviewer and the current situation rather than the religious content.

Search for evidence to support or disconfirm the hypothesis.

- *Tests malingering by noting affect and spontaneity of response*
- *Interprets patient's ability to focus on present situation; sees it as a positive evidence for paranoid schizophrenia (functional), and negative for posttoxic reaction (organic)*

DR. N: Um-hmm.

MR. R: Unless they're voices I *should* hear.

DR. N: Okay. How have you been sleeping recently?

MR. R: *Perfectly.* I can relax now that I know all my friends can *sleep* well, so can I. And if any doctor here can honestly administer that drug to me knowing full well that I have been too an *addict,* and *believe me,* I am *cured,* I have no cravings for anything.

16:00

DR. N: Have you taken drugs in the past?

MR. R: Oh yeah. Oh yeah. And the amounts I've taken should have *killed* me.

DR. N: What kinds of drugs have you taken?

MR. R: Name drugs that you know and they're probably there. Amphetamines, cocaine,
16:30 heroin, morphine, dilaudid, opium, valium, reserpine – no, I've never taken reserpine,
but I know what it is. Thorazine, mellaril, now you know. Any drug that just about you
can name I have had.

DR. N: When was the last time you took any drugs?

MR. R: That I took any on my own?

DR. N: Yes.

17:00 MR. R: A few nights ago, and I really didn't take it on my own, it was offered to me.

DR. N: What was the drug that you took then?

MR. R: Cocaine.

DR. N: How much did you take?

MR. R: I can't say for sure.

DR. N: Have you been taking that regularly?

MR. R: No.

DR. N: When was the last time before then that you took cocaine?

MR. R: The last time that it was offered to me.

DR. N: Approximately how long ago?

MR. R: Only three or four days before that.

DR. N: I see. And have you taken other drugs in the last few weeks?

17:30 MR. R: Pot. I've always smoked pot.

DR. N: Yes.

MR. R: Well, not always. I guess since I started smoking, I've always smoked it.

DR. N: Yes. What about amphetamines or speed?

*#13. This data about drugs is, of course,
highly unreliable, but the patient obviously has
some knowledge about drug names. The patient is not toxic now; and even if this is a
posttoxic schizophreniform state, it would still
be likely that the patient had early signs of
schizophrenia and the drug precipitated the
state. It does not seem to be an amphetamine
psychosis, although time and observation
would perhaps differentiate that from a
paranoid schizophrenic reaction.*

1. *Refine hypotheses if new evidence
   warrants it*
   - *Notes that drug knowledge does not
     invalidate hypothesis of paranoid
     schizophrenia*
   - *Suggests that drugs may have precipitated
     disorder*
   - *Implicitly contrasts chronic vs. reactive
     schizophrenia*
2. *Develop an inquiry plan*
   - *Notes similarity of behavior in
     amphetamine psychosis and paranoid
     schizophrenia and suggests method of
     differentiation*

MR. R: Don't do it. Best course, gave it up.

DR. N: Angel Dust?

MR. R: Don't do it.

DR. N: Tried that?

MR. R: Oh, yeah. PCP.

DR. N: How long ago?

MR. R: Huh?

DR. N: Yes.

MR. R: How long ago was the last time?

DR. N: Yes.

MR. R: I don't know. But I do know I have taken PCP for sure. Horse tranquilizers, whatever you want to call it. I have had it.

18:00

DR. N: Yes.

MR. R: And I have put it all into my veins at one time, believe me. All of it.

DR. N: But you've taken nothing into your veins recently?

MR. R: No.

DR. N: How long since . . .

MR. R: *Look,* the only mark I have right there is where they took blood from me today.

DR. N: I see.

MR. R: You know, I mean I am *here* for you to test. (*He stretches out his arms to show his cubital fossae.*)

DR. N: I know. You're clean. I can see that.

MR. R: Okay? There's no scars there, are there?

DR. N: No.

MR. R: But believe me, there *should* be. At one time I must have done this before I can say it, at least maybe thirty times a day sometimes, at least. Now, I'm not saying as the absolute truth because, you know, I think.

DR. N: How long ago was that that you took drugs intravenously?

MR. R: I think the last time I stuck a needle in my arm (*pause*) . . . I don't know, but I *do* know that I am *not* an addict and I will *never, ever* put a shaft of *steel* into my arm again.

19:00

DR. N: How long since you've done it? Approximately.

MR. R: A year and a half, 2 years.

DR. N: Quite a long time.

MR. R: Oh, yeah.

DR. N: Have you ever had treatment to cure an addiction?

MR. R: Yes, yes, I *surely* have.

DR. N: Where was that?

MR. R: Umm, at ——— House, a halfway house in ———, Massachusetts. Okay? ——— House, halfway house in ———, Massachusetts. Okay? Those are the only two halfway houses that I really believe were something like ———.

DR. N: Umm.

MR. R: The original.

DR. N: Did they help you there?

MR. R: Oh, yeah. But they didn't cure me.

DR. N: What cured you? What got you off the stuff?

MR. R: I don't know.

DR. N: Belief?

MR. R: Any belief.

DR. N: Just yourself?

MR. R: Yeah, myself. And believe me, all of my friends that know that I have been an addict know, too, that I can stop whenever I want. They've witnessed it. The seizure that you have on record that I had, you might not know, but it is on medical record here. I

20:00

suffered a seizure in front of my friend David, who witnessed it. Okay? And at that time, I had a vision, I don't remember it. But I said, "Oh, My God!" and I ran into the street and fell and had that seizure. And when I came up here, a neurosurgeon, mind you, said there was no residual effect.

DR. N: When was this seizure that you had? How long ago was that?

MR. R: I don't know. *He* knows the day, *you* know the day, too, because it's *documented.*

Dr. N: I haven't yet read the document.

Mr. R: Okay, but I can't tell you what I *don't* know and you *know* that.

Dr. N: Approximately.

Mr. R: Oh, a year ago maybe. Year and a half, maybe two years ago. That's how unsure I am of that.

Dr. N: Had you had any convulsions before that point?

21:00   Mr. R: Oh, yeah. Ah, the last time I put all my trust into a *doctor.* Okay? And I mean *all* my trust was in that man. I had so much trust in that man that even when I knew that he was killing me, that I left the hospital because I didn't, you know, they kicked me out of the hospital in ——. Kicked *me* out because he had me on so many drugs that they didn't want me to die in their bed.

22:00   Dr. N: I see. But you were in the hospital because of convulsions?

Mr. R: No, I was in the hospital because I was bleeding from my ulcer.

Dr. N: I see. Let's come to that in a moment because you mention convulsions, and you had one about a year ago?

Mr. R: Right. And I've never had another again.

Dr. N: And you've had none since that time?

Mr. R: No.

Dr. N: No attacks of unconsciousness?

Mr. R: No.

Dr. N: Or blankness where your mind switches off?

Mr. R: No.

Dr. N: No fainting attacks?

Mr. R: No, no.

Dr. N: No unusual movements with your head or body?

#14. Review of systems is so unreliable it only raises the possibility that a full neurological exam with EEG, CT scan, as well as medical records from other hospitals (if indeed the patient was there), and history from relatives and friends are necessary to document past medical psychiatric history.

Develop an inquiry plan with routine and discretionary lines of inquiry.
- *Concludes that unreliable data necessitate neurological examination and past history from other sources*

Mr. R: No.

Dr. N: No headaches?

Mr. R: No.

Dr. N: So, nothing at all of that nature for about 1 year.

Mr. R: Well, yeah, about. I won't say what I can't know is true.

Dr. N: About a year?

Mr. R: About a year, year and a half, maybe.

Dr. N: Now, prior to that convulsion a year ago, approximately a year ago, had you had any previous convulsions?

Mr. R: Oh, yeah, those are all documented, too, at —— State Hospital.

Dr. N: How many convulsions have you had?

Mr. R: *I* don't know. *They* can tell you.

Dr. N: When did they start? How old were you when they first began?

Mr. R: Ah, when my dear friend, Dr. ——, in —— called me one day and said,

23:00   "Matthew, you're going cold turkey." Click. Buzzzzz. Three days later, I was hallucinating. When the first seizure came upon me, I don't know.

DR. N: So you had seizures when you were withdrawing from drugs. What drug were you withdrawing from?

MR. R: Okay. Here you go: 40 milligrams of Valium every four hours; 1500 milligrams of placidyl at bedtime; 40–50 milligrams talwin tablets guaranteed supplied every 2 days; 150 milligrams of sinequan a day.

DR. N: So you've stopped those like that and it has controlled . . .

MR. R: It has controlled the seizures, yes.

DR. N: So the only times you've really had seizures were when you were withdrawing from that medication.

MR. R: Yeah. Oh, I will have the seizures, you know, if I have to take the drug again. I don't want to have to do anything I don't *have* to.

DR. N: Yes. And you had seizures as a child?

MR. R: No.

DR. N: No. Now, you mentioned an ulcer.

24:00   MR. R: Uh-hmm.

DR. N: You have a peptic ulcer?

MR. R: It was called duodenal when it was found by (who was it?), Dr. ———— at the State Hospital in ———— sent me. He was the only man to believe that I could've had an ulcer.

DR. N: Yes.

MR. R: Okay? Everybody before that said, "No; rest assured; you don't have an ulcer." And they did check it and it didn't appear, okay?

DR. N: Yes.

MR. R: But it did appear that time, plain and clear.

DR. N: Where was it diagnosed?

MR. R: In ———— State Hospital.

DR. N: On X-ray?

MR. R: On X-ray, yes. They do have it, okay?

DR. N: Um-hmm.

MR. R: And you can take an X-ray now and I don't know if it's there or not, I don't feel it is.

DR. N: Um-hmm.

MR. R: So it might not be, but I won't say that unless it's true either.

DR. N: So you haven't had any symptoms from that recently?

MR. R: No, I don't.

DR. N: No pain?

MR. R: No.

DR. N: No bleeding?

MR. R: No.

DR. N: No vomiting?

MR. R: No.

DR. N: No indigestion?

MR. R: No.

DR. N: Okay. Have you had any other physical symptoms recently?

#15. Patient smiles in a rather secretive, private way, and I think I might even ask him about that again, to get at affect rather than history of such questionable reliability.

Design management plan.
• Notes unreliable data but finds them useful for evaluating affect

MR. R: No.

DR. N: No dizziness?

MR. R: No.

DR. N: No pains and aches anywhere in your body?

MR. R: No.

25:00   DR. N: No attacks of numbness or loss of feeling?

MR. R: Oh, I don't have any feeling in this hand; but, yes, I felt that. (*Touches hand.*) And that's documented, too. Dr. ———, a very good surgeon, one of the best, sewed that hand when I cut it to the bone. I shall not feel in that hand, right?

DR. N: I see.

MR. R: And yet, you can lay in my hand right now anything you want and without a doubt I hope it comes up, I can tell you the exact weight.

DR. N: I see.

MR. R: Okay?

DR. N: And you cut your wrist at one time.

MR. R: Oh, yes.

DR. N: How did that come about?

MR. R: I guess I hated myself. I must have hated myself still for some reason.

DR. N: When was that?

MR. R: Umm, December, 29, 19--. December 29, I don't know. Check in ——— at the hospital, please, for *God's* sake, do that (*inaudible*).

DR. N: Around about how long ago?

26:00   MR. R: Oh, about 2 years ago, 3, no. . . . It's 1979, right? Roll back 4 years. Around '75.

DR. N: Has there been any other attempt at suicide apart from that?

MR. R: Oh, yeah. But not that I really knew it was suicidal, it's kinda, well, "nobody cares about me" – you know what I mean?

DR. N: Sort of an OD.

MR. R: Yeah.

DR. N: But you didn't really mean to kill yourself?

MR. R: I didn't think so. Ahh, yeah, I did, you know, I wanted to die, man, I wanted out. I didn't understand *anything* that was happening to me or why. Not at all. All I knew I was *Matthew,* a *man,* I *never* wanted my hair cut, I *always* wanted a beard on my face, but I didn't know why. I had to grow and develop into what I am before I could be sitting here now and saying, "Yes, I am *Christ* in the *flesh* and if I come again, I will spare *no one.*"

27:00   DR. N: Okay. Could I ask you a few questions about your earlier childhood? Are your parents alive still?

MR. R: Oh, yes, they live in ———.

DR. N: How old are they?

MR. R: Umm, Dad's probably 56 now, going on 60. My mother is 48, 50; I don't know. Around, I'm telling ya, around.

DR. N: Are your parents in good health?

MR. R: As far as I know. I know my father has high blood pressure, has suffered a couple of heart attacks, you know. But as far as I know, he's still alive unless he's died and I don't know it.

DR. N: Yes. Have you been out of touch with them?

MR. R: Oh, yes.

DR. N: How long since you've seen them?

MR. R: Four months, maybe now 5 months since the last time I saw them, yeah.

DR. N: Why so out of touch?

28:00 MR. R: Well, I don't know. I know I want them again with me.

DR. N: Did you have some estrangement from them?

MR. R: Umm. All this came about really weird, man; like I can remember I was about 7 at the time, and my mother in very plain English said it so that I could understand; anyhow, at the time, with what knowledge I had, that she was threatening to kill all of us children. Okay?

DR. N: Um-hmm.

MR. R: And now I know, too, why I suffered insomnia for a good 3 years after that. And the only one I could turn to was my older sister, Helen, because I had no faith left in either of my parents. Why, I don't know.

DR. N: She threatened to kill her children?

MR. R: And herself.

DR. N: Do you understand why?

MR. R: No.

DR. N: She must have been very unhappy.

MR. R: Um-hmm. But she'll be happier as soon as she knows who I am. Because she told

29:00 me also at one time in ——— only 3 or 4 years ago now, "Matthew, you're the only child I ever really wanted."

DR. N: Umm.

MR. R: And so I know she'll be relieved to know who I am.

DR. N: Yes. But when you were younger, you didn't really have too much faith in either of them, huh?

MR. R: No.

DR. N: Why not in your father?

MR. R: Oh, I never had reason to doubt my father; it was my mother, remember, who made that threat.

DR. N: Yes, yes.

MR. R: And I guess all I ever wanted to know was that my father loved me.

DR. N: Did he show you that?

MR. R: Oh, yes. And that happened, documented once again, ——— Hospital, ———, Massachusetts. I had a car accident there. I left my body. I died at that time, I came back. When I came back, you see these two scars on my head; do you see *them*? (*points to scars on forehead*)

DR. N: I do.

MR. R: Can you see *these*? (*points to scars on forehead*)

DR. N: Okay.

30:00 MR. R: Those scars were my assurance that I wasn't the *Antichrist*. But I don't know that, either why. . . .

#16. Irrespective of reliability, some of this content does begin to suggest some psychodynamic formulations about the delusional scheme. The perception of a threatening mother and a father who might be dead (but who also supposedly was not to be doubted) might well fit with a fear of men and more comfort with warm and maternal women.

Revise interpretations or hypotheses if new evidence warrants it, by adding to the array.
 • *Notes unreliability of patient's data but suggests psychodynamic hypothesis for family interaction and its impact*

DR. N: I don't understand how the scars show you that.

MR. R: No, but they *do, believe* me.

DR. N: In what way?

MR. R: In the belief that I always believed that Satan had horns.

DR. N: Oh, I see.

MR. R: *Now,* do you see? Okay? Now, I know my horns, if they ever were there, aren't there now.

DR. N: They've been removed by the accident if ever they were there?

MR. R: Right. If *ever* they were there. Right, and I don't believe they were now.

DR. N: All right. What work did your father do when you were a kid?

MR. R: Ah, he was *devoted* to the Army.

DR. N: He was in the military?

MR. R: Yes.

DR. N: He must have moved around quite a bit.

MR. R: Oh, yeah.

DR. N: What rank did he achieve?

MR. R: Sergeant, first class.

DR. N: And he was very devoted to that job?

MR. R: Oh, yes. He's . . . he's always been devoted to his occupation, whatever it was.

DR. N: What does he do now?

MR. R: Drives taxi, which is exactly what he likes to do.

DR. N: I see. How many brothers and sisters do you have?

MR. R: By those parents?

DR. N: Yes.

31:00 MR. R: I have four other brothers: John, Mark, Patrick, and James. I have two sisters: Helen and Beth.

DR. N: Um-hmm. Okay. Where do you come in the family?

MR. R: Third.

DR. N: Has anybody in your family had any nervous problems or emotional disorders?

MR. R: Yes, yes.

DR. N: Who were they?

MR. R: Well, the one that has had them all the time is my mother.

DR. N: Yes. Has she ever had to go to hospital with her nervous problem?

MR. R: I don't think she ever went. I don't know if she had, I know she's had to, whether she went or not for it, I don't know. I do know I found her overdosed many a times, or just once I could say for sure. But I do know she's overdosed many times to wake up to, but I found her once.

32:00 DR. N: Do you know why she used to take those overdoses? Did you have any inkling why?

MR. R: Maybe she wanted out, too, *I* don't know.

DR. N: Did she say that?

MR. R: No, she never said that to me.

DR. N: Only once.

MR. R: Huh?

DR. N: You mentioned she wanted to get rid of her children and herself on one occasion?

MR. R: Well, that's what she said to me.

DR. N: Yes.

MR. R: And my sisters and brothers have they heard plainly what I heard, they, too. . . .

DR. N: Umm. Did your father have any nervous or emotional problems?

MR. R: No, he's always been calm as far as I know.

DR. N: Was he a drinking man?

MR. R: Oh, yes. He was an alcoholic who he, himself, cured himself.

DR. N: When you were younger?

MR. R: No, he never was an alcoholic that I knew him as, as just my father.

DR. N: I see. So by the time you came along, he'd cured his own alcoholism.

MR. R: Now you understand why he never could understand my addiction.

DR. N: I see. Did your mother and father get on well together?

MR. R: No, not really.

DR. N: What was the problem?

MR. R: I'm not sure. Only *they* know.

DR. N: Do you know what came between them?

33:00   MR. R: No.

DR. N: Did they argue?

MR. R: Oh, *constantly.*

DR. N: Did they ever split up?

MR. R: Not that I know of.

DR. N: What would they argue about?

MR. R: Money. Mostly money.

DR. N: I see. Did your mother ever attempt suicide after arguments with your father?

MR. R: Not that I know of.

DR. N: Umm. What about your brothers and sisters? Have any of them had any nervous problems?

MR. R: Oh, yes. Helen had a nervous breakdown. At least that's what *she* told *me,* now. Okay? And I know that it must have happened if she told me. She's never lied to me.

DR. N: Do you know what form the breakdown took?

MR. R: No, I don't. All I know is that it, too, is documented at —— of ——.

DR. N: Um-hmm.

MR. R: *Check* the clinics *there.* They have it on record. Helen R. appeared there, and if they don't, it didn't happen and she, *too,* must have lied to me.

34:00   DR. N: Yes. What about your other brothers and sister?

MR. R: Oh, yes. John. He too went to —— State Hospital in ——, Massachusetts, for whatever reason he was there for, I'm not sure. But he was there, too.

DR. N: I see. Is he well now?

MR. R: I believe he is. I don't know.

DR. N: Yes. Any other brothers or sisters had any problems?

MR. R: Not so far as I know of, but there's – you mean that they sought professional help?

DR. N: Yes.

MR. R: Not that I know of.

#17. Again, the history is unreliable, but the possibility of siblings with "nervous breakdowns," and parental alcoholism and/or depression, and suicide attempts in the mother raises the possibility that this is a schizophrenic reaction or major affective disorder. But no other interview data support the major

Revise hypotheses if fresh evidence warrants it, by adding and refining.
- *Notes family history suggests affective disorder vs. schizophrenic reaction*
- *Reconsiders paranoid schizophrenia complicated by toxic drug intake*

affective disorder. The possibility of a familial
pattern of drug/alcohol abuse may indicate or
support the possibility of this being a posttoxic
psychosis. But the strongest diagnostic impres-
sion is that of paranoid schizophrenia with
drugs and alcohol contributing to further
thought disruptions.

DR. N: Have any of your brothers and sisters had any addiction problems?

MR. R: Umm. Mark, my next one down as far as brothers go – no; Beth is placed between him – but Mark, well, he drinks. I don't know if he's an alcoholic or not. You see,
I don't know because he hasn't been cured, and I don't know if he's cured and I don't
know if he's strung out. All I know is he's still alive.

35:00 DR. N: I see. So, you were brought up mostly in Massachusetts, then, umm?

MR. R: Yes.

DR. N: But you lived in a number of other places?

MR. R: Yes.

DR. N: And you came to Vermont with your parents, perhaps, or is that why you came
here originally?

MR. R: No. Oh, yeah, I did. That's right. They moved first. I was in the halfway house,
——— House.

DR. N: Um-hmm.

MR. R: Okay. And when I got out of there, there were two people, ah, ———, and
———, who now reside in ———, Massachusetts, who kinda took me in. I don't know
why, I have no understanding of this. But I've always accepted them as my second set of
parents.

DR. N: I see.

MR. R: Okay? And I know deep down that they *love* me, too, just as they always *should*
have.

DR. N: How far did you go in school, Mr. R.?

MR. R: Ninth grade education.

36:00 DR. N: And what happened then? Did you . . .

MR. R: I was so strung out I couldn't, couldn't do anything but be a slave to drugs.

#18. The patient's vocabulary has been such
that he is at least normal and above normal in-
telligence. If this history of ninth grade educa-
tion is accurate, then it may reflect early
disruption of thinking or behaviors in such a
way that he could not continue in school.

Search for evidence to support or disconfirm the
hypotheses.
- *Notes school history as positive evidence for*
  early thought disorder
- *Implicitly evaluates chronic vs. reactive*
  psychosis

DR. N: I see. So you dropped out because of drugs at that time?

MR. R: Oh, yeah.

DR. N: What drugs were you on at that time?

MR. R: Amphetamines mostly.

DR. N: I see.

MR. R: And acid, or LSD, whichever way you want me to say it. LSD 25, whatever –
lysergic acid diethylamide, whichever.

DR. N: What jobs have you had since that time?

MR. R: Umm, since I dropped out of school?

DR. N: Yes.

MR. R: I'm not sure all of them. I know I've worked, you know, and I know every time I worked, my Social Security number went down. So, please, I can't assure you of 'em with just that number. Get my work records.

DR. N: What kind of work did you do usually?

37:00   MR. R: Just about anything manual, you know. Anything I had to do to become who I am, I guess.

DR. N: When was the last time you had a job?

MR. R: Umm. Oh, ———, ———, Vermont. I worked there for, happily, mind ya, for what, 3, 3½ months, then I did this to my wrist and they fired me because, "Hey, you're not supposed to be here."

DR. N: What were you doing there? What kind of work?

MR. R: Oh, I was a bucket setter in which, I can't describe it, but you take two rings, you set 'em down and, you know, the staves that go into a bucket? (*makes the hand movements of weaving cane*) They become a bucket.

DR. N: Okay. That's a very graphic description. All right. Umm, look, I want to change the subject a bit and ask a few routine questions . . .

MR. R: Surely.

DR. N: that I ask everybody I see.

MR. R: Okay.

DR. N: First of all, what's the date today?

MR. R: Fifteenth of June. (*correct*)

DR. N: Year?

38:00   MR. R: 1979. (*correct*)

DR. N: Where are you now?

MR. R: I'm sitting here in the studio in ———, Vermont.

DR. N: Right. Umm. I'm going to tell you a proverb. I'm sure you've done this before . . .

MR. R: Sure.

DR. N: . . . and I would like you to explain the meaning of this proverb to me in your own words.

MR. R: Okay, go ahead.

DR. N: Take this proverb: "A rolling stone gathers no moss"; have you heard that proverb before?

MR. R: Sure have.

DR. N: What does it mean?

MR. R: It means that if you continue to move and always move and always, always follow yourself though, don't follow anyone, you won't ever have a parasite grow on you. You will never have the evil one in you. Okay? And is that clear?

DR. N: That's clear. Excellent. Now, let me put another one to you.

MR. R: Okay.

DR. N: Umm, but tell me if you've heard it, because if you haven't heard it, it's meaningless: "People in glass houses should not throw stones." Have you heard that one?

MR. R: Sure have.

39:00   DR. N: Tell me what you think.

MR. R: It means that those who know what has been seen, I mean that they have done, and none has been seen, believe me, it's all been seen, they too shouldn't do it. Remember, "Let him who is without sin cast the first stone"?

#19. Response to the first two proverbs are personalized, partially concretized, partially abstracted, but highly personalized with some overinclusiveness and dissociated responses which compare fairly accurately with the interview data and support the diagnosis of a schizophrenic reaction.

Search for evidence to support or disconfirm the hypothesis.

* *Uses Mental Status Examination to support dissociation of thinking as positive evidence for schizophrenia*

DR. N: Um-hmm.

MR. R: Okay, that's what I believe it means.

DR. N: I must admit, I don't quite follow that. Let me put the question or proverb again and you explain it.

MR. R: *(inaudible)*

DR. N: ''People in glass houses should not throw stones.''

MR. R: Maybe it just means that people in glass houses who do throw stones ought to expect one to come back to shatter the glass that they live in.

DR. N: Um-hmm.

MR. R: Is that clear?

DR. N: Sort of retaliation?

MR. R: Um-hmm.

DR. N: Okay.

MR. R: Was that what you wanted?

40:00 DR. N: Fine. One more question. Umm, ''Strike while the iron is hot.'' What does that mean?

MR. R: It just means that while the moment is at hand, please, take what you must and do with it what you must.

DR. N: Good. Okay, let me ask you some questions about, oh, about calculations, first of all. How are you at figures?

MR. R: I don't know. I know basic math, but I . . .

DR. N: Taken 7 from 100.

MR. R: 93.

DR. N: Okay. Keep going back in 7's.

MR. R: Okay. I want your assurance that I'm right, if I'm not right. *(inaudible)*

DR. N: Yes. I'll tell you if you're not right.

MR. R: Okay. 93, 86,

DR. N: Yes.

MR. R: 79,

DR. N: Yes.

MR. R: 72,

DR. N: Yes.

MR. R: 65? 65.

DR. N: That's, that's correct. Okay. Just a few other questions about the general situation. Who's the president now?

MR. R: Carter.

DR. N: And, can you tell me who the previous three Presidents have been?

41:00 MR. R: Gerald Ford.

DR. N: Yes.

MR. R: Richard Nixon.

DR. N: Right.

MR. R: Lyndon Baines Johnson.

DR. N: Fine. Okay. And before that?

MR. R: John Fitzgerald Kennedy . . .

DR. N: Good. How many . . .

MR. R: Dwight D. Eisenhower before that,

DR. N: Right.

MR. R: Harry Truman before that,

DR. N: Keep going.

MR. R: Franklin Delano Roosevelt before him.

DR. N: Yes.

MR. R: That's all I *need* to say. I *know* what I *know.*

DR. N: You're doing pretty well. How far back could you go beyond that?

MR. R: I don't know.

DR. N: Who was before Roosevelt, do you recall?

MR. R: Umm, before Roosevelt? Now, you see, when I don't *need* to know, I *won't* know.

DR. N: All right. He's a bit before your time, I think, huh?

MR. R: Oh, he sure was, now you know for a fact I was born January 1st, 1955, but I am here on time again, people (*turns to the camera*). Let's hope *you* all are.

DR. N: Okay. You feel this time you're on time?

42:00   MR. R: Oh, yes. I just hope the rest of the world is ready 'cause I don't want to have to walk out of here to die, and you know that, too. I don't understand it, I'll *never* understand why anyone has to die.

DR. N: You mean you have to die when you leave here?

MR. R: It's not that I *have* to. I don't *fear* it, okay? And I *don't* have to.

DR. N: No.

MR. R: Right?

DR.N: No. You don't have to.

MR. R: *You know* I don't and *I* know I don't, now let's hope *everybody else* gets the message.

DR. N: But you're concerned that you might be crucified when you leave here?

MR. R: Oh, no. I know I won't be crucified again.

DR. N: What do you plan to do, then. What do you think will happen when you . . .

MR. R: When I leave here? I'll go to school. I'll become a *psychiatrist.*

DR. N: And then what will you do with that knowledge?

MR. R: I'll cure the people that I trust with that knowledge.

DR. N: And you decided to do that only recently, since you've been in the hospital?

43:00   MR. R: No, that was something that kinda came to me a little at a time, you know; I've been through all the institutions and things as you know; I well just kinda, well, that's what I want to do now. And in my heart, I will do it if I am allowed to leave here when Paul comes for me.

DR. N: Okay. Do you have any other plans beyond that?

MR. R: No, none at all.

DR. N: How are things going for you in the hospital? Are people cooperating here?

MR. R: They sure are.

DR. N: The staff are cooperative?

MR. R: They sure are.

DR. N: Okay. I think we should now – I should ask you – if you have any questions you'd like to ask me before we close, because our time is drawing short.

MR. R: Okay, can you believe all that you've been *led* to believe?

DR. N: By you?

MR. R: Yeah, by me.

DR. N: Yes, I do. I believe you've told me the truth.

MR. R: Okay. Let *no one* deceive you, including *me*.

DR. N: I could have no doubt of your integrity.

44:00 MR. R: And when the time comes, you, too, in your own *heart* will deliver me a *Bible*, I won't deliver it to you, and *you* will get your final message just as surely as *anybody* who will watch this tape and see my *face*. When the time comes, they will hand it to *me* and I'll read it to *them*, too, okay?

DR. N: What we should do now, I think, is to both of us look at this tape and see if you think it's okay.

MR. R: I know it will be, so long as your *camera* is what it should be.

DR. N: The camera will be okay.

MR. R: Okay, and you know you're seeing me do this, right.

DR. N: Yes.

MR. R: Okay, well, can we witness what . . .

44:28 DR. N: Thank you very much.

#20. The tentative diagnosis is paranoid schizophrenia, chronic, with toxic factors or other organic factors to be ruled out by appropriate tests for organicity. The plans, as stated earlier, are to develop a relationship with the patient, to gather data from all other possible sources, and engage whatever social support system the patient has to structure his life to prevent recurrent hospitalizations, perhaps maximize his capacity for relating to others. The sense of playfulness at the end of the tape raises the possibility that this is a man who still is malingering. This can only be ruled out by observing him with friends and in situations in which he feels he does not have to put on a front of "craziness."

1. *Reach a conclusion about which hypothesis is best supported by the evidence.*
2. *Formulate a comprehensive diagnosis.*
   - *Concludes with a strong provisional diagnosis and a differential*
     a. *Provisional: paranoid schizophrenia, chronic.*
     b. *Differential: Rule out toxic factors and other organic factors.*
     c. *Test for malingering.*
3. *Design a management plan based on goals derived from the comprehensive diagnosis.*
   - *Proposes a two-part plan:*
     a. *Inquiry.*
        a. *Other family information.*
        b. *Tests of biologic function.*
     b. *Management.*
        a. *Engage social support systems.*
        b. *Maximize relating to others.*

Tactics of an experienced clinician's reasoning: a flowchart (Figure I.1)

The flowchart illustrated in Figure I.1 provides a graphic summary of the interactions among evidence, inquiry, and hypothesis-testing in Dr. McKegney's

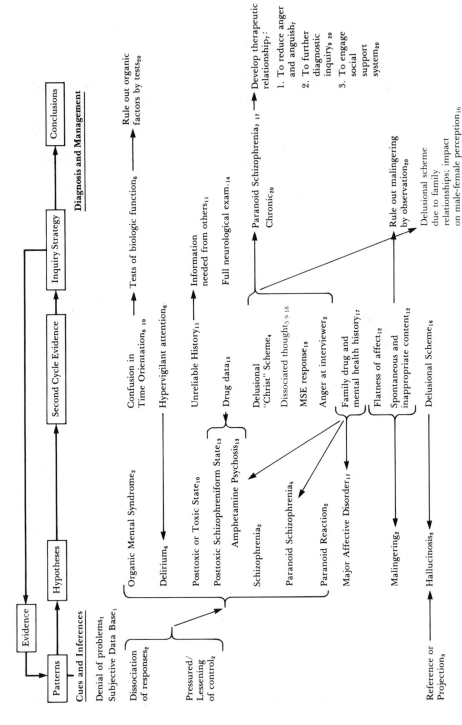

FIGURE I.1

Tactics of an experienced clinician's reasoning: a flowchart

658

diagnosis of the case of Mr. R. This format is similar to the flowchart illustrated in chapter 27 (Figures 27.7 and 27.8), where it was recommended as a teaching technique. Figure 27.8 contains the group deliberations of a class of medical students who analyzed the videotaped case of Mr. R. In this appendix, Figure I.1 displays the content of the same process as it appears in Dr. McKegney's type-scripted responses.

To understand this figure fully, the reader should be aware of these flowchart characteristics:

1. The flowchart's major categories are designated in boxes across the top of the chart. They include patterns (cues and inferences), hypotheses, second-cycle evidence, inquiry strategy, and conclusions (diagnosis and management). Arrows indicate a flow of interaction among these categories. Relevant units of information present in Dr. McKegney's comments are grouped below the appropriate category.

2. Numerical subscripts following each unit of information indicate the response number of Dr. McKegney's comments in the typescript. The reader can thus refer to the original typescript in this appendix to verify the context of the information.

3. Arrows are drawn within the flowchart to indicate directional impact when a unit of information affects decision-making regarding a unit of information in another category. For example, reference or projection is a pattern that clearly contributes to the generation of the hypothesis, *hallucinosis*, from response #3. *Flatness of affect* and *spontaneous and inappropriate content* (second-cycle evidence) in response #12 are used to rule out malingering as an active hypothesis.

4. The reader should follow the flowchart from left to right to observe the evidence involved in the development of a hypothesis, its validation, and the conclusion whether to accept or reject it. The reader can thus evaluate the accumulation of evidence throughout the videotaped case leading to the final diagnostic decision(s).

The reader can study similarities and differences in the diagnostic reasoning of novices versus experienced clinicians by comparing Figures 27.8 and I.1.

Hypothesis tracing by an experienced clinician (Figure I.2)

Figure I.2 presents a schematic form of hypothesis-tracing. By referring to this figure, the reader can follow the generation and evaluation of each hypothesis mentioned by Dr. McKegney during the course of his observation of the videotaped case of Mr. R.

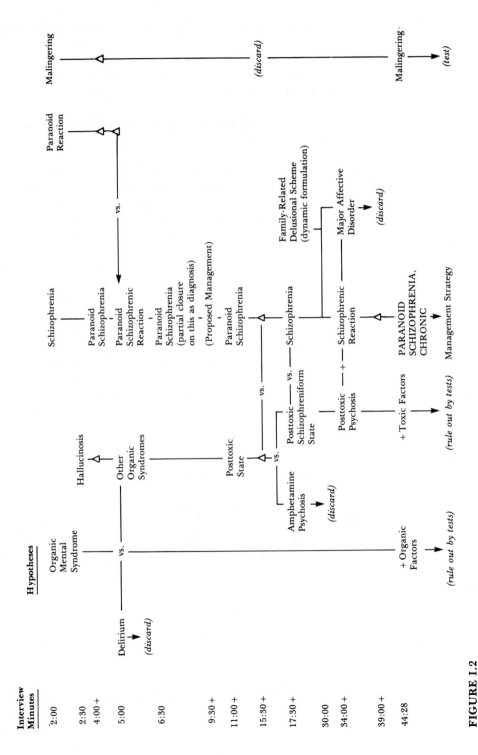

FIGURE I.2
Case of Mr. R. Hypothesis tracing by an experienced clinician

660

The figure is designed to display specific information in matrix form:

1. The number of videotape minutes and seconds elapsed at the time Dr. McKegney considered any diagnostic hypothesis is listed in sequence on the left vertical axis.

2. The discrete hypotheses Dr. McKegney generated are arrayed by categorical name on a horizontal axis beginning at the top of the figure. The reader can follow each hypothesis from generation to acceptance or rejection, by reading downward on the vertical axis.

    Each time a hypothesis is modified, the new categorical hypothesis is specified on the vertical axis. If the hypothesis is simply reviewed, a triangle codes the review. The reader can note the timing of each consideration by referring to the minutes designated on the parallel axis to the left.

    For example, *organic mental syndrome, schizophrenia, paranoid reaction,* and *malingering* all appear at 2:00 minutes during Dr. McKegney's second response. While following this category through the time sequence, the reader will see that various forms of *schizophrenia* are considered during the 45-minute videotape.

3. Subordinate (more specific) categorical hypotheses that have been derived from superordinate (more general) hypotheses are shown by an hierarchical-branching line on the vertical axis of the original hypothesis.

    For example, *organic mental syndrome* is refined to include *delirium* (5:00 minutes); later in the same family of hypotheses, *posttoxic state* (11:00 + minutes) is subdivided into *amphetamine psychosis* and *posttoxic schizophreniform state* (17:30 + minutes).

4. Contrasting hypotheses are indicated by a connecting line and the term *versus* (vs.); *in addition to* is indicated by a plus sign (+).

    For example, *paranoid reaction* is specifically combined with schizophrenic reaction at 5:00 minutes, and *schizophrenic reaction* is contrasted with *major affective disorder* at 34:00 + minutes.

5. Decisions regarding the outcome of specific hypotheses are indicated by comments enclosed in brackets; these include conclusions to discard, rule out, and proposed management.

6. The major diagnosis is indicated in upper-case letters, and two differential diagnoses are noted with the term *plus* (+) at 44:28 minutes. Proposed management strategies, including further inquiry, are specified beneath each diagnosis.

Conclusion

The following comments summarize Dr. McKegney's diagnostic reasoning for the case of Mr. R.:

1. He considers two families of diagnoses: *functional* and *organic psychosis*. All hypotheses are implicitly adumbrated by these two groups (responses #2, 6, 10, 13, and 17).

    He generates the first hypotheses very early, at 2 minutes. As the interview proceeds, he refines major hypotheses in more explicit categorical terms, specifying subordinate hypotheses in each diagnostic family (responses #3, 6, 10, and 13; responses #5 and 20).

2. He implicitly contrasts *chronic* and *reactive psychoses* (responses #13 and 18). He evaluates the role of toxic drugs both in precipitating *reactive psychosis* and in contributing to the recurrence of a chronic disorder. This evaluation can be observed in the latter part of the interview (response #17), as he suggests that the patient's *posttoxic state* may have contributed to the *schizophrenic behavior* seen in the interview.

3. He regularly evaluates the objectivity and reliability of the patient's responses (responses #1, 11, 14, 15, 16, and 17). Finding contradictions and confusion in these responses, he suggests the immediate establishment of a therapeutic relationship to relieve the patient of some of the more serious characteristics of his behavior, such as anguish and anxiety (response #7). Dr. McKegney does not, however, engage in premature closure. He avoids this by continuing to consider other hypotheses and by stating that a therapeutic relationship could aid further diagnostic inquiry (response #9).

Dr. McKegney's reasoning is an excellent example of hypothetico-deductive thought. He systematically generates and tests multiple diagnostic hypotheses. As the case progresses, he uses fresh evidence to evaluate these hypotheses, revising and refining them as new information becomes available. He uses the tactics that are set forth in this textbook in a natural and efficient manner. His strategy is also consistent with that recommended in this book.

Finally, Dr. McKegney differs from the novice clinician in particular ways that seem to be a function of knowledge and experience:

1. He moves from cues to inferences immediately. Most of his hypothetico-deductive reasoning is based on higher-level inferences rather than on concrete cues; however, he regularly tests the validity of the inferences.

2. He generates an array of hypotheses relatively early in the interview.

3. By choice, he places a somewhat greater emphasis on management than on inquiry in this particular patient. His rationale for doing so is implicit in his comments questioning the validity of the patient's responses. This does not, however, diminish his efforts systematically to analyze the patient's disorder.

II

Child and Adolescent Mental Status Rating Scales

Rating

Each of the following items represents a phenomenon or set of phenomena that could be important to diagnosis. When evaluating the item, the rater should keep in mind the norm for other subjects of the same age, social class, and ethnicity.

Apart from height and weight, the intensity of each item in sections A and B is to be rated on a four-point scale: 0 (not present), 1 (uncertain or doubtful), 2 (mildly or moderately evident), and 3 (markedly evident). If an item is rated 2 or 3, the interviewer should give details under the heading *Describe*. If uncertain, the interviewer should score 1, give details, and check at a later date, if possible.

The items in section C (12) represent fantasy themes and are to be rated 0 (absent) or 1 (present).

Glossary

The glossary in appendix III defines each item in the scale.

Rating scales

A. Appearance and behavior

	Not Present	Doubtful	Moderate	Marked
1. Appearance				
1.1 Height _____ cm _____ percentile	0	1	2	3
1.2 Weight _____ kg _____ percentile				
1.3 Precocious physical maturation	0	1	2	3
*Describe:*_____				
1.4 Delayed physical maturation	0	1	2	3
*Describe:*_____				
1.5 Abnormality of skin	0	1	2	3
*Describe:*_____				
1.6 Abnormality of head, facies, or mouth	0	1	2	3
*Describe:*_____				
1.7 Abnormality of physique	0	1	2	3
*Describe:*_____				
1.8 Lack of personal hygiene	0	1	2	3
*Describe:*_____				
1.9 Untidiness of dress	0	1	2	3
*Describe:*_____				
1.10 Inappropriateness of dress	0	1	2	3
*Describe:*_____				
1.11 Attachment to inanimate object	0	1	2	3
*Describe:*_____				
1.12 Other abnormality of appearance	0	1	2	3
*Describe:*_____				

		Not Present	Doubtful	Moderate	Marked
2. Motor behavior					
2.1	Hyperkinesis	0	1	2	3
	Describe:				
2.2	Hypokinesis	0	1	2	3
	Describe:				
2.3	Bradykinesis	0	1	2	3
	Describe:				
2.4	Abnormality of posture	0	1	2	3
	Describe:				
2.5	Abnormality of gait	0	1	2	3
	Describe:				
2.6	Impairment of balance	0	1	2	3
	Describe:				
2.7	Impairment of coordination	0	1	2	3
	Describe:				
2.8	Impairment of power	0	1	2	3
	Describe:				
2.9	Abnormality of tone	0	1	2	3
	Describe:				
Abnormal movements					
2.10	Tremor	0	1	2	3
	Describe:				
2.11	Twitching	0	1	2	3
	Describe:				

		Not Present	*Doubtful*	*Moderate*	*Marked*
2.12	Tics	0	1	2	3
	Describe:				
2.13	Fidgeting	0	1	2	3
	Describe:				
2.14	Choreiform movements	0	1	2	3
	Describe:				
2.15	Athetoid movements	0	1	2	3
	Describe:				
2.16	Ballismus	0	1	2	3
	Describe:				
2.17	Mirror movements and motor overflow	0	1	2	3
	Describe:				
2.18	Motor impersistence	0	1	2	3
	Describe:				
2.19	Torticollis	0	1	2	3
	Describe:				
2.20	Pronounced startle response	0	1	2	3
	Describe:				
2.21	Mannerisms	0	1	2	3
	Describe:				
2.22	Rituals	0	1	2	3
	Describe:				

		Not Present	Doubtful	Moderate	Marked
2.23	Echopraxia	0	1	2	3
	Describe:_____				
2.24	Stereotyped movements	0	1	2	3
	Describe:_____				
2.25	Repetitive habits	0	1	2	3
	Describe:_____				
2.26	Lack of sphincter control	0	1	2	3
	Describe:_____				
2.27	Self-mutilation	0	1	2	3
	Describe:_____				
2.28	Other abnormality of motor behavior	0	1	2	3
	Describe:_____				

3. Sensation

3.1	Abnormality of somatic sensation	0	1	2	3
	Describe:_____				
3.2	Itching or paresthesia	0	1	2	3
	Describe:_____				
3.3	Synesthesia	0	1	2	3
	Describe:_____				
3.4	Abnormality of special sense	0	1	2	3
	Describe:_____				

		Not Present	Doubtful	Moderate	Marked
3.5	Abnormality of body image	0	1	2	3
	Describe:_____				
3.6	Abnormality of time sense	0	1	2	3
	Describe:_____				

4. Voice, speech, and language

4.1	Absence of speech	0	1	2	3
	Describe:_____				
4.2	Unusual accent	0	1	2	3
	Describe:_____				
4.3	Abnormality of amplitude	0	1	2	3
	Describe:_____				
4.4	Abnormality of pitch or tone	0	1	2	3
	Describe:_____				
4.5	Abnormality of tempo	0	1	2	3
	Describe:_____				
4.6	Abnormality of phonation	0	1	2	3
	Describe:_____				
4.7	Abnormality of rhythm	0	1	2	3
	Describe:_____				
4.8	Abnormality of articulation	0	1	2	3
	Describe:_____				
4.9	Abnormal use of words	0	1	2	3
	Describe:_____				

	Not Present	Doubtful	Moderate	Marked
4.10 Obscenity or profanity	0	1	2	3
Describe:				
4.11 Abnormality of syntax	0	1	2	3
Describe:				
4.12 Babbling	0	1	2	3
Describe:				
4.13 Idioglossia	0	1	2	3
Describe:				
4.14 Echolalia	0	1	2	3
Describe:				
4.15 Impairment of expressive language	0	1	2	3
Describe:				
4.16 Impairment of comprehension	0	1	2	3
Describe:				
4.17 Talks to self in public	0	1	2	3
Describe:				
4.18 Other abnormality of voice, speech, or language	0	1	2	3
Describe:				

5. Interaction with interviewer

	Not Present	Doubtful	Moderate	Marked
5.1 Aversion of gaze	0	1	2	3
Describe:				
5.2 Distant focus of gaze	0	1	2	3
Describe:				

		Not Present	Doubtful	Moderate	Marked
5.3	Staring	0	1	2	3
	Describe:				
5.4	Unresponsive	0	1	2	3
	Describe:				
5.5	Tense	0	1	2	3
	Describe:				
5.6	Impulsive	0	1	2	3
	Describe:				
5.7	Other abnormality of interaction	0	1	2	3
	Describe:				

B. Inferences about attitudes, affect, cognition, and thought

6. Relationship to interviewer

		Not Present	Doubtful	Moderate	Marked
6.1	Bewildered	0	1	2	3
	Describe:				
6.2	Boastful	0	1	2	3
	Describe:				
6.3	Clinging	0	1	2	3
	Describe:				
6.4	Clowning	0	1	2	3
	Describe:				
6.5	Demanding	0	1	2	3
	Describe:				

		Not Present	Doubtful	Moderate	Marked
6.6	Evasive *Describe:*	0	1	2	3
6.7	Fearful *Describe:*	0	1	2	3
6.8	Hostile *Describe:*	0	1	2	3
6.9	Impudent *Describe:*	0	1	2	3
6.10	Indifferent *Describe:*	0	1	2	3
6.11	Ingratiating *Describe:*	0	1	2	3
6.12	Invasive *Describe:*	0	1	2	3
6.13	Loquacious *Describe:*	0	1	2	3
6.14	Overcompliant *Describe:*	0	1	2	3
6.15	Preoccupied *Describe:*	0	1	2	3
6.16	Seductive *Describe:*	0	1	2	3

		Not Present	Doubtful	Moderate	Marked
6.17	Shy	0	1	2	3
	Describe:				
6.18	Suggestible	0	1	2	3
	Describe:				
6.19	Suspicious	0	1	2	3
	Describe:				
6.20	Uncooperative	0	1	2	3
	Describe:				
6.21	Withdrawn	0	1	2	3
	Describe:				
6.22	Other characteristic of interaction	0	1	2	3
	Describe:				

7. Affect and mood

		Not Present	Doubtful	Moderate	Marked
7.1	Anger	0	1	2	3
	Describe:				
7.2	Anhedonic	0	1	2	3
	Describe:				
7.3	Anxious	0	1	2	3
	Describe:				
7.4	Apathetic	0	1	2	3
	Describe:				
7.5	Depressed	0	1	2	3
	Describe:				

			Not Present	Doubtful	Moderate	Marked
7.6	Euphoric		0	1	2	3
	Describe:					
7.7	Flat affect		0	1	2	3
	Describe:					
7.8	Guilty		0	1	2	3
	Describe:					
7.9	Histrionic		0	1	2	3
	Describe:					
7.10	Inappropriate affect		0	1	2	3
	Describe:					
7.11	Labile affect		0	1	2	3
	Describe:					
7.12	Resigned		0	1	2	3
	Describe:					
7.13	Restricted affect		0	1	2	3
	Describe:					
7.14	Silly		0	1	2	3
	Describe:					
7.15	Other abnormality of affect or mood		0	1	2	3
	Describe:					

8. Information processing
8.1	Disoriented		0	1	2	3
	Describe:					

			Not Present	Doubtful	Moderate	Marked
8.2	Inattentive		0	1	2	3
	Describe:					
8.3	Distractible		0	1	2	3
	Describe:					
8.4	Impairment of recent memory		0	1	2	3
	Describe:					
8.5	Impairment of remote memory		0	1	2	3
	Describe:					
8.6	Deficiency in general knowledge		0	1	2	3
	Describe:					
8.7	Impairment of comprehension		0	1	2	3
	Describe:					
8.8	Impairment of spatial reasoning		0	1	2	3
	Describe:					
8.9	Impairment of social judgment		0	1	2	3
	Describe:					
8.10	Impairment of conceptual capacity		0	1	2	3
	Describe:					

9. Thought processes
  9.1 Blocking   0   1   2   3
    Describe:

		Not Present	Doubtful	Moderate	Marked
9.2	Circumlocution	0	1	2	3
	Describe:				
9.3	Circumstantiality	0	1	2	3
	Describe:				
9.4	Concretistic thinking	0	1	2	3
	Describe:				
9.5	Defect in memory	0	1	2	3
	Describe:				
9.6	Distractibility	0	1	2	3
	Describe:				
9.7	Flight of ideas	0	1	2	3
	Describe:				
9.8	Incoherence	0	1	2	3
	Describe:				
9.9	Looseness of associations	0	1	2	3
	Describe:				
9.10	Paralogia	0	1	2	3
	Describe:				
9.11	Perseveration	0	1	2	3
	Describe:				
9.12	Poverty of thought	0	1	2	3
	Describe:				

	Not Present	Doubtful	Moderate	Marked
9.13 Slowing of thought *Describe:*	0	1	2	3
9.14 Tangential thinking *Describe:*	0	1	2	3
9.15 Other disturbance in thought processes *Describe:*	0	1	2	3

10. Thought content

	Not Present	Doubtful	Moderate	Marked
10.1 Anergia *Describe:*	0	1	2	3
10.2 Compulsion *Describe:*	0	1	2	3
10.3 Confabulation *Describe:*	0	1	2	3
10.4 Déjà vu *Describe:*	0	1	2	3
10.5 Delusion *Describe:*	0	1	2	3
10.6 Depersonalization *Describe:*	0	1	2	3
10.7 Derealization *Describe:*	0	1	2	3

		Not Present	Doubtful	Moderate	Marked
10.8	Dissociation	0	1	2	3
	Describe:_____				
10.9	Fabrication	0	1	2	3
	Describe:_____				
10.10	Hallucination	0	1	2	3
	Describe:_____				
10.11	Illusion	0	1	2	3
	Describe:_____				
10.12	Impulsion	0	1	2	3
	Describe:_____				
10.13	Malingering	0	1	2	3
	Describe:_____				
10.14	Obsession	0	1	2	3
	Describe:_____				
10.15	Phobia	0	1	2	3
	Describe:_____				
10.16	Preoccupation with identity issues	0	1	2	3
	Describe:_____				
10.17	Preoccupation with own mental functioning	0	1	2	3
	Describe:_____				
10.18	Preoccupation with past or future	0	1	2	3
	Describe:_____				

			Not Present	Doubtful	Moderate	Marked
10.19	Preoccupation with personal competence		0	1	2	3
	Describe:					
10.20	Self-consciousness		0	1	2	3
	Describe:					
10.21	Suicidal ideation		0	1	2	3
	Describe:					
10.22	Trance state		0	1	2	3
	Describe:					

C. Fantasy

11. Quality of fantasy

		Not Present	Doubtful	Moderate	Marked
11.1	Bizarreness	0	1	2	3
	Describe:				
11.2	Decreased productivity	0	1	2	3
	Describe:				
11.3	Increased productivity	0	1	2	3
	Describe:				

12. Salient themes in fantasy

		Absent	Present
12.1	Achievement	0	1
	Describe:		
12.2	Acquisition	0	1
	Describe:		

			Absent	*Present*
12.3	Affiliation		0	1
	Describe:			
12.4	Affliction		0	1
	Describe:			
12.5	Aggression		0	1
	Describe:			
12.6	Alienation		0	1
	Describe:			
12.7	Antisocial		0	1
	Describe:			
12.8	Anxiety		0	1
	Describe:			
12.9	Autonomy		0	1
	Describe:			
12.10	Avoidance of blame		0	1
	Describe:			
12.11	Change		0	1
	Describe:			
12.12	Compensation		0	1
	Describe:			
12.13	Conflict		0	1
	Describe:			
12.14	Creativity		0	1
	Describe:			

	Absent	Present
12.15 Curiosity	0	1
Describe: _____		
12.16 Death	0	1
Describe: _____		
12.17 Deference	0	1
Describe: _____		
12.18 Dominance	0	1
Describe: _____		
12.19 Exhibition	0	1
Describe: _____		
12.20 Exposition	0	1
Describe: _____		
12.21 Fantasy	0	1
Describe: _____		
12.22 Failure	0	1
Describe: _____		
12.23 Guilt	0	1
Describe: _____		
12.24 Injury	0	1
Describe: _____		
12.25 Inferiority	0	1
Describe: _____		
12.26 Lack	0	1
Describe: _____		

		Absent	*Present*
12.27	Loneliness	0	1
	*Describe:*_____		
12.28	Loss	0	1
	*Describe:*_____		
12.29	Nurturance	0	1
	*Describe:*_____		
12.30	Optimism	0	1
	*Describe:*_____		
12.31	Pessimism	0	1
	*Describe:*_____		
12.32	Play	0	1
	*Describe:*_____		
12.33	Preoccupation with body function	0	1
	*Describe:*_____		
12.34	Preoccupation with mental function	0	1
	*Describe:*_____		
12.35	Recognition	0	1
	*Describe:*_____		
12.36	Rejection	0	1
	*Describe:*_____		
12.37	Relaxation	0	1
	*Describe:*_____		
12.38	Resignation	0	1
	*Describe:*_____		

		Absent	Present
12.39	Retention	0	1
	*Describe:*_____		
	_____		
	_____		
12.40	Revenge	0	1
	*Describe:*_____		
	_____		
	_____		
12.41	Seclusion	0	1
	*Describe:*_____		
	_____		
	_____		
12.42	Self-pity	0	1
	*Describe:*_____		
	_____		
	_____		
12.43	Sexuality	0	1
	*Describe:*_____		
	_____		
	_____		
12.44	Shame	0	1
	*Describe:*_____		
	_____		
	_____		
12.45	Succor	0	1
	*Describe:*_____		
	_____		
	_____		
12.46	Suicide	0	1
	*Describe:*_____		
	_____		
	_____		
12.47	Understanding	0	1
	*Describe:*_____		
	_____		
	_____		
12.48	Vindication	0	1
	*Describe:*_____		
	_____		
	_____		
12.49	Other salient theme	0	1
	*Describe:*_____		
	_____		
	_____		

D. Insight

			Not Present	Doubtful	Moderate	Marked

13. Insight

13.1 Lack of understanding of reason for interview   0   1   2   3
    *Describe:*_____
    _____
    _____

13.2 Lack of understanding of nature of problems   0   1   2   3
    *Describe:*_____
    _____
    _____

13.3 Lack of desire for help   0   1   2   3
    *Describe:*_____
    _____
    _____

III

Glossary for the Child and Adolescent Mental Status Rating Scales

A. Appearance and behavior

1. Appearance
   1.1 Height _____ cm _____ percentile
   1.2 Weight _____ cm _____ percentile
   1.3 *Precocious physical maturation:* Above the 10th percentile in height, with muscular development and other primary and secondary sexual development characteristic of an older child of the same sex.
   1.4 *Delayed physical maturation:* Below the 10th percentile in height, with physical proportions and primary and secondary sexual development characteristic of a younger child of the same sex.
   1.5 *Abnormality of skin:* Scar, rash, or other abnormality of exposed skin surface other than the face.
   1.6 *Abnormality of head, facies, or mouth:* Scar, rash, baldness, dental caries, deformity, asymmetry, or other abnormality of head, facies, or mouth.
   1.7 *Abnormality of physique:* Deformity, asymmetry, or other abnormality of body or limbs.

1.8 *Lack of personal hygiene:* Unclean skin, hair, and clothes; poor grooming; unclean teeth and/or mouth or odor suggesting inadequate attention to hygiene.

1.9 *Untidiness of dress:* Ill-fitting, unkempt costume; for example, with buttons or laces undone and shirt hanging out.

1.10 *Inappropriateness of dress:* Wears clothing unsuited to or socially out of keeping with the situation in that it is more formal, casual, or revealing than would be expected, or more appropriate for a person of the opposite sex.

1.11 *Attachment to inanimate object:* Carries and may resist the removal of a particular object or objects, such as a doll, rubber pipe, or piece of string.

1.12 *Other abnormality of appearance*

2. Motor behavior

2.1 *Hyperkinesis:* Restless. Has difficulty sitting for longer than a few minutes. Moves around the room, going from object to object, at a rate that may vary from moderately overactive to tumultuous.

2.2 *Hypokinesis:* Underactive. Sits or lies down. Makes little attempt to explore the surroundings.

2.3 *Bradykinesis:* Perceptible slowing of all movement.

2.4 *Abnormality of posture:* Stands, sits or lies in an unusual physical position; for example, stooping; swayback; with bilateral, unilateral, or localized stiffness; or with lack of tone.

2.5 *Abnormality of gait:* Walks in an unusual way; for example, on a wide base, with high steps, on tiptoe, circumducting one leg, limping, or stiff-legged.

2.6 *Abnormality of balance:* Tends to topple over when pushed or bumped or when upright with eyes closed. May be unable to remain upright with eyes open.

2.7 *Abnormality of coordination:* Lacks dexterity in executing gross or fine movements. Has more difficulty than would be expected in a child of that age; for example, in dressing, tying laces, doing buttons, using a pencil, hopping, catching or throwing a ball.

2.8 *Impairment of power:* General, local, or regional muscular weakness or paralysis.

2.9 *Abnormality of tone:* Bilateral, unilateral, or regional increase or decrease of muscle tone, associated with stiffness or flaccidity.

2.10 *Tremor:* A persistent, rhythmical, coarse or fine movement usually of the head, mouth, tongue or outstretched hands and fingers.

2.11 *Twitching:* The sudden involuntary fasciculation of a muscle or part thereof, particularly around the eyes or mouth, in the cheek, or in the upper extremities.

2.12 *Tics:* The intermittent repetitive, involuntary, purposeless contraction of a circumscribed muscle group, particularly in the eyes, face, vocal cords, head, neck, or shoulders. Can be inhibited voluntarily, but not completely; and can often be demonstrated by the patient at will.

2.13 *Fidgeting:* Squirminess. Inability to sit still without constant, diffuse, random, fine, spasmodic, or wriggling movement.

2.14 *Choreiform movements:* Sudden, unpredictable, phasic, arrhythmic, and purposeless contraction of different groups of muscles producing displacement of body parts, especially face, tongue, and extremities. Increased in stress and diminished in repose. Cannot be voluntarily inhibited, but the subject may attempt to conceal movements by merging them into common gesture of grooming or postural adjustment.

2.15 *Athetoid movements:*   Constant, repetitive, involuntary, slow, writhing movements of limbs and/or trunk.

2.16 *Ballismus:*   Persistent, involuntary, wild jactitations, usually of one limb or one side of the body.

2.17 *Mirror movements and motor overflow:*   Involuntary, adventitious, symmetrical movements that appear with lesser amplitude in an extremity that is opposite one in volitional movement, or that appear in the tongue and mouth when the subject is involved in a concentrated manual operation, such as writing.

2.18 *Motor impersistence:*   The inability of a child over 7 years of age to maintain any of the following fixed postures for more than 20 seconds: keeping the eyes closed, protruding the tongue, or keeping the mouth open.

2.19 *Torticollis:*   Wry-neck; the involuntary contraction of neck muscles, producing a fixed lateral rotation and flexion of the head.

2.20 *Pronounced startle response:*   The subject is surprised by sudden stimuli, especially noises, and responds with spasmodic movement and autonomic discharge.

2.21 *Mannerisms:*   Characteristic, repetitive, purposeful, automatic but controllable actions usually involving speech, gesture, or grooming movements; for example: stroking the forelock, pulling the earlobe, clearing the throat. Often accentuated at times of tension, such as during a public exhibition.

2.22 *Rituals:*   Repetitive activities of which the subject is consciously aware, usually undertaken at a special time such as going to bed, for the purpose of self-consolation, atonement, or warding off misfortune.

2.23 *Echopraxia:*   A tendency to imitate the interviewer's gestures, movements, or actions.

2.24 *Stereotyped movements:*   Fragments of actions, or fully executed, repetitive actions, the purpose of which is obscure or symbolic or related to stimulus deprivation due to blindness, deafness, or mental retardation.

2.25 *Repetitive habits:*   Nail-biting, finger-sucking, nose-picking, lip-chewing, lip-licking, hair- or eyebrow-pulling, object sucking, object smelling, pica, picking, masturbation, scratching, head-rocking, body-rocking, humming, or yawning.

2.26 *Lack of sphincter control:*   Passes gas or needs to go to the toilet during the interview. Loses control of bladder or bowel during the interview.

2.27 *Self-mutilation:*   Damages or mutilates the skin by self-inflicted cutting, lacerating, tattooing, bruising, or damaging with chemicals.

2.28 *Other abnormality of motor behavior*

3. Sensation

   3.1 *Abnormality of somatic sensation:*   Generally or regionally deficient, absent, or accentuated temperature, pain, touch, deep pressure, or position sensation.

   3.2 *Itching or paresthesia:*   A superficial itching or tingling sensation that may be persistent or intermittent and fixed or shifting in location.

   3.3 *Synesthesia:*   A perceptual response in one sensory modality as a result of the stimulation of another sensory modality; for example, seeing colors while listening to music.

   3.4 *Abnormality of special sense:*   Absent, deficient, altered, or accentuated sense of hearing, vision, olfaction, or taste.

   3.5 *Abnormality of body image:*   Absent, deficient, exaggerated, or aberrant sense of body image.

3.6 *Abnormality of time sense:* A disruption of the perception of time involving slowing, acceleration, alternation, or other distortion.

4. Voice, speech, and language
   4.1 *Absence of speech:* Little or no speech detected during the interview.
   4.2 *Unusual accent:* Has an idiosyncratic or ethnic mode of pronunciation and idiom that would be unusual in the peer group with whom the subject is associated.
   4.3 *Abnormality of amplitude:* Abnormally quiet or loud voice throughout the interview.
   4.4 *Abnormality of pitch or tone:* Unusually deep or high-pitched speech or unusually modulated speech; for example: croaking, squeaking, squawking, piping, falsetto, or monotone.
   4.5 *Abnormality of tempo:* Decelerated or accelerated speech, characteristic of the subject throughout the interview.
   4.6 *Abnormality of phonation:* Absent, weak, or deviant phonation; for example: whispering, hoarseness, nasality, or whining.
   4.7 *Abnormality of rhythm:* Irregularity of vocal rhythm and meter, leading to hesitancy, syllable or word repetition, stuttering, cluttering, slurring, or scanning speech.
   4.8 *Abnormality of articulation:* Indistinct enunciation of speech due to the elision, insertion, omission, or substitution of sounds; for example: lisping, burring, lalling, or infantile speech.
   4.9 *Abnormal use of words:* A tendency to use words in an unusual or inappropriate way that is more than an incidental slip of the tongue; for example: malapropisms, metaphoric language, neologisms, punning, rhyming associations, and pronominal reversal.
   4.10 *Obscenity or profanity:* Swearing or blaspheming. May be incidental and stylistic or associated with antagonism to the interviewer.
   4.11 *Abnormality of syntax:* Consistent grammatical errors; for example in tense, case, or number. Often encountered as an aspect of infantile language pattern, in association with articulation defect, or in foreign or nonstandard speech and grammar.
   4.12 *Babbling:* Infantile vocalization, often of repetitive nature, that may have the intonation of speech but contains no recognizable language pattern.
   4.13 *Idioglossia:* Aberrant language that has communicative content but is idiosyncratic in vocabulary and syntax. Usually understood only by a parent or sibling.
   4.14 *Echolalia:* The tendency to repeat the interviewer's words, especially the last word or phrase in a question or comment.
   4.15 *Impairment of expressive language:* A consistent difficulty in finding or meaningfully combining words, not due to emotional arousal or inhibition.
   4.16 *Impairment of comprehension:* A consistent difficulty in understanding conversation, not due to emotional arousal or inhibition.
   4.17 *Talks to self in public:* Mutters, speaks, or remonstrates with self regardless of the presence of others.
   4.18 *Other abnormality of voice, speech, or language*

5. Interaction with interviewer

5.1 *Aversion of gaze:* Makes only fleeting or intermittent eye contact with the interviewer, or deliberately averts gaze when the interviewer seeks eye contact.

5.2 *Distant focus of gaze:* Eyes appear to be focused on a distant scene, with attention partly or completely distracted for the interviewer. May appear to look through the examiner.

5.3 *Staring:* Fixes the interviewer with intent, persistent, hypervigilant, or hostile gaze.

5.4 *Unresponsive:* Deficient or absent response to the interviewer's social overtures.

5.5 *Tense:* Hypervigilance revealed by increased tone in facial, body, or limb musculature; wide shining eyes; dilated pupils; skin pallor and sweating; altered vocal pattern; and motor restlessness.

5.6 *Impulsive:* Prone to act without reflection or deliberation; for example, with abrupt movements, thoughtless comments, or such uninhibited emotional response as exaggerated laughter, weeping, or combativeness.

5.7 *Other abnormality of interaction*

B. Inferences about attitudes, affect, cognition, and thought

6. Relationship to interviewer

6.1 *Bewildered:* Although there is no evidence of clouding of consciousness, seems less able to grasp the purpose of the interview and to be more confused by the interviewer's questions than would be expected at this age.

6.2 *Boastful:* Flaunts superior strength, beauty, intelligence, achievement, possessions, family, home, or friends.

6.3 *Clinging:* Persistently holds on to or nestles into another person who is usually a parent or guardian and has difficulty separating sufficiently to be engaged in conversation or play.

6.4 *Clowning:* Attempts to divert the interviewer with buffoonery involving exaggerated facial expression, body movement, and conversation, sometimes in imitation of a well-known comedian or actor.

6.5 *Demanding:* Makes direct demands on the interviewer to satisfy personal needs. Orders the interviewer to perform certain actions or to desist from others.

6.6 *Evasive:* Avoids answering questions without explicitly refusing to do so. Gives incomplete, irrelevant, or patently false answers to queries about personal matters.

6.7 *Fearful:* Expresses alarm about or terror of the interview, in facial expressions, posture, or conversation. Shrieks or weeps in a frightened manner. May attempt to escape from the interview room.

6.8 *Hostile:* Expresses dislike of or animosity toward the interviewer in words and open resistance to social overtures. May deliberately test the limits of the interviewer's patience. Rails at the interviewer in derogatory terms.

6.9 *Impudent:* Relates to the interviewer in a provocatively disdainful, contemptuous, or insolent manner.

6.10 *Indifferent:* Exhibits by bored facial expression, posture, and/or verbal response a conspicuous lack of interest in the interview, interviewer, and surroundings.

6.11 *Ingratiating:* Relates to the interviewer in an exceptionally complaisant, affable, or tactful manner with the apparent intent of placating or disarming the interviewer.

6.12 *Invasive:* Stands too close to the interviewer, interferes with the interviewer's possessions, or asks inappropriate personal questions.

6.13 *Loquacious:* Relates to the interviewer in a chatty, garrulous manner, in extreme cases so incessantly as to prevent the interviewer from asking questions or responding appropriately.

6.14 *Overcompliant:* Unusually polite and deferential. Passively yields or submits to whatever the interviewer wants done or defers to whatever the interviewer says to a degree beyond what would be expected.

6.15 *Preoccupied:* Unable to attend fully to the interviewer or play materials because something else seems to be on the subject's mind.

6.16 *Seductive:* Relates to the interviewer in such a way as to attract attention to personal sexuality and arouse the interviewer erotically; for example, by suggestive facial expression, eye or body movement, posture, or provocative dress.

6.17 *Shy:* Relates to the examiner in a timid, reserved, or diffident manner and is thus difficult to engage in conversation or play.

6.18 *Suggestible:* Can be influenced or persuaded by the interviewer to alter an account of an event, to accept or deny symptoms, or to adopt or reject ideas.

6.19 *Suspicious:* Relates to the examiner in a mistrustful manner. Replies to questions guardedly or evasively. May question the true purpose of the interview and the interviewer's good will and imply or suggest a hidden purpose for the proceedings.

6.20 *Uncooperative:* Performs tasks in a grudging or perfunctory manner. Actively opposes the interviewer by refusing to answer questions or comply with the interviewer's requests. May obstruct the interviewer's conversation by persistently interjecting.

6.21 *Withdrawn:* Difficult or impossible to engage in conversation or play. Remote and apparently self-involved. Apparently oblivious to the examiner, with little or no eye contact and little or no response to social overtures.

6.22 *Other characteristic of interaction*

7. Affect and mood

7.1 *Angry:* Sullen, ill-humored, touchy, or intemperate. May be sarcastic or otherwise hostile in conversation. May erupt into accusatory shouting or tantrum.

7.2 *Anhedonic:* Apparently unable to gain pleasure from or develop an interest in activities most children enjoy. Loss of pleasure from or interest in activities formerly pleasurable or interesting.

7.3 *Anxious:* Eyes, facies, posture, skin, movement, and speech display hypervigilance and autonomic discharge. Conscious preoccupation and conversation express unfocused subjective disturbance that can vary from mild discomfort to panic. May be of such intensity that concentration is impaired and the interview impeded.

7.4 *Apathetic:* Lack of concern about or indolent responses to matters expected to be of significance.

7.5 *Depressed:* Looks morose and feels dejected, sad, or despondent. May be pessimistic or self-deprecatory and feel lonely. May be concomitantly irritable, agitated, withdrawn, weepy, or fatigued and slowed in movement, speech, and ideation.

7.6 *Euphoric:* In expansive good spirits. Elated, ebullient, optimistic, and suffused with well-being to an exaggerated or inappropriate extent.

7.7 *Flat affect:* Expresses a limited range of affect, apparently due to impoverishment of inner emotional life and lack of emotional sensitivity and responsiveness. May be manifest as coldness, callousness, apathy, or emotional dullness.

7.8 *Guilty:* Persistent distressing preoccupation with a past event or events involving the transgression of a moral standard.

7.9 *Histrionic:* Dramatically expressive presentation of symptoms, personal history, or impersonations, apparently with the intent of captivating the interviewer.

7.10 *Inappropriate affect:* Lack of congruence between facial expression, emotions, and the subject of conversation. For example, smiles or giggles while discussing a serious matter.

7.11 *Labile affect:* Fluctuations in mood. Veers abruptly from calm, silly, or euphoric to sullen, angry, tearful, or morose. Easily reduced to tears or tantrums.

7.12 *Resigned:* Unusually fatalistic. Appears to have given up the struggle against difficult circumstances.

7.13 *Restricted affect:* The subject is not insensitive to the interviewer's feelings but expresses a limited range of affect, apparently due to exaggerated control of emotional expression.

7.14 *Silly:* Inappropriately giddy or playful. Laughs or giggles persistently.

7.15 *Other abnormality of affect or mood*

8. Information processing

8.1 *Disoriented:* Uncertain or confused about the time of day, the date, current whereabouts, the route between home and present location, personal identity, home address, telephone number, or the identity/function of the interviewer. Stipulate whether the disorientation affects time, place, or person.

8.2 *Inattentive:* Unable to sustain concentration on a particular activity or topic. Prone to move from object to object or topic to topic. In mild form, may be inattentive only when the activity or topic is not self-selected.

8.3 *Distractible:* Attention is readily diverted from an activity or topic by random environmental stimuli (e.g., visual, auditory, olfactory) or internal factors (e.g., visceral sensations, mental associations, auditory hallucinations).

8.4 *Impairment of recent memory:* Relative inability to recall the immediate or recent past as revealed, for example, by the inability to repeat digits forwards and backwards or to recall events, names, addresses, or telephone numbers that have been part of daily experience during the previous week.

8.5 *Impairment of remote memory:* Relative inability to recall events, names, places, dates, or addresses from the distant past; that is, from a period more remote than one week before the examination. Stipulate whether the impairment is general or limited to a particular period of time.

8.6 *Deficiency in general knowledge:* A relative lack of awareness of current events, history, geography, or popular science that cannot be explained on the basis of memory defect or inadequate education.

8.7 *Impairment of comprehension:* Relative inability to grasp the meaning, implication or import of written, oral or visual communication.

8.8 *Impairment of spatial reasoning:* The relative inability to solve problems that involve manipulating objects in space; for example, jigsaw puzzles, constructing models, or mechanical repairs.

8.9 *Impairment of social judgment:* When presented with a social situation requiring a response, the subject behaves in a socially inappropriate manner that is not due to a lack of awareness of the relevant social conventions.

8.10 *Impairment of conceptual capacity:* When presented with objects, events, or ideas, the subject shows a relative inability to discern principles, patterns, or rules; or the relative inability to apply principles or rules to actual problems

9. Thought processes

9.1 *Blocking:* Sudden interruptions in the train of thought, lasting from seconds to a minute or more in duration, following which the subject takes up the conversation where it was left off or begins on a different subject.

9.2 *Circumlocution:* Takes a long time to get to the point. Gives more specific examples to illustrate a general idea than should be required to convey meaning and seems out of touch with the listener's impatience.

9.3 *Circumstantiality:* Conversational flow rendered tedious by the unnecessary description of details that would ordinarily be left for the listener to understand implicitly.

9.4 *Concretistic thinking:* The subject has difficulty generalizing from specific instances and is unusually literal in interpreting the interviewer's questions.

9.5 *Defect in memory:* The subject has a relative or absolute amnesia for a past event or events from the recent or remote past.

9.6 *Distractibility:* The subject is readily diverted from a train of thought or activity by random sensory stimuli.

9.7 *Flight of ideas:* An acceleration of thinking manifest in the subjective perception of racing thoughts and rapid, pressured speech. Conversation is disorganized by the subject's tendency to link ideas on the basis of playful or irrelevant acoustic or semantic associations.

9.8 *Incoherence:* Conversation difficult or impossible to understand because the subject does not associate ideas normally, use appropriate syntax, or choose appropriate words.

9.9 *Looseness of association:* The logical connection between ideas is deficient. Apparently disparate themes are linked, the subject's ideational flow being organized by a private logic, by metaphor, or by the similarity between words and sounds rather than by the need to communicate clearly.

9.10 *Paralogia:* Gives incorrect but predictably approximate answers to questions, saying, for example, that a cow has five legs or that $2 + 2 = 3$.

9.11 *Perseveration:* The subject persists with a point or theme after it has been dealt with exhaustively, even after the interviewer has tried to change the subject. The repetitious theme may reappear periodically after conversation has moved to another topic.

9.12 *Poverty of thought:*   Paucity of ideation manifest in poor verbal production; elementary, sometimes repetitious, fantasy themes; or apparent inability to fantasize.

9.13 *Slowing of thought:*   Retardation in thinking revealed by latency of response to questions and sluggish conversational flow.

9.14 *Tangential thinking:*   A particular form of associational looseness in which the subject's conversation is diverted from its apparent goal and digresses in a seemingly irrelevant or only vaguely relevant direction.

9.15 *Other disturbance in thought process*

10. Thought content

10.1 *Anergia:*   Persistent, subjective lack of energy and concentration and excessive fatigue.

10.2 *Compulsion:*   Persistent, repetitive actions that stem from obsessional thinking and are usually performed, despite subjective awareness of their irrationality, to check for omissions, make reparation for transgressions, or to ward off danger; for example, touching doorknobs, handwashing, checking the gas, or performing bedtime rituals.

10.3 *Confabulation:*   Prone to rely on sensational or wish-fulfilling fantasies to substitute for reality or to resolve real problems to such a degree that the subject believes the stories.

10.4 *Déjà vu:*   A sudden uncanny perception that the precise event, situation, or conversation being currently experienced has occurred in the past.

10.5 *Delusion:*   A false belief not susceptible to argument and inconsistent with the subject's sociocultural background. Delusions are characteristically of persecutory, grandiose, referential, somatic, erotic, jealous, or nihilistic nature or about thought insertion, withdrawal, or broadcasting.

10.6 *Depersonalization:*   A perception or alteration of the self in that the subject feels alienated from or like a spectator of the self.

10.7 *Derealization:*   A perception that the external world has changed in that it has become unreal, vague, or remote.

10.8 *Dissociation:*   A psychological fragmentation of mental life varying in intensity from swooning, to amnesia, and to multiple personality.

10.9 *Fabrication:*   Deliberate lying usually intended to evade blame or punishment, gain notoriety, take revenge by getting others into trouble, or enjoy the consequences of mischief.

10.10 *Hallucination:*   A false perception occurring in the waking state in the absence of a stimulus and carrying a sense of conviction. May be of auditory, visual, tactile, olfactory, visceral, or genital nature.

10.11 *Illusion:*   Sensory stimulation given a false interpretation. Perception is commonly distorted in accordance with a mental preoccupation (for example of hunger, fear, or anger).

10.12 *Impulsion:*   An episodic urge, which may or may not be resisted, to engage in a particular dangerous or forbidden activity, such as theft, fighting, speeding, drinking, or sexual misbehavior.

10.13 *Malingering:*   The deliberate assumption of false physical or mental symptoms designed to convey that the subject is physically or mentally ill.

10.14 *Obsession:*   A persistent, repetitive idea, image, desire, doubt, phrase, or fragment of music that cuts across consciousness and that the subject appreciates is senseless or repugnant but that can be resisted only with mounting anxiety.

10.15 *Phobia:* A morbid fear of a specific person, object, situation, or event. The subject may know the fear is both irrational and exaggerated. Typical phobias include being alone, leaving home for school, animals, insects, enclosures, heights, elevators, embarrassment in public places, using public transport, or contracting a disease.

10.16 *Preoccupation with identity issues:* A persistent, distressing uncertainty and rumination about gender identity, friendship, sexual morality, orientation, group loyalties, religion, career choice, or long-term goals.

10.17 *Preoccupation with own mental functioning:* An excessive concern for the integrity of mental functioning, usually manifest as a fear of going crazy or a conviction of being mentally ill.

10.18 *Preoccupation with past or future:* Excessive concern for past events. Unwarranted worry about a future untoward event or events that may or may not be specified.

10.19 *Preoccupation with personal competence:* A persistent fear or conviction of being unable to function at a desired level of competence in a particular area, such as scholastic competition, sport, or the ability to attract a sexual partner.

10.20 *Self-consciousness:* A proneness to embarrassment or humiliation in social situations, combined with exaggerated need for reassurance.

10.21 *Suicidal ideation:* Has considered the possibility of suicide during the past month. May be currently preoccupied with or determined to commit suicide.

10.22 *Trance state:* A state of altered consciousness in which the subject is partly or completely unaware of the interviewer and may seem abstracted, remote, or ecstatic.

C. Fantasy

11. Quality of fantasy
    11.1 *Bizarreness:* The subject's fantasy is highly unusual or eccentric in that it deals with very private, tabooed, magical, grotesque, or grossly immature themes or with ideas connected in a highly unusual manner.

    11.2 *Decreased productivity:* Sparse fantasy is produced despite the interviewer's attempts to evoke it.

    11.3 *Increased productivity:* Exuberant fantasy produced spontaneously or in response to the interviewer's questions.

12. Salient themes in fantasy
    12.1 *Achievement:* Working towards a self-selected goal.
    12.2 *Acquisition:* Making money or acquiring possessions.
    12.3 *Affiliation:* Making friends, being befriended, enjoying company, relating to one's family.
    12.4 *Affliction:* Physical or mental disease or disorder in self or others.
    12.5 *Aggression:* Verbal or physical attack, assault, torture, injury.
    12.6 *Alienation:* Lack of emotional contact with others due to voluntary or involuntary emotional distance.

12.7   *Antisocial:*   Illegal activity involving cheating, theft, burglary, assault, rape, homicide, arson, forgery, vandalism, gang activity, illicit drug taking, and so on.

12.8   *Anxiety:*   Worry, apprehension, fretfulness.

12.9   *Autonomy:*   The need for independence, freedom, or escape from restraint.

12.10   *Avoidance of blame:*   The need to resist temptation or avoid criticism.

12.11   *Change:*   The need to move from place to place, seek new friends, or have new experiences.

12.12   *Compensation:*   Overcoming weakness, defect, or obstacles.

12.13   *Conflict:*   Uncertainty, perplexity, indecision.

12.14   *Creativity:*   Inventing, producing, creating, or generating things, art, or ideas.

12.15   *Curiosity:*   Interest in exploring or investigating places, things, or ideas.

12.16   *Death:*   The demise or possible demise of a person or persons not as a result of suicide.

12.17   *Deference:*   Admiring, following, pleasing, or hero-worshipping another person.

12.18   *Dominance:*   One person influencing, controlling, or leading another or others.

12.19   *Exhibition:*   A person or group of persons attracting, exciting, amusing, or entertaining another or others.

12.20   *Exposition:*   Explaining, relating, or making a verbal judgment.

12.21   *Fantasy:*   Daydreaming, night dreaming, using the imagination.

12.22   *Failure:*   The conviction of having fallen short of a desired goal.

12.23   *Guilt:*   The conviction of having transgressed internal standards and deserving punishment.

12.24   *Injury:*   Physical harm, hurt, damage, wounding, or crippling.

12.25   *Inferiority:*   The conviction of being less able, less beautiful, or less strong than another or others.

12.26   *Lack:*   A sense of the current and/or past insufficiency of material possessions, food, money, friends, or affection.

12.27   *Loneliness:*   The desire for but the inability to find friends.

12.28   *Loss:*   The sense of having lost an important person, object, money, affection, prestige, or ideal.

12.29   *Nurturance:*   Giving or receiving sympathy, consolation, protection, child-rearing, or parental affection.

12.30   *Optimism:*   Elation, confidence in the future.

12.31   *Pessimism:*   Pessimism, disappointment, a sense of inability to influence an adverse future.

12.32   *Play:*   Enjoyment of amusement, recreation, play, sport, or entertainment.

12.33   *Preoccupation with body function:*   Hypochondriasis; concern with body physiology.

12.34   *Preoccupation with mental function:*   Concern about mental function; fear of mental illness.

12.35   *Recognition:*   Seeking honor, fame, or appreciation.

12.36   *Rejection:*   Ignoring, rejecting, abandoning another person or persons; or being ignored, rejected, or abandoned by another or others.

12.37   *Relaxation:*   Enjoyment of ease and such sensual pleasures as eating and drinking.

12.38   *Resignation:*   Resigning oneself to defect, loss, or defeat.

12.39   *Retention:*   Frugality. Preventing loss by careful husbanding of resources. Preventing theft.

12.40   *Revenge:*   Seeking redress for slight, harm, or injury.

12.41 *Seclusion:*   The desire to be alone or for privacy or inconspicuousness.

12.42 *Self-pity:*   Feeling sorry for one's self.

12.43 *Sexuality:*   Erotic relationships or interaction.

12.44 *Shame:*   Humiliation, embarrassment, public failure.

12.45 *Succor:*   Seeking or offering aid in distressful situations.

12.46 *Suicide:*   Planning or attempting to kill self or actually doing so.

12.47 *Understanding:*   Seeking knowledge or truth.

12.48 *Other salient theme.*

D. Insight

13. Insight

13.1 *Lack of understanding of reason for interview*

13.2 *Lack of understanding of nature of problems*

13.3 *Lack of desire for help*

IV

Child Information Form

CHILD INFORMATION FORM

This form completed by —————————————   Date —————————————
Relationship to child   —————————————

A. Identification data
    Child's full name ————————————— Sex ———— Race ————
    Date of birth ————————————— Current age ———— years ———— months
    Person with legal custody ————————— Relationship to child —————
    Address of child ————————————————— Phone —————
    Is child covered by any health insurance (including Medicaid)? Yes ———— No ————
    Amount deductible ————— Extent of psychiatric coverage —————
    Name of insurance company —————————————————
    Estimated family income (to determine sliding scale fee) —————————
    Who referred you to our clinic? ————————————————
    Name

    —————————————————————   —————————————
    Address   *Phone*

B. Family composition
    1. Natural father (Is he living?   Yes _ No _) (Is he living with child?   Yes _ No _)
        Name ————————————————————— Age —————
        Address —————————————————————————
        Occupation ————————————— Work hours —————
        Place of work ————————————— Work phone —————
        Highest grade completed in school ————— Religion —————
        Date of marriage to child's mother —— Any other marriages? Yes ——— No ———
        Any children from other marriages? Yes ———— No ———— Number —————

    2. Natural mother (Is she living? Yes _ No _) (Is she living with child? Yes _ No _)
        Name ————————————————————— Age —————
        Address —————————————————————————
        Occupation ————————————— Work hours —————
        Place of work ————————————— Work phone —————
        Highest grade completed in school ————— Religion —————
        Any other marriages? Yes ———— No ————
        Any children from other marriages? Yes ———— No ———— Number —————

    3. Are child's natural parents currently living together? Yes ———— No ————
        If no, a. date of separation ————————————— Child's age —————
               b. date of divorce ————————————— Child's age —————

    4. Siblings *(Please list here child's full brothers and sisters only)*

Name	Date of birth	Age	Sex	Place where living
————	————	——	——	————
————	————	——	——	————
————	————	——	——	————
————	————	——	——	————

C. Living situation for child
1. With whom does child live? Both natural parents _____ Adoptive parents _____
Foster parents _____ Other _____

2. Adults living in child's current home *(other than natural parents living with child)*

Name	Age	Sex	Relationship to child	Occupation
_____	___	___	_____	_____
_____	___	___	_____	_____
_____	___	___	_____	_____
_____	___	___	_____	_____

3. Other children presently living in the child's current home *(if not listed above)*

Name	Date of birth	Age	Sex	Relationship to child
_____	_____	___	___	_____
_____	_____	___	___	_____
_____	_____	___	___	_____
_____	_____	___	___	_____

4. Home setting. *(Check any that apply)*

Large house   _____   Rural   _____
Medium house _____   Suburban _____
Small house   _____   Urban   _____
Apartment   _____
Other   _____

D. Child's pediatrician _____ _____
                              Name   *Address*
Last complete checkup _____ Outcome _____

E. Child's school _____
Grade _____ Teacher(s) _____

F. 1. What concerns you about your child? _____

_____

How long have these problems existed? _____
Have you sought previous help for these problems?   No _____ Yes _____
If yes, name _____ place _____ date _____
        name _____ place _____ date _____
        name _____ place _____ date _____

2. Do any of your other children have learning, behavior, or other problems?
_____ No   _____ Yes (If yes, supply information requested below.)

Name	Date	Problem	Treatment
_____	_____	_____	_____
_____	_____	_____	_____

G. Child's medical history

1. _____

   Birthplace

<table>
<tr><td></td><td colspan="2">*Hospital*</td><td></td></tr>
<tr><td></td><td>No</td><td>Yes</td><td>Describe</td></tr>
<tr><td>2. Did mother have medical problems during pregnancy? (For example, bleeding, infections, high blood pressure, high blood sugar, convulsions, large weight gain, operations, X-rays, hospitalization, etc.)</td><td>____</td><td>____</td><td>_____</td></tr>
<tr><td>3. Did mother take medications during pregnancy?</td><td>____</td><td>____</td><td>_____</td></tr>
<tr><td>4. Did mother or father drink much alcohol during pregnancy?</td><td>____</td><td>____</td><td>_____</td></tr>
<tr><td>5. Did mother have other problems during pregnancy? (For example, problems with spouse, job, money, or living arrangements, etc.)</td><td>____</td><td>____</td><td>_____</td></tr>
<tr><td>6. Did mother or child have problems during labor or delivery? (For example, prolonged bleeding, etc.)</td><td>____</td><td>____</td><td>_____</td></tr>
<tr><td>7. Was child born premature?</td><td>____</td><td>____</td><td>_____</td></tr>
</table>

8. Birthweight: ____ pounds
   ____ ounces

<table>
<tr><td>9. Did child have problems during newborn period? (For example, yellow jaundice or blue colored, difficulty feeding, seizures, infections, or birth defects, etc.)</td><td>____</td><td>____</td><td>_____</td></tr>
<tr><td>10. Was child difficult to care for as a baby?</td><td>____</td><td>____</td><td>_____</td></tr>
<tr><td>11. Has child had any severe illnesses?</td><td>____</td><td>____</td><td></td></tr>
</table>

Illness	Age	Treatment	Doctor
_____	____	_____	_____
_____	____	_____	_____

	No	Yes	Describe

12. Has child had repeated medical problems? (For example, earaches, infection, or headaches) ____ ____ _____ Ages____
    _____ Ages____

13. Has child had any operations? ____ ____ _____ Age____
    _____ Age____

14. Has child had any serious accidents or injuries? (Especially head injury or unconsciousness)? ____ ____ _____ Age____
    _____ Age____

15. Has child been prescribed a medication for behavior problems? ____ ____

Type	Date	Doctor	Result
_____	____	_____	_____
_____	____	_____	_____

	No	Yes	

16. Is child on medication now? ____ ____

Type	Dose	Its purpose	Its effect
_____	____	_____	_____

	No	Yes	Describe

17. Is child allergic to any medication? ____ ____ _____

18. Does child have any other allergies? ____ ____ _____

19. Is there anything else about your child's health that concerns you? ____ ____ _____

H. Child's developmental history
   1. Did you notice any problems with your child's development? ____ ____ _____

   2. Did your child have any difficulty in any of the following areas (for example, were any of

	No	Yes	Describe

these areas especially hard for the child or was the child slower to do them than you would expect?)

a. Walking alone   ____ ____ _____

b. Saying words   ____ ____ _____

c. Speaking phrases   ____ ____ _____

d. Bowel training   ____ ____ _____

e. Bladder training   ____ ____ _____

f. Dry at night   ____ ____ _____

g. Writing alphabet   ____ ____ _____

h. Reading words   ____ ____ _____

i. Riding a bicycle   ____ ____ _____

j. Tying shoelaces   ____ ____ _____

3. While your child was growing up, did you notice any difficulties in the following areas?

a. Discipline   ____ ____ _____

b. Temper tantrums, fighting   ____ ____ _____

c. Moods   ____ ____ _____

d. Relationships with others   ____ ____ _____

e. Sex play   ____ ____ _____

f. School problems   ____ ____ _____

g. Other behavior problems   ____ ____ _____

h. Has raising your child presented many difficulties?   ____ ____ _____

I. The child's temperament

1. Is your child overactive?   ____ ____ _____

2. Does your child have trouble paying attention?   ____ ____ _____

3. Does your child have trouble staying with one activity – jumping around from one thing to another or failing to finish things?   ____ ____ _____

4. Does your child fluctuate from happy to sad quickly with little apparent cause?   ____ ____ _____

5. Does your child get frustrated easily?   ____ ____ _____

	No	Yes	Describe
6. Does your child get upset by abrupt changes in his or her life?	____	____	_____
7. Are your child's emotional responses generally unpredictable?	____	____	_____
8. Does it take your child a long time to warm up to a new situation or people?	____	____	_____
9. Does your child react strongly to physical pain?	____	____	_____
10. Does your child react strongly to things?	____	____	_____

J. Child's family history
Has anyone in the family had the following?

	No	Yes	Describe who
1. Neurological disease, such as seizures, fits, weaknesses, etc.	____	____	_____
2. Medical disease, such as diabetes, thyroid disease, heart disease, etc.	____	____	_____
3. Mental illness, such as schizophrenia, manic-depressive disease, depression, etc.	____	____	_____
4. Mental retardation	____	____	_____
5. Learning problems	____	____	_____
6. Behavior problems	____	____	_____
7. Excessive use of alcohol	____	____	_____
8. Excessive use of drugs	____	____	_____
9. Trouble with the law	____	____	_____
10. Trouble holding a job	____	____	_____

K. Current living situation   No   Yes   Describe
1. Does your present marriage
dissatisfy you?
   ____   ____   _____

2. Does your present work situation dissatisfy you?
   ____   ____   _____

3. Do your present living circumstances dissatisfy you?
   ____   ____   _____

4. Has anyone else in your family
seen a psychologist, psychiatrist,
or other mental-health worker?
   ____   ____   _____

5. Have there been recent major
changes or stresses in your living
situation or family?
   ____   ____   _____

L. Summary:
1. Do you have any ideas about why your child is having behavior problems now?
_____

2. What are your child's strengths?
_____

3. Is there anything else we should know about your child or his or her life?
____ No   ____ Yes
If yes, describe: _____
_____

Thank you

References

Abrams, H. S. The psychiatrist, the treatment of renal failure, and the prolongation of life: 3. *American Journal of Psychiatry,* 1972, *128,* 1534-1538. (19)

Abroms, E. M. Beyond eclecticism. *American Journal of Psychiatry,* 1983, *140,* 740-745. (12)

Abroms, G. M. Setting limits. *Archives of General Psychiatry,* 1968, *19,* 113-119. (18)

Achenbach, T. M. DSM-III in light of empirical research on the classification of child psychopathology. *Journal of the American Academy of Child Psychiatry,* 1980, *19,* 395-412. (23)

—*Developmental psychopathology* (2nd ed.). New York: Wiley, 1982. (21, 22, 24, 25)

Achenbach, T. M., & Edelbrock, C. *Manual for the Child Behavior Checklist and Revised Behavior Profile.* Burlington, Vt.: Queen City Printers, 1983. (11, 21, 23, 26)

Adams, G. L., Brochstein, J. R., Cheney, C. C., Friese, J. H., & Tristan, M. P. A. Primary care mental health training and service mode. *American Journal of Psychiatry,* 1978, *135,* 121-123. (20)

Adams, P. L. *A primer of child psychotherapy.* Boston: Little, Brown, 1982. (25)

Akiskal, H. S. Dysthymic disorder: Psychopathology of proposed subtypes. *American Journal of Psychiatry,* 1983, *140,* 11-20. (10, 12)

Akiskal, H. S., & McKinney, W. T., Jr. Overview of recent research in depression. Integration of ten conceptual models into a comprehensive clinical frame. *Archives of General Psychiatry,* 1975, *32,* 285-305. (5)

Allal, L. K. Training of medical students in a problem-solving skill: The generation of diagnostic problem formulations. Unpublished doctoral dissertation. East Lansing: Michigan State University, 1973. (27)

Als, H., Tronick, E., & Brazelton, T. B. Stages of a sighted infant and of a blind infant in interaction with their mothers. In T. M. Fields, D. Stern, A. Sostek, &

S. Goldberg (Eds.), *Interactions of high-risk infants and children: Disturbances and interventions.* New York: Academic Press, 1980. (21)

Anderson, O. Health services systems in the United States and other countries – critical comparisons. *New England Journal of Medicine,* 1963, *269,* 839–843; 896–900. (3)

Anderson, R., Francis, A., Lion, J., & Dougherty, V. S. Psychologically related illness and health services utilization. *Medical Care,* 1977, *25*(Suppl.), 59–73. (3, 20)

Anderson, W. H. The emergency department. In T. P. Hackett & N. H. Cassem (Eds.), *Handbook of general psychiatry.* St. Louis: Mosby, 1978. (17)

—The physical examination in office practice. *American Journal of Psychiatry.* 1980, *137,* 1188–1192. (10)

Andreason, N. V. C., Tsuang, M. T., & Canter, A. The significance of thought disorder in diagnostic evaluations. *Comprehensive Psychiatry,* 1974, *15,* 27–34. (9)

Anstett, R. Patient discussion groups in the training of family practice residents. *Journal of Family Practice,* 1980, *10,* 143–144. (19)

Argyle, M. *The psychology of interpersonal behavior.* Harmondsworth, Middlesex: Penguin, 1967. (9)

Arkes, H. R. Impediments to accurate clinical judgment and possible ways to minimize their impact. *Journal of Consulting and Clinical Psychology,* 1981, *49,* 323–330. (27)

Axline, V. M. *Play therapy* (Rev. ed.). New York: Ballantine, 1969. (25)

Bachrach, L. L. General hospital psychiatry: Overview from a sociologic perspective. *American Journal of Psychiatry,* 1981, *138,* 879–887. (18)

Baldessarini, R. J. *Biomedical aspects of depression and its treatment.* Washington, D.C.: American Psychiatric Press, 1983. (10)

Balint, M. *The doctor, his patient, and the illness.* New York: International Universities Press, 1957. (3, 20)

Barrows, H. S. An overview of medical problem solving. Paper presented at conference, The Role of Problem Solving in Medicine, Smugglers Notch, Vt.; October, 1979. (27)

Barrows, H. S., & Abrahamson, S. The programmed patient: A technique for apprising student performance in clinical neurology. *Journal of Medical Education,* 1964, *39,* 802–805. (27)

Barrows, H. S., & Bennett, K. Experimental studies on the diagnostic (problem solving) skill of the neurologist: Their implications for neurological training. *Archives of Neurology,* 1972, *26,* 273–277. (27)

Barsky, A. J. Application of psychiatry to primary care medicine. In A. Lazare (Ed.), *Outpatient psychiatry: Diagnosis and treatment.* Baltimore: Williams & Wilkins, 1979. (20)

Barsky, A. J. Hidden reasons some patients visit doctors. *Annals of Internal Medicine,* 1981, *94,* 492–498. (3, 20)

Bartlett, F. C. *Thinking.* London: Allen & Unwin, 1958. (27)

Barton, G., & Friedman, R. (Eds.). *Psyhciatric emergency care: A task force report of the American Psychiatric Association.* Washington, D.C.: American Psychiatric Association, 1982. (17)

Bartrop, R. W., Luckhurst, E., Lazarus, L., Kiloh, L. G., & Penny, R. Lymphocyte function after bereavement. *Lancet,* 1977, *1,* 834–836. (3)

Beck, A. T. *Cognitive therapy and the emotional disorders.* New York: International Universities Press, 1976. (12, 20)

Beecher, H. *Measurement of subjective responses.* New York: Oxford University Press, 1959. (3)

Beitman, B. D., Williamson, P., Featherstone, H., & Katon, W. Resistance to physician use of the biopsychosocial model. *General Hospital Psychiatry,* 1982, *4,* 81–84. (3, 14)

Bellak, L., & Bellak, S. S. *Children's apperception test* (6th rev. ed.). Larchmont, N.Y.: C.P.S., Inc., 1974. (22)

Bemporad, J. R. (Ed.). *Child development in normality and psychopathology.* New York: Brunner/Mazel, 1980. (24)

Benson, D. F., & Blumer, D. *Psychiatric aspects of neurological disease.* New York: Grune & Stratton, 1975. (10)

Berkman, L. F., & Syme, S. L. Social networks, host resistance, and mortality: A nine-year follow-up study of Alameda County residents. *American Journal of Epidemiology,* 1979, *109,* 186–204. (3)

Bernstein, J. G. *Handbook of drug therapy in psychiatry.* Boston: John Wright · PSG Inc., 1983. (12)

Bernstein, L., Bernstein, R. S., & Dana, R. H. *Interviewing: A guide for health professionals* (2nd ed.). New York: Appleton-Century-Crofts, 1974. (8)

Bernstein, R. A., & Dreyfus, D. Medical and surgical consultations to a general hospital psychiatric unit. *General Hospital Psychiatry,* 1980, *2,* 267–270. (18)

Bianchi, G. N. Patterns of hypochondriasis: A principal components analysis. *British Journal of Psychiatry,* 1973, *122,* 544–548. (3)

Billowitz, A., & Freidson, W. Are psychiatric consultants' recommendations followed? *International Journal of Psychiatry in Medicine,* 1978–79, *9,* 179–189. (19)

Billowitz, A., Freidson, W., & Schubert, D. S. Liaison psychiatry on a burns unit. *General Hospital Psychiatry,* 1980, *2,* 300–305. (18)

Bleuler, E. *Dementia praecox oder die Gruppe der Schizoprenien.* Liepzig: Deuticke, 1911. (9)

—*Dementia Praecox or the group of schizophrenias* (J. Zinkin, trans.). New York: International Universities Press, 1950. (9)

Bloch, S., Crouch, E., & Reibstein, J. Therapeutic factors in group psychotherapy. A review. *Archives of General Psychiatry,* 1981, *38,* 519–526. (12)

Blois, M. S. Clinical judgment and computers. *New England Journal of Medicine,* 1980, *303,* 192–197. (27)

Borghi, J. Premature termination of psychotherapy and patient–therapist expectations. *American Journal of Psychotherapy,* 1968, *22,* 460–473. (16)

Borus, J. F., & Casserly, M. K. Psychiatrists and primary care physicians: Collaborative learning experiences in delivering primary care. *Hospital and Community Psychiatry,* 1979, *30,* 686–689. (20)

Borysenko, M., & Borysenko, J. Stress, behavior and immunity: Animal models and mediating mechanisms. *General Hospital Psychiatry,* 1982, *4,* 59–68. (3, 5)

Brady, J. P. Psychotherapy by a combined behavioral and dynamic approach. *Comprehensive Psychiatry,* 1968, *9,* 536–543. (12)

Braestrup, C., & Nielsen, M. Neurotransmitters and CNS disease: Anxiety. *Lancet,* 1982, *2,* 1030–1034. (5)

Brazelton, T. *Neonatal Behavior Assessment Scale.* Philadelphia: Lippincott, 1973. (21)

Breger, L., and McGaugh, J. L. Critique and reformulation of "learning theory" approaches to psychotherapy and neurosis. *Psychological Bulletin,* 1965, *63,* 338–358. (12)

Bruner, J. S., Goodnow, J. J., & Austin, G. A. *A study of thinking.* New York: Wiley, 1956. (27)

Brunswik, E. Representative design and probabilistic theory in a functional psychology. *Psychological Review,* 1955, *62,* 193–217. (27)

Buck, J. N. *The House-Tree-Person Technique* (Rev. manual). Beverly Hills, Calif.: Western Psychological Services, 1966. (22)

Burns, B. J., Scott, J. E., Burke, J. K., & Kessler, L. G. Mental health training of primary care residents: A review of recent literature (1974–1981). *General Hospital Psychiatry,* 1983, *5,* 157–170. (20)

Burns, D. D. *Feeling good: The new mood therapy.* New York: Morrow, 1982. (12)

Cameron, N. Reasoning, regression and communication in schizophrenics. *Psychological Monographs,* 1938, *50(1),* 221. (9)

Cannon, W. B. *Bodily changes in pain, hunger, fear, and rage.* New York: Appleton, 1934. (3)

Caplan, G. *Principles of preventive psychiatry.* London: Tavistock, 1964. (4, 12)

Carlson, N. R. *Physiology of behavior* (2nd ed.). Boston: Allyn & Bacon, 1981. (5)

Carroll, B. J., Feinberg, M., and Greden, J. F. A specific laboratory test for the diagnosis of melancholia. *Archives of General Psychiatry,* 1981, 38, 15–22. (10)

Cassano, G. B., Maggini, C., & Akiskal, H. S. Short-term, subchronic, and chronic sequelae of affective disorders. In H. S. Akiskal (Ed.), *Diagnosis and treatment of affective disorders. Psychiatric Clinics of North America,* 1983, *6,* 55–68. (16)

Cassata, D. M., & Kirkman-Liff, B. L. Mental health activities of family physicians. *Journal of Family Practice,* 1981, *12,* 683–692. (20)

Cavanaugh, S. The prevalence of emotional and cognitive dysfunction in a general medical population: Using the MMSE, GHQ, and BDI. *General Hospital Psychiatry,* 1983, *5,* 15–24. (10, 19)

Cawte, J. E. *Medicine is the law.* Honolulu: University Press of Hawaii, 1974. (3)

Close, J. Scored neurological examination in the pharmacotherapy of children. *Psychopharmacology Bulletin,* special issue: *Psychopharmacology of children,* 1973, 142–148. (22)

Cohen, H. *The nature, method and purpose of diagnosis.* Cambridge: Cambridge University Press, 1943. (11)

Colby, K. M. *A primer for psychotherapists.* New York: Ronald, 1951. (8)

Cooper, J. R., Bloom, F. E., & Roth, R. H. *The biochemical basis of neuropharmacology.* New York: Oxford, 1982. (5)

Cox, T. *Stress.* Baltimore: University Park Press, 1978. (3)

Craig, T. J. An epidemiological study of a psychiatric liaison service. *General Hospital Psychiatry,* 1982, *4,* 131–137. (19)

Crick, F., & Mitchison, G. The function of dream sleep. *Nature,* 1983, *304,* 111–114. (5)

Davis, J. M., Dysken M. W., Matuzas, W. M., & Nasr, S. J. Some conceptual aspects of laboratory tests in depression. *Journal of Clinical Psychiatry,* 1983, *44,* 21–26. (10, 16)

Davis, J. M. Anti-psychotic drugs. In A. M. Freedman, H. I. Kaplan, & B. J. Sadock (Eds.), *Comprehensive textbook of psychiatry* (3rd ed.). Baltimore: Williams & Wilkins, 1980. (12)

Davis, M. S. Variation in patients' compliance with doctors' advice: An empirical analysis of patterns of communication. *American Journal of Public Health,* 1968, *58,* 274–288. (6)

DeGowin, E. L., & DeGowin, R. L. *Bedside diagnostic examination* (3rd ed.). New York: Macmillan, 1976. (27)

DeGroot, A. D. *Thought and choice in chess.* The Hague: Mouton, 1965. (27)

Detre, T. P., & Kupfer, D. J. Psychiatric history and mental status examination. In A. M. Freedman, H. I. Kaplan, & B. J. Sadock (Eds.), *Comprehensive textbook of psychiatry* Vol. 1 (2nd ed.). Baltimore: Williams & Wilkins, 1975. (8)

Devaul, R. A., & Hall, R. C. W. Hallucinations. In R. C. W. Hall (Ed.), *Psychiatric presentation of medical illness.* New York: Spectrum, 1980. (10)

Diagnostic and statistical manual of mental disorders: DSM-III (3rd ed.). Washington, D.C.: American Psychiatric Association, 1980. (9, 11, 14, 23)

Dollard, J., & Miller, N. E. *Personality and psychotherapy.* New York: McGraw-Hill, 1950. (12)

Donlon, P. T., Hopkin, J., & Tupin, J. P. Overview: Efficacy and safety of the rapid neuroleptization method with injectable haloperidol. *American Journal of Psychiatry,* 1979, *136,* 273–278. (12)

Doyle, A. C. "The Adventure of the Speckled Band." In *The Complete Sherlock Holmes* (Vol. 1). Toronto: Coles, 1980. (7)

Dunn, L. M., & Dunn, L. M. *Peabody Picture Vocabulary Test – Revised.* Circle Pines, Minn.: American Guidance Service, 1981. (21)

Eaton, J. W., & Weil, R. J. The mental health of the Hutterites. *Scientific American,* 1953, *189,* 31–37. (3)

Eddy, D. M., & Clanton, C. H. The art of diagnosis: Solving the clinico-pathological exercise. *New England Journal of Medicine,* 1982, *306,* 1263–1268. (27)

Edelbrock, C., & Achenbach, T. M. A typology of child behavior profile patterns: Distribution and correlates in disturbed children aged 6 to 16. *Journal of Abnormal Child Psychology,* 1980, *8,* 444–470. (21)

Edwards, W. Conservation in human information processing. In B. Kleinmuntz (Ed.), *Formal representation of human judgment.* New York: Wiley, 1968. (27)

Eisenberg, L. What makes persons "patients" and patients well? *American Journal of Medicine,* 1980, *69,* 277–286. (3)

Elliott, G. R., & Eisdorfer, C. *Stress and human health.* New York: Springer, 1982. (3)

Ellis, A. *Reasons and emotion in psychotherapy.* New York: Lyle Stuart, 1962. (12, 17)

Elstein, A. S. Clinical judgment: psychological research and medical practice. *Science,* 1976, *194,* 696–700. (27)

Elstein, A. S., & Bordage, G. Psychology of clinical reasoning. In G. Stone, F. Cohen, & N. Adler (Eds.), *Health psychology – a handbook.* San Francisco: Jossey-Bass, 1979. (27)

Elstein, A. S., Shulman, L. S., & Sprafka, S. A. *Medical problem solving: An analysis of clinical reasoning.* Cambridge: Harvard University Press, 1978. (27)

Enelow, A. J., & Swisher, S. N. *Interviewing and patient care.* New York: Oxford University Press, 1972. (8)

Engel, G. L. Psychogenic pain and the pain-prone patient. *American Journal of Medicine,* 1959, *26,* 899–910. (3)

—The need for a new medical model: A challenge for biomedicine. *Science,* 1977, *196,* 129–136. (3, 12, 14)

—The need for a new medical model: A challenge for biomedicine. In G. U. Balis (Ed.), *Dimensions of behavior: The psychiatric foundations of medicine.* London: Butterworth, 1978. (1, 14)

—The clinical application of the biopsychosocial model. *American Journal of Psychiatry,* 1980, *137,* 535–544. (3, 12, 14)

—Sounding board. The biopsychosocial model and medical education. Who are to be the teachers? *New England Journal of Medicine,* 1982, *306,* 802–805. (20)

Erikson, E. *Childhood and society.* New York, Norton, 1950. (24)

Exner, J. E. *The Rorschach: A comprehensive system* (Vol. 2). New York: Wiley-Interscience, 1978. (10, 22)

Eysenck, H. J., & Eysenck, S. B. G. *Manual for the Eysenck Personality Inventory.* San Diego: Educational and Industrial Testing Service, 1963. (22, 25)

Fauman, M. A. The emergency psychiatric evaluation of organic mental disorders. In S. M. Soreff (Ed.), *Emergency psychiatry. Psychiatric Clinics of North America.* 1983, *6,* 223–258. (17)

Feighner, J. P., Robins, E., Guze, S. B., Woodruff, R. A., Winokur, G., Munoz, R. Diagnostic criteria for use in psychiatric research. *Archives of General Psychiatry,* 1972, *26,* 57–63. (11)

Feightner, J. W., Norman, G. R., Barrows, H. S., & Neufeld, V. R. A comparison of the clinical methods of primary and secondary care physicians. Paper presented at symposium sponsored by the Association of American Medical Colleges, Washington, D.C., November, 1975. (27)

Feinstein, A. R. *Clinical judgment.* Baltimore: Williams & Wilkins, 1967. (27)

—An analysis of clinical reasoning: 1. The domains and disorders of clinical macrobiology. *Yale Journal of Biology and Medicine,* 1973a, *46,* 212–232. (27)

—An analysis of clinical reasoning: 2. The strategy of intermediate decisions. *Yale Journal of Biology and Medicine,* 1973b, *46,* 264–283. (27)

—An analysis of clinical reasoning: 3. The construction of clinical algorithms. *Yale Journal of Biology and Medicine,* 1974, *47,* 5–32. (27)

—A critical overview of diagnosis in psychiatry. In V. M. Rakoff, H. C. Stancer, & H. B. Kedward (Eds.), *Psychiatric diagnosis.* New York: Brunner/Mazel, 1977. (13)

Feussner, J. R., Lintors, E. W., Blessing, C. L., & Starmer, C. F. Computed tomography brain scanning in alcohol withdrawal seizures. *Annals of Internal Medicine,* 1981, *94,* 519–522. (10)

Fish, F. T. *Clinical psychopathology: Signs and symptoms in psychiatry.* Bristol: Wright, 1967. (9)

Fitzhenry-Coor, I., & Nurcombe, B. Assessing clinical reasoning: The development of a new test in psychiatric education. *Journal of Psychiatric Education,* 1983, *7,* 183–196. (27)

Folstein, M. F., Folstein, S. E., & McHugh, P. R. Mini mental state: A practical method for grading the cognitive state of patients for the clinician. *Journal of Psychiatric Research,* 1975, *12,* 189–198. (9, 19)

Fordyce, W. E., Fowler, R. S., Lehmann, J. F., & DeLateur, B. J. Some implications of learning in problems of chronic pain. *Journal of Chronic Disease,* 1968, *21,* 179–190. (3)

Frank, J. D. Some problems of research in group psychotherapy. *International Journal of Group Psychotherapy,* 1975, *25,* 141–145. (12)

Freedman, A. M., Kaplan, H. I., & Sadock, B. J. *Comprehensive textbook of psychiatry,* Vol. 3 (3rd ed.) Baltimore: Williams & Wilkins, 1980. (18)

Freeman, A. M., & Sack, R. L. Contributions of psychiatry to primary care medicine. In A. M. Freeman, R. L. Sack, & P. A. Berger (Eds.), *Psychiatry for the primary care physician.* Baltimore: Williams & Wilkins, 1979. (20)

Freeman, A. M., Sack, R. L., & Berger, P. A. *Psychiatry for the primary care physician.* Baltimore: Williams & Wilkins, 1979. (20)

Friedman, M., Thousen, C. E., Gill, J. J., Ulmer, D., Thompson, L., Powell, L., Price, V., Elek, S. R., Rabin, D. D., Breall, W. S., Piaget, G., Dixon, T., Bourg, E., Levy, R. A., & Tatso, D. L. Feasibility of altering type A behavior after myocardial infarction. Recurrent coronary project prevention study methods, baseline results, and preliminary findings. *Circulation,* 1982, *66,* 83–92. (12)

Gallagher, R. M. Aggressive behavior in the disabled. In D. Bishop (Ed.), *Behavior problems in the disabled.* Baltimore: Williams & Wilkins, 1980. (17)

—The biopsychosocial grid in consultation-liaison psychiatry. Paper presented at the International Congress of Psychosomatic Medicine, Montreal, October 1982. (20)

Gallagher, R. M., & Chapman, R. The medication seminar and primary care education. *General Hospital Psychiatry,* 1981, *3,* 16–23. (3, 20)

Gallagher, R. M., McKegney, F. P., & Gladstone, T. Psychiatric interventions in spinal cord injury. *Psychosomatics,* 1982, *23,* 1153–1167. (19)

Gardner, E. A. Emotional disorders in medical practice. *Annals of Internal Medicine,* 1970, *73,* 651–653. (20)

Gardner, R. A. *Therapeutic communication with children: The mutual storytelling technique.* New York: Science House, 1971. (21)

Gauron, E. F., & Dickinson, J. K. Diagnostic decision making in psychiatry: I. Information usage. II. Diagnostic styles. *Archives of General Psychiatry,* 1965, *14;* 225–232; 233–277. (27)

Gazda, T., Gallagher, R. M., Little, D., & Sproul, M. S. The group practice seminar: A Balint-type group in a family practice residency program. *Family Medicine,* 1984, *16,* 54–58. (3, 20)

Gehi, M., Strain, J. J., Weltz, R. N., & Jacob, J. Is there a need for admission and discharge cognitive screening of the medically ill? *General Hospital Psychiatry,* 1980, *2,* 186–191. (19)

Gelenberg, A. Lithium and the kidney. *Massachusetts General Hospital Newsletter: Biological Therapies in Psychiatry,* 1981, *4,* 25. (12)

—(Ed.). Lithium-related skin reaction. *Massachusetts General Hospital Newsletter: Biological Therapies in Psychiatry,* 1982, *5,* 39. (12)

—Laboratory tests for patients taking psychotropic drugs. *Massachusetts General Hospital Newsletter: Biological Therapies in Psychiatry,* 1983b, *6,* 5–7. (a) (12)

—Lithium may suppress respiration in chronic lung disease. *Massachusetts General Hospital Newsletter: Biological Therapies in Psychiatry,* 1983c, *6,* 19. (b) (12)

—The DST in perspective. *Massachusetts General Hospital Newsletter: Biological Therapies in Psychiatry,* 1983a, *6,* 1–2. (10)

Gerson, S., & Bassuck, E. Psychiatric emergencies: An overview. *American Journal of Psychiatry,* 1980, *137,* 1–11. (17)

Gesell, A., & Amatruda, C. S. *Developmental diagnosis.* New York: Hoeber, 1947. (21)

Ginsburg, H., & Opper, S. *Piaget's theory of intellectual development: An introduction.* Englewood Cliffs, N.J.: Prentice-Hall, 1969. (24)

Glaser, K., & Clemmens, R. L. School failure. *Pediatrics,* 1965, *35,* 128–141. (21)

Glick, I., & Kessler, D. R. *Marital and family therapy* (2nd ed.). New York: Grune & Stratton, 1980. (21, 25)

Goldberg, S. C., Schooler, N. R., Hogarty, G. E., & Roper, M. Prediction of relapse in schizophrenic outpatients treated by drugs and sociotherapy. *Archives of General Psychiatry,* 1977, *34,* 171–184. (12)

Golden, C. J., Hammeke, T., & Purisch, A. Diagnostic validity of a standardized battery derived from Luria's neuropsychological tests. *Journal of Consulting and Clinical Psychology*, 1978, *46*, 1258–1265. (22)

Gonda, T. A. The relation between complaints of persistent pain and family size. *Journal of Neurology, Neurosurgery and Psychiatry*, 1962, *25*, 277–281. (3)

Gori, G., & Ritker, B. J. Macroeconomics of disease prevention in the United States. *Science*, 1978, *20*, 1124–1130. (3)

Graham, F. K., & Kendall, B. S. Memory-for-designs test: Revised general manual. *Perceptual and Motor Skills*, 1960, *11*, 147–188. (22)

Grant, R. L., & Maletzky, B. Application of the Weed system to psychiatric records. *Psychiatric Medicine*, 1972, *3*, 119–129. (13)

Greenspan, S. I. *The clinical interview of the child*. New York: McGraw-Hill, 1981. (a) (21)

—*Psychopathology and adaptation in infancy and early childhood*. New York: International Universities Press, 1981. (b) (21, 24)

Greenspan, S. I., & Pollock, G. H. *The course of life: psychoanalytic contributions toward understanding personality development* (2 vols.). Washington, D.C.: U.S. Department of Health & Human Services, 1980. (24)

Greer, S., Morris, T., & Pettingale, K. W. Psychological response to breast cancer: Effect on outcome. *Lancet*, 1979, *13*, 785–787. (3)

Greist, J. H., Eischens, M. S., Klein, M. H., & Faris, J. W. Antidepressant running. *Psychiatric Annals*, 1979, *9*, 23–33. (12)

Greist, J. H., Jefferson, J. W., & Spitzer, R. L. (Eds.). *Treatment of mental disorders*. New York: Oxford, 1982. (12)

Group for the Advancement of Psychiatry. *Psychopathological disorders in childhood: Theoretical considerations and a proposed classification*. New York: GAP Report No. 62, 1966. (23)

—*From diagnosis to treatment in child psychiatry*. New York: Jason Aronsen, 1974. (25)

Groves, P., & Schlesinger, K. *Introduction to biological psychiatry*. Dubuque, Ia.: William Brown, 1979. (5)

Guidano, V. F., & Liotti, G. *Cognitive processes and emotional disorders*. New York: Guilford, 1983. (4)

Guggenheim, F. G., & O'Hara, S. Peer counseling in a general hospital. *American Journal of Psychiatry*, 1976, *133*, 1197–1199. (12, 19)

Guttman, H. A. Symposium on psychosomatics and the family: Introduction. *General Hospital Psychiatry*, 1983, *5*, 37–39.

Hackett, T. P., & Cassem, N. H. (Eds.). *Handbook of general hospital psychiatry*. St. Louis: Mosby, 1978. (19)

Haley, J. The perverse triangle. In G. Zuk & I. Boszormenyi-Nagy (Eds.), *Family therapy and disturbed families*. Palo Alto, Calif.: Science and Behavior Books, 1967. (12)

Hall, R. C. W. Anxiety. In R. C. W. Hall (Ed.), *Psychiatric presentation of medical illness*. New York: Spectrum, 1980. (a) (10)

—Depression. In R. C. W. Hall (Ed.), *Psychiatric presentation of medical illness*. New York: Spectrum, 1980. (b) (10)

Hall, R. C. W., Popkin, M. K., & Devaul, R. A. Physical illness presenting as psychiatric disease. *Archives of General Psychiatry*, 1978, *35*, 1315–1320. (10)

Hamburg, D. A., Elliott, G. R., & Parron, D. L. (Eds.). *Health and behavior: Frontiers of research in the biochemical sciences*. Washington, D.C.: National Academy Press, 1982. (3)

Hammond, K. R. Probabilistic functioning and the clinical method. *Psychological Review*, 1955, *62*, 255–262. (27)

Hathaway, S. R., & McKinley, J. C. *The Minnesota Multiphasic Personality Inventory.* New York: Psychological Corp., 1943. (10)

Haynes, R. B., Sackett, D. L., & Taylor, D. W. How to detect and manage low patient compliance in chronic illness. *Geriatrics,* 1980, *35,* 96–97. (3)

Herjanic, B., & Campbell, W. Differentiating psychiatrically disturbed children on the basis of a structured interview. *Journal of Abnormal Child Psychology,* 1977, *5,* 127–134. (21)

Herskowitz, J., & Rosman, N. P. *Pediatrics, neurology and psychiatry – common ground: Behavioral, cognitive, affective and physical disorders in childhood and adolescence.* New York: Macmillan, 1982. (22)

Hilgard, E. R., Atkinson, R. L., & Atkinson, R. C. *Introduction to psychology* (7th ed.). New York: Harcourt, Brace & Jovanovitch, 1979. (4)

Hillman, D. *Family assessment procedure.* Unpublished manuscript. Burlington, Vt.: University of Vermont, 1982. (21)

Hinsie, L. E., & Campbell, R. J. *Psychiatric dictionary* (4th ed.). London: Oxford University Press, 1970. (9)

Hinton, J., & Withers, E. The usefulness of clinical tests of the sensorium. *British Journal of Psychiatry,* 1971, *119,* 9–18. (9)

Hobson, J. A., & McCarley, R. W. The neurobiological origins of psychoanalytic dream theory. *American Journal of Psychiatry,* 1977, *134,* 1211–1221. (a) (5)

—The brain as a dream state generator: An activation–synthesis hypothesis of the dream process. *American Journal of Psychiatry,* 1977, *134,* 1335–1348. (b) (5)

Hollinshead, A., & Redlich, R. C. *Social class and mental illness.* New York: Wiley, 1958. (3)

Holmes, D. J. *The adolescent in psychotherapy.* Boston: Little, Brown, 1964. (21, 25)

Holt, R. R. Clinical and statistical prediction: A reformulation and some new data. *Journal of Abnormal and Social Psychology,* 1958, *56,* 1–12. (27)

Horowitz, M. J. Intensive repetitive thoughts after experimental stress: A summary. *Archives of General Psychiatry,* 1975, *32,* 1457–1463. (3)

Horowitz, M. J., & Wilner, N. Stress, emotion and cognitive response. *Archives of General Psychiatry,* 1976, *30,* 1339–1344. (3)

Houpt, J. L., Orleans, C. S., George, L. K., & Brodie, K. H. The role of psychiatric and behavioral factors in the practice of medicine. *American Journal of Psychiatry,* 1980, *137,* 37–47. (3, 20)

Houts, P. K., & Scott, R. A. *Individualized goal planning.* Hershey, Pa.: Mental Health Rehabilitation, 1976. (15)

Hull, C. L. *Essentials of behavior.* New Haven: Yale University Press, 1950. (12)

Hutt, M. L. *The Michigan Picture Test – Revised.* New York: Grune & Stratton, 1980. (22)

Ireton, H., & Thwing, E. *Manual for the Minnesota Child Development Inventory.* Minneapolis: Behavior Science Systems, 1972. (21)

Issacs, B., & Kennie, A. T. The set test as an aid to the detection of dementia in old people. *British Journal of Psychiatry,* 1973, *123,* 467–470. (9)

Iverson, L. L. Neurotransmitters and CNS disease: Introduction. *Lancet,* 1982, *2,* 914–918. (5)

Jackson, D. D. The question of family homeostasis. *Psychiatric Quarterly,* 1957, *31*(suppl.), 79–90. (12)

Jacobs, J. W., Bernhard, M. R., Delgado, A., & Strain, J. J. Screening for organic mental syndromes in the medically ill. *Annals of Internal Medicine,* 1977, *86,* 40–46. (19)

Jakobsen, R. *Kindersprache, Aphasie und Allgemeine Lautgesetze.* Uppsala, Sweden: Almquist and Wiksell, 1941. (24)

Jaspers, K. *Allgemeine psychopathologie* (5th ed.). Berlin & Heidelberg: Springer, 1948 (originally published 1913.) [*General psychopathology*] (J. Hoenig & M. W. Hamilton, trans.) Manchester: Manchester University Press, 1962. (9)

Jastak, J. F., & Jastak, S. R. *Wide Range Achievement Test.* Wilmington, Del.: Jastak Associates, 1978. (22)

Jensen, P. S. The doctor patient relationship: Headed for impasse or improvement? *Annals of Internal Medicine,* 1981, *95,* 769–771. (19)

Jessell, T. M. Neurotransmitters and CNS disease: Pain. *Lancet,* 1982, *2,* 1084–1088. (5)

Jolly, W., Froom, J., & Rosen, M. G. The genogram. *Journal of Family Practice,* 1980, *10,* 251–255. (20)

Kagan, N. *Influencing human interaction.* East Lansing: Instructional Media Center, Michigan State University, 1971. (27)

Kahana, R. J., & Bibring, J. L. Personality types in medical management. In N. Zinberg (Ed.), *Psychiatry and medical practice in a general hospital.* New York: International Universities Press, 1964, 108–123. (3)

Kahn, R. L., Goldfarb, A. I., Pollack, M., & Peck, A. Brief objective measures for the determination of mental status in the aged. *American Journal of Psychiatry,* 1960, *117,* 326–328. (9)

Kahneman, D., Slovic, P., & Tversky, A. *Judgment under uncertainty: Heuristics and biases.* Cambridge: Cambridge University Press, 1982. (27)

Kandell, E. R. Psychotherapy and the single synapse. *New England Journal of Medicine,* 1979, *301,* 1028–1037. (5)

Kannell, W. B. Role of blood pressure in cardiovascular morbidity and mortality. *Progress in Cardiovascular Disorder,* 1974, *17,* 5–24. (3)

Kaplan, H. S. The new sex therapy. In H. S. Kaplan (Ed.), *The new sex therapy.* New York: Brunner/Mazel, 1974. (12)

Karasu, T. K. Psychotherapy and pharmacotherapy: Toward an integrative model. *American Journal of Psychiatry,* 1982, *139,* 1102–1113. (12)

Karmer, A. D., Cayne, J. C., Schaefer, C., & Lapanes, R. S. Comparison of two modes of stress management: Daily hassles and uplifts versus major life events. *Journal of Behavioral Medicine,* 1981, *4,* 1–39. (3)

Kaufman, D. M., Weinberger, M., Strain, J. J., & Jacobs, J. W. Detection of cognitive deficits by a brief mental status examination: The cognitive capacity screening examination, a reappraisal and a review. *General Hospital Psychiatry,* 1979, *1,* 247–255. (9)

Keefe, F. J., & Blumenthal, J. A. (Eds.). *Assessment strategies in behavioral medicine,* New York: Grune & Stratton, 1982. (19)

Kendell, R. E. Psychiatric diagnoses: A study of how they are done. *British Journal of Psychiatry,* 1973, *122,* 437–445. (27)

—*The role of diagnosis in psychiatry.* London: Blackwell, 1974. (11)

Kimball, C. P. (Ed.). Liaison psychiatry. *Psychiatric Clinics of North America,* 1979, *2,* 191–416. (19)

—*The biopsychosocial approach to the patient.* Baltimore: Williams & Wilkins, 1981. (19)

Kiresuk, T. J., & Sherman, G. E. Goal attainment scaling: A general method for evaluating comprehensive community mental health programs. *Community Mental Health Journal,* 1968, *6,* 443–453. (15)

Kirk, S. A., McCarthy, J. J., & Kirk, W. D. *Illinois Test of Psycholinguistic Ability.* Urbana: University of Illinois Press, 1968. (22)

Klein, D. F., Gittelman, R., Quitkin, F., & Rifkin, A. *Diagnosis and drug treatment of psychiatric disorders: Adults and children.* Baltimore: Williams & Wilkins, 1980. (25)

Kleinmuntz, B. *Clinical information processing by computer.* New York: Holt, 1969. (27)

Klerman, G. L. Psychotherapies and somatic therapies in affective disorder. In H. S. Akiskal (Ed.), Diagnosis and treatment of affective disorders. *Psychiatric Clinics of North America,* 1983, *6,* 85–103. (12)

Knox, E. G. Multiphasic screening. *Lancet,* 1974, *2,* 1434–1436. (10)

Koppitz, E. M. *Psychological evaluation of children's human figure drawings.* New York: Grune & Stratton, 1968. (21, 22)

—*The Bender Gestalt Test for Young Children* (2 vols.). New York: Grune & Stratton, 1975. (22)

—*The Visual Aural Digit Span Test.* New York: Grune & Stratton, 1977. (22)

Koran, L. M., Moos, R. H., Moos, B., & Zasslow, M. Changing hospital work environments: An example of a burn unit. *General Hospital Psychiatry,* 1983, *5,* 7–13. (19)

Koranyi, E. K. Morbidity and rate of undiagnosed physical illness in a psychiatric clinic population. *Archives of General Psychiatry,* 1979, *36,* 414–419. (10)

Kovacs, M., & Beck, A. T. An empirical-clinical approach toward a definition of childhood depression. In J. G. Schulterbrand & A. Raskin (Eds.), *Depression in childhood: Diagnosis, treatment and conceptual models.* New York: Raven, 1977. (23)

Kovacs, M., Rush, J. A., Beck, A. T., & Hollon, S. D. Depressed outpatients treated with cognitive therapy or pharmacotherapy: One year follow-up. *Archives of General Psychiatry,* 1981, *38,* 33–39. (12)

Kraepelin, E. *Lectures in clinical psychiatry* (2nd rev. ed.). (T. Johnstone, trans.). New York: Hafner, 1968. (9)

Kristian, M. M., Arnold, C. R., & Wynden, K. L. Health economics and preventive care. *Science,* 1977, *195,* 457–462. (3)

Kuhn, T. *The structure of scientific revolutions* (2nd. ed.). International encyclopedia of unified science (vol. 2) 2. Chicago: University of Chicago Press, 1970. (13)

Kupfer, D. J., Gillen, J. C., & Coble, P. A. REM sleep, naps, and depression. *Psychiatry Research,* 1981, *5,* 195–203. (10)

Kupfer, D. J., & Thase, M. E. The use of the sleep laboratory in the diagnosis of affective disorders. In H. S. Akiskal (Ed.), Diagnosis and treatment of affective disorders. *The Psychiatric Clinics of North America,* 1983, *6,* 3–26. (10)

Laing, R. D. *The divided self: A study of sanity and madness.* London: Tavistock, 1960. (9)

—*Sanity, madness and the family.* London: Tavistock, 1964. (11)

—*The politics of experience and the bird of paradise.* New York: Random House, 1967. (11)

Lamb, D. *Psychotherapy with adolescent girls.* San Francisco: Jossey-Bass, 1978. (21, 25)

Laqueur, H. P. Multiple family therapy and general systems theory. *International Journal of Psychiatry Clinics,* 1970, *7,* 99–124. (12)

Larkin, J., McDermott, J., Simon, D. P., & Simon, H. Expert and novice performance in solving physics problems. *Science,* 1980, *208,* 1335–1342. (27)

Larson, E. B., Mach, L. A., Watts, B., & Cromwell, L. D. Computerized tomography in patients with psychiatric illness: Advantage of a ''rule-in'' approach. *Annals of Internal Medicine,* 1981, *95,* 360–364. (10)

Lazare, A. The psychiatric examination in the walk-in clinic: Hypothesis generation and hypothesis testing. *Archives of General Psychiatry,* 1976, *33,* 981–996. (7)

—*Outpatient psychiatry: Diagnosis and treatment.* Baltimore: Williams & Wilkins, 1979. (6, 12, 16)

Lazare, A., & Eisenthal, S. Patient requests in a walk-in clinic: Replication of a factor analysis in an independent sample. *Journal of Nervous and Mental Diseases,* 1977, *165,* 330–340. (16)

Lazare, A., Eisenthal, S., & Wasserman, L. The customer approach to patienthood: Attending to patient requests in a walk-in clinic. *Archives of General Psychiatry,* 1975, *32,* 553–558. (16)

Lazarus, A. A. *The practice of multimodal therapy.* New York: McGraw-Hill, 1981. (12)

Leitenberg, H. (Ed.). *Handbook of behavior modification and behavior therapy.* Englewood Cliffs, N.J.: Prentice-Hall, 1976. (25)

Leiter, R. G. *Leiter International Performance Scale.* Chicago: Stoelting, 1948. (22)

Lewis, J. M., & Usdin, G. *Treatment planning in psychiatry.* Washington, D.C.: American Psychiatric Association, 1982. (12)

Lewis, M. *Clinical aspects of child development.* Philadelphia: Lea & Febiger, 1982. (24)

Lipowski, Z. J. Physical illness, the individual, and the coping process. *Psychiatry in Medicine,* 1970, *1,* 91–102. (3)

—Consultation-liaison psychiatry: An overview. *American Journal of Psychiatry,* 1974, *131,* 623–630. (19)

—Consultation-liaison psychiatry: Past failures and new opportunities. *General Hospital Psychiatry,* 1979, *1,* 3–10. (19)

—Discussion: Liaison psychiatry and the quest for new knowledge. *General Hospital Psychiatry,* 1983, *5,* 111–114. (a) (19)

—Transient cognitive disorder (delirium, acute confusional states) in the elderly. *American Journal of Psychiatry,* 1983, *140,* 1426–1436. (b) (19)

Lipowski, Z. J., Lipsitt, D. R., & Whybrow, P. C. (Eds.). *Psychosomatic medicine.* New York: Oxford, 1977. (19)

Lippman, H. S. *Treatment of the child in emotional conflict.* New York: McGraw-Hill, 1962. (21, 25)

Lipsitt, D. R., & Lipsitt, M. P. The family in consultation psychiatry. *General Hospital Psychiatry,* 1981, *3,* 231–236. (19)

Lishman, W. A. *Organic psychiatry.* London: Oxford University Press, 1978. (10)

Locke, S. E. Stress, adaptation, and immunity: Studies in humans. *General Hospital Psychiatry,* 1983, *4,* 49–58. (3, 5)

London, P., & Klerman, G. L. Evaluating psychotherapy. *American Journal of Psychiatry,* 1982, *139,* 709–717. (12)

Lovitt, R. Psychological testing and consultation-liaison psychiatry. *General Hospital Psychiatry,* 1982, *4,* 233–240. (19)

Luce, B. R., & Schitzer, H. O. Smoking and alcohol abuse: A comparison of their economic consequences. *New England Journal of Medicine,* 1978, *298,* 569–571. (3)

Ludwig, A. M. *Principles of clinical psychiatry.* New York: The Free Press, 1980. (9, 10, 11, 13)

Lusted, L. B. *Introduction to medical decision making.* Springfield, Ill.: Thomas, 1968. (27)

MacKenzie, T., & Popkin, M. Organic anxiety syndrome. *American Journal of Psychiatry,* 1983, *140,* 342–344. (10)

Mahler, M. S., Pine, F., and Bergman, A. *The psychological birth of the human infant.* New York: Basic Books, 1975. (24)

Main, T. F. The ailment. *British Journal of Medical Psychology,* 1957, *30,* 144–145. (18)

Marmor, J. Systems thinking in psychiatry: Some theoretical and clinical implications. *American Journal of Psychiatry,* 1983, *140,* 833–838. (12)

Marmor, J., & Woods, S. M. *The Interface between the psychodynamic and behavioral therapies.* New York: Plenum, 1980. (12)

Marsden, C. D. Neurotransmitters and CNS disease: Basal ganglia disease. *Lancet,* 1982, *2,* 1141–1147. (5)

Maslow, P., Frostig, M., Lefever, D. W., & Whittlesey, J. R. B. The Marianne Frostig developmental test of visual perception in 1963 standardization. *Perceptual and Motor Skills,* 1964, *19,* 463–499. (22)

Maxmen, J. S., Tucker, G. J., & LeBow, M. D. *Rational hospital psychiatry: The reactive environment.* New York: Brunner/Mazel, 1974. (18)

McCarthy, D. *McCarthy Scales of Children's Abilities.* New York: Psychological Corporation, 1972. (22)

McIntyre, J. S., & Romano, J. Is there a stethoscope in the house (and is it used)? *Archives of General Psychiatry,* 1977, *34,* 1147–1151. (10)

McKegney, F. P., & Beckhardt, R. M. Evaluation research in consultation-liaison psychiatry: Review of the literature. *General Hospital Psychiatry,* 1982, *4,* 197–218. (19)

McKegney, F. P., McMahon, T., & King, J. The use of DSM-III in a general hospital consultation-liaison service. *General Hospital Psychiatry,* 1983, *5,* 115–121. (19)

McMahon, T., Gallagher, R. M., & Little, D. N. Psychiatry-family practice liaison: A collaborative approach to clinical training. *General Hospital Psychiatry,* 1983, *5,* 1–6. (20)

Mechanic, D. Religion, religiosity and illness behavior: The special case of the Jews. *Human Organization,* 1963, *22,* 202–208. (3)

—The influence of mothers on their children's health attitudes and behavior. *Pediatrics,* 1964, *33,* 444–453. (3)

—*Medical Sociology.* New York: Free Press, 1968. (3, 6)

—Social psychologic factors affecting the presentation of bodily complaints. *New England Journal of Medicine,* 1972, *286,* 1132–1139. (3)

—Effects of psychological distress on perceptions of physical health and use of medical and psychiatric facilities. *Journal of Human Stress,* 1978, *4,* 26–32. (3)

Meehl, P. E. *Clinical versus statistical prediction.* Minneapolis: University of Minnesota Press, 1954. (27)

—*Psychodiagnosis: Selected papers.* Minneapolis: University of Minnesota Press, 1974. (27)

Meeks, J. E. *The fragile alliance: An orientation to the outpatient psychotherapy of the adolescent.* Huntington, N.Y.: Kreiger, 1980. (21, 25)

Meissner, W. W., Mack, J. E., & Semrad, E. V. Classical psychoanalysis. In A. M. Freedman, H. I. Kaplan, & B. J. Sadock (Eds.), *Comprehensive textbook of psychiatry,* Vol. 3 (2nd ed.). Baltimore: Williams & Wilkins, 1975. (4)

Mellinger, G. D., Balter, M. B., Manheimer, D. I., Cisin, I. H., & Parig, H. J. Psychic distress, life crisis, and use of psychotherapeutic medications: National household survey data. *Archives of General Psychiatry,* 1978, *35,* 1045–1052. (12)

Menninger, K. Changing concepts of disease. *Annals of Internal Medicine,* 1948, *29,* 318–325. (11)

Merskey, H., & Spear, F. G. The concept of pain. *Journal of Psychosomatic Research,* 1967, *11,* 59–67. (a) (3)

—*Pain: Psychological and psychiatric aspects.* London: Balliere, Tindall & Cassell, 1967. (b) (3)

Miller, J. G. *The living system.* New York: McGraw-Hill, 1978. (12)

Milstein, V., Small, J. G., & Small, I. F. The subtraction of serial sevens test in psychiatric patients. *Archives of General Psychiatry,* 1972, *26,* 439–441. (9)

Minuchin, S. *Families and family therapy.* London: Tavistock, 1974. (21, 25)

Mitchell, J. E., & Mackenzie, T. B. Cardiac effects of lithium therapy in man: A review. *Journal of Clinical Psychiatry,* 1982, *43,* 47–51. (12)

Modell, J. Principles of ordering laboratory tests for diagnosis and management. Personal communication to R. M. Gallagher, 1 December, 1983. (10, 18)

Mohl, P. C. What model of liaison psychiatry meets whose needs? *General Hospital Psychiatry,* 1983, *5,* 213–215. (19)

Money, J., & Ehrhardt, A. A. *Man and woman, boy and girl: The differentiation and dimorphism of gender identity from conception to maturity.* Baltimore: Johns Hopkins University, 1972. (24)

Moore, D. P. Rapid treatment of delirium in critically ill patients. *American Journal of Psychiatry,* 1977, *134,* 1431–1432. (12)

Morgan, W. P. Anxiety reduction following acute physical activity. *Psychiatric Annals,* 1979, *9,* 36–45. (12)

Moyer, K. E. *The physiology of hostility.* Chicago: Markham, 1971. (17)

Murray, G. R. Violent behavior. In A. Lazare (Ed.), *Outpatient psychiatry.* Baltimore: Williams & Wilkins, 1979. (17)

Murray, H. A. *Thematic Apperception Test.* Cambridge: Harvard University Press, 1943. (10, 22)

Mussen, P. H., Conger, J. J., & Kagan, J. *Child development and personality* (5th ed.). New York: Harper & Row, 1979. (24)

Neill, J. R. Once more into the breach: Doubts about liaison psychiatry. *General Hospital Psychiatry,* 1983, *5,* 205–208. (19)

Nelson, W. H., Orr, W. W., & Stevenson, J. Hypothalamic-pituitary-adrenal axis activity and tricyclic response in major depression. *Archives of General Psychiatry,* 1982, *39,* 1033–1036. (10)

Newell, A., & Simon, H. A. Computer simulation of human thinking. *Science,* 1961, *134,* 2011–2017. (27)

Newell, A., & Simon, H. A. *Human problem solving.* Englewood Cliffs, N.J.: Prentice-Hall, 1972. (27)

Newman, G. Intermittent recurring psychosis. In R. C. W. Hall (Ed.), *Psychiatric presentation of medical illness.* New York: Spectrum, 1980. (10)

Nicholi, A. M. History and mental status. In A. M. Nicholi (Ed.), *The Harvard guide to modern psychiatry.* Cambridge: Harvard University Press, 1978. (8)

Nurcombe, B., & Fitzhenry-Coor, I. How do psychiatrists think? Clinical reasoning in the psychiatric interview: A research and education project. *Australian and New Zealand Journal of Psychiatry,* 1982, *16,* 13–24. (27)

Offer, D., & Offer, J. Three developmental routes through normal male adolescence. In S. C. Feinstein & P. L. Giovacchini (Eds.), *Adolescent Psychiatry,* Vol. 4. New York: Aronsen, 1975. (24)

Opler, M. K., & Singer, J. L. Ethnic differences in behavior and psychopathology: Italian and Irish. *International Journal of Social Psychiatry,* 1956, *2,* 11–22. (3)

Parsons, T. Illness and the role of the physician: A sociologic perspective. *American Journal of Orthopsychiatry,* 1951, *21,* 452–460. (3)

Pavlov, I. D. *Conditioned reflexes.* London: Oxford University Press, 1927. (12)

Pfeiffer, E. A short portable mental status questionnaire for the assessment of organic brain deficit in elderly patients. *Journal of the American Geriatrics Society,* 1975, *13,* 443–451. (9, 19)

Pilowsky, I. The diagnosis of abnormal illness behavior. *Australian and New Zealand Journal of Psychiatry,* 1971, *5,* 138–139. (3)

—A general classification of abnormal illness behaviors. *British Journal of Medical Psychology,* 1978, *51,* 131–137. (3)

Pilowsky, I., Spence, N. D., & Waddy, J. L. Illness behavior and coronary artery by-pass surgery. *Journal of Psychosomatic Research,* 1978, *23,* 39–44. (3)

Pincus, J., & Tucker, G. *Behavioral neurology.* New York: Oxford, 1974. (10)

Prakash, R., Kelwala, S., & Ban, T. A. Neurotoxicity with combined administration of lithium and a neuroleptic. *Comprehensive Psychiatry,* 1982, *23,* 567–571. (12)

Prusoff, B. A., Weissman, M. M., Klerman, G. L., & Rounsanville, B. J. Research diagnostic criteria subtypes of depression as predictors of differential response to psychotherapy and drug treatment. *Archives of General Psychiatry,* 1980, *37,* 796–801. (12)

Pucees, H. A., Strain, J. J., Houpt, J. L., & Gise, L. H. Models of mental health training in primary care. *Journal of the American Medical Association,* 1983, *249,* 3065–3068. (20)

Rahe, R. H., & Arthur, R. J. Life change and illness studies: Past history and future directions. *Journal of Human Stress,* 1978, *4,* 3–15. (3)

Rahe, R. H., Ryman, D. H., & Ward, H. W. Simplified scaling for life change events. *Journal of Human Stress,* 1980, *6,* 22–27. (3)

Rapoport, J. L. Congenital anomalies, appearance and body build. In M. Rutter (Ed.), *Scientific foundations of developmental psychiatry.* Baltimore: University Park Press, 1981. (22)

Rapoport, J. L., Quinn, P. O., Burg, C., & Bartley, C. Can hyperactives be identified in infancy? In R. L. Trites (Ed.), *Hyperactivity in children.* Baltimore: University Park Press, 1979. (22)

Raven, J. C. *Progressive matrices.* New York: Psychological Corporation, 1960. (22)

Regier, D. A., Goldberg, I. D., & Taube, C. A. The de facto U.S. mental health service system. *Archives of General Psychiatry,* 1978, *35,* 684–693. (16, 20)

Reiser, D. E., & Schroder, A. K. *Patient interviewing: The human dimension.* Baltimore: Williams & Wilkins, 1980. (8)

Reiser, M. F. Changing theoretical concepts in psychosomatic medicine. In M. F. Reiser (Ed.), *American Handbook of Psychiatry,* Vol. 4. New York: Basic Books, 1975, 477–500. (12)

Reisman, J. M. *Principles of psychotherapy with children.* New York: Wiley, 1973. (25)

Reitan, R. M., & Davison, L. A. (Eds.). *Clinical neuropsychology: Current status and applications.* Washington, D.C.: Winston, 1974. (10, 22)

Reynolds, C. F., Coble, P. A., & Kupfer, D. J. Application of the multiple sleep latency test in disorders of excessive sleepiness. *EEG Clinical Neurophysiology,* 1982, *53,* 443–452. (10)

Ripley, H. S. Psychiatric interview. In A. M. Freedman, H. I. Kaplan, & B. J.

Sadock (Eds.), *Comprehensive textbook of psychiatry*, Vol. 1 (2nd ed.). Baltimore: Williams & Wilkins, 1975. (8)

Rogers, C. R. *Client-centered therapy: Its current practice, implications and theory*. Boston: Houghton Mifflin, 1951. (8, 21, 25)

Rogers, M. P., Dubey, D., & Reich, P. The influence of the psyche and brain on immunity and disease susceptibility: A critical review. *Psychosomatic Medicine*, 1979, *41*, 147–164. (3, 5)

Rose, S. D. *Treating children in groups: A behavioral approach*. San Francisco: Jossey-Bass, 1972. (25)

Rosen, B. M., Locke, B. Z., Goldberg, I. D., & Babigian, H. M. Identification of emotional disturbance in patients seen in general medical clinics. *Hospital and Community Psychiatry*. 1972, *23*, 364–370. (20)

Rosenhan, D. L. On being sane in insane places. *Science*, 1973, *179*, 250–258. (11)

Rossor, M. N. Neurotransmitters and CNS disease: Dementia. *Lancet*, 1982, *2*, 1200–1204. (5)

Ruoff, P. *The Child Information Form*. Unpublished questionnaire. Burlington, Vt.: University of Vermont, 1980. (21)

Russell, E. W. The pathology and clinical examination of memory. In C. W. M. Whitty & O. L. Zangwill (Eds.), *Amnesia*. London: Butterworth, 1977. (5)

Rutter, M., & Graham, P. The reliability and validity of the psychiatric assessment of the child: 1. Interview with the child. *British Journal of Psychiatry*, 1968, *114*, 563–579. (21)

Rutter, M., & Hersov, L. (Eds.). *Child psychiatry: Modern approaches*. Oxford: Blackwell, 1977. (25)

Ryback, R. S., Longabaugh, R., & Fowler, D. R. *The problem-oriented record in psychiatry and mental health care* (rev. ed.). New York: Grune & Stratton, 1981. (13, 15)

Salzman, C. Psychologic drug use and polypharmacy in a general hospital. *General Hospital Psychiatry*, 1981, *3*, 1–9. (19)

Sandifer, M. G., Hordern, A., & Green, I. M. The psychiatric interviews: The impact of the first three minutes. *American Journal of Psychiatry*, 1970, *126*, 968–973. (27)

Scadding, J. G. Diagnosis: The clinician and the computer. *Lancet*, 1967, *2;* 877–882. (11)

Schachter, S., & Singer, J. E. Cognitive, social and physiological determinants of emotional state. *Psychological Reviews*, 1962, *69*, 379–399. (6)

Scharfetter, C. [*General psychopathology: An introduction*] (H. Marshall, trans.). Cambridge: Cambridge University Press, 1980. (Originally published as *Allgemeine Psychopathologie*, 1976). (9)

Scheff, T. J. The role of the mentally ill and the dynamics of mental disorder: A research framework. *Sociometry*, 1963, *26*, 436–453. (11)

—Users and non-users of a student psychiatric clinic. *Journal of Health and Human Behavior*, 1966, *7*, 114–121. (3)

Schilgen, B., & Tolle, R. Partial sleep deprivation as therapy for depression. *Archives of General Psychiatry*, 1980, *37*, 267–271. (12)

Schleifer, S. J., Keller, S. E., McKegney, F. P., & Stein, M. Bereavement and lymphocyte function. Paper presented at annual meeting, American Psychiatric Association, San Francisco, May 1980. (3)

Schneider, K. *Klinische Psychopathologie* (8th ed.). Stuttgart: Thieme, 1967. (9)

Scott-Henderson, S. Social relationships, adversity and neurosis: An analysis of prospective observations. *British Journal of Psychiatry*, 1981, *138*, 391–398. (3)

Sederer, L. I. (Ed.). *Inpatient psychiatry: Diagnosis and Treatment.* Baltimore: Williams & Wilkins, 1983. (18)

Segraves, R. T., & Smith, R. C. Concurrent psychotherapy and behavior therapy. *Archives of General Psychiatry,* 1976, *33,* 756–763. (12)

Seligman, M. E. P. *Helplessness: On depression, development and death.* San Francisco: Freeman, 1975. (23)

Seligson, D., & Gallagher, R. M. The psychiatric team on a spinal cord injury service. *Psychosomatics,* 1982, *23,* 1152–1159. (19)

Shaffer, D. Soft neurological signs and later psychological disorder. *Journal of Psychology, Psychiatry and Allied Disciplines,* 1978, *19,* 63–65. (22)

Shafii, M., & Shafii, S. L. *Pathways of human development: Normal growth and emotional disorders in infancy, childhood and adolescence.* New York: Thieme-Stratton, 1982. (24, 25)

Shapiro, M. F., Lehman, D. F., & Greenfield, S. Biases in the laboratory diagnosis of depression in medical practice. *Archives of Internal Medicine,* 1983, *143,* 2085–2088. (10)

Shaw, J., & McKegney, F. P. Problem-oriented record. In A. M. Freedman, H. I. Kaplan, & B. J. Sadock (Eds.), *Comprehensive textbook of psychiatry,* Vol. 3 (3rd ed.). Baltimore: Williams & Wilkins, 1980. (13)

Shectman, F. A. Operant conditioning and psychoanalysis. *American Journal of Psychotherapy,* 1975, *29,* 72–78. (12)

Sheehan, D. V. Current views on the treatment of panic and phobic disorders. *Drug Therapy,* 1982a, *10,* 74–93. (20)

Sheehan, D. V. Answer to questions in R. J. Shader (Ed.), Panic disorders: Current perspectives. *Journal of Clinical Psychopharmacology,* 1982b, *6*(suppl.), 18–195. (12, 16, 18, 19)

Sheehan, D. V., Ballinger, J., & Jacobson, G. The treatment of endogenous anxiety with phobic, hysterical, and hypochondriacal symptoms. *Archives of General Psychiatry,* 1980, *37,* 51–59. (20)

Shepherd, M., Oppenheim, A. N., & Mitchell, S. Childhood behavior disorders and the child guidance clinic: An epidemiologic study. *Journal of Child Psychology, Psychiatry and Allied Disciplines,* 1966, *7,* 39–52. (3)

Shepherd, M., & Zangwill, O. L. (Eds.). *Handbook of psychiatry I: General psychopathology.* Cambridge: Cambridge University Press, 1983. (9)

Shulman, L. S., & Elstein, A. S. Studies of problem solving, judgment and decision making: Implications for educational research. In F. N. Kerlinger (Ed.), *Review of research in education.* Itasca, Ill.: Peacock, 1975. (27)

Siegman, A. Review of interview research. In G. U. Balis, L. Wurmser, E. McDaniel, & R. G. Grenell (Eds.), *The behavioral and social sciences and the practice of medicine. The psychiatric foundations of medicine,* Vol. 2. Boston: Butterworth, 1978. (8)

Simmons, J. E. *Psychiatric examination of children* (3rd. ed.). Philadelphia: Lea & Febiger, 1981. (21, 25)

Simpson, G. M., & May, P. R. A. Schizophrenic disorders. In J. H. Greist, J. W. Jefferson, & R. L. Spitzer (Eds.), *Treatment of mental disorders.* New York: Oxford, 1982. (12)

Skinner, B. F. *The behavior of organisms: An experimental analysis.* New York: Appleton-Century-Crofts, 1957. (12)

Slavson, S. R., & Schiffer, M. *Group psychotherapies for children: A textbook.* New York, International Universities Press, 1975. (25)

Slosson, R. L. *Slosson Intelligence Test for Children and Adolescents.* Los Angeles: Western Psychological Services, 1975. (22)

Smith, A. The serial sevens subtraction test. *Archives of Neurology,* 1967, *17,* 78–80. (9)

Snyder, S. H. Neurotransmitters and CNS disease: Schizophrenia. *Lancet,* 1982, *2,* 970–974. (5)

Soreff, S. M. *Management of the psychiatric emergency.* New York: Wiley, 1981. (17)

Soreff, S. M. (Ed.). Emergency psychiatry. *Psychiatric Clinics of North America,* 1983, *6,* 211–362. (17)

Spitzer, R. L. More on pseudoscience in science and the case for psychiatric diagnosis: A critique of D. L. Rosenhan's "On being sane in insane places" and "The contextual nature of psychiatric diagnosis." *Archives of General Psychiatry,* 1976, *33,* 459–470. (11)

Spitzer, R. L., Endicott, J., & Robbins, E. Research diagnostic criteria: Rationale and reliability. *Archives of General Psychiatry,* 1978, *35,* 773–782. (12)

Sproul, M. S., & Gallagher, R. M. The genogram as an aid to crisis intervention. *Journal of Family Practice,* 1982, *14,* 959–960. (20)

Sternbach, R., & Tursky, B. Ethnic differences among housewives in psychophysical and skin potential responses to electric shock. *Psychophysiology,* 1965, *1,* 241–246. (3)

Steward, R. B., & Cluff, L. E. A review of medication errors and compliance in ambulant patients. *Clinical Pharmacology Therapy,* 1972, *13,* 463–468. (3)

Stone, L. A. Residential treatment. In S. I. Harrison (Ed.), *Basic handbook of child psychiatry,* Vol. 3. *Therapeutic interventions.* New York: Basic Books, 1979. (25)

Strain, J. J. (Ed.). The medically ill patient. *Psychiatric Clinics of North America,* 1981, *4,* 199–425. (19)

—Liaison psychiatry and its dilemmas. *General Hospital Psychiatry,* 1983, *5,* 209–212. (19)

Suchman, E. A. Sociomedical variations among ethnic groups. *American Journal of Sociology,* 1964, *70,* 319–331. (3)

—Social patterns of illness and medical care. *Journal of Health and Human Behavior,* 1965, *6,* 2–16. (a) (3)

—Stages of illness and medical care. *Journal of Health and Human Behavior,* 1965, *6,* 114–128. (b) (3)

Szasz, T. S. *The myth of mental illness: Foundations of a theory of personal conduct.* New York: Harper & Row, 1961. (3, 11)

—*Law, liberty and psychiatry: An inquiry into the social uses of mental health practices.* New York: Macmillan, 1963, (3, 11)

Talbott, J. A. *The death of the asylum: A critical study of state hospital management, services and cases.* New York: Grune & Stratton, 1978. (18)

Tallman, J. F., Paul, S. M., Skolwoch, P., & Gallagher, D. W. Receptors for the age of anxiety: Pharmacology of the benzodiazepines. *Science.* 1983, *207,* 274–281. (12)

Taylor, G., & Doody, K. Psychiatric consultations in a Canadian general hospital. *Canadian Journal of Psychiatry.* 1979, *74,* 717–723. (19)

Temoshok, L., Van Dyke, C., & Zegans, L. S. *Emotions in health and illness, theoretical and research foundations.* New York: Grune & Stratton, 1983. (3)

Terman, L. M., & Merrill, M. A. *Stanford-Binet Intelligence Scale. Manual for the third revision, form L-M.* Boston: Houghton Mifflin, 1973. (22)

Tessler, R., Mechanic, D., & Diamond, M. The effect of psychological distress on physician utilization: A prospective study. *Journal of Health and Social Behavior,* 1976, *17,* 353–364. (3)

Thomas, A., Chess, S., & Birch, H. G. *Temperament and behavior disorders in children.* New York: New York University Press, 1968. (21, 22, 24)

Tversky, A., & Kahneman, D. Judgment under uncertainty: Heuristics and biases. *Science,* 1974, *185,* 1124–1131. (27)

—The framing of decisions and the psychology of choice. *Science,* 1981, *211,* 453–458. (27)

Usdin, E., Kvetnansky, R., & Kapin, I. J. (Eds.), *Catecholamines and stress: Recent advances.* New York: Elsevier/North-Holland, 1980. (3)

van Praag, H. M. Neurotransmitters and CNS disease: Depression. *Lancet,* 1982, *2,* 1259–1264. (5)

Von Bertalanffy, L. *General systems theory.* New York: Braziller, 1968. (3, 12)

Waldrop, M., Pederson, F. A., & Bell, R. O. Minor physical anomalies and behavior in pre-school children. *Child Development,* 1968, *39,* 391–400. (22)

Waring, E. M. Marriages of patients with psychosomatic illness. *General Hospital Psychiatry,* 1983, *5,* 49–53. (19)

Waring, E. M., & Russell, L. Family structure, marital adjustment, and intimacy in patients referred to a consultation-liaison service. *General Hospital Psychiatry,* 1983, *3,* 198–203. (19)

Wechsler, D. *The measurement and appraisal of adult intelligence* (4th ed.). Baltimore: Williams & Wilkins, 1958. (10)

—*Wechsler Preschool and Primary Scale of Intelligence.* New York: Psychological Corporation, 1967. (22)

—*Wechsler Intelligence Scale for Children – Revised.* New York: Psychological Corporation, 1974. (10, 22)

—*Wechsler Adult Intelligence Scale – Revised.* New York: Psychological Corporation, 1981. (22)

Weed, L. L. *Medical records, medical education and patient care.* Cleveland, Ohio: Case Western Reserve University Press, 1969. (13)

Weiner, H. *Psychobiology and human disease.* New York: Elsevier, 1977. (3)

Weinstein, M. C., Fineberg, H. V., Elstein, A. S., Frazier, H. S., Neuhauser, D., Neutra, R. R., & McNeil, B. J. *Clinical decision analysis.* Philadelphia: Saunders, 1980. (27)

Weisman, M. M. The psychological treatment of depression: Research evidence for the efficacy of psychotherapy alone, in comparison and in combination with pharmacotherapy. *Archives of General Psychiatry,* 1979, *36,* 1261–1269. (12)

Weiss, P. A. From cell to molecule. In J. M. Allen (Ed.), *The molecular control of cellular activity.* New York: McGraw-Hill, 1962. (3)

Wells, C. E. Diagnostic evaluation and treatment in dementia. In D. E. Wells, (Ed.), *Dementia* (2nd ed.). Philadelphia: Davis, 1977. (12)

Wells, C. E., & Duncan, G. W. *Neurology for psychiatrists.* Philadelphia: Davis, 1980. (9)

Werner, H. *Comparative psychology of mental development.* Chicago: Follett, 1948. (24)

Werry, J. S. (Ed.). *Pediatric psychopharmacology: The use of behavior modifying drugs in children.* New York: Brunner/Mazel, 1978. (25)

Werry, J. S., & Aman, M. G. The reliability and diagnostic validity of the physical and neurological examination for soft signs (PANESS). *Journal of Autism and Childhood Schizophrenia,* 1976, *6,* 253–262. (22)

Wing, J. K., Birley, J. L., & Cooper, J. E. Reliability of a procedure for measuring and classifying "present mental state." *British Journal of Psychiatry,* 1967, *113,* 499–508.

Winnicott, D. W. Child therapy: A case of anti-social behavior. In J. G. Howells (Ed.), *Modern perspectives in child psychiatry.* Edinburgh: Oliver & Boyd, 1965. (21)

Withers, E., & Hinton, J. Three forms of the clinical tests of the sensorium and their reliability. *British Journal of Psychiatry,* 1971, *119,* 1–8. (9)

Wolman, B. B. (Ed.) *Handbook of developmental psychology.* Englewood Cliffs, N.J.: Prentice-Hall, 1982. (24)

Wolpe, J. *Psychotherapy by reciprocal inhibition.* Palo Alto, Calif.: Stanford University Press, 1958. (12)

Wolsten, E., & Lipowski, Z. J. Liaison psychiatry: Referral patterns and their stability over time. *American Journal of Psychiatry,* 1981, *138,* 1608–1611. (19)

Woodcock, R. W., & Johnson, M. B. *Woodcock-Johnson Psychoeducational Battery.* Hingham, Mass.: Teaching Resources Corporation, 1977. (22)

Woodruff, R. A., Jr., Goodwin, D. W., & Guze, S. B. *Psychiatric diagnosis.* New York: Oxford University Press, 1974. (11)

Wooley, S. C., Blackwell, B., & Winget, M. A.: A learning theory model of chronic illness behavior: Theory, treatment, and research. *Psychosomatic Medicine,* 1978, *40,* 379–401. (3)

Yarrow, M. R., Schwartz, C. G., Murphy, H. S., & Deasy, L. C. The psychological meaning of mental illness in the family. *Journal of Social Issues,* 1955, *11;* 12–24; 33–48. (3)

Young, M., Bernard, B., & Wallis, G. The mortality of widowers. *Lancet,* 1963, 454–456. (3)

Zborowski, M. Cultural components in responses to pain. *Journal of Social Issues,* 1952, *8,* 16–30. (3)

Zinn, D. Hospital treatment of the adolescent. In S. I. Harrison (Ed.), *Basic handbook of child psychiatry,* Vol. 3. *Therapeutic interventions.* New York: Basic Books, 1979. (25)

Zola, I. K. Studying the decision to see a doctor. *Advances in Psychosomatic Medicine,* 1972, *8,* 216–236. (3)

Author index

Subject index